PSYCHOSOCIAL CONCEPTUAL PRACTICE MODELS *in* OCCUPATIONAL THERAPY

Building Adaptive Capability

PSYCHOSOCIAL CONCEPTUAL PRACTICE MODELS *in* OCCUPATIONAL THERAPY

Building Adaptive Capability

Moses N. Ikiugu, PhD, OTR/L
Associate Professor and Director of Research
Department of Occupational Therapy
University of South Dakota
Vermillion, South Dakota

CONTRIBUTOR
Elizabeth A. Ciaravino, PhD, OTR/L
Licensed Occupational Therapist, Licensed Psychologist
Department of Occupational Therapy
The University of Scranton
Scranton, Pennsylvania

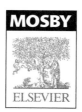

MOSBY

ELSEVIER

MOSBY
ELSEVIER

11830 Westline Industrial Drive
St. Louis, Missouri 63146

Psychosocial Conceptual Practice Models in Occupational Therapy:
Building Adaptive Capability
Copyright © 2007 by Mosby, Inc., an affiliate of Elsevier Inc.

ISBN-13:978-0-323-04182-9
ISBN-10:0-323-04182-5

Notice

Neither the Publisher nor the Author assumes any responsibility for any loss or injury and/or damage to persons or property arising out of or related to any use of the material contained in this book. It is the responsibility of the treating practitioner, relying on independent expertise and knowledge of the patient, to determine the best treatment and method of application for the patient.

The Publisher

ISBN-13:978-0-323-04182-9
ISBN-10:0-323-04182-5

Publishing Director: Linda Duncan
Editor: Kathy Falk
Developmental Editor: Melissa Kuster Deutsch
Publishing Services Manager: Pat Joiner
Senior Project Manager: David Stein
Designer: Kimberly Denando

Printed in the United States
Last digit is the print number: 9 8 7 6 5 4 3 2 1

Working together to grow
libraries in developing countries

www.elsevier.com | www.bookaid.org | www.sabre.org

ELSEVIER   BOOK AID
International   Sabre Foundation

This work is dedicated to my mother Elizabeth and my
two wonderful children Ivan and Nora

REVIEWERS

Rebecca Argabrite-Grove, MS, OTR/L
Special Education Supervisor
Loudoun County Public Schools
Ashburn, Virginia

Jeanenne Dallas, MA, OTR/L, CPRP
Instructor and Clinical Specialist
Department of Occupational Therapy
Washington University
St. Louis, Missouri

Yolanda Griffiths, OTD, OTR/L, FAOTA
Associate Professor
Department of Occupational Therapy
Creighton University Medical Center
Omaha, Nebraska

Linda Kelly, MS
Occupational Therapy Assistant Program
Delgado Community College
New Orleans, Louisiana

Janice Robinson, MS, OTR/L
Staff Occupational Therapist
AnMed Health
Anderson, South Carolina

Preface

A new occupational therapy paradigm has recently emerged, one that has been described in the Occupational Therapy Practice Framework and that has also been particularly well articulated by Gary Kielhofner, a leading scholar in the profession. In this new paradigm, theory-based, occupation-based, client-centered, collaborative, and evidence-based practice is emphasized. This textbook/laboratory manual is designed to fulfill the mandate of this newly evolved professional paradigm.

Many occupational therapists are familiar with the complaint among professionals that theory-based practice is impractical, because client problems do not fit theoretical frameworks taught in university programs. As many practitioners often put it, theories taught in occupational therapy schools do not work in the "real world." One reason many therapists hold such a sentiment is that there is a scarcity of resources designed to assist them in pragmatically and experientially bridging theory and practice. This book is designed to facilitate establishment of this bridge by clearly defining theoretical constructs in such a manner that they can be applied and then providing specific exercises in a laboratory manual to help the therapist apply those constructs in clinical practice. The book therefore effectively meshes theory and practice in order to facilitate effective theory-based practice.

This book is designed to be applicable to different levels of knowledge and practice skills in occupational therapy. It is meant for entry-level occupational therapy students who want to master the basic assumptions, principles, and values of the profession; for practicing clinicians wishing to deepen their theoretical understanding of what they are doing as occupational therapy practitioners; and for post-professional (advanced) masters and doctoral level students who want to understand the profession's conceptual basis at a deeper level. To meet those multileveled needs, an Instructor's Resource Manual, based on Bloom's taxonomy of knowledge development, is available on the instructor's portion of the Evolve Resources website. This manual will help the instructor create educational experiences based on this textbook and the laboratory manual so that they are optimally useful to students, irrespective of their level of knowledge of occupational therapy principles.

Finally, the reader will notice that many case examples in this book are derived from Africa (Kenya in particular). This is because my experience in psychosocial practice is largely based on my practice in the Kenyan mental health system. These examples are also meant to appeal to the international readership of this textbook. Although occupational therapy textbooks portray case examples from the United States and several other parts of the world, Africa is largely under-represented. The examples used in this textbook are an attempt to help occupational therapists worldwide develop an awareness of the African psychosocial occupational therapy experience, albeit drawn from only one African nation, Kenya. If after reading this book, potential or practicing occupational therapists become more reflective about how they apply theory in practice, about how they use available empirical evidence to support their clinical decisions, and about occupational therapy experiences from other parts of the world, including Africa, then I will have achieved my objective.

Rationale

This textbook/laboratory manual is intended for use in psychosocial rehabilitation courses in occupational therapy. As I embarked on this work, I was aware that there are numerous textbooks in psychosocial occupational therapy already in the market. Therefore I had to ask myself: "Why write this book? What does it add to the already available fund of knowledge in this area of practice?" In answer to the above questions, I realized that the book was a result of my experience teaching courses on psychosocial rehabilitation.

For many years, I struggled with the process of seeking information from varied sources, then trying to organize it so that it makes sense and meets the requirements of the course. Moreover, since psychosocial rehabilitation is a practice course, I found myself scrambling in search of activities and exercises for use in the laboratory sections. Sometimes I had to devise my own exercises because I could not find published ones that met the requirements of my students. As I continued in this manner, it occurred to me that other instructors might be having a similar struggle. I then thought, "Would it not be nice if most of the course information that my students needed to access was available in one textbook? And would it not also be nice if there was a laboratory manual–somewhat analogous to a laboratory manual in basic sciences such as anatomy–with systematically developed exercises and activities that students could use to practice and develop their skills in translating the textbook's theoretical concepts into practice? This textbook/laboratory manual was born out of the above thoughts and desires.

As I was developing an outline for the book/laboratory manual, I imagined myself or a close relative being treated by an occupational therapist who had taken my psychosocial rehabilitation course. What kind of therapist would I like to work with in such a context? In answer to the question, I realized that I would like a therapist treating my loved one or me (1) to have a clear identity as a professional, to be comfortable with the theoretical principles guiding his or her therapeutic interventions, and to be clear about their historical origins and about how occupational therapy is different from other services that my loved one or I may be receiving, (2) to convince me about the value of occupational therapy for my loved one's or my rehabilitation, (3) to explain the theoretical principles underlying therapeutic interventions being received in such a way that they are easily understandable, (4) to translate those principles into simple, easily applicable interventions that are effective, (5) to use procedures and techniques effectively to implement interventions, and (6) to provide me with research evidence demonstrating that his or her planned interventions have been found to be effective.

This textbook/laboratory manual was designed in an attempt to help produce an occupational therapist with the above-listed characteristics. It was also written to meet the needs of entry-level occupational therapy students (by providing clear, practical guidelines for practice with case examples) as well as higher level advanced professionals (e.g., doctoral level students) who desire to deepen their knowledge of the profession (the in-depth philosophical and theoretical discussions and the critique of models, for example, were written with these professionals in mind).

Organization

To best explain how this vision was translated into a book, I will use an architectural analogy. Imagine that the profession of occupational therapy is a residential building complex. Psychosocial occupational therapy may be viewed as one phase of the building complex's development with several housing units (e.g., direct practice with clients who have a variety of diagnoses, addressing psychosocial issues of clients with physical disabilities, working with clients' families, working with community agencies). The historical development of the profession is comparable to the process of leveling the ground so that there is adequate support for the entire complex, through all its phases (e.g., psychosocial rehabilitation, physical disabilities, geriatrics, home health, pediatrics).

The philosophy (which I argue is primarily pragmatism) and scientific framework (which I propose to be complexity/chaos theory) constitute the foundation. This foundation is laid on firm ground leveled by a clear understanding of the historical evolution of concepts that are at the basis of the profession so that it is adequately supported. The specific practice techniques and procedures (e.g., skillful use of everyday occupations, use of groups and group processes, clinical reasoning, ethical decision making) form the building blocks of clinical practice. Active listening and effective communication constitute the mortar that binds together those therapeutic building blocks, and the therapeutic relationship makes the finishing décor that gives the professional structure its aesthetic appearance and elegance. Conceptual practice models provide columns and beams that support the entire weight of the structure and transmit this weight to the supporting foundation of philosophy and scientific framework. Management, consultation, and team building skills form the roof that provides shelter to the contents of the structure (clients and therapists).

Bearing in mind the aforementioned structural analogy, the book is divided into five parts. In Part I, *Background,* the historical origin of occupational therapy, from the moral treatment movement up to the present, is discussed. I have gone to great lengths to explicate the social and intellectual context within which the profession developed. The history as presented is meant to level the ground and make it firm through a clear understanding of our origins and our rich intellectual heritage in preparation for laying the professional foundation. Psychological theories that have contributed to the development of psychosocial occupational therapy are also discussed as the hard core that provides reinforcement in preparation for laying the foundation.

In Part II, *Contemporary Conceptual Foundations of Psychosocial Occupational Therapy,* conceptual foundations of the profession are discussed, as are the role of the philosophy of pragmatism and the complexity/chaos theoretical framework as a basis for occupational therapy practice. Finally, the newly evolved professional paradigm is articulated. This part of the book forms what I see as the foundation of the profession, supporting all psychosocial occupational therapy practice.

In Part III, *General Practice Considerations in Psychosocial Occupational Therapy,* general practice considerations are discussed. These include client evaluation, use of therapeutic relationship, use of groups and group techniques, clinical reasoning, cultural considerations in therapy, and ethical decision making. This part constitutes the building blocks as well as the décor of the profession, providing professional aesthetics. It constitutes elements of practice that have been referred to by some occupational therapy scholars as the art of practice. A therapist who is skillful in the use of those building blocks is admired for his or her elegance in practice.

Part IV, *Specific Interventions: Application of Conceptual Models of Practice in Occupational Therapy,* is concerned with select conceptual practice models used by psychosocial occupational therapists. For each model, the theoretical core and guidelines for evaluation and intervention are discussed. Its consistency with the foundation of the profession (the philosophy of pragmatism and chaos/complexity theory) is critiqued. Recommendations on how to make the model more consistent with this foundation and research evidence illustrating clinical usefulness of the model are presented. Part IV may be comparable to the structural framework of a building, with each of the conceptual practice models constituting a column or beam that supports the weight of our professional house.

In Part V, *Application of Psychosocial Occupational Therapy Across the Continuum of Care,* application of occupational therapy across the continuum of care, ranging from consideration of age and developmental stages to application of psychosocial occupational therapy principles in the community is discussed. This is comparable to the landscaping that enhances the beauty of our profession.

Language and Style

This book is written with the need to help therapists conduct occupation-based, collaborative, client-centered, theory and evidence-based practice in mind. Care has been taken to carefully reduce abstract concepts into practical intervention guidelines that can be easily applied in clinical practice. Case examples have been used throughout the book to illustrate how the discussed concepts are applied.

Regarding the use of language, I am aware that since the development of phenomenology by the philosopher Edmund Husserl (1857-1938) and subsequent application in psychology by phenomenologists such as Martin Heidegger (1889-1976), there has been increasing support of the view that there is no true separation between the observer and the observed, the subjective and the objective. (Assumption of objectivity has for a long time been the basis of scientific inquiry, which up until very recently required scientific discourses to be written in the third person so as to be perceived to be objective.)

This trend culminated in the view articulated by Thomas Kuhn (see Chapter 4) that every scholar necessarily brings into scientific inquiry his or her subjective perceptions of the phenomenon being observed. As such, true objectivity is really a myth. The publication manual of the American Psychological Association now recognizes this reality, as indicated by its recommendation that writers use the first person because using the third-person pronoun when referring to yourself "is ambiguous and may give the impression that you did not take part in your own study" (pp. 37-38). However, because some readers are annoyed by too frequent use of the pronoun "I," in this book it has been limited to the following situations: (1) addressing the reader directly when I share personal experiences; in these instances I am trying to connect with the reader in a personal way, which I believe makes the experiences in the book real and alive, and (2) when I want to make clear that the ideas being presented are my own opinions and not necessarily based on consensus derived from literature.

I think that use of language in this manner allows the reader to differentiate between my own ideas and opinions, ideas and opinions derived from interpretation and synthesis of literature, and factual information reported from literature. This makes it easier to judge opinions and agree or disagree with them on their own merit, while still finding value in information reported or synthesized from literature. Finally, I realize that in the information age, in which new information is rapidly being generated and ideas are transformed constantly, it is difficult for any one person to be an authority in an area as extensive as psychosocial occupational therapy practice. I therefore welcome ongoing constructive criticism that will help me refine and improve this work on an ongoing basis.

Acknowledgments

Many people have made this book possible. My deceased father, Joseph Ikiugu, and my mother, Elizabeth Kathuni Ikiugu, sacrificed much to ensure that I acquired my education. I owe all my achievements to them.

My sisters Angelica, Pilippina, Paulina, Justah, and Micheline, and their husbands contributed to my success in many ways, both financially and in their undying faith in my abilities. They encouraged me to be all that I can be.

My friends Arnie and Amy Mindell and the entire process-oriented psychology community demonstrated to me what true friendship and generosity mean. I could not have achieved what I have without their support.

My dear friends Susanna Davila and Dick Curtis are particularly responsible for making my immigration into the United States and my doctoral education possible. I consider them my adopted United States parents and am forever grateful for their love, friendship, and immense generosity.

I want to acknowledge my doctoral advisers, Drs. Sally Schultz, Jeanette Schkade, and Jack Sibley for pointing me in the direction of lifelong scholarly curiosity and inquiry.

My psychosocial rehabilitation students at the University of Scranton and the University of South Dakota provided me with a chance to explore and develop ideas used in this book. I learned from them as much, if not more than I taught them.

My editors Kathy Falk and Melissa Kuster and the entire Elsevier publication team deserve special mention for their professionalism and support. They made this task more painless than I could have ever expected. It was a pleasure working with all of them.

I would like to acknowledge in a special way all my clients in both Kenya and the United States. They were a crucial source of the experiences that provided the material for this book. I consider them my valuable teachers.

I want also to acknowledge my colleagues at the University of South Dakota, Department of Occupational Therapy: Barbara Brockevelte, Stacy Smalfield, Angela Anderson, Lynne Anderson, and Connie Twedt for their unqualified acceptance, warmth, friendship, and collegiality. Without their support, I could not have accomplished this task.

I am grateful to Dr. Elizabeth A. Ciaravino of the University of Scranton for contributing a chapter in this book. Through the chapter, her expertise in the treatment of clients with substance abuse disorders became available to occupational therapists who will read this book.

Finally, and not in any way the least, I want to thank my partner Marie Anne Ben for her love and unwavering support. She is the reason that I was able to complete this project without going crazy. I am indebted to her forever.

CONTENTS

APPENDIX

Part I consists of three chapters. In Chapters 1 and 2, the history of occupational therapy in mental health is discussed. Chapter 1 begins with the rise of the moral treatment movement in the late eighteenth century and continues through the arts and crafts movement era at the end of the nineteenth century and extends into the beginning of the twentieth century. Chapter 2 deals with the evolution of occupational therapy from its formal founding at the turn of the twentieth century to the present. Why devote two entire chapters to the history of occupational therapy, especially when the subject is discussed elsewhere in occupational therapy literature?

The answer to the above question is simply that this textbook will cover the profession's history in a manner different from other sources. In one of the most quoted phrases in occupational therapy literature, Mary Reilly stated in her Slagle lecture that, "One of the greatest ideas in 20th century medicine is that man, by use of his own hands, as they are directed by the mind and energized by the will, can affect the state of his own health" (p. 2).[3] It is put forth in this book that to understand this great twentieth century idea, and to come to the full realization of its potential benefits, we must have a clear and insightful understanding of its origin. What Roberts proposed for psychology holds true for occupational therapy: "the lessons of the past have to be well studied" (p. 12).[4]

Chapters 1 and 2 are necessary to trace the origin of occupational therapy from the moral treatment movement in Europe. In this historical account, it will be demonstrated that moral treatment was primarily part of a wider social reform effort. To understand the origin and development of the profession in a meaningful way, occupational therapists need to appreciate the social and intellectual context within which that reform took place. Understanding this context is essential if we wish to learn what may have remained stable and what has changed over time as our profession has evolved, and it will provide insights that are crucial as we chart our future with authority, self-knowledge, and confidence. As Detweiller and Peyton argue, a chronotopic study of professions (based on Bakhtin's[1] constructs of *chronos* [time] and *topos* [place]) allows professions to keep in view their "stability or transhistorical qualities, as well as their context-sensitivity or their specific reinterpretations in new times and places of use" (p. 425).[2] By keeping in view the stability and transhistorical qualities, professionals can develop "shared understandings" (p. 429).[2]

The first two chapters of this book are spirited attempts to help occupational therapists keep in view the stability and transhistorical qualities of their profession, and to help them develop shared understandings that have trickled through history to the present, and which help us maintain our identity and integrity as a profession. I want to make my contribution toward helping every individual occupational therapist understand that which has remained constant through history even as our profession has evolved over time, so that every therapist in turn can make insightful contributions toward the realization of that great twentieth century idea that Reilly visualized in 1962. Obviously, two chapters cannot do justice to an in-depth discussion of the history of occupational therapy. However, an effort will be made to discuss as fully as possible, in the limited space, the rise of the moral treatment movement and the social and intellectual context in which it was founded, the development of the moral treatment movement in the United States, the influence of the arts and crafts movement to the development of occupational therapy, the mental hygiene movement, the community mental health models, and the current community support movement. To help the reader understand the multiple interacting contexts of this development, the historical account is summarized in a diagram (see Figure 1-1).

Also in Chapter 2, considerable space has been devoted to a discussion of the philosophy of pragmatism. This is considered necessary to help the reader understand the philosophical constructs of the profession and where they might have originated from. This is part of

facilitating appreciation of the profoundness of the basic premises of our profession. In Chapter 3, psychosocial theories that have contributed to the development of psychosocial occupational therapy are presented.

REFERENCES

1. Bakhtin M: *The dialogic imagination*, Austin, TX, 1981, University of Texas Press.
2. Detweiler J, Peyton C: Defining occupations: a chronotopic study of narrative genres in a health discipline's emergence, *Written Communication* 16:412-468, 1999.
3. Reilly M: Occupational therapy can be one of the great ideas of 20th century medicine, *Am J Occup Ther* 16:1-9, 1962.
4. Roberts N: *Mental health and mental illness*, New York, 1967, The Humanities Press.

Chapter 1

Formal Therapeutic Use of Occupations: The Moral Treatment Movement and the Arts and Crafts Movement

Preview Questions

1. Why is it necessary to be conversant with the history of occupational therapy?
2. Discuss the rise and development of the moral treatment movement in Europe and the United States by answering the following questions:
   a. How did the moral treatment movement rise in Europe?
   b. Explain the social and intellectual events that led to rise of the moral treatment movement.
   c. Describe the introduction of moral treatment principles in institutions in the United States.
   d. How did moral treatment principles guide therapeutic interventions in mental health in the United States?
   e. What led to the decline of the moral treatment movement in Europe and in the United States?
3. Describe the rise of the arts and crafts movement, and explain how its principles were used in hospitals to guide therapeutic interventions and in social institutions as a means of meliorating cultural alienation.

In Chapters 1 and 2, we will explore the genesis of occupational therapy. Figure 1-1 illustrates this genealogy by showing how the age of enlightenment emerged from the philosophy of empiricism. Based on enlightenment and the religious work of the Quakers, the moral treatment movement was founded. The arrow suggests that the religious principles of the Quakers contributed to the rise of moral treatment. This connection is not intended to suggest that Pinel's version of moral treatment was influenced by the Quaker religion. Rather, it is meant to illustrate the influence of Quaker ideas to the movement's development in the United States.

The theory of evolution, in combination with enlightenment, contributed to the philosophy of pragmatism. Enlightenment also contributed to the rise of the arts and crafts movement. From pragmatism and the arts and crafts movement emerged the mental hygiene movement. The mental hygiene, arts and crafts, and moral treatment movements contributed to the formal founding of occupational therapy. The mental hygiene movement in turn evolved into the community mental health and community support movements. Events of World War I, World War II, and the medical and psychological advances contributed to occupational therapy's adoption of the reductionistic paradigm. Systems theory and the second industrial revolution (advent of information technology) led to professional self-questioning. In response to the self-questioning, supported by the community support movement and development of qualitative research methodologies, a new occupational therapy paradigm was articulated. A more in-depth discussion of the history follows.

3

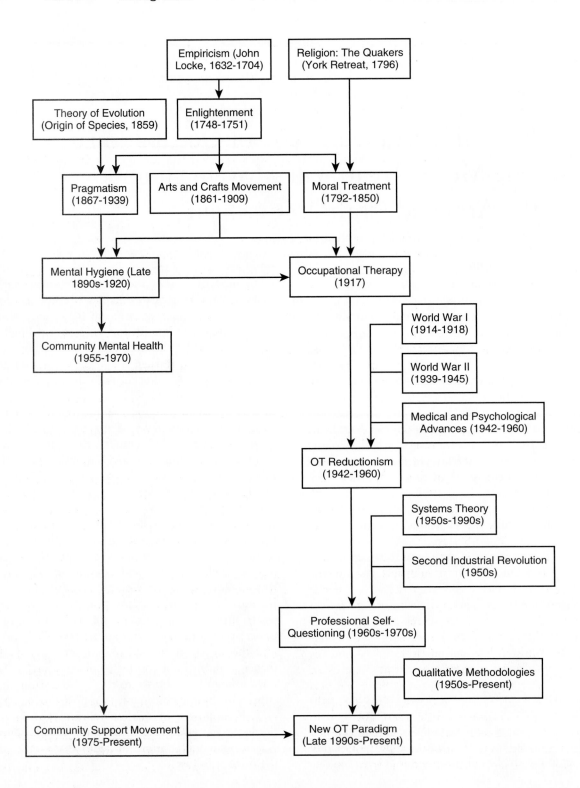

Figure 1-1.   Illustration of the genealogy of occupational therapy.
Note: Dates presented in the figure are approximations derived from the following sources: Brigham A: The moral treatment of insanity [electronic version], *Am J Insanity,* 1847. Retrieved March 2006, from http:// www.disabilitymuseum.org/lib/docs/1246.htm?page=print; Columbia University: *Encyclopedia: Locke, John,* 2006. Retrieved March, 2006, from http:// education.yahoo.com/ reference/encyclopedia/entry/Locke-Jo; Darwin C: *The origin of species,* New York, 1985, Penguin Books; Friends Hospital: *A history of Friend's Hospital,* 2000. Retrieved March 2006, from http:// www.friendshospitalonline.org/ History.htm; Hooker R: *The European enlightenment: the philosophes,* 1999. Retrieved March 2006, from http:// www.wsu.edu/~dee/ENLIGHT/PHIL.HTM; McColl MA, Law M, Stewart D, et al, eds: *Theoretical basis of occupational therapy,* ed 2, Thorofare, NJ, 2002, Slack; National Mental Health Association: *NMHA and the history of the mental health movement,* 2006. Retrieved March 2006, from http:// www.MoreAboutNMHAHistoryofMentalHealth.html; Samuel B: *Quaker tour of England, page 19 of 22: the retreat mental hospital,* 2002. Retrieved March 2006, from http:// www.quakerinfo.com/qt_retr.shtml; and United States Surgeon General: *Mental health: a report of the Surgeon General,* 2005. Retrieved May 2005 from http:// www.surgeongeneral.gov/ library/mentalhealth/home.html.

Rise of the Moral Treatment Movement in Europe

The moral treatment movement in Europe was a reform effort in mental health care that was spearheaded by two individuals. Philippe Pinel, often referred to as the "striker of chains,"[12] started the reform in France. In 1792, he was appointed director of asylum de Becetre. Pinel was appalled by the condition in which patients were kept. As was common regarding the treatment of the mentally ill at that time, they were "often chained and kept safely away from all public contact" (p. 2).[8] Other methods of treatment included cutting to induce bleeding in hope of expelling demons that were believed to cause mental illness, flogging, spinning, and using cold douches, straight waistcoats, emetics, and purges.[12,31,39] Patients were not given enough food. Other forms of treatment included exorcism to expel demons, torture to induce repentance, and burning at stake under the accusation of being witches.[31,37]

It is important to note that moral treatment, in Pinel's sense, was not conceived to have religious moral connotations.[8,43] Rather, it was an application of psychologically-oriented therapy to help patients regain reason. The French term for the kind of therapy he proposed was *traitement moral,* which translates into the idea of regaining a sense of well-being or morale.[22] In other words, he conceptualized mental illness as resulting from diminished morale and decreased sense of well-being. To counteract this loss of morale, restore the sense of well-being, and help patients regain a sense of reason, he proposed that they be treated kindly, with therapy consisting in part of a regular routine of daily activities including self care, recreation, religious observances, and labor or work.[4,12,17]

In England, William Tuke, a Quaker merchant, was similarly moved by the plight of the mentally ill. He proposed to the Society of Friends the need to establish an asylum at York, England, where the mentally ill could be treated humanely and the virtues of quietness and solitude could be instilled in a place where unhappy patients could find refuge.[9] At first, the Society of Friends opposed his proposal on the basis that not enough Quakers were afflicted with mental illness to warrant the retreat.[35] However, with persistence he established the retreat and became the administrator. Tuke's grandson Samuel and then his great grandson Daniel ran the retreat in later years.[8]

At the York Retreat, Tuke sought to begin treatment early because he believed that early intervention was the most effective strategy to save patients from a life of insanity.[17,43] He also believed that the mentally ill could respond to reinforcements (such as praise and blame) as a means of getting them to change behavior.[39] As such, there was no need for restraint. Instead, he proposed that they be treated with kindness, "in pleasant surroundings and with sufficient diversions to relieve their boredom" (p. 2). He aimed at helping patients to divert their minds from the "favorite but unhappy musings, by bodily exercise, walks, conversation, reading, and other innocent recreations" (pp. 151-152).[42]

The moral treatment movement, as founded by Pinel in France and Tuke in England, was therefore an attempt to reform mental health practice. In this reform, therapy was conceived to consist of a regular routine of activities, using occupations that included both work and recreation. They both proposed that patients be treated with kindness, and prohibited use of restraint and other cruel forms of treatment. In this approach to therapy, the environment was perceived to play a crucial role.[8,13,14] Both Tuke[42] and Pinel[30] emphasized the need to treat patients in a suitable environment approximating as much as possible a loving family, with the therapist playing the role of a gentle, yet firm parent. The goal was to remove "the insane from their environments that drove them insane" and provide them with "counseling, recreation, physical labor, and religion" (p. 4).[8]

Social and Intellectual Events

In order to understand the reason for the rise of the moral treatment movement, it is necessary to understand how poorly individuals with mental illness were treated before the age of enlightenment. In addition, one should consider the intellectual beliefs that influenced social thinking about mental illness, its cause, and how to treat those who were afflicted. At the time the moral treatment movement was founded, an intellectual revolution was taking place in Europe (with a measure of social revolution as well). This revolution began in England with the pivotal philosophical doctrine of John Locke.

Before Locke, many philosophers, beginning with Plato, believed in innatism.[12,23] This was the idea that humans had innate knowledge with which they were born. This group of philosophers in general became known as idealists (referring to their belief in innate ideas). Extending the argument of innatists, rationalists such as Descartes, Liebniz, and Spinoza (who believed that knowledge can be acquired only through reasoning to uncover innate ideas)[23] argued that we cannot be sure of the reality of our experiences. What we perceive through our senses, they asserted, was often different from what it seemed. Furthermore, what we believed were the circumstances of our existence (e.g., when we think we are doing something) often turned out to be wrong. They concluded therefore that the only certain source of knowledge was reason. Such knowledge was perceived to have mathematical certainty because it was based on irrefutable, simple, self-evident premises, and derived through simple, logical, irrefutable steps. In other words, rationalists deemphasized, even denigrated, sense experience as fallible and unreliable as a source of knowledge.

According to innatists and rationalists, social classes were justified by the belief that people were born with innate capabilities. The very notion of innate ideas contributed to the stability of religion, morality, and natural law in England and other parts of Europe.[49] In a world dominated by those ideas, the mentally ill were treated almost like outcasts. As mentioned earlier, it was generally believed that they were possessed by evil spirits, or their illness was punishment for their sins or their parents' or grandparents' sins. Such people were the way they were by divine design, which meant that there was no attempt or hope of improving their lot. This explains the cruel treatment meted to the mentally ill at that time.

John Locke's work was a reaction to the rationalists' doctrine of the indubitable knowledge derived from reason with subsequent deemphasis of sense experience. It was also a reaction to the idea of innate superiority of some people over others by virtue of social status. By his denial of innate ideas, he attacked institutions of authority whose very justification was based on the doctrine. Locke was a firm believer in common sense. Even when common sense compelled him to give up a favorite idea, he did so without reservation.[23] He argued that everything humans knew came from their consciousness, and the content of consciousness was derived directly from experiences. In this postulation, he directly challenged the rationalists' contention that the only irrefutable source of knowledge was reasoning. To him, the only knowledge of a thing consisted of its observable characteristics, apprehended through the senses. Beyond those characteristics, a thing could not be known. Thus he asserted: "As subjects of knowledge and experience all we can ever find within ourselves are the contents of our awareness, our experiences of every kind: what that entity is, the self or whatever it is, that has these experiences, is unknowable to us" (p. 106).[23]

Because all knowledge was seen as coming to us through our senses, Locke believed that the environment to which one was exposed was an important determinant, among other things, of how one turned out to be. His basic premise was that when one was born, the mind was a *tabula rasa* or blank slate.[41] As soon as one was born the environment began to write on this blank slate. Ideas began to be formed in the mind in the form of sensation and reflection, which provided the basic material of ideas. According to Locke, what humans became depended on the experiences to which they were exposed and inductive reasoning through which they developed a sense of general principles based on those experiences. It followed that since we all come into this world with minds that are blank slates, "then no one is superior by birth than anyone else in this regard: everything for the individual depends on how he or she is educated" (p. 105).[23] This conclusion was a vindication of the mentally ill and other unfortunate members of the human species. They could not be blamed for their circumstances. Their mental illness could to a large

extent be attributed to exposure to pernicious environmental circumstances. Locke's doctrine also denoted the need to pay close attention to environmental cues, as accessed through the senses, and to arrive at conclusions about the environment through reasoning based on facts. Locke's philosophical system became known as empiricism.[23,46]

Empiricism was superimposed on Descartes' rationalism and Newtonian view of the universe to found what came to be known in France as the Age of Enlightenment.[23,32] Condillac, for instance, carried Locke's refutation of innatism to its logical conclusion and asserted that even perception was transformed sensation. Voltaire propounded John Locke's principle that "the confidence we have in our beliefs needs to relate to the evidence that exists in their support" (pp. 122-123).[23] Thus this era was characterized by emphasis on the following[32]:

- The particular rather than the general
- Observable facts rather than principles
- Experience rather than rational speculation

In this sense, enlightenment was based on a belief of the need to educate people to think for themselves and to make informed decisions based on reason rather than speculation or institutional authority.[8,23,32] Emphasis was on reason and science. In other words, the age of enlightenment was characterized by logical reasoning based on facts; a new world view based on Newtonian science and Lockean empirical philosophy; scientific methods of experimentation, observation, hypothesis formation, and testing; a belief that anything is possible if reason is properly applied to processing of experiential facts; acceptance of varying ways of life; freedom of thought that precludes prejudice; and mass education. It was within this intellectual and social atmosphere that Philippe Pinel and William Tuke began their reform of mental health.

At the same time, King George III of England was afflicted with bipolar disorder. This helped change public opinion regarding mental illness.

It was then evident that mental illness was not only for the lowly but could afflict anyone. This helped spur sympathy for patients because they were seen as victims rather than villains. All of the above events help explain the emphasis by moral treatment proponents on environmental modification to facilitate recovery, treatment of the mentally ill with kindness and understanding, and in particular, Pinel's commitment to the idea that "observations proceed theory" (p. 3)[8] and his careful daily observation and recording of patients' behavior.[8,30]

Introduction of Moral Treatment Principles In the United States

According to the report of the U.S. Surgeon General (USSG),[43] the history of mental health in the United States may be divided into five eras: the precolonial era, the moral treatment movement, the mental hygiene movement, the community mental health movement, and the community support movement. It is important for an occupational therapist to understand this historical perspective since it is clear that, as Bockoven[1] asserts, the history of moral treatment is the same as the history of occupational therapy. Since the moral treatment movement was central to the mental health reform that took place in both Europe and North America in the late eighteenth and early to mid-nineteenth centuries, it follows that we cannot separate the history of the reform from that of occupational therapy. We will discuss the era of the arts and crafts movement in the history, although review of the literature indicates that it is not clearly distinguished from the mental hygiene movement. All the same, the philosophical principles underlying the arts and crafts movement contributed significantly to the development of occupational therapy and therefore deserve mention in this book.

The Precolonial Era

During the precolonial era, families took care of their mentally ill members at home.[10,43]

However, with increased urbanization, families were broken as people migrated to cities and there was no one to take care of the mentally ill patients. Consequently, states had to confront the problem. They responded by building mental health institutions known as asylums. Mental health patients were subsequently placed either in these asylums or in almshouses (homes for the poor), or workhouses. Similar to what was happening in Europe before the reforms by Pinel and Tuke, these asylums, almshouses, and workhouses often resembled torture chambers. Patients were manacled, whipped, treated to cold douches, purges, restrained with strait waistcoats, and generally treated like beasts.[22,39] It was in these circumstances that the moral treatment movement was introduced in the United States toward the end of the eighteenth century, soon after the Revolutionary War.[43]

The Moral Treatment Movement (1800-1850)

The moral treatment movement was introduced in the United States by mental health workers who either had studied or had visited Europe where they became acquainted with moral treatment principles. However, unlike Pinel's version of the moral treatment movement, which made no reference to religious morality, in the United States it was a unique "fusion of enlightenment philosophy with American protestant piety" (p. 2),[40] modeled along the principles used at the York Retreat. Chief among those who spearheaded introduction of the moral treatment movement in the United States were Benjamin Rush, Dorothea Lynde Dix, Thomas Scattergood, and Thomas Story Kirkbride.

Benjamin Rush was a physician and also Surgeon General of the Continental Armies.[47] He is also recognized today as the father of American psychiatry. He was well acquainted with enlightenment philosophy and moral treatment ideas. He was remarkably influential in American politics having signed the Declaration of Independence.[38] Consistent with moral treatment principles, Rush "made the first systematic effort to classify patients and improve their behavior through recreation and humane discipline" (p. 3).[8]

Rush indicated his disdain for cruel treatment of the mentally ill by his concern for the "slender and inadequate means that have been employed for ameliorating the condition of mad people" and his dissatisfaction with the "slow progress of humanity in its efforts to relieve them" and the tendency for them to be treated "like criminals, or shunned like beasts of prey" (p. 1).[47] He set out to reform these conditions for the mentally ill. As a result, Rush led an effort to construct the earliest hospital in the United States to be devoted exclusively to the humane treatment of the insane. This hospital was called the Friends Asylum and was constructed in Frankford, Pennsylvania.

Dorothea Lynde Dix was influenced by the works of Rush, Pinel, and Tuke.[8] Dix had a difficult childhood, with an alcoholic father and a frail, invalid mother. At age 12, she left home to live with her paternal grandmother in Boston. At age 14, she opened a school for children and thus began an education career. At age 39, she volunteered to teach Sunday school to women at the East Cambridge Jail in Massachusetts. She was dismayed by the conditions under which patients were kept. She saw "prostitutes, drunks, criminals, retarded individuals, and the mentally ill all housed together in unheated, unfurnished and foul smelling quarters, huddling together and shivering" (p. 1).[8] When she inquired about why patients were kept in those conditions, she was told that the mentally ill did not need heat because they did not feel cold, and that her concerns were futile. She was enraged with this lack of concern for these patients and thus began her crusade for the improvement of mental health institutions, a crusade that led her eventually to England and a meeting with Queen Victoria and Pope Pius IX.[35]

Dix's crusade led to expansion of mental health institutions and other reforms. She also promoted the use of moral treatment principles as taught by Benjamin Rush, Philippe Pinel, and William Tuke, for whom she had much respect. Dix had a nervous breakdown in 1836 and was treated at the York Retreat in England, where she recovered.[8] She was impressed with the moral treatment methods used there, and in her crusade for reform of mental health facilities, she strongly advocated the use of their methods.

Thomas Scattergood was a tanner by profession and later felt a calling to be a minister.[47] He was given to frequent bouts of melancholy that earned him the nickname "the mournful prophet" among his contemporaries. In 1794, he went to Europe where he remained for the next six years. While at York, he met William Tuke, who described to him the York Retreat and acquainted him with moral treatment principles. Upon his return to the United States, he presented a proposal to the Society of Friends to establish a mental asylum. After a while, Thomas Scattergood, along with Benjamin Rush, spearheaded the construction of the Friends Asylum, whose doors opened for the first time in 1817. Its physical structure and the methods of treatment were modeled along the York Retreat.

Thomas Story Kirkbride studied medicine under Dr. Nicholas Belleville of Trenton, New Jersey, and later at Pennsylvania Hospital, receiving his medical degree in 1832.[2] During his medical education, he had studied Benjamin Rush's *Rush on the Mind* and was impressed with his ideas (which indicated that humane treatment of the insane could lead to their cure). As a resident physician, he spent some time at the Friend's Asylum where he participated in instituting the treatment techniques used there. Later, when he became the superintendent of Pennsylvania Hospital in 1840,[21] he became a strong advocate of moral treatment philosophy. He expressed his belief that "patients responded to greater freedom with better behavior."[44]

Later, Kirkbride became the founding member of the Association of Medical Superintendents of American Institutions for the Insane (AMSAII), which later became the American Psychiatric Association (APA).[21] Through his leadership, he helped spread the use of moral treatment principles in most of the mental health institutions in the United States.

The above brief historical account indicates that mental health reform leaders in the United States were closely allied and were influenced by moral treatment principles. Leading among these reformers were the Quakers, and their efforts were to a large extent guided by principles developed by William Tuke in England. Thomas Scattergood visited the York Retreat and experienced moral treatment techniques firsthand, and Dorothea Lynde Dix experienced the actual therapeutic benefits of moral treatment principles. We will explore how these principles precisely influenced treatment of the mentally ill in the United States.

Use of Moral Treatment Principles as a Guide to Therapeutic Interventions

The goal of moral treatment was early intervention and prevention of chronicity among the mentally ill.[43] As part of this endeavor, treatment consisted of environmental modification (to remove environmental stresses that caused mental illness), humane and kind treatment of patients, and use of productive occupations and leisure.[2,8,39,47] The influence of moral treatment principles on therapeutic interventions in mental health institutions in the United States and Europe were well summarized by van Atta and her colleagues.[47] Such principles included an optimistic view of patients, acceptance, use of occupation as a means of restoring health, and instilling a sense of responsibility in patients.

Optimistic View of Patients

The Quakers believed that irrespective of how insane one was, there was always residual rationality.[40,47] Thus "The faculties that remained intact during bouts of insanity were thought to be dormant but able to be reawakened by the right kind of therapy" (p. 3).[40] Since, as Pinel argued,[14,30] rationality distinguished man from beast, the first principle of

moral treatment was to bring the patient back to reason and therefore to a modicum of control of his or her disorder. Thus proponents of moral treatment in the United States proposed that "it was the job of the Asylum staff to expose and strengthen that healthy portion of the patient's mind; to 'cherish every ray of returning reason'" (p. 7).[47] Without this optimistic belief in the potential of patients, many moral treatment techniques such as gentleness and use of mentally challenging occupations such as reading would not have made sense.

Acceptance

Consistent with the enlightenment perspective as discussed earlier, the Quakers and all moral treatment advocates believed in accepting all people, including mentally ill patients, as individuals and treating them with dignity. This belief was the basis of the second principle of moral treatment, that "within the limitations of their illnesses, the patients were given the opportunity to become stable and productive members of the community" (p. 7).[47] Patients were not only to be accepted as equals in the community, but efforts were made to make them productive so that they could be equals in reality. In accordance with this principle, patients and staff members worked together on the farm in the asylum, ate meals together, and resided in the same building. This principle is the basis of the rehabilitation efforts to date, where efforts are made to reintegrate and make patients productive members of society as they recover from illness.

Use of Occupation

All advocates of moral treatment emphasized occupation, including productive labor as well as leisure, as a central tenet of therapy. For example, Pinel[29] prescribed both "physical exercises and manual occupations" (p. 63) for all patients in mental hospitals. Similarly, Kirkbride[20] and Rush[34] opposed the use of restraints, physical abuse, and seclusion, and they encouraged regular exercise; healthy amusements; good, balanced meals; and manual labor (including gardening, mentally challenging games, reading, and other literary endeavors). All mental health facilities where moral treatment principles were used had "a variety of crafts rooms, gardens, and recreation areas designed to provide clients with an active schedule of productive, creative, and recreational occupations" (p. 59).[36] Thus the third principle was that every patient needed to be engaged in some form of occupation. Consistent with this principle, "Every patient at the Friends Asylum was expected to make at least an attempt at some form of occupation: the men usually working outdoors on the farm and the women sewing or cooking" (p. 8).[47] Indeed, "The success of the entire treatment program was often believed to have been a direct result of the acceptance, by the patient, of this work ethic, and the methods used to convince him to work were numerous" (p. 8).[47]

Instilling a Sense of Responsibility in Patients

As mentioned earlier, one of the principles of the moral treatment movement was acceptance of patients as equals. As part of this acceptance, patients had to demonstrate a certain sense of responsibility. The superintendent of the Friends Asylum, for example, "saw this as a two-way commitment and expected his patients to understand what that commitment implied" (p. 8).[47] Consequently, efforts were made to encourage patients to recognize consequences of their behavior: "A patient who became violent, for example, would be removed from the rest of the patients and staff and placed in a room by himself. When he composed himself, he would then be allowed to rejoin the group" (p. 8).[47]

The above principles necessitated that asylum residents be treated in small patient-to-staff ratios so that each patient could be observed carefully and treated with dignity, engaged in carefully structured occupations, and shown consideration and acceptance as an individual. However, with the success of moral treatment methods, more patients were admitted in mental health asylums. Furthermore, physicians started arguing that the

basis of mental illness was abnormality of the brain structure rather than the environment as argued by advocates of moral treatment. One of the physicians argued that "that which...has its foundation in a definite physical cause must have its cure in the production of physical change" (p. 2).[39] Moral treatment began to be considered nonmedical. Furthermore, early treatment failed to prevent chronicity as promised by moral treatment advocates.[43] Overcrowding in mental health institutions and subsequent deterioration in patient care, along with change in attitudes regarding etiology and treatment of mental illness, led to a decline of the moral treatment movement. Shortly after the American Civil War, moral treatment significantly declined in the United States.

The Rise of the Arts and Crafts Movement

According to the USSG,[43] the mental hygiene movement followed the decline of the moral treatment movement. However, as mentioned earlier, the arts and crafts movement became prominent at around the same time. It is unclear as to whether arts and crafts ideas influenced the mental health reform efforts of the mental hygiene movement. Nevertheless, we will discuss the arts and crafts movement as a separate event owing to its crucial role in the development of occupational therapy.

The arts and crafts movement began in England in the second half of the nineteenth century (in the 1860s).[6,33,45] This was soon after the American Civil War, when moral treatment had waned. The movement was based largely on the philosophy of John Ruskin, who was among the philosophers at the forefront of social reform at this time. Generally, Ruskin and other reform philosophers believed that the medieval world was purer than the postrenaissance industrialized world, because people in medieval times were more closely linked to nature. He believed that industrialization, which was associated with mechanization, alienated humans from themselves and from nature, causing discontent. In his view, the machine "dehumanized the worker and led to a loss of dignity because it removed him from the artistic process and thus, nature itself" (p. 1).[45]

It is evident that Ruskin's ideas originated from a wider social movement led by reformers in postrenaissance Europe such as Karl Marx. Marx had appropriated the dialectical philosophical arguments of Wilhelm Friedrich Hegel, under whom he had studied.[18,19] Hegel had used Plato and Aristotle's syllogistic method to argue that ideas as well as social institutions evolved through the process of thesis (existing status quo), antithesis (challenging ideas), and synthesis (combining the best of the status quo with the best of new challenging ideas to come up with a superior hybrid of ideas or social institutions).[7] Therefore he was concerned with evolution of ideas rather than practical application of philosophy to solve social problems.

Marx agreed with this dialectical approach to social evolution, having studied the history of the French Revolution that resulted from enlightenment ideas[19,26] but divulging from Hegel's teaching, he believed that "philosophy ought to be employed in practice to change the world" (p. 1).[19] He proposed that social problems in industrial Europe could be characterized by the inherent struggle between two social classes: the capitalistic class (bourgeoisie or owners of means of production), and the workers (proletariat).[18,19,24,25] Marx believed that the struggle between these two classes characterized the dialectical process that would lead to social evolution and result in a classless society.

Marx saw labor in this dialectically conflicted industrial society as objectified into a commodity that could be bought and sold in a marketplace. In this sense, it became external to the worker, who became separated from that which was once his or her very life (labor). The worker was also separated from the product of his or her labor, which now existed independently of him or her;

from the natural world that supplied the raw materials used to make the product; and from other workers. Labor became a meaningless activity in which workers engaged begrudgingly. He referred to this separation as alienation, which he saw as an inevitable consequence of industrialization and which was the source of class conflicts and revolutions (such as the French revolution), which were the result of the ongoing dialectical process of social evolution.

Ruskin borrowed the concept of alienation primarily from Marx. William Morris, a British poet, artist, and architect, used Ruskin's philosophical ideas to found the arts and crafts movement. He and other proponents of the movement saw engagement in artistic endeavors as part of social reform. This reform was aimed at reducing alienation of humanity in the industrial world by making labor more meaningful, reconnecting the worker with nature, and thus restoring harmony. As Sabonis-Chafee and Hussey[35] state,

> In reaction to the expanding use of tools and machines, a contingency of proponents of the arts and crafts developed. They were opposed to the production of items by machine, believing this alienated people from nature. It was believed that using one's hands to make items connected people to their work, physically and mentally, and thus was healthier. (p. 20)

This view was well illustrated in Morris' address to the Trades' Guild of Learning in which he stated that "everything made by man's hands has a form, which must be either beautiful or ugly; beautiful if it is in accord with Nature, and helps her; ugly if it is discordant with Nature, and thwarts her; It cannot be indifferent" (p. 2).[28] In other words, he saw beauty as being not only utilitarian but also consistent with harmonious intercourse with nature. The reader should note how similar this idea is to the statement by Meyer later, where he proposed that good health is tantamount to a state of harmony with nature, which he saw as adaptive (see Chapter 2 for a discussion of Meyer and the pragmatists).[27] Morris stated,

…but now only let the arts we are talking of ornament our labor, and be widely spread, intelligent, well understood both by the maker and user, let them grow on one word popular, and there will be pretty much an end of dull work and its wearing slavery; and no man will any longer have an excuse for talking about the curse of labour, no man will any longer have an excuse for evading the blessing of labour.[28]

In this statement, it is apparent that Morris believed that artistic endeavors connect the human with his or her labor, with nature, with those who enjoy the product of the labor, and thus engage the body and mind in labor. In Morris's view, this was the source of enjoyment of one's labor, which would reduce the alienation that Ruskin, Marx, and others perceived to be a problem in the industrial world. In this sense, the arts and crafts movement was clearly part of a larger social reform, similar and in fact continuous with the reform that had resulted from enlightenment and that propelled mental health reform during the moral treatment movement. It is not surprising therefore that the arts and crafts movement was seen as a useful tool for continuation of mental health reform that had begun with the moral treatment movement (which had declined in the second half of the nineteenth century). Indeed, these arts and crafts movement ideas would continue to influence mental health practice well into the early twentieth century.[6,31]

It was in these circumstances that Herbert J. Hall, a physician who had graduated from Harvard Medical School, borrowed the principles of the arts and crafts philosophy and sought to apply them in medicine.[35] Hall was working with clients diagnosed with neurasthenia (a nervous condition characterized by severe weakness), who were mostly female, at a facility in Mablehead, Massachusetts. At the time, the typical prescription for clients with this condition was "rest cure." Hall[11] saw this condition as being a result of alienation from life. In 1904, instead of prescribing rest cure to these clients, he engaged them in arts and crafts[35] as part

of re-engaging them with life, decreasing their alienation, and helping them begin their journey toward recovery.[11]

Hall had clients engage in bedside activities (which he then graded as they improved), leading to weaving, ceramics, and other crafts in workshops.[35] He combined principles from the arts and crafts movement with ideas from the moral treatment movement. He insisted that the 24 hours for each client be divided into periods of work, rest, and recreation, and that clients receive plenty of air, sufficient and nutritious food, counseling, and medical treatment as indicated. He saw this kind of treatment as a kind of industrial therapy.[11]

As discussed earlier, work, rest, recreation, plenty of fresh air, and good food were all emphasized by proponents of the moral treatment movement. Here, we can see that Hall endeavored to marry the moral treatment movement with the arts and crafts movement. At the same time, Jane Addams and Julia Lanthrop at the Hull House in Chicago were using arts and crafts to help poor immigrants from Europe stay connected to their cultural roots and transition to the new culture in the United States.[3,48] Indeed, Jane Addams, the founder of Hull House, was involved in the establishment of the Chicago Arts and Crafts Society.[16] As noted in Chapter 2, Hull House was to play a major role in the development of occupational therapy in the early twentieth century.[3,13,15,48] At this juncture, the use of arts and crafts was introduced to occupational therapy.

To deepen your insight regarding the historical, intellectual, and social contexts of occupational therapy and articulation of the new professional paradigm, complete Lab Manual Exercise 2-1 in your laboratory manual.

SUMMARY

In this chapter, we saw that the history of formal therapeutic use of occupation developed from the rise of moral treatment movement in Europe (which was part of the mental health reform).

The moral treatment ideas spread in the United States and subsequently declined after the American Civil War. It has been demonstrated that the moral treatment movement was a psychologically oriented therapy aimed at helping patients regain a sense of well-being or morale by treating them kindly and using a daily routine consisting of self care, recreation, religious observances, and manual labor. The milieu in which therapy took place was also considered important, and it was proposed that it needed to consist of a homelike atmosphere, plenty of clean air, and pleasant surroundings.

Mental health reform (of which moral treatment was a part) comprised a larger social reform whose momentum was supported by the empirical philosophical principles of John Locke and their translation into enlightenment principles in France. Owing to a variety of factors, the moral treatment movement declined in the second half of the nineteenth century. Later, the rise of the arts and crafts movement (part of another social reform movement) was based on the idea that industrialization alienated the worker from the self, the product of his or her labor, other workers, and nature. Doing arts and crafts was a way of ameliorating this sense of alienation, therefore leading to good health. Arts and crafts ideas combined with moral treatment principles provided a rationale for the use of arts and crafts as therapeutic media. The reader should be clear by now of the context in which occupation became part of therapy in mental health, and particularly of how arts and crafts entered the therapeutic scene in our professional history.

REFERENCES

1. Bockoven JS: Occupational therapy: a historical perspective. Legacy of moral treatment 1800s to 1910, *Am J Occup Ther* 25:223-225, 1971.
2. Bradford SS: *Kirkbride's hospital: also known as institute of Pennsylvania hospital placed on the national register of historic places July 24, 1975*, 2005. Retrieved June 2005 from http:// www.uchs.net/HistoricDistricts/kirkbride.html.
3. Breines E: *Origins and adaptations: a philosophy of practice*, Lebanon, NJ, 1986, Geri-Rehab.
4. Bruce MA, Borg B: *Psychosocial frames of reference: core for occupation-based practice*, Thorofare, NJ, 2002, Slack.
5. Burrows JR & Company: *Art, design, and visual thinking: the arts and crafts movement*, 2005. Retrieved May 2005 from http://char.txa.cornell.edu/art/decart/artcraft.htm.
6. Detweiler J, Peyton C: Defining occupations: a chronotopic study of narrative genres in a health discipline's emergence, *Written Communication* 16:412-468, 1999.
7. Dewey J: *Reconstruction in philosophy*, Boston, 1957, Beacon Press.
8. Foley A: "Dorothea Lynde Dix (1802-1887): humanitarian reform and its contribution to the history of psychology," Simon Frasier University, 2000. Retrieved May 2005 from http://www.sfu.ca/~wwwpsyb/issues/2000/summer/foley.htm.
9. Gollaher D: *Voice for the mad: the life of Dorothea Dix*, Toronto, 1995, The Free Press.
10. Grob GN: *Mental illness and American society, 1875-1940*, Princeton, 1983, Princeton University Press.
11. Hall HJ: Work-cure: a report of 5 years experience at an institution devoted to the therapeutic application of manual work, *J Am Med Assoc* 55:12-13, 1910.
12. Hergenhahn BR: *An introduction to the history of psychology*, Pacific Grove, Calif, 1997, Brooks/ Cole.
13. Ikiugu MN: The philosophy and culture of occupational therapy (doctoral dissertation, Texas Woman's University, 2001), *Dissertation Abstracts International*, 62(12B), 5678.
14. Ikiugu MN: Instrumentalism in occupational therapy: an argument for a pragmatic conceptual model of practice, *Internat J Psychosocial Rehabil* 8:109-117, 2004.
15. Ikiugu MN, Schultz S: An argument for pragmatism as a foundational philosophy of occupational therapy, *Canad J Occup Ther* 73(2):86-97, 2006.
16. Jackson Lears TJ: *No place of grace: antimodernism and the transformation of American culture, 1880-1920*, New York, 1981, Pantheon Books.
17. Jimenez MA: *Changing faces of madness*, London, 1987, University Press of New England.
18. Kemerling G: *Marx and Engels: communism*, 2001. Retrieved June 2005 from http://www.philosophypages.com/hy/5o.htm.
19. Kemerling G: *Karl Marx (1818-1883)*, 2002. Retrieved June 2005 from http://www.philosophypages.com/ph/marx.htm.
20. Kirkbride TS: *On the construction, organization, and general arrangements of hospitals for the insane*, Philadelphia, 1948, Lindsay & Blakiston.
21. Kirkbride Buildings: *Dr. Thomas Story Kirkbride*, 2005. Retrieved June 2005 from http://www.kirkbridebuildings.com/about/kirkbride.html.

22. Lightner DL: *Asylum, prison, and poorhouse*, Carbondale, 1999, Southern Illinois University Press.

23. Magee B: *The story of thought: the essential guide to the history of Western philosophy*, New York, 1998, DK Publishing.

24. Marx K: *Economic and philosophical manuscripts: first manuscript: wages of labor* [electronic version], 1844. Retrieved July 2005, from http://eserver.org:16080/marx/1944-ep.manuscripts/1st.manuscript/1-labor.wages.txt.

25. Marx K, Engels F: *Manifesto of the communist party* [electronic version], 1848. Retrieved July 2005, from http://eserver.org/marx/1848-communist.manifesto/cm1.txt.

26. Marxists Internet Archive: *Footnotes for volume 4 of Marx-Engels collected works*. Retrieved June 2005 from http://www.marxists.org/archive/marx/works/cw/volume04/footnote.htm.

27. Meyer A: The philosophy of occupation therapy, *Arch Occup Ther* 1:1-10, 1922.

28. Morris W: *The decorative arts, their relation to modern life and progress: an address delivered before the Trades' Guild of Learning*, December 4, 1877. Retrieved May 2005 from http://www.burrows.com/dec.html.

29. Pinel P: *Traite medico-philosophique sur palienation mentale, ou la manie* [Medical philosophical treaties on mental alienation], Paris: Chez Richard, Caille et Ravier. Excerpts reprinted in *Occupational Therapy and Rehabilitation* 26, 63–68, 1947.

30. Pinel P: *A treatise on insanity*, New York, 1962, Hafner.

31. Quiroga VA: *Occupational therapy: the first 30 years— 1900 to 1930*. Bethesda, MD, 1995, American Occupational Therapy Association.

32. Rempel G: *Age of the enlightenment*, 2005. Retrieved June 2005 from http:// mars.acnet.wnec.edu/_grempel/courses/wc2/lectures/enlightenment.html.

33. Research Machines PLC: *Arts and crafts movement*, 2005. Retrieved May 2005 from http://www.tiscali.co.uk/reference/encyclopedia/hutchinson/m0018503.html.

34. Rush B: *Medical inquiries and observations, upon the disease of the mind*, Philadelphia, 1947, Kimber & Richardson.

35. Sabonis-Chafee B, Hussey SM: *Introduction to occupational therapy*, ed 2, St Louis, 1998, Mosby.

36. Schwartz KB: The history and philosophy of psychosocial occupational therapy. In Cara E, McRae A, eds: *Psychosocial occupational therapy: a clinical practice*, Clifton Park, NY, 2005, Delmar, pp. 57-79.

37. Stein F, Cutler SK: *Psychosocial occupational therapy: a holistic approach*, ed 2, Albany, NY, 2002, Delmar.

38. Stevens G, Gardner S: *The women of psychology*, Cambridge, Mass, 1982, Schenkman.

39. Sutherland S: Books: the most solitary of afflictions: madness and society in Britain, 1700–1900 [electronic version]. *The Guardian*, p. NOPGCIT, July 15, 1993.

40. Taubes T: "Healthy avenues of the mind": psychological theory building and the influence of religion during the era of moral treatment [electronic version], *Am J Psychiatry* 155(8):1001-1009, 1998.

41. Tipton IC: *Locke on human understanding: selected essays*, Oxford, 1977, Oxford University Press.

42. Tuke S: *Description of the retreat: an institution near York for insane persons of the Society of Friends containing an account of its origin and progress, the mode of treatment, and a statement of cases*, London, 1964, Dawsons of Pall Mall.

43. United States Surgeon General: *Mental health: a report of the Surgeon General*, 2005. Retrieved May 2005 from http://www.surgeongeneral.gov/library/mentalhealth/home.html.

44. University of Pennsylvania Health System: *Dr. Thomas Story Kirkbride*, 2005. Retrieved June 2005 from http://www.uphs.upenn.edu/paharc/timeline/1801/tline14.html.

45. University of Toledo: *The noble craftsman we promote: The arts and crafts movement in the American North West: Roots of arts and crafts*, 1999. Retrieved May 2005 from http:// www.cl.utoledo.edu/canaday/artsandcrafts/ roots.html.

46. Uzgalis W: John Locke. In *Stanford Encyclopedia of Philosophy*, 2001. Retrieved June 2005 from http://plato.stanford.edu/entries/locke/.

47. van Atta K, Roby DS, Roby RR: *Friends hospital: an account of the events surrounding the origin of Friends hospital and a brief description of the early years of Friends Asylum 1817–1820*, 1988. Retrieved June 2005 from http://www.freindshospitalonline.org/eventsaccount.htm.

48. Wilcock AA: *An occupational perspective of health*, Thorofare, NJ, 1998, Slack.

49. Yolton J: *John Locke and the way of ideas*, Oxford, 1956, Oxford University Press.

Chapter 2

The Formal Founding of Occupational Therapy and Its Evolution from 1900 to the Present

Preview Questions

1. Discuss the formal founding of occupational therapy as a profession at the turn of the twentieth century.
2. What social and intellectual influences guided the early years of occupational therapy development?
3. Explain paradigmatic changes that led to the professional identity crisis of the 1930s to the 1960s.
4. Discuss the profession's struggle with identity beginning in the 1960s and leading to the emergence of a new professional paradigm in the late 1990s to early 2000s.

In 1917, George Barton and Thomas Bessel Kidner (architects), Eleanor Clarke Slagle (a social worker), William Rush Dunton Jr. (a physician), Susan Cox Johnson (a teacher), and Isabel Newton (a secretary and later Barton's wife) met at the Consolation House in Clifton Springs, New York, and founded the National Society for the Promotion of Occupational Therapy (NSPOT).[89,106] Herbert J. Hall, although not present, became a member and was the organization's president from 1920 to 1923.[89] Susan Tracy was also not present but was an active member of the organization.

According to Quiroga, the profession was formed by threading ideas from "nursing, teaching, medicine, psychiatry, arts and crafts, reha-

bilitation, self-help, orthopedics, mental hygiene, social work, and more, enriching occupational therapy's professional depth and breadth" (p. 14).[81] In this chapter, we will discuss some of these intellectual and social influences—the arts and crafts and mental hygiene movements, the philosophy of pragmatism, and Charles Darwin's theory of evolution, among others. We will also discuss other social influences such as World War I and World War II, the Great Depression, various scientific and technological advances, the discovery of various drugs, and the development of psychological theories. We will also cover the profession's history from its founding in 1917 to the present within the context of these intellectual and social influences.

Influence of the Arts and Crafts Movement

As mentioned in Chapter 1, the arts and crafts movement was an attempt at social reform to decrease the sense of alienation that was perceived to be a consequence of industrialization. Herbert J. Hall applied its principals to treat clients suffering from neurasthenia. At the same time, arts and crafts were used at the Chicago School of Philanthropy, and particularly at the Hull House to help integrate poor immigrants from Europe into the American culture.[9,92,106] Many of the early founders of occupational therapy including Tracy, Barton, and Dunton used arts and crafts in therapeutic interventions. All the founders "were profoundly influenced by arts and crafts, efficiency, mental hygiene, antituberculosis, and women's philanthropy and reform movements of the early 20th century" (p. 32).[81]

For example, George Barton "studied in London under the leader of Britain's arts and crafts movement. Later, he returned to Boston to incorporate the Boston Society of arts and crafts" (p. 21).[89] Susan Cox Johnson, another founding member of the NSPOT, was an arts and crafts teacher. Similarly, Susan Tracy, a charter member of the newly founded profession, "was an occupational nurse involved in the arts and crafts movement and in the training of nurses in the use of occupations" (p. 23).[89] Her book, *Studies in Invalid Occupations,*[96] was a guide to prescription and selection of arts and crafts for the treatment of patients. As Detweiller and Peyton[19] suggest, the arts and crafts movement was the basis of the principles that were used to provide a rationale for therapeutic use of arts and crafts activities. Engagement in arts and crafts was seen as a way of capturing "productive and meaningful life experiences" (p. 39)[81] and in that way counteracting the problem of alienation due to industrialization.

The Mental Hygiene Movement

The concept of mental hygiene dates back in American history to the period soon after the American Civil War.[59] Concerned about the effects of unsanitary conditions, Dr. J.B. Gray, a psychiatrist, suggested community mental hygiene, similar to the concept of physical hygiene in public health. This concept denoted the use of community-based mental health efforts through education, social culture, religion, and civil involvement. Mental hygiene was therefore a social reform movement that could be understood within the wider context of public health,[58] characterized by advocacy for public involvement in the promotion of health.

As Dr. C. Winslow states, "The mental hygiene movement...bears the same relation to psychiatry that public health movement, of which it forms a part, bears to medicine in general" (p. 7).[58] Later, *mental hygiene* was defined as the art of preservation of the mind and intellect in the face of assault from pernicious environmental conditions. This could be achieved by controlling passions and cultivating intellectual discipline through management of physical bodily functioning by exercising, eating well, getting enough rest, dressing appropriately, maintaining a comfortable environment, and so on.[59]

At the turn of the twentieth century, the mental hygiene movement was given impetus by the work of Clifford Beers, a former mental patient who was also a graduate of Yale University.[59,95] Beers had published a book detailing his firsthand experiences of the deplorable conditions in mental health institutions. As an example of how this publication influenced the spread of mental hygiene, Julia Lanthrop read the book while attending a Mental Hygiene Association (MHA) meeting in Connecticut in 1908. The contents of the book moved her so much that she was determined to help initiate mental health reform when she returned to Chicago.[81] The work of Beers and others led to the founding of the National Committee for Mental Hygiene (NCMH) in 1909.

The reader may notice that the principles of mental hygiene were consistent with those of the arts and crafts movement. Since mental hygiene was part of the public health social reform effort, naturally (as is the case with the moral treatment movement before it) it was based on the belief that mental illness was a result of environmental factors and therefore it was preventable. If no measures were taken to prevent the malady, it would continue to get progressively worse. The belief among proponents of arts and crafts that industrialization caused alienation thus was consistent with the principles of mental hygiene. Alienation was an environmental factor causing mental illness. Therefore, the arts and crafts movement, based on the idea that eliminating alienation was the way to good mental health, was a means by which mental hygienists could achieve their goals.

Mental hygiene advocates proposed early treatment of mental illness with one of the objectives as prevention of chronicity.[98] Chief among the mental hygienists was Adolf Meyer.[59,89,92,93,106] Meyer was a psychiatrist from Zurich, Switzerland, who had migrated to the United States, and was working at an asylum for the insane at Kankakee, Illinois. He developed what he called the *psychobiological approach* in psychiatry, which was based on the premise that life experiences were central to the etiology of mental illness. His acquaintance with arts and crafts principles was apparent in his conviction that "industrialization and urbanization were undermining human potential for continuous adaptability and constructive activity" (p. 1).[59] Like arts and crafts enthusiasts, he argued that mental health could be attained and maintained through education and environmental modification.

Meyer was also influenced by American pragmatism and the psychology of functionalism that was espoused by William James and John Dewey,[106] as well as by Darwin's theory of evolution.[81] Functionalism was the American version of German structuralism, developed by Wundt.[36] One argument within functionalism was that the sole purpose of the mind was to enable individuals to pursue personal interests and goals. As such, adherents to this school of thought proposed that the study of the mind should not be through introspection but through practical situations of everyday life. One of the pragmatists, George Herbert Mead, developed an entire philosophical discourse based on this idea, which he called the *philosophy of the act*.[64] Based on the principles of arts and crafts philosophy, the mental hygiene movement, pragmatic philosophy, and the psychology of functionalism, Dewey proposed that " 'doing, action, and experience are being' and that the activities expressed in living demonstrate mind-body synthesis" (p. 173).[106] These were the ideas behind

Meyer's further proposal that the problems of persons with mental illness were problems of adaptation and that work was a valuable tool for treatment of those problems. He stated that "The proper use of time in some helpful and gratifying activity appeared to me a fundamental issue in the treatment of any neuropsychiatric patient" (p. 639).[65]

Consistent with the doctrines of pragmatism, functionalism, and Darwinian evolutionism, Meyer saw the therapeutic use of occupation as justifiable through an understanding of mental illness as a problem of living. In this view, personality was fundamentally determined by performance. He thus conceptualized the human as an organism that organized and maintained itself by acting in temporal harmony with its environment. He argued that through this kind of activity, the human actualized his or her existence by putting his or her mark in the environment. Meyer's idea that performance equals being (combined with his theory that patients needed help to develop sound habits consistent with healthy, adaptive living)[106] was close to James'[43] proposition that action aimed at establishing proper habits was necessary, and that humans needed to cultivate these habits in order to make their nervous system an ally instead of an enemy.

In this regard, James conceived the whole purpose of education as an endeavor to make an individual's nervous system an ally rather than an enemy. This endeavor, he argued, could be achieved by cultivating appropriate habits (referred to in this book as *adaptive habits*) early in life and guarding against developing those that are disadvantageous (*maladaptive habits*). He argued that by allowing adaptive habits to guide most of our moment-to-moment decisions (so that we did not have to deliberate about every action we took in our lives), our higher powers of the mind would be appropriately released to engage in creative endeavors.

These were the ideas upon which Meyer's psychobiological principles, and Slagle's "habit training" program at the Phipps clinic were based.[106] In other words, Meyer derived his principles from three sources: (1) the arts and crafts postulation that industrialization caused alienation and mental illness, (2) the mental hygiene principle that the cause of mental illness was environmental and could be alleviated through education and community action, and (3) the pragmatic and functionalist principle that proper habits of action resulted in adaptiveness and good health. The mental hygiene movement, with Meyer at the helm, was a significant influence in American psychiatry for at least the first 20 years of the twentieth century.

Influence of the Four American Pragmatists

It has been suggested in literature that the foundational philosophy of occupational therapy is American pragmatism.[9,18,37,41] This assertion is likely to be correct considering that pragmatism is particularly an American philosophy. According to Fisch, it matured during "the classic period in American philosophy" (p. 1).[32]

Charles Sanders Peirce

The philosophy of pragmatism was founded by Charles Sanders Peirce. He began developing his ideas at a time when there was continuing rebellion in modern science and philosophy against middle age authoritarianism as discussed in Chapter 1. This revolt was led by the enlightenment movement and was based on the major themes of humanism, freedom, naturalism, Epicureanism, historiography, religious tolerance, science based on experimentation, and de-Christianization of philosophy. Peirce was caught up in this rebellion. In this historical context, and because of his training as a scientist, he attempted to develop a philosophy based on the methods of scientific experimentation rather than idle speculation.

Peirce refuted the tendency in philosophy at the time to use authority as justification of speculative propositions. He was of the opinion that authority was an institutional tool of fixing belief, which had been used for ages, but which was often erroneous. He agreed with Bacon that belief about knowledge should be based on experience "as something which must be open to verification and re-examination" (p. 55).[78] By making propositions that were open to verification rather than being accepted on the basis of institutional authority, Peirce was proposing to develop what could be seen as "laboratory philosophy" (p. 363).[72] The primary argument in this philosophy was that "reasoning is good if it be such as to give true conclusions from true premises, and not otherwise" (p. 57).[78] We can only draw true conclusions from true premises if the premises and conclusions are soundly grounded in fact. The validity of reasoning is, therefore, a matter of fact.

The second argument in Peirce's philosophical doctrine was that the mind could exist in one of two states: doubt or belief. Doubt caused irritation and belief a settlement of the mind. Belief was the state toward which the mind tended and was the basis of habits that determined our actions as human beings. In practice, "Our beliefs guide our desires and shape our actions" (p. 59).[77] Belief, action, and habit were central constructs in the philosophy of pragmatism. Peirce saw the essence of belief as establishment of habit.[73] He proposed that the way to distinguish beliefs was to examine the mode of action to which they gave rise. If beliefs perceived to be different appeased doubt by giving rise to the same mode of action, then by all intent and purpose, they constituted the same belief, analogous to playing the same note on different keys on a piano. Peirce's argument can be logically interpreted to mean that since habits constitute repeated modes of action, beliefs can be distinguished by the habits to which they give rise, and if different beliefs give rise to the same habit, then they constitute the same belief.

In this argument, Peirce established two core propositions: (1) belief is a rule for action, which means that belief without action is meaningless and (2) action is a method of verifying belief. Furthermore, the consequences of actions emanating from a belief are the yardstick by which the truth of that belief is measured. In this regard, Peirce[76] proposed that to clarify our conception of an object (our beliefs about the essential characteristics of an object), we only need to examine the practical implications of our conception, and that would inform us about the perceived nature of the object. Peirce's ideas were infused into occupational therapy by latter-day pragmatists such as William James, John Dewey, and George Herbert Mead as will be apparent later in this chapter.

William James

Peirce's ideas were popularized by his longtime friend William James, although he did not agree entirely with James' interpretation of his philosophical arguments. At one time, he declared that he would drop use of the term *pragmatism* in favor of *pragmaticism,* a term "ugly enough to be safe from kidnappers" (p. 4).[5] He was referring to James and others, whom he thought had misinterpreted the concept. The cause of disagreement between Peirce and James was based on two factors.

James seemed to have been unaware of Peirce's change of thought as his philosophy evolved. In his earlier work, he saw the pragmatic method of discounting doubt and settling belief as consisting of the practical consequences of holding the belief.[75] For example, if you believe that an object on the floor is a solid obstacle in your path, you will act accordingly by walking around the object to get to the other side. If, however, you find that it is a mirage, as is the case in 3-D motion pictures, you will experience doubt regarding the validity of your belief, and that will be the motivation for further investigation of the object.

James' notion of belief was consistent with this premise.[32] However, in his mature thought Peirce had changed this notion and considered practical consequences as unnecessary as a test of belief. Rather, intellectual consequences, including the expectation of action based on the belief, even though not acting in present, would suf-

fice as verification of the belief.[11] Thus, if you believed that the object in front of you is solid and you had the expectation that you would need to walk around it in order to get to the other side, this would be verification enough for your belief. James seemed to be unaware of this change in Peirce's thought and continued to insist that the test for belief consisted of the practical consequences of acting on the belief.

James, unlike Peirce, went beyond the realm of factual verification of belief to theism. In this move, he wanted to make it possible for a pragmatist to include within his or her domain the moral and religious aspects of belief.[5,32,61,71] James began this endeavor by defining belief as a hypothesis,[46] or a theory that things are a certain way. Also, he saw beliefs as dead or alive. A dead belief was one that a person was not ready to act on. A live belief was one on the basis of which a person was likely to act. Defined that way, a live belief had real, practical consequences because a person was likely to act based on it.

In this sense, religious and moral beliefs on the basis of which people were likely to act became, by definition, verifiable beliefs in the pragmatic sense. This notion was beyond Peirce's intention in founding pragmatism, considering that his philosophy was in part a rebellion against religious authoritarianism. These two factors are the reason that Peirce believed that the "pragmatism" construct had been kidnapped and was being used in ways that were different from his intentions.[32]

Following is a summary of central themes in James' thought, which were evidently applied in occupational therapy. First, James believed in the creative energy of humans.[61] This ability to create, he believed, made humans unique because, along with God, they engendered truth on the reality of the world and therefore were its co-creators.[45] He saw this creativity as *existence through doing,* which was the tendency for human beings. In other words, through doing, one was creative, and in being creative, one existed. Thus, James saw the universe as the context of human activity, whereby humans were co-creators in its continual evolvement. This theme was not present in Peirce's thought. James' emphasis on existence through creativity by doing is obvious in occupational therapy's focus on doing throughout the profession's history.

The second central theme in James' propositions, similar to Peirce's philosophy, was the centrality of experience as a source of human knowledge and activity.[44,61] He went as far as calling his doctrine "radical empiricism,"[44] by which he meant "a radically new account of how the self penetrates and is penetrated by the world" (p. xxx).[61] In this view, he saw the human as not apart from nature or above nature, but as being inextricably bound to nature. He conceptualized the mind as an instrument or tool for adaptation to the environment. In this sense, James agreed with Dewey (discussed below), that all activities of the mind are instrumental. This idea is best illustrated in the statement that in the pragmatic method, "Theories thus become instruments, not answers to enigmas, in which we can rest" (p. 28).[45] This focus on human interaction with nature (the environment) is another central theme in occupational therapy that originated from the moral treatment movement and was strengthened by the principles of the philosophy of pragmatism. For example, Meyer, in his theory of psychobiology, was of the opinion that the purpose of the mind was to "enable individuals...to pursue specific interests and achieve specific goals" (p. 173).[106]

The third central theme in James' philosophy was the importance of habit in human functioning. The idea of habit of action and thinking was actually a continuation of Peirce's argument that in an attempt by the mind to settle doubt and establish belief, there is "The presence of regularity and novelty, synechistically conjoined" (p. xxxii).[61] James went further and analyzed habit from a physiological perspective. In his *Principles of Psychology*,[42] he proposed that habit developed from neural pathways that were repeatedly etched out in the human brain by repeated experience. He considered habit to be essential to proper human functioning and adap-

tation because it made it possible to perform acts efficiently without consciously having to think about every single action. He proposed that it was important to develop appropriate habits that were advantageous to survival as early as possible and to "guard against the growing into ways that are likely to be disadvantageous to us, as we should guard against the plague" (p. 17).[43]

This theme was evident in the principles of habit training, articulated by Meyer and applied by Slagle in occupational therapy.[9,89,106] Meyer saw lack of adaptation as the reason for clients' habit deterioration and proposed a regimen of habit training as a remedy, while Slagle visualized the role of occupational therapy as that of substituting healthy work habits for invalid ones to facilitate clients' adaptation.[81] Thus, the philosophy of James significantly influenced the development of occupational therapy in the early years, under the influence of the mental hygiene movement.

John Dewey

While Peirce initiated the philosophy of pragmatism and James popularized it, Dewey applied it in education and solution of social issues. This preoccupation with application was based on his belief that philosophy should be context-based and should deal with prominent social and cultural issues of the day.[32,103] Having been highly influenced by Wilhelm Friedrich Hegel's philosophical emphasis on the historical, social, and cultural context,[20,62] he viewed philosophy as an "intellectual expression of a conflict in culture. Its function is to locate the sources of these conflicts, and to offer a broad and general solution for them" (p. 327).[32]

In order to understand Dewey's philosophical propositions, it is important to understand his intellectual influences. As mentioned earlier, Hegel greatly influenced Dewey's thought. He "stresses the significance...as 'a permanent deposit' in his thinking" (p. 1).[62] Hegel impressed Dewey not only because of his historical contextualization of philosophy, but even more importantly, because of his attempts to dissolve all kinds of dualisms by synthesizing, for example, the "subject and object, matter and spirit, the divine and the human," and so on (p. 7).[20] Dewey referred to his experience of discovering Hegel as "an immense release, a liberation" (p. 7).[20] This influence by Hegel explains his preoccupation with meliorism of social issues. Hegel had advanced a dialectic method of evolution of not only intellectual ideas, but also of social institutions.[36] In his dialectic approach, ideas, cultures, political systems, and so on, evolved through the process of antitheses that challenged the theses (status quo), and led to synthesis (emergence of a superior hybrid of the old and the new). This process of evolution was teleological, tending toward perfection, which he referred to as the *absolute*. Thus one can understand how Dewey saw his work as an attempt to facilitate this process of social evolution.

Another great influence on Dewey's thought was James. He stated the following about the effect that James had on him: "As far as I can discover, one specifiable philosophic factor which entered into my thinking so as to give it a new direction and quality, it is this one (referring to James' philosophy)" (p. 10).[20] He explained that what was attractive was James' psychological theory, which brought objectivity to the question of consciousness, "having its roots in a return to the earlier biological conception of the *psyche* but a return possessed of a new force and value due to the immense progress made by biology since the time of Aristotle" (p. 11).[20] He was particularly fond of James' idea of life "in terms of life in action" (p. 11).[20] James' psychological theory probably influenced Dewey's formulation of the doctrine of instrumentalism (discussed later).

The third influence, as is the case with all the other pragmatists, was Darwin's theory of evolution. Beginning with Peirce, the theory of evolution was central to the philosophy of pragmatism. Peirce considered Darwin's theory to be a great breakthrough in the advance of science because "Mr. Darwin proposed to apply

the statistical method to biology" (p. 7),[75] thus doing away with the last fixity advanced by religious dogmas, the fixity of biological species. Similarly, in his discussion of habits and the origin of instincts, James[43] considered Darwin's concepts of adaptation and natural variation as foregone conclusions among his intellectual contemporaries. On his part, Dewey[22] was of the opinion that by explaining the principle of transition of life through the phenomenon of adaptation and natural variation, Darwin had freed a new logic that could be applied to the mind, morals, and life in general. In other words, questions could at last be asked about the nature of the mind, morality, and life in general, which could be answered through experimental investigation.

In fact, Dewey's whole notion of instrumentalism, which was based on a central premise of "interaction of the human organism with nature or with the environment" (p. xxv),[62] may be understood to emanate in large part from the principles of the theory of evolution. He viewed even social institutions as instruments that humans created using intelligence and which they used to help them adapt and survive, in the Darwinian sense. Among these institutions, in his view, was politics, which he conceptualized as a "struggle to construct an optimum environment for the realizing and sanctioning of the aesthetic processes of living" (p. xxv).[62] He argued that "creative intelligence" should be geared toward achieving "optimum possibilities in the never-ending moral struggle to harmonize the means-end relationship for the purpose of enhancing human life and achieving growth" (pp. xxv-xxvi).[62]

Finally, there is evidence that Dewey was influenced by John Ruskin's and William Morris' principles of arts and crafts philosophy. One hint of this influence is the fact that Dewey was associated with the Hull House, where arts and crafts ideas were in part the guiding principles.[106] Even more compelling are some of the statements in his writings that indicated that like Ruskin and other social reformers, he saw modern life as alienating human beings and arts and crafts as one way of reconnecting humanity to nature. In his essay, *The Living Creature,* Dewey[23] expressed the opinion that originally art was part of human life, or in other words, contextualized. However, in modern society, walls had been built between the artistic and ordinary lives. In this sense, he saw art as having been alienated from the life that gave it meaning. He wrote that "When artistic objects are separated from both conditions of origin and operation in experience, a wall is built around them that renders almost opaque their general significance, with which esthetic theory deals" (p. 526).[23]

Having examined some influences on Dewey's philosophy, some of his core themes and their relationship to occupational therapy will now be discussed. Dewey's entire philosophy may be understood as a discourse on human experience. He expounded on the structure of experience as lived experience.[62] His view of experience was conceived in the spirit of experimentalism. Like Peirce, he saw himself as an experimentalist.[73] He argued that philosophy should emulate science in its methodology rather than being antagonistic to it. In this sense, he saw experience as a grasp of what had already taken place. He asserted that experienced things were "things had before they are things cognized" (p. 68).[73] He proposed that experience preceded cognition. Furthermore, consistent with James' idea "of life in terms of life in action" (p. 11),[20] he proposed that an organism experienced by trying things out, or in other words, by experimentation, on the basis of inferred consequences of actions.

This view of experience and how it was experimentally used by the organism led to the second and what may be seen as the central theme in Dewey's philosophy. Based on James' psychology, grounded on naturalistic, biological basis of behavior, Hegel's integrative dialectical method with a primary focus on resolving social and cultural tensions, and Darwin's theory of evolution, he saw philosophy as a method of "locating and interpreting the more serious of the conflicts that

occur in life, and a method of projecting ways of dealing with them: a method of moral and political diagnosis and prognosis" (p. 343).[24] This was the premise of his melioristic philosophy.

Therefore, "All of his writings are devoted to this purpose, to show how we may apply our intelligence to every primary concern of life" (p. 335).[48] This conscious application of the mind to the solution of personal and social problems he named *instrumentalism*. In other words, he saw "The method of intelligence [as] the pragmatic or instrumentalist method...[of] testing the meaning and worth of ideas, customs, in the light of their consequences, not just the immediate personal consequences, but their broad social consequences, [leading] to the conception of a new society" (p. 334).[48]

This instrumental view of the mind was based on the premise derived from Darwin that a human organism interacts with the environment in an attempt to adapt. This was clear in his proposition that an organism often falls out of harmony with its environment.[23] If it recovers through its own action and effort, it functions at a higher level, having been enriched by ensuing challenges (a phenomenon that may be understood as adaptation). However, if the challenges are too overwhelming, the gap between the organism and its environment becomes too large and cannot be bridged, in which case it dies.

To understand the influence of Dewey's philosophy on the early development of occupational therapy, bear in mind that he not only had connections with leading occupational therapists through his work at the Hull House,[9,106] but also that a similarity exists between the above statement and Meyer's assertion in his *Philosophy of Occupation Therapy* that "Our conception of man is that of an organism that maintains and balances itself in the world of *reality* and *actuality* by being in active life and active use, that is, using and living and acting its *time* in harmony with its own nature and the nature about it" (p. 641).[65]

Meyer continued to emphasize that in order to remain healthy, the human organism had to work, play, rest, and sleep so as to remain in balance and in harmony with the environment. Meyer likely borrowed this emphasis on balance and harmony directly from Dewey's view of an organism adapting by interacting with the environment and using the mind or intelligence instrumentally in order to be in balance and in harmony with its surroundings.

Furthermore, in his conceptualization of the instrumental nature of intelligence and the mind, Dewey perceived practical application of the mind as being through learning. Learning in this sense was nothing more than an instrumental function to help humans adapt to their environment and survive, through "reconstruction of experience" (p. 450).[21] This kind of learning was understood to occur through involvement in one's life context, or "doing." He saw intellectual processes as resulting "from action" and devolving "for the sake of better control of action. What we term *reason* is primarily the law of orderly or effective action" (p. 450).[21] In other words, there was no intellectual process devoid of physical action. One can see how this idea was applied in occupational therapy. Beginning with Dunton, and throughout the profession's history, learning by doing has been the hallmark of the profession.[4,9,89]

Dewey's conceptualization of a live, growing organism interacting with the environment also hinted at the latter-day complexity/chaos theory. He argued that when the organism fell out with its environment, its "recovery is never mere return to a prior state, for it is enriched by the state of disparity and resistance which it has successfully passed" (p. 535).[23] In this statement, Dewey seemed to anticipate the principle of chaos/complexity theory that increased self-organization emerges as the organism interacts dynamically with its environment.[38,40] Incidentally, currently there is increased advocacy for the use of complexity as a theoretical framework for occupational therapy.[38-40,54,88] Dewey's philosophy, therefore, not only influenced the development of occupational therapy in the early years of the profession, but its principles were futuristic and may be found extremely useful in the profession today.

George Herbert Mead

George Herbert Mead worked with John Dewey with whom he was quite close.[73] Both were involved in social programs such as Jane Addams' Hull House.[103] His philosophical ideas were therefore influenced by Dewey, and one may assume also by James through Dewey. Also like Dewey, Mead was influenced by Hegelian philosophy, which he saw as the philosophy of evolution. Similarly, Darwin's theory of evolution had a significant effect on his thinking.[64] To Mead, Darwin's theory of evolution was a scientific revolution that made possible the explanation of all aspects of life, including thought as a process and the individual as a member of the community. We will now discuss Mead's core philosophical propositions as they relate to occupational therapy.

Based on Hegelian dialectics and the theory of evolution, Mead conceptualized all forms as being in a state of evolution and continual emergence. Thus, his focus was on temporality, since he thought that emergence, whether evolutionary or otherwise, involved passage of time. He considered classical physical theories such as Newtonian physics as inadequate in explaining this emergence, because they reduced the Universe into particles and failed to adequately take into account passage of time.[63] Thus to him, Einstein's theory of relativity was closest to life processes as explicated in the theory of evolution. This was because in the theory of relativity, everything was reduced to energy and historicity, which was a crucial component of evolution. It was in terms of historicity that to Mead, emergence made sense.

In view of his relativistic and evolutionary perspective, Mead conceived reality to exist only in the present, based on events. In other words, to him reality was marked by appearance and disappearance, or the past and the future. Since we live in a world of events, the present was marked by current events as they unfolded in time. Through those events, the present was conditioned by and emerged from the past.[63,72] This conditioning nature of the past was evolutionary. To survive, the organism related to and adjusted to the environment through time. In the case of humans, development of higher centers of the brain enabled them to reflect on the past. From this reflection, they were able to make predictions of the future in order to make essential adjustments necessary for survival. To Mead, the human ability to reflect constituted what he perceived as conscious intelligence. In a nutshell, his philosophy was close to Dewey's instrumentalism. Both emphasized that life process constituted conscious intelligence through whose reflective action it was maintained by enhancing compatibility between the organism and its environment.[72]

By using reflective intelligence, humans made the present a condition for adjustment to the environment. Past experiences became subjective reinterpretations of the present in order to determine the future. The past conditioned the present, and through actions of the present, the emerging future was determined. For living organisms, these adaptive actions were geared toward meeting the need for food. Humans, like other organisms were in this struggle for food in order to survive. However, rather than waiting for new organs to develop through evolution so they could meet their nutrition needs like other life forms, humans used the scientific method to solve problems and attain necessary nutrition. Thus the scientific method was a conscious manifestation of the evolutionary process. Science was a process of using intelligence to solve human problems to enable humans to take control of the environment. Mead postulated this to be the basis of all human activity.[82]

Mead saw human action as a process of perceiving and relating to the environment, where objects in the environment were manipulated and consummated to meet needs.[64] It follows then, that his focus, similar to Dewey's, was human adaptive interaction with the environment with the mind as the instrument making possible

this interaction. We have already discussed how Meyer used this principle of instrumentalism to develop his psychobiological theory of psychiatry, which was the intellectual basis of Slagle's habit-training programs.

It is evident that the philosophical propositions of the four leading pragmatists (Charles Sanders Peirce, William James, John Dewey, and George Herbert Mead) influenced the mental hygiene movement, and consequently occupational therapy. Through pragmatism, ideas from Darwin's theory of evolution infiltrated the profession. Pragmatism and Darwinism might have been the basis of the view in occupational therapy of humans as active agents interacting with the environment through action, and mental health as balance and harmony with that environment. The role of habit in this adaptive interaction through activity also became prominent.

Influence of the Moral Treatment Movement

A discussion of the intellectual influences that shaped the early development of the formally founded profession of occupational therapy would not be complete without expounding the effects of the moral treatment movement. The influence of moral treatment principles on the founders, and therefore the early development of occupational therapy, is most apparent in the work of William Rush Dunton Jr. Dunton studied treatment strategies of Pinel and Tuke, founders of the moral treatment movement, and was interested in implementing similar programs consisting of a structured environment and occupations such as arts and crafts.[89] He believed that occupational therapy was a continuation of the moral treatment movement as indicated by his historical account of the use of occupations as therapy. In this account, he stated that "Philippe Pinel was probably the first to express the more modern viewpoint in 1791, in that part of his *Treatise on Moral Treatment of Insanity*" (p. 5).[28] He also referred to the work of Benjamin Rush, one of the psychiatrists who implemented moral treatment principles in the United States. Considering that Dunton formulated the first set of occupational therapy principles, this is probably why Bockoven states that "It appears almost conspicuously evident that moral treatment could be reasonably described in philosophy and practice as comprehensive occupational therapy program" (p. 223).[7]

Character of the Newly Founded Occupational Therapy

Such then, was the intellectual context within which occupational therapy was formally established as a profession. The character of the new profession was derived from the moral treatment, arts and crafts, and mental hygiene movements, and the philosophy of pragmatism, particularly the philosophical propositions of James, Dewey, and Mead. Intellectual building blocks of the profession from these influences can be discerned in the principles developed by Dunton[29] and presented to the national association of the new profession:

1. *Work should be carried on with cure as the main object.* This principle probably originated from Dunton's education as a physician. In his professional role, he was influenced by the primary goal of medicine, which is to cure diseases. To him, occupation was a curative agent, similar to drugs. This was the position also taken by Barton[6] in his proposition about prescription and grading of occupations as patients improved.
2. *The work should be interesting.* This principle could have originated from either the moral treatment movement or pragmatism. Pinel[79] had proposed that occupations used as therapy should appeal to the intelligence with the goal of restoring rationality, which he perceived to be the distinguishing factor between humans and animals. He directed that occupation be chosen that appealed to the patient's intelligence, which may be deduced to mean that it had to be interesting enough to appeal to the individual's intellect.

Dewey, in his pedagogical philosophy, similarly emphasized that "Education, therefore, must begin with a psychological insight into the child's capacities, *interests,* and habits" (p. 445, emphasis mine).[21]

3. *The patient should be carefully studied.*
4. *One form of occupation should not be carried to the point of fatigue.* The previous two principles were derived from Pinel's principles. Drawing from John Locke's empiricism with its doctrine of the value of observation and experience as a source of knowledge, Pinel[79] emphasized that every patient had to be observed carefully before a treatment program consistent with his or her needs was planned. It was only through such careful observation that fatigue, frustration, and so on, could be detected early, as Dunton directed, before becoming counterproductive to the patient's well being.
5. *It should have some useful end.* This principle could have been derived from pragmatism with its insistence on actions that have real, practical consequences. However, it could also have originated from the principles of the arts and crafts movement, which supported "the idea that meaning and wellness could come from working with one's hands to produce an item having aesthetic value" (p. 259).[35] Incidentally, principles of arts and crafts and of pragmatism were sometimes intertwined given that pragmatists such as Dewey and Mead were active in the arts and crafts movement both in their individual work as exemplified in Dewey's writings[23] and through their association with the Hull House in Chicago.[9,106]
6. *Preferably, it should lead to an increase in the patient's knowledge.* This seems to be a principle derived from Dewey's instrumentalism.
7. *It should be carried on with others.* This was a principle of the moral treatment movement requiring that mentally ill patients be engaged in occupations, preferably in the company of others of sound mind.[79,97] This principle was also exemplified in the work of the Quakers

in asylums in the United States where patients and staff worked together on the farm, ate meals together, and resided in the same dwellings.[99]

8. *All possible encouragement should be given the worker.* This principle was strongly expounded in the early asylums in which moral treatment principles were used. In these asylums, all efforts were made to encourage patients to engage in occupations, take responsibility, and recognize and acknowledge consequences of their behavior.[99]

9. *Work resulting in a poor or useless product is better than idleness.* This principle suggests adoption of the arts and crafts value of aesthetically beautiful things made by humans. The movement conceived such things as those that were consistent with nature and useful to humanity. In other words, similar to the arts and crafts movement,[66] this principle expressed a preference for fashioning out sound, useful products. However, it was also consistent with the principles of pragmatism that emphasized action as preferable to idleness, even when that action led to products that were not aesthetically beautiful or useful.

The above analysis indicates that the first principles of occupational therapy, as developed by Dunton, were derived from the moral treatment movement, the arts and crafts movement, pragmatism, and medicine. We have also seen that the mental hygiene movement had a significant influence on the profession through the work of Meyer and Slagle. These were the intellectual ideas that helped inform the early character of the profession of occupational therapy. Having established the profession's intellectual basis, we will trace its subsequent development, focusing particularly on its paradigmatic changes.

Early Development of the Profession (1910-1920)

Occupational therapy developed rapidly during this decade. This development was given impetus by several factors, chief among which was World War I. The major goal of the orthopedic department in the military then was to establish a reconstruction program for soldiers either injured at war or suffering from neurosis, so that they could return to active duty or be prepared for an economically productive civilian life.[10,35,57] This was the beginning of the rehabilitation movement and of occupational therapy's venture into physical rehabilitation. The reconstruction program was modeled on a rehabilitation framework in England, which was based on the following assumptions:

> that soldiers with disabilities could undergo a process of orthopedic rehabilitation that would make them fit for either continued military duty or, if discharged, civilian employment—thus mitigating the economic strain on the country of having to provide financially for pensioned soldiers with disabilities...and that the nation had a higher social responsibility or moral obligation to assist soldiers with disabilities in becoming independent 'wage earning happy citizens' rather than 'boastful, idle derelicts' (p. 257).[35]

The workers charged with the responsibility of facilitating attainment of the above goals of the program were physiotherapists (who used media such as electrotherapy, hydrotherapy, mechanotherapy, and exercises), and occupational therapists (who used a variety of arts and crafts).[34,57] These civilian workers were collectively called *reconstruction aides,* a name derived from the *reconstruction program* or what might today be referred to as a *rehabilitation program.*

Initially, reconstruction workers were directed by orthopedic surgeons who "sought to create a large corps of 'specially trained masseurs' who could treat joint and muscle conditions, and to organize these workers into some official position" (p. 45).[34] They insisted on overseeing all reconstruction activities.[35] They sought to establish occupational therapy as "a curative application whose primary role was to supplement the orthopedists' own work with continued exercising of muscles and ranging of joints through activity" (p. 259).[35] However, physiotherapists challenged the attempt by orthopedic surgeons to control reconstruction aides, leading to their transfer to the Division of Physical Reconstruction (p. 45). The aides, who were placed in the military in 1917, served in the "Division of Orthopedic Surgery and specialized in application of physical agents, occupational therapy, and dietetics" (p. 53).[35]

The medical control of the work of occupational therapists, however, did not begin with reconstruction aides during World War I. Physicians initiated the profession, and it was their intention to maintain tight control of the activities of the new discipline.

Dunton for example, advanced a definition of occupational therapy as "any activity, mental or physical, *definitely prescribed and guided for the distinct purpose of contributing to and hastening recovery from disease*" (p. 4, emphasis mine).[28] He continued to identify the responsibility of prescribing and guiding occupational therapy as that of the physician by stating that: "If the physician is sufficiently informed to indicate the specific activity desired this may also be written on the prescription" (p. 29).[29]

Thus, Dunton was responsible, to a large extent, for establishing the tradition of occupational therapists working under physicians and the adoption of the medical model in which therapists needed a physician's referral and prescription in order to work with a client.[34] He proposed the idea that the occupational therapist be regarded as a technical assistant similar in status to the relationship between the nurse and physician. This was the basis of the long reliance of the profession on medicine for leadership. This control of occupational therapy by medicine would later create dissonance between the profession's holistic foundations and medicine's reductionism as will be discussed later.

Although the military was at first reluctant to accept the civilian women reconstruction workers in their midst,[35] the effectiveness of their work eventually led to a high demand for them. This led to hasty development and expansion of short-term training programs. It was an advantage that generally these workers were well-educated, and many of them were college graduates.[57] To prepare for shipment overseas to engage in the work of reconstruction, they received about six weeks of instruction in "arts and crafts, medical lectures, and hospital etiquette as well as practical experience in a hospital or clinic" (p. 28).[89]

Other factors that led to high demand for reconstruction aides and the venture of occupational therapy into physical rehabilitation included advances in medicine (with the discovery of x-rays, new types of medication such as the polio vaccine in 1916, and improved surgical methods), which led to saving the lives of those who would otherwise have died.[10,108] Many of those who recovered from conditions that were hitherto fatal were physically disabled or developed chronically debilitating conditions. Also, increased automation and industrialization, use of the automobile, and so on, led to an increased number of accidents that left many victims physically disabled. All of these factors increased the demand for reconstruction aides to help these individuals lead a decent, productive life.

It is also important to note that while occupational therapists (reconstruction aides) began treating individuals with physical disabilities for the first time, their focus remained on mental health. They saw their role in part as "to teach various forms of simple hand craft to patients in military hospitals and other sanitary formations of the army...in the orthopedic and surgical wards" as well as those *"suffering from nervous or mental diseases"* (p. 38, emphasis mine).[57] As J.F. Low stated, their charge was "to provide treatment to enable *physically sound men suffering from war neurosis to return to duty as quickly as possible*" (p. 38, emphasis mine).[57] A director of the Red Cross Institute for Crippled and Disabled Men was hired by the military to study worldwide programs for reeducation of soldiers. He expressed the opinion that "The soldier's state of mind had to be considered if the soldier was to be brought back into civilian life as a complete man" (p. 153).[81] Also, according to the Surgeon General's Office, "Occupational therapy 'prepare[d] the mind for subsequent vocational treatment'" (p. 159).[81]

Continued emphasis on the psychosocial ramifications of disorders emanating from the battlefield was probably due to the fact that the mental hygiene movement was supportive of reconstruction programs. Such support was evident in the movement's editorial in 1919 that detailed the effect of a reconstruction program for patients with *functional nervous disorders* treated at Base Hospital 117.[30] The report indicated that 65 percent of these patients returned to duty within a short time. It is also important to note that the arts and crafts movement had a significant influence on reconstruction aides. Most of them had an arts and crafts background. For example, Myers, who was a leader of one group of reconstruction aides, had studied arts and crafts at Columbia University and taught history of art.[57] Similarly, Ora Ruggles, another pioneer, had taught manual arts before attending a reconstruction aides training program. Besides, an advertisement for an opening for reconstruction aides in the war department specified that "Applicants must have a theoretical knowledge of the following crafts and a practical training in at least three of them: Basketry, weaving (hand and bead looms including simple forms of rugs and mat making), simple wood carving, block-printing (paper and textiles), knitting, needlework" (p. 39).[57]

The above factors led to the fast development of the new profession of occupational therapy between 1910 and 1920. However, following the end of World War I, the demand for reconstruction aides declined, and many training programs were closed.[57,89] Many of the aides who had been occupational therapists left the field. According to the U.S. Surgeon General,[98] this decline was precipitated in part by the fact that the mental hygiene movement (the leading supporter of occupational therapy) fell short of the promise to prevent chronicity of mental illness, although the length of stay for newly admitted patients began to decline.

Continued Developments (1920-1929)

Notable developments during this decade included changing the name of the National Society for the Promotion of Occupational Therapy (NSPOT) to the American Occupational Therapy Association (AOTA) in 1921,[89] organizing occupational therapy schools, and establishing the *Essentials for Professional Education* by the AOTA and the Council on Medical Education of the American Medical Association (AMA) in 1923.[108] One may observe that this determination of occupational therapy education standards by the AMA only served to entrench the medical control of the profession. Also in 1923, the Federal Industrial Rehabilitation Act was legislated mandating that any industrial accident hospitalization was entitled to occupational therapy.[87] This legislation led to significant expansion of occupational therapy services in institutions catering to chronic conditions.

It was also during this decade that medicine generally accepted the germ theory of disease with subsequent development of a variety of vaccines. At the same time, psychological theories such as Freud's psychoanalysis and Pavlov's behaviorism matured.[10] The influence of the medical model on the profession continued to be ingrained so that in the last 5 years of this decade, "The first reference to physical rehabilitation and matching the activity to disease" was made (p. 31).[10] Because of sensitivity to labor abuse due to the work of social reformers such as Karl Marx, many hospitals shied away from engaging patients in arts and crafts activities or work. This trend continued until the stock market crash in 1929.

Effects of the Stock Market Crash: The Depression Years (1929-1941)

The stock market crash in October 1929 drastically halted the growth of occupational therapy,[87] as it did that of the entire North American Society.[10] Everyone was preoccupied with survival, jobs were scarce, and people did not have adequate means of earning a livelihood. To make matters worse, there was a drought. Many Americans were left destitute.

Faced with these hardships, spending money on medical care was not a priority for many people.[87] This was the beginning of the weakening of medical ethics (the avowed commitment, in the Hippocratic oath, to avail medical care to all who need it). This repudiation of ethics was evident in the following example: West Virginia hospitals refused to take patients unless the bill was guaranteed. In 1934, the Nassau County Medical Society suggested that any code of medical ethics should provide that "...free medical care is a charity which is the privilege of the physician to bestow...it is not a commodity which can be demanded" (p. 232).[87]

Under these circumstances, it became more and more difficult for the AOTA to implement the new occupational therapy standards, so they sought help from the AMA for protection and implementation of the standards. At this point, "occupational therapy thereby formally became a medical ancillary" (p. 232).[87] The profession then began to strive earnestly for recognition as a legitimate medical discipline, resulting in "the debate...over diversionary versus therapeutic activity, and one of the original tenets of occupational therapy—that diversionary activity was therapeutic—was temporarily lost."[10] Considering that the later identity crisis lasted for decades, one may wonder whether this loss was temporary.

In 1935, the profession developed ties with the AMA's Medical Education and Hospitals branch through which a mechanism for accreditation of occupational therapy schools was established.[34] This raised the status and stability of the profession within the medical field. Later, occupational therapy became allied to the American Hospital Association (AHA), which meant that subordination to medical specialty decreased but the profession relied more and more on physicians and AHA members for leadership. At the same time, occupational

therapy adhered increasingly to the mechanistic, reductionistic medical model (in the struggle for recognition by the medical community), and departed from mental health. This departure was so acute that in 1937, some occupational therapists "suggested that occupational therapy should expand beyond physical activities into the psychosocial field" (p. 32),[10] seemingly forgetting that the roots of the profession were in mental health.

The Rehabilitation Movement and Adoption of Reductionism (1942-1960)

The Great Depression ended with the attack at Pearl Harbor on Sunday, December 7, 1941.[87] The following day, President Franklin D. Roosevelt declared war, and the United States officially joined World War II. This event put every employable person to work. A new demand for occupational therapists arose. However, there were few therapists employed by the military because the reconstruction aides did not have military status and therefore had left once World War I had ended. According to Gritzer and Arluke, "By 1939 there were fewer than a dozen occupational therapists on duty in the military" (p. 104).[34] Through a concerted campaign by the AOTA, occupational therapy was eventually recognized in the military, and occupational therapists were commissioned as military officers.

The War Department initiated emergency occupational therapy courses in mid-1944, which signified the profession's recognition by the military medical corps. Consequently, "By the end of the war, there were 447 graduate occupational therapists and 452 apprentices working in the military medical system" (p. 106).[34] This recognition also tended to entrench occupational therapy's identification with the medical model and subordination and control by medicine. At the time, "Most occupational therapists welcomed adoption of the medical model and increased subservience to medicine" (p. 107)[34] in return for the safety that medicine provided to the profession.

One significant event during the 1940s was the rapid development of the rehabilitation movement.[67] Large numbers of veterans of the armed forces who were physically disabled in the war helped to accelerate this growth. Of course, rehabilitation was not a new concept in occupational therapy. Even the founders of the profession had espoused the values of this movement. Both Barton[6] and Dunton,[27] for instance, emphasized the need to make patients productive members of society in order to help them reclaim their humanity to the fullest. Also, the philosophy of pragmatism, which we have demonstrated was the philosophical foundation of occupational therapy, was always of the view that contribution to society is an ethical obligation for every human. This was one of the basic premises of pragmatic social activism in Chicago, as seen in the work of pragmatists such as Emil Hirsch, Jane Addams, and John Dewey.[9] Furthermore, we have seen that the reconstruction program during World War I was really a rehabilitation program whose model was borrowed from England. During and after World War II, rehabilitation advocacy became a formal movement affiliated with medicine, with physicians taking firm control of rehabilitation programs.[67]

Other factors that facilitated rapid growth of the rehabilitation movement included failure of institutions to take care of the injured and disabled, and evidence that disabled persons could become more independent, therefore proving that there was an economic advantage.[67] Also, continued development of more effective medical procedures allowed disabled persons to live longer. Furthermore, due to increased urbanization, families could not care for their disabled members, requiring the need for professionals to take that role. In mental health, discovery of neuroleptics changed the course of psychiatric treatment.[89]

Psychotropic drugs were used to control psychotic symptoms, and many patients were discharged. This eventually led to a nationalized plan to release most of the patients from custodial care, a process that was dubbed *deinstitutionalization*. This necessitated the rise of what came to be known as *community mental health*: "Borrowing some ideas from the mental hygienists and capitalizing on the advent of new drugs for treating psychosis and depression, community mental health reformers argued that they could bring mental health services to the public in their communities" (p. 6).[98] One of the shortcomings of the community mental health movement, however, was that the policy of deinstitutionalization was implemented without much evidence of its ability to work.[98] Thus, many patients with debilitating mental illnesses were released into the community without much support. Many of them became homeless.

The discovery of neuroleptics also led to the ability to manage patients' symptoms using psychotropic drugs, therefore making them amenable to psychotherapeutic interventions.[10] In this atmosphere, occupational therapists attempted to fit in the rehabilitation movement by developing skills consistent with the reductionistic view of expertise prevalent in the medical model at the time. Their focus became intervention to enhance performance of activities of daily living, vocational and prevocational assessment and training, training in the use of orthotics and prosthetics, and psychological guidance.[10,67]

The idea of health through integrated function in a balanced occupational repertoire, which was the main stay of the moral treatment movement and early occupational therapy, was lost. Occupational therapists borrowed techniques from other disciplines such as psychodynamic techniques from psychology and biomechanical techniques from medicine. Their focus became treatment of specific diseases with an emphasis on techniques rather than principles underlying the use of occupation. According to Kielhofner,[52] the profession adopted the mechanistic, reductionistic paradigm of the medical model, with its emphasis on the internal intrapsychic, neurologic, and kinesiologic mechanisms as they influenced function. By *paradigm* here is meant an integrating culture in a profession as determined by "core themes or ideas that members of the profession see as their basic concerns" (p. 16).[52]

The effect of this change was that the significance of arts and crafts in occupational therapy declined. There was a shift toward basic sciences[67] because "the therapeutic reasons for asking patients to weave baskets or hand tool leather became increasingly unclear as professional education became more standardized and as the arts and crafts movement waned in public importance" (p. 431).[19] As mentioned earlier, the negative effect of this development was that occupational therapy became an ancillary of medicine rather than a primary treatment method, with occupational therapists functioning as technicians rather than professionals.[67] For example, occupations were used in psychiatry as a means of assisting the psychiatrist to diagnose patients' unconscious feelings and motives through interpretation of the meaning of colors, themes, and so forth.[12,55,56,104] In physical rehabilitation, occupational therapists tried to use activities to achieve specific movements[52] and eventually, in some cases, dropped activities altogether in favor of rote exercises claiming that such exercises were more therapeutically efficient.[105]

When the use of activities was retained, they often were not meaningful to the patient. During the early years of occupational therapy, the principles of the profession dictated that occupations used in therapy be interesting and meaningful, and have personal and cultural relevance to the patient.[6,28] With reductionism, *purposefulness* (goal-directedness of the activity) was substituted for *meaningfulness*.[52] In this sense, moving a sander up and down an inclined plane was seen as a purposeful activity, because it was effective in achieving the goal of increasing upper-extremity range of motion. The meaningfulness of the activity was not considered, thus the profession's fundamental view of the human and therapy changed significantly.

Professional Crisis and Call to Return to the Roots (1960s and 1970s)

One consequence of adopting the reductionistic paradigm was *role blurring*. It became increasingly difficult to differentiate between occupational therapists and physical therapists, or psychotherapists.[19] Consequently there was a sense of conflict and self-doubt in the professional ranks.[10] As Gritzer and Arluke state, "In the 1940s, actual problems did exist among occupational therapy, physical therapy, and vocational rehabilitation. These struggles were reflected in calls for intergroup coordination and conflict resolution in individual work situations" (p. 108).[34] Thus the stage was set for professional self-appraisal.

Also, the intellectual and social atmosphere of the time supported this questioning and self-appraisal. The 1960s were characterized by accelerated technological growth. The moral treatment movement emerged from the industrial revolution of the Renaissance period in the late eighteenth century. The second half of the twentieth century was similarly a time of industrial revolution, this time in information technology.[25] The United States landed a person on the moon during this era. At the same time, there was civil unrest, not only in the United States but all over the world. Minorities in the United States were demanding equal rights. Similarly, much of Africa (e.g., Kenya, Ghana) was embroiled in a struggle for independence from colonialism. There was also a counterculture in the United States that challenged the status quo and presented alternative ways of living (the hippie culture). These social dynamics led to civil rights legislation. Later, these rights were extended to patients in hospitals and other health care institutions, leading to an antipsychiatry movement.

Scientific advances also posed a challenge to the pre-existing scientific paradigm. It became increasingly clear that the Newtonian scientific model of cause-and-effect relationships was inadequate in explaining many human phenomena. Systems theory was presented as an alternative.[100,102] In this scientific framework, the environment was considered to be connected to every part of human discourse. The framework was therefore more holistic and friendly to the original, holistic tenets of occupational therapy. It was within this sociopolitical and intellectual context that a number of occupational therapists called upon their colleagues to reconsider their professional identity.

The professional self-appraisal began with a pivotal call to occupational therapists to return to their professional roots to a practice based on the basic premise that *"man, through the use of his hands as they are energized by mind and will, can influence the state of his own health"* (p. 2).[84] This rallying call by Reilly in her Slagle lecture in 1961 has become one of the most often quoted statements in occupational therapy, and deservedly so, because it marked the turning point of the profession. In her lecture, Reilly described this concept as perhaps the greatest idea in twentieth century medicine and went on to suggest that the time to test the idea was then, and the United States, with her propensity for action, was the right place to test it. She concluded that occupational therapy, from its roots, offered a vital service to humankind: that of meeting the human need for occupation. She worried that if occupational therapists failed to fulfill that need, someone else would come up to do it, since it is so vital.

The challenge by Reilly was soon echoed by other occupational therapy scholars such as Yerxa.[110] Shannon claimed that occupational therapy had been derailed and suggested that we needed to arrest the process of derailment by reconstructing our paradigm so as to "reinstate the paradigmatic values and beliefs on which the profession was founded" (pp. 233-234).[94] This initiative was necessary because derailment meant that our professional "paradigm is incompatible with the needs/wants of the population it serves" (p. 233).[94] Gillette and Kielhofner[33] argued that specialization in occupational therapy, which originated in the reductionistic paradigm of the 1950s and 1960s as an attempt to cope with rapid technological development, had led to loss of identity and role confusion, throwing the profession into what Thomas Kuhn called a *state of crisis.* They suggested that occupational therapists come to a consensus through which a new professional paradigm would be established, to avoid prolonging the state of crisis in the profession.

West[105] followed with the admonition that the profession needed to reestablish its identity rooted in its founding philosophy. These scholars and many others called for a return to professional practice grounded on the premise of occupation as a healing phenomenon; focus on adaptation of patients after dysfunction; a return to concepts of original founders such as habit training as advanced and practiced by Slagle, Haas, and Marsh; and engagement in a serious study of human achievement, life space, lifestyle occupations and choice, and job satisfaction.[85]

A New Occupational Therapy Paradigm (1980s to Present)

Since the 1980s, much has occurred in the occupational therapy practice in the United States and other parts of the world. In the United States, there was legislation such as the Balanced Budget Act, introduction of Managed Care, and the Prospective Pay System. Throughout the world, there has been an increasing demand for proof of efficacy of interventions using research evidence (evidence-based practice). However, in keeping with the scope of this book, the events during this time are summarized with a primary focus on illustrating the emergence of a new occupational therapy paradigm.

Beginning in 1975, the latter part of the twentieth century has been characterized by a tendency toward an increased value of the dignity of the individual person, and of the person's subjective experiences. In the 1980s, qualitative methods of research were developed due to this recognition of the importance of subjectivity.[60] Combined with the influence of the scientific framework of systems theory, these methods enabled occupational therapists to study occupation, not only as an objective phenomenon, but also as a subjectively felt experience of a person engaged in a dynamic interaction with the environment. At the same time, in psychiatry, the community support movement was established to meet the shortcomings of the community care initiative, which resulted in psychiatric patients being discharged to the community without support.[98]

The community support movement emphasized the social welfare needs of clients who had been discharged from mental health institutions. It was argued that "individuals could once again become citizens of their community, if given support and access to mainstream resources such as housing and vocational opportunities" (p. 7).[98] This view was supported by development of a newer generation of more effective psychotropic drugs such as Selective Serotonin Reuptake Inhibitors (SSRIs) and more effective psychological interventions such as assertive community treatment, which made it possible for discharged mental health patients to function more effectively. The community support movement was therefore closely allied to the independent living movement, which helped shift focus of dysfunction from the individual to the environment.[60] According to this movement, disability did not occur because of the victim's inability to function. Rather, it was a function of an environment created with a bias in favor of able-bodied persons. It was therefore argued that intervention should be aimed at eliminating environmental barriers that make it difficult for physically and psychologically impaired people to function optimally.

In the latter part of the twentieth century, the systems theory evolved into the complex, dynamic, adaptive systems/chaos theory.[38,40,88,101] This theory challenges the hierarchical perspective of the older systems theory and instead emphasizes complex interaction between systems and subsystems as an organism dynamically interacts with its environment, leading to self-organization characterized by emergence of more effective adaptive behavior. This perspective has led to a revision of how occupational therapists view occupational performance, human development, and so on.[80] This theoretical framework also makes it possible to integrate and scientifically explain the founding principles of occupational therapy as influenced by the intellectual perspectives of the time, such as the concepts of learning by doing and adaptation introduced to occupational therapy by the pragmatists, and the personality organizing capacity of occupation as proposed by the moral treatment, arts and crafts, and mental hygiene movements.

Within this social and intellectual context, occupational therapists began the work of arresting derailment of their profession.[94] This has been the preoccupation of many occupational therapy scholars in the last two decades of the twentieth century. Mosey,[68] for example, suggested a biopsychosocial model that would account for the patient's physical needs (such as increasing range of motion, strengthening, and so on), psychological needs related to normal human growth and development, and social need for a person to live meaningfully in a community. She suggested that this would systematize our knowledge and practice. Breines[9] suggested that the profession was founded on the philosophy of pragmatism, and that its principles could provide a framework for organizing occupational therapy knowledge and providing the profession with a unique identity.

Other scholars offered new ways of conceptualizing and carrying out therapy. Reilly[86] developed an occupational behavior model focusing more on play as an aspect of the play-work continuum. She analyzed play from the perspectives of evolution, anthropology, and psychology. Reilly saw play as a means of adaptation to the environment in which a child learns the rules of the how and why of objects in the environment and subsequently develops skills leading to competency and mastery of the real world. Extending Reilly's model of occupational behavior, Kielhofner,[49] one of her former students at the University of Southern California, developed the temporal adaptation conceptual framework based on Meyer's[65] statement that the natural rhythms of life organize human behavior so that the human organism can live in harmony and balance with its environment. With this perspective of balance in mind, Kielhofner argued that "occupational therapy should view patients within the context of time through the unfolding of their daily lives" (p. 235).[49] This view would make occupational therapists the caretakers of activities of daily living (ADLs) rather than simply using ADLs as a checklist for self care.

Later, Kielhofner incorporated the temporal adaptation framework into the Model of Human Occupation (MOHO).[50,51,53] This model was created in an attempt to reaffirm the principles of occupational therapy espoused by early founders of the profession by emphasizing the use of occupation as a health-maintaining medium, habit training, and occupational role maintenance. Based on the systems theory, Kielhofner perceived the human as a system consisting of *input* (taking in information and energy), *throughput* (processing information), *output* (in terms of occupational performance), and a *feedback loop.*

This view was hierarchical with the volitional subsystem (consisting of values, interests, and personal causation) of throughput, assuming the role of guiding all other subsystems of occupational performance such as the habituation subsystem (consisting of habits and roles) and performance subsystem. *Note:* The reader should be aware that this model has changed as theoretical concepts have evolved. Currently, its constructs are stated differently (more consistent with the current dynamical systems theory). See Chapter 12 for a detailed discussion of the model as it currently exists Many other conceptual models were developed along these lines, such as occupational adaptation,[90,91] the ecology of human performance,[26] and client-centered practice.[13]

Another response to Reilly and others' call to return to the roots of the profession was a concerted effort to define occupation, flesh out its unique qualities, and distinguish it from other forms of activity. In this endeavor, Engelhardt, for example, found problems with the AOTA's definition of occupational therapy as "the art and science of directing man's participation in selected activity to restore, reinforce, and enhance performance, facilitate learning of those skills and functions essential for adaptation and productivity, diminish or correct pathology and to promote and maintain health" (p. 667).[31] He felt that this definition was not unique to occupational therapy as it could pertain to medicine, physical therapy, or social work. Instead, drawing from the historical emphasis of the profession as found in the moral treatment and the principles advanced by Meyer, he proposed that the profession adopt a *praxial* model that captures the "doing, a transaction, the progress of a business, an action" and therefore "an accent on persons as whole entities living in the tasks they do" (p. 670).[31]

Breines proposed that role identity conflicts in the profession at the time resulted from the fact that therapists defined their practice by the tools they used rather than by the process of engagement by clients. Drawing on philosophical principles of John Dewey, she suggested that the problem may be resolved by defining purposeful activity in terms of "the unique directions of individual patients and the enabling of patients toward enhanced growth and development, and by involvement and organization of self and environment, both structural and personal" (p. 544).[8] Breines also proposed that the definition include the therapists' responsibility to enlist the patient's will and choice of activities, and to facilitate integration of choices into automatic behaviors. Other occupational therapy scholars offered a variety of definitions of occupation, and tried to explain its characteristics and its difference from other forms of activity.[*] These collective efforts culminated in the founding of the discipline of occupational science by the faculty and students of the occupational therapy depart-

---

*References 1,14,15,47,69,74,83,107.

ment at the University of Southern California,[16] as a scientific discipline whose purpose was a systematic "study of the form, function, and meaning of occupation" (p. 13).[17]

The newly conceived discipline was seen as a venue where a multidisciplinary knowledge of occupation could be generated.[111] This knowledge could in turn be employed in the service of the profession of occupational therapy. Although there was some opposition to this idea, with some scholars claiming that being an applied profession, occupational therapy did not need a basic science discipline,[70] eventually the idea held. Occupational science thrived. A journal dedicated to the discipline (*Journal of Occupational Science*) was founded in 1993. Considerable research has been generated in the discipline to date.

The New Occupational Therapy Paradigm

Activities in the late twentieth century led to the emergence of a new occupational therapy paradigm that became clearly articulated in the first few years of the twenty-first century.[52] As mentioned earlier, the term *paradigm* is used as borrowed by Kielhofner from Kuhn, to refer to unifying core concepts and themes that are arrived at by consensual agreement in a profession. In this new paradigm, the profession has returned to a focus on occupation, a holistic viewpoint emphasizing interdependence between mind, body, and the environment, and an integrating framework provided by a dynamic, adaptive systems perspective that proposes that there is order in the whole that "transcends the parts of which the system is composed" (p. 66).[52]

Based on the dynamic systems perspective, the human is seen as "an integrated, self-organizing system" (p. 66).[52] In this paradigm, "occupational therapy provides individuals with opportunities to reshape their performance and their lives into new patterns that meet personal needs and desires" (p. 66).[52] The role of occupational therapists in this paradigm is to do the following:

- Provide clients with opportunities for occupational performance
- Modify the environment to facilitate optimal occupational performance
- Provide assistive/technical devices to enable occupational performance in spite of dysfunction
- Provide education/counseling geared toward facilitating occupational performance

The objective of therapy, ultimately, is client participation in life through engagement in meaningful occupations, and consequent maintenance of a good quality of life and, therefore, a healthy state of being.

This new paradigm is aptly captured and expressed in the new *Occupational Therapy Practice Framework*.[4] In order to understand how this framework has evolved in tandem with professional evolution, it is important to outline briefly its historical genesis. In 1979, in response to the Education for All Handicapped Children Act (Public Law 94-142, 1975, which required practitioners to provide a reporting system for all departments in hospitals for reimbursement purposes), the AOTA developed the *Uniform Terminology for Occupational Therapy* to provide a common language for reporting occupational therapy services.[3] The resulting document replaced the product output reporting system developed earlier. The *Uniform Terminology for Occupational Therapy* (second edition) defined occupational performance areas and components, and as such, focused more on performance components (which was consistent with the reductionistic, mechanistic perspective of the biomedical model).

Later, the *Uniform Terminology for Occupational Therapy* (third edition) was developed. This document expanded focus to reflect practice at the time. It incorporated contextual aspects (social/environmental) of practice, and it defined the domains of concern of the profession. It was updated and revised recently to incorporate the language of International Classification of Function (ICF) developed by the World Health

Organization (WHO).[109] The resulting document was the *Occupational Therapy Practice Framework: Domain and Process*.[4] The relationship between the framework and the new paradigm is apparent in its focus, which is as follows:

- Collaborative, client-centered intervention with all interventions focusing on client priorities. The client is encouraged to be an active participant in therapy, rather than a passive recipient of interventions.
- Occupation-based practice in which occupation is the basis of the entire therapeutic process.
- Definition of the role of the occupational therapist as therapeutic use of self, therapeutic use of occupations and activities (providing opportunities for participation in occupations), consultation on issues of participation in meaningful occupations, and education about the value and process of participation in occupation.
- Engagement in occupation to support participation in life as the desired outcome of therapy

The framework adopts Clark and colleagues'[16] definition of occupation as activity of everyday life that can be named, organized, and valued by self and culture. Activity is specifically distinguished from occupation by defining it as simply goal-directed human action(s). Furthermore, the framework emphasizes that occupations are meaningful because they are chosen, named, and valued by the individual, and are therefore motivating, personally meaningful, and require active participation on the part of the client. The overarching objective of therapy as guided by the vision provided in the framework is community/social participation to enhance engagement in occupation necessary to support participation in life. The framework, therefore, articulates a new professional paradigm that, according to Detweiler and Peyton, "link physiological function, psychological processes, and human

agency" or what they call the "*psychological narrative*" genre (p. 438).[19]

To deepen your insight regarding the historical intellectual and social context of occupational therapy and articulation of the new professional paradigm, complete exercise 2-1 in your laboratory manual.

SUMMARY

In this chapter, we discussed the historical evolution of occupational therapy in the twentieth century. We also covered the social and intellectual contexts in which this evolution took place. Of particular importance were the intellectual influences of the moral treatment, arts and crafts, mental hygiene, community mental health, and community support movements, and the philosophy of pragmatism. Other influences included World War I and World War II, the social and industrial revolution of the 1960s, the social systems theory, qualitative research methods, and more recently, the dynamical systems/chaos theory. Within the context of these influences, we discussed the history of the profession, with special emphasis on paradigmatic changes that have occurred (with adoption of the mechanistic, reductionistic paradigm of the medical model in the 1940s, 1950s, and 1960s resulting in a call by leaders in the profession for a return to the roots). We also discussed how the call to "return to the roots" led to a concerted activity by occupational therapy scholars that resulted in a new paradigm that was articulated well in the new *Occupational Therapy Practice Framework*.

REFERENCES

1. Allen CK: Activity: occupational therapy's treatment method, *Am J Occup Ther* 41:563-575, 1987.
2. American Occupational Therapy Association: The philosophical base of occupational therapy, *Am J Occup Ther* 33:785, 1979.
3. American Occupational Therapy Association: *Uniform terminology system for reporting occupational therapy services,* Rockville, MD, 1979, AOTA.

4. American Occupational Therapy Association: Occupational therapy practice framework: domain and process, *Am J Occup Ther* 56(6):609-639, 2002.

5. Ayer AJ: *The origins of pragmatism: studies in the philosophy of Charles Peirce and William James*, San Francisco, 1968, Freeman Cooper.

6. Barton GE: *Teaching the sick*, Philadelphia, 1980, WB Saunders.

7. Bockoven JS: Legacy of the moral treatment: 1800s to 1910, *Am J Occup Ther* 25:223-225, 1971.

8. Breines E: An attempt to define purposeful activity, *Am J Occup Ther* 38:543-544, 1984.

9. Breines E: *Origins and adaptations: a philosophy of practice*, Lebanon, NJ, 1986, Geri-Rehab.

10. Bryden P, McColl MA: The concept of occupation 1900 to 1974. In McColl MA, Law M, Stewart D, et al, eds: *Theoretical basis of occupational therapy*, Thorofare, NJ, 2003, Slack, pp. 27-37.

11. Buchler J, ed: *Philosophical writings of Peirce*, New York, 1955, Dover Publications.

12. Buck RE, Provancher MA: Magazine picture collages as an evaluative technique, *Am J Occup Ther* 26: 36-39, 1972.

13. Canadian Association of Occupational Therapists: *Occupational therapy: guidelines for the client-centered practice*, Toronto, ON, 1983, CAOT ACE.

14. Christiansen C: Defining lives—occupation as identity: an essay on competence, coherence, and the creation of meaning, *Am J Occup Ther* 53:547-558, 1999.

15. Clark F: Occupation embedded in a real life: interweaving occupational science and occupational therapy, *Am J Occup Ther* 47:1067-1078, 1993.

16. Clark F, Parham D, Carlson ME, et al: Occupational science: academic innovation in the service of occupational therapy's future, *Am J Occup Ther* 45:300-310, 1991.

17. Clark F, Wood W, Larson EA: Occupational science: occupational therapy's legacy for the 21st century. In Neistadt ME, Crepeau EB, eds: *Willard and Spackman's occupational therapy*, ed 9, Philadelphia, 1998, Lippincott-Raven, pp. 13-21.

18. Cutchin MP: Using Deweyan philosophy to rename and reframe adaptation-to-environment, *Am J Occup Ther* 58:303-312, 2004.

19. Detweiler J, Peyton C: Defining occupations: a chronotopic study of narrative genres in a health discipline's emergence, *Written Communication* 16(4):412-468, 1999.

20. Dewey J: From absolutism to experimentalism. In McDermott JJ, ed: *The philosophy of John Dewey*, Chicago, 1981, Chicago University Press, pp. 1-13.

21. Dewey J: My pedagogical creed. In McDermott JJ, ed: *The philosophy of John Dewey*, Chicago, 1981, Chicago University Press, pp. 442-454.

22. Dewey J: The influence of Darwinism on philosophy. In McDermott JJ, ed: *The philosophy of John Dewey*, Chicago, 1981, Chicago University Press, pp. 31-41.

23. Dewey J: The live creature. In McDermott JJ, ed: *The philosophy of John Dewey*, Chicago, 1981, Chicago University Press, pp. 525-540.

24. Dewey J: The influence of Darwinism on philosophy. In Fisch MH, ed: *Classic American philosophers*, New York, 1996, Fordham University Press, pp. 336-344.

25. Diasio K: The modern era—1960 to 1970, *Am J Occup Ther* 25:237-242, 1971.

26. Dunn W, Brown C, McClain L, et al: The ecology of human performance: a contextual perspective on human occupation. In Royeen CB, ed: *AOTA self-study series: the practice of the future: putting occupation back into therapy* (Module I), Rockville, MD, 1994, American Occupational Therapy Association.

27. Dunton WR: The training of occupational teachers and directors, *Maryland Psychiatric Quarterly* 7:8-23, 1917.

28. Dunton WR: History of occupational therapy. In Dunton WR, Licht S, ed: *Occupational therapy: principles and practice*, Springfield, IL, 1957, Charles C. Thomas, pp. 3-13.

29. Dunton WR: The prescription. In Dunton WR, Licht S, ed: *Occupational therapy: principles and practice*, Springfield, IL, 1957, Charles C. Thomas, pp. 29-52.

30. Editorial, *Mental Hygiene* 3:1-3, 1919.

31. Engelhardt HT: Defining occupational therapy: the meaning of therapy and the virtues of occupation, *Am J Occup Ther* 31:666-672, 1977.

32. Fisch MH: *Classic American philosophers*, New York, 1996, Fordham University Press.

33. Gillette N, Kielhofner G: The impact of specialization on the professionalization and survival of occupational therapy, *Am J Occup Ther* 33:20-28, 1979.

34. Gritzer G, Arluke A: *The making of rehabilitation: a political economy of medical specialization, 1890–1980*, Los Angeles, 1985, University of California Press.

35. Gutman SA: Influence of the U.S. military and occupational therapy reconstruction aides in World War I on the development of occupational therapy, *Am J Occup Ther* 49:256-262, 1995.

36. Hergenhahn BR: *An introduction to the history of psychology*, Pacific Grove, CA, 1997, Brooks/Cole.

37. Ikiugu MN: Instrumentalism in occupational therapy: an argument for a pragmatic conceptual model of practice, *Internat J Psychosocial Rehabil* 8:108-117, 2004.

38. Ikiugu MN: Instrumentalism in occupational therapy: a theoretical core for the pragmatic conceptual model

of practice, *Internat J Psychosocial Rehabil* 8: 150-162, 2004.

39. Ikiugu MN: Meaningfulness of occupations as an occupational-life-trajectory attractor, *J Occup Sci* 12: 102-109, 2005.

40. Ikiugu MN, Rosso HM: Understanding the occupational human being as a complex, dynamical, adaptive system, *Occup Ther in Health Care* 19(4):43-65, 2005.

41. Ikiugu MN, Schultz S: An argument for pragmatism as a foundational philosophy of occupational therapy, *Canadian J Occup Ther* 73(2):86-97, 2006.

42. James W: *The principles of psychology* (2 vols.), New York, 1980, Henry Holt.

43. James W: Habit: Its importance for psychology. In McDermott JJ, ed: *The writings of William James: a comprehensive edition*, Chicago, 1977, University of Chicago Press, pp. 9-21.

44. James W: Necessary truths and the effects of experience. In McDermott JJ, ed: *The writings of William James: a comprehensive edition*, Chicago, 1977, University of Chicago Press, pp. 74-133.

45. James W: *Pragmatism,* Indianapolis, 1981, Hackett.

46. James W: The will to believe. In Fisch MH: *Classic American philosophers,* New York, 1996, Fordham University Press, pp. 136-148.

47. Katz N: Occupational therapy domain of concern reconsidered, *Am J Occup Ther* 39:518-524, 1985.

48. Kennedy G: John Dewey: introduction. In Fisch MH: *Classic American philosophers,* New York, 1996, Fordham University Press, pp. 327-335.

49. Kielhofner G: Temporal adaptation: a conceptual framework for occupational therapy, *Am J Occup Ther* 31:235-242, 1977.

50. Kielhofner G: *A model of human occupation: theory and applications,* Baltimore, 1985, Williams & Wilkins.

51. Kielhofner G: *Model of human occupation,* ed 3, Philadelphia, 2002, Lippincott Williams & Wilkins.

52. Kielhofner G: *Conceptual foundations of occupational therapy,* ed 3, Philadelphia, 2004, FA Davis.

53. Kielhofner G, Burke J: A model of human occupation, part 1: conceptual framework and content, *Am J Occup Ther* 34:572-581, 1980.

54. Lazzarini I: Neuro-occupation: the nonlinear dynamics of intention, meaning and perception, *Br J Occup Ther* 67(8):342-352, 2004.

55. Lerner C, Ross G: The magazine picture collage: development of an objective scoring system, *Am J Occup Ther* 31:156-161, 1977.

56. Llorens IA, Young GG: Fingerpainting for the hostile child, *Am J Occup Ther* 14:306-307, 1960.

57. Low JF: The reconstruction aides, *Am J Occup Ther* 46:38-43, 1992.

58. MacLennan D: Beyond the asylum: professionalization and the mental hygiene movement in Canada, 1914–1928, *CBMH/BCHM* 4:7-23, 1987.

59. Mandell W: *Mental health: history—the realization of an idea* [Electronic version], Baltimore, 2005, Johns Hopkins University. Retrieved May 2005, from http://www.jhsph.edu/Dept/MH/History/.

60. McColl MA: The concept of occupation 1975 to 2000. In McColl MA, Law M, Stewart D, et al, eds: *Theoretical basis of occupational therapy,* Thorofare, NJ, 2003, Slack, pp. 39-61.

61. McDermott JJ, ed: *The writings of William James: a comprehensive edition,* Chicago, 1977, University of Chicago Press.

62. McDermott JJ, ed: *The philosophy of John Dewey,* Chicago, 1981, University of Chicago Press.

63. Mead GH: *The philosophy of the present,* Chicago, 1932, Open Court.

64. Mead GH: *The philosophy of the act,* Chicago, 1967, University of Chicago Press.

65. Meyer A: The philosophy of occupation therapy, *Am J Occup Ther* 31:639-642, 1977. (Originally published in the *Archives of Occupational Therapy* 1:1-10, 1922.)

66. Morris W: *The decorative arts, their relation to modern life and progress: an address delivered before the Trades' Guild of Learning,* December 4, 1877. Retrieved May 2005 from http://www.Burrows.com/dec.html.

67. Mosey AC: Involvement in the rehabilitation movement: 1942–1960, *Am J Occup Ther* 25:234-236, 1971.

68. Mosey AC: An alternative: the biopsychosocial model, *Am J Occup Ther* 28:137-140, 1974.

69. Mosey AC: *Occupational therapy: configuration of a profession,* New York, 1981, Raven Press.

70. Mosey AC: Partition of occupational science and occupational therapy, *Am J Occup Ther* 46:851-853, 1992.

71. Mounce HO: *The two pragmatists: from Peirce to Rorty,* New York, 1997, Routledge.

72. Muelder WG, Sears L, Schlabach AV, eds: *The development of American philosophy: a book of readings,* ed 2, Boston, 1990, Houghton Mifflin.

73. Murphy JP: *Pragmatism from Peirce to Davidson,* San Francisco, 1990, Westview Press.

74. Nelson D: Occupation: form and performance, *Am J Occup Ther* 42:633-641, 1988.

75. Peirce CS: The fixation of belief. In Buchler J, ed: *Philosophical writings of Peirce,* New York, 1955, Dover, pp. 5-22.

76. Peirce CS: How to make our ideas clear. In Buchler J, ed: *Philosophical writings of Peirce,* New York, 1955, Dover, pp. 23-41.

77. Peirce CS: The scientific attitude and fallibilism. In Buchler J, ed: *Philosophical writings of Peirce,* New York, 1955, Dover, pp. 42-59.

78. Peirce CS: The fixation of belief. In Fisch MH, ed: *Classic American philosophers,* New York, 1996, Fordham University Press, pp. 54-70.

79. Pinel P: *A treatise on insanity,* New York, 1962, Hafner.

80. Pollock N, McColl MA: How occupation changes. In McColl MA, Law M, Stewart D, et al, eds: *Theoretical basis of occupational therapy,* Thorofare, NJ, 2003, Slack, pp. 63-80.

81. Quiroga VA: *Occupational therapy: the first 30 years—1900 to 1930,* Bethesda, MD, 1995, AOTA.

82. Reck AJ, ed: *Mead: selected writings,* New York, 1964, Bobbs-Merril.

83. Reed K: Tools of practice: heritage or baggage? *Am J Occup Ther* 40:597-605, 1986.

84. Reilly M: Occupational therapy can be one of the great ideas of 20th century medicine, *Am J Occup Ther* 16(1):1-9, 1962.

85. Reilly M: The modernization of occupational therapy, *Am J Occup Ther* 25:243-246, 1971.

86. Reilly M, ed: *Play as exploratory learning: studies in curiosity behavior,* Beverly Hills, 1974, Sage.

87. Rerek MD: The depression years—1929 to 1941, *Am J Occup Ther* 25:231-233, 1971.

88. Royeen C: Chaotic occupational therapy: collective wisdom for a complex profession, *Am J Occup Ther* 57:609-624, 2003.

89. Sabonis-Chafee B, Hussey SM: *Introduction to occupational therapy,* ed 2, St Louis, 1998, Mosby.

90. Schkade JK, Schultz S: Occupational adaptation: toward a holistic approach for contemporary practice, part 1, *Am J Occup Ther* 46:829-837, 1992.

91. Schultz S, Schkade JK: Occupational adaptation: toward a holistic approach for contemporary practice, part 2, *Am J Occup Ther* 46:917-925, 1992.

92. Schwartz KB: The history of occupational therapy. In Crepeau EB, Cohn EC, Schell BA, eds: *Willard and Spackman's occupational therapy,* ed 10, New York, 2003, Lippincott Williams & Wilkins, pp. 5-13.

93. Schwartz KB: The history and philosophy of psychosocial occupational therapy. In Cara E, MacRae A, eds: *Psychosocial occupational therapy: a clinical practice,* ed 2, Clifton Park, NY, 2005, Thomson Delmar Learning, pp. 57-79.

94. Shannon PD: The derailment of occupational therapy, *Am J Occup Ther* 31:229-234, 1977.

95. Stein F, Cutler SK: *Psychosocial occupational therapy: a holistic approach,* ed 2, Albany, NY, 2002, Delmar.

96. Tracy SE: *Studies in invalid occupations,* Boston, 1910, Whitcomb & Barrows.

97. Tuke S: *Description of the retreat: an institution near York for insane persons of the Society of Friends containing an account of its origin and progress, the mode of treatment, and a statement of cases,* London, 1964, Dawsons of Pall Mall.

98. United States Surgeon General: *Mental health: a report of the Surgeon General,* 2005. Retrieved May 2005, from http://www.surgeongeneral.gov/library/mentalhealth/home.html.

99. van Atta K, Roby DS, Roby RR: *Friends hospital: an account of the events surrounding the origin of Friends Hospital and a brief description of the early years of Friends Asylum 1817-1820,* 1988. Retrieved June 2005 from http://www.freindshospitalonline.org/eventsaccount.htm.

100. von Bertalanffy L: General systems theory and psychiatry. In Arieti S, ed: *American handbook of psychiatry,* vol 3, New York, 1966, Basic Books, pp. 705-721.

101. Waldrop MM: *Complexity: the emerging science at the edge of order and chaos,* New York, 1992, Simon & Schuster.

102. Weiss P: Living nature and the knowledge gap, *Saturday Review* 56:19-22, 1969.

103. West C: *The American evasion of philosophy,* Madison, WI, 1989, University of Wisconsin Press.

104. West W: *Psychiatric occupational therapy,* New York, 1959, AOTA.

105. West W: A reaffirmed philosophy and practice of occupational therapy, *Am J Occup Ther* 38:15-23, 1984.

106. Wilcock AA: *An occupational perspective of health,* Thorofare, NJ, 1998, Slack.

107. Wood W: The warp and weft of occupational therapy: an art and science for all times, *Am J Occup Ther* 49:44-52, 1995.

108. Woodside HH: The development of occupational therapy 1910–1929, *Am J Occup Ther* 25:226-230, 1971.

109. World Health Organization: *International classification of functioning, disability and health,* Geneva, 2001, WHO.

110. Yerxa EJ: Authentic occupational therapy, *Am J Occup Ther* 21:1-9, 1967.

111. Zemke R, Clarke F, eds: *Occupational science: the evolving discipline,* Philadelphia, 1996, FA Davis.

Chapter 3

Psychological Theories that have Contributed to the Development of Occupational Therapy Practice

Preview Questions

1. List at least five psychological theories that have contributed to the development of psychosocial occupational therapy.
2. Compare and contrast the core constructs and propositions of the following psychological schools:
   a. Freudian and Neo-Freudian psychoanalysis
   b. Behavioral psychology
   c. Cognitive/behavioral psychology
   d. Cognitive/learning theories
   e. Humanistic psychology
   f. Developmental psychology
3. Explain how constructs from each of the psychological schools listed in # 2 above have informed occupational therapy psychosocial practice.

As discussed in Chapter 2, the intellectual foundations of occupational therapy can be traced back to American pragmatism, particularly to the philosophy of William James, John Dewey, and George Herbert Mead. We saw that occupational therapy borrowed concepts from the psychology of functionalism subscribed to by both William James and John Dewey.[37,90] Functionalism was based on the belief that the mind should be studied by observing practical actions of individuals as they pursue their interests rather than through introspection, as suggested by structuralists.

In this chapter, we will examine two psychological schools that are considered to have been major influences on occupational therapy in the late nineteenth and early twentieth centuries.[15,49] These are *behaviorism,* which also originated in the German school of functionalism,[37,63,77] and *psychoanalysis*. Other psychological orientations that have contributed to the development of occupational therapy such as humanistic and cognitive theories borrowed constructs and techniques from psychoanalysis and behaviorism to varying degrees. Psychoanalysis and behaviorism were at their peak in the 1950s and 1960s.[37] Therefore they influenced occupational therapy at a time when the profession was trying to align itself with medicine. Psychoanalysis and behaviorism contributed to its adoption of the mechanistic, reductionistic, medical model.[21,47,59] However, these theoretical perspectives also provided the profession with constructs that continue to be used in practice today.

In this chapter, we will discuss the psychological theories in question (behaviorism and psychoanalysis) and other theories derived from them (humanistic psychology, developmental psychology, cognitive/behavioral psychology, and learning theories). We will give a brief overview of the background of each, and explain its basic arguments, core constructs, and application in occupational therapy. Refer to Lab Manual Exercises 6-1 through 6-5 to learn how to apply these constructs in practice.

Classical Freudian Psychoanalysis

Background

Unlike other psychological systems that evolved from academia, such as structuralism, functionalism, and subsequently behaviorism, psychoanalysis originated from clinical practice.[37] The motivation to found psychoanalysis was a desire to understand the cause of psychopathology and how to alleviate it. Furthermore, it was the only school of thought at the time to focus exclusively on the unconscious motivation of behavior. The leader of this movement was Sigmund Freud.

Social/Intellectual Context

Freud grew up and developed psychoanalysis at a time when scientific innovations were numerous.[82] When Freud was 3 years old, Charles Darwin published his theory of evolution. Around the same time, Gustav Fechner began work on what he called *scientific psychology*, which was founded on the idea that the study of psychology should be based on the methods of physiology, with emphasis on behavior that could be observed and measured, rather than introspection.[37,82] Herman von Helmholtz, a proponent of functionalism, published a paper in 1847 entitled *The Conservation of Force* that outlined his *principle of conservation of energy*.[37] In this principle, he considered energy in living organisms to be similar to physical energy (as in physics). The principle therefore stated that "energy is never created or lost in a system but is only transformed from one form to another" (p. 208).[37] This principle was later to play a significant role in Freud's formulation of his theory of psychic energy.

Psychic Energy

From Helmholtz's principle of conservation of energy, Freud came up with the idea that psychic energy was a closed energy system.[82] This meant that if some of it was used to meet a certain need (e.g., to repress strong emotions that a person perceived to be inappropriate), there was less energy left to devote to meeting other needs of the organism, such as logical reasoning to solve problems, because psychic energy could neither be created nor destroyed. It stayed the same throughout and was only transformed into various forms to meet needs. At first, Freud conceptualized this energy to be sexual in nature. The idea of sexual desire as motivation for behavior originated from Freud's clinical work with clients who had hysteria. From these clinical cases, he concluded that "Whatever case and whatever symptom we take as our point of departure, *in the end we infallibly come to the field of sexual experience*. So here for the first time, we seem to have discovered an aetiological precondition for hysterical symptoms" (p. 259).[55]

Freud called this sexual/psychic energy the *libido,* a Latin word meaning "lust." However, later he used the term *libidinal energy* to refer to all instinctual drives, including hunger, thirst, and sex.[37]

Structure of the Psyche

The word *psyche* has its roots in the Greek language. The literal translation of the word is "butterfly."[71] In order to understand Freud's view of the structure of the psyche, and therefore human personality, we need to understand the following terms: *id, primary process, ego, cathexis, secondary process, superego, ego defense mechanisms, anticathexis, eros,* and *death instinct*.[28,29,37] We will discuss each of these terms in the context of the structure of the mind as understood in Freudian psychoanalysis.

The Id

According to Freud, the psyche consisted of conscious and unconscious components. The relationship between these two parts of the mind was analogous to an iceberg. The conscious part was the tip of the iceberg, and the unconscious part was comparable to the massive part of the iceberg, which was underwater and therefore invisible. The Latin word *id* (*das es* in German) means "the it." According to Freud, this was the original driving energy of the human psyche. When one is born, he postulated, the id constitutes the whole of the psyche. It is the desire to attain pleasure and avoid discomfort. Thus, when an infant is hungry, he or she wants to satiate the hunger. Thus he argued that the id operated on the basis of the *pleasure principle*. Furthermore, the pleasure principle sought immediate satisfaction of needs. There was no concept of delayed gratification. Gratification of needs took place either through reflex action (e.g., the infant instinctively reaching for the nipple of the mother's breast when hungry), or through imagination of objects that might satisfy the need (e.g., when the mother is not available, the infant conjures up the image of the mother's breast when hungry). Thus this type of need fulfillment occurred through wishful thinking.

Freud referred to activities of the id as the *primary process* because they occurred before the person had experience in the external environment, and therefore they were primary and provided the foundation for personality. The primary process was part of the unconscious and was illogical. That is why there was no concept of delayed gratification. There was no logical mediation to give an individual the idea that objects for need gratification may not always be immediately available, or that sometimes it may not be appropriate to satisfy certain needs immediately.

The Ego

The Latin word *ego* (*das ich* in German) means "the I." Its purpose was postulated by Freud to mediate between the id and the external environment. In other words, the id perceived a need, such as hunger. The ego invested psychic energy in pursuit of objects, such as food, to gratify the need (satiation of hunger). The investment of libidinal energy in thought about the object of need gratification was referred to as *cathexis*, from the Greek word, *"kathexo,"* meaning "to occupy." Because the ego mediated between the

primary process and the external world of reality, it operated on the *reality principle* and was the logical part of the psyche. It was the part of the psyche that examined data, processed it, and solved problems in order to help the id gratify needs. Activities of the ego occurred through the *secondary process*, which consisted of a logical, conscious, thinking process.

The Superego

If needs of the id were to be met all the time, there would be no civilization. Imagine, for example, people having sex any time they feel like it, even in public, irrespective of who was watching. Or imagine what life would be like if there were no laws and whenever you liked something, you could grab it from anybody with or without their permission. Life would be very difficult. That is why, as a child grows up, he or she has to be socialized. The purpose is to create order in society and protect everybody. This socialization process takes place by teaching the child that some things are good and ought to be done while others are wrong and must not be done. Through this process, the child learns the concept of right and wrong, which is the basis of value formation. Initially, the values adopted are those of the parents. However, with time, they become internalized and the child makes them his or her own. Freud conceptualized the purpose of the superego as to ensure that one did not do things that went against those values.

The Latin word *superego* (*das uberich* in German) means the "over I." The superego, according to Freud, was the moral part of the psyche that exerted control over personality. If one engaged or even thought of engaging in acts that went against internalized values, one felt a sense of guilt because of expectation of punishment, which was based on previous experience where the child was punished for engaging in similar acts. This fear of punishment is what Freud conceptualized as the *conscience*. On the other hand, the child had past experiences where he or she was rewarded for engaging in certain acts (e.g., saying "thank you," studying hard and attaining good grades). These experiences formed another part of the superego that Freud called the *ego-ideal*. Engagement in actions that went against internalized values caused a sense of anxiety because of one's conscience based on past experiences of being punished for engaging in those acts. Engaging in ego-ideal tasks led one to feel good about oneself.

With the development of the superego, the task of the ego became more complicated. It had to find objects to fulfill needs of the id while at the same time staying within the superego's regulation. When the ego sensed a danger of being overrun by needs of the id and therefore unable to control them, one suffered what Freud called *neurotic anxiety*. This was the anxiety associated with the feeling that one was getting out of control (e.g., when one felt as if he or she could not help acting in such a way as to inevitably shame him or herself). On the other hand, when one acted or even thought of acting in such a way that an internalized value was likely to be violated, one felt a sense of what Freud referred to as *moral anxiety*.

Ego Defense Mechanisms

According to Freud, when a person acted, or desired to act in such a way that internalized values would be violated, there was a sense of anxiety because the ego perceived a threat. To alleviate the anxiety and therefore protect the ego, defense mechanisms were used. These mechanisms operated at an unconscious level. The primary defense mechanism was *repression*. Any time an idea that threatened the integrity of the *ego* formed, it was pushed down into the unconscious. Other defense mechanisms were *displacement, sublimation, substitution, suppression, regression, introjection, projection, rationalization, reaction formation,* and *denial,* among others.[37,68]

Displacement

Displacement occurred when an object prohibited by the superego was desired and the desire was redirected to another object that was perceived to be more acceptable. For example, a child who was angry with his or her mother directed the anger to a cat because the mother was too powerful, and it was unacceptable to express that emotion toward her.

Sublimation

Sublimation occurred when, instead of displacing the energy invested in unacceptable desired object, one would substitute the object for another that was more acceptable. For example, painting or writing poetry would be substituted for strong sexual urges. It was more acceptable, and one could even be rewarded for painting, while one was likely to be punished for engaging in illicit sex. We will see later that this defense mechanism played a big role in occupational therapy at some point in the profession's history.

Substitution

This defense mechanism was used when a valued but relatively unattainable goal or object was unconsciously replaced by another that had similar characteristics but was more attainable. For example, someone who wanted to be a doctor could opt to be a nurse because nursing had similar characteristics to medicine, but took less time to attain and was cheaper. This decision could be conscious or unconscious. When it happened unconsciously, it constituted substitution.

Suppression

Suppression was voluntary relegation of unacceptable impulses into the preconscious, or conscious forgetting. This mechanism required a strong ego.

Regression

During regression, a person reversed to a less mature stage of development where he or she felt most secure in the past when faced with challenges. For example, when a new baby was born, a 5-year-old sibling who now lost the status and attention of being the baby in the family would regress and begin wetting the bed and soiling himself so that he could be taken care of and feel secure again.

Introjection

During introjection, an individual assimilated a loved or hated person's values, attitudes, and standards as one's own. Unacceptable tendencies such as anger, aggressiveness, or sexuality were turned against oneself. The person criticized him or herself for these tendencies and felt guilty. This was common in conditions such as depression.

Projection

Projection was the opposite of introjection. In this case, the person attributed thoughts, feelings, motives, or desires that were perceived to be unacceptable to others, and accused them of those attributes. For example, a preacher who had strong sexual desires would see others as immoral, and preach to them about impending punishment for their improprieties. Sometimes, what was projected to other people would be projected back. We tend to project only to individuals who are likely to accept our projections, and these individuals are likely to project back to us. According to Carl Gustav Jung,[44] projection was the cause of political and social scapegoating. Sometimes what was projected to others could also be positive. A person who lacked self-confidence would project skills perceived to be lacking to others. For example, someone who felt lacking intellectually would project intellectual capacity (which was really inherent in him or her) to others and then idealize those people (this may be the basis of hero worship).

Rationalization

During rationalization, painful experiences were explained away because the person did not want to get in touch with those experiences. In other words, events that were perceived to be painful were justified with rational explanations. For example, a person who felt guilty about breaking a social rule would explain how it was not his or her fault because the situation could not

be avoided. He or she would even blame other people as bad influences on him or her, thus incorporating other defense mechanisms such as projection.

Reaction Formation

During reaction formation, behaviors and characteristics were developed that were the opposite of impulses and inclinations perceived as unacceptable. For example, a person who was afraid of physically being hurt could portray absolute bravery in the face of danger to cover up for characteristics he perceived as cowardice.

Denial

The existence of experiences too painful to accept was denied. The person behaved as if those experiences did not exist. An extreme example would be someone who refused to accept the fact that she was divorced and continued to plan an upcoming wedding anniversary.

Theory of Personality Development

Freud developed a theory of personality development based on psychosexual stages.[37,68] In his theory, psychological development was complete in the first 5 or 6 years of life. The stages of development were: *oral, anal, phallic (oedipal), latency,* and *genital.* This conceptualization was based on what he thought were the *erogenous zones,* or areas of focus in pursuit of pleasure, at different points in one's life.

Oral Stage

During this stage (0 to 18 months of age), the libidinal focus was on the oral region. Gratification was achieved first through sucking on satisfying objects, such as the mother's breast, then later as the infant grew, actively seeking oral pleasure (oral aggressive phase). In adulthood, the residual of this stage was seen in activities such as kissing, oral caressing of breasts, and so on. Deprivation during early years led to fixation at this stage. An adult who was fixated at the oral stage was pessimistic, suspicious, self-belittling, passive, and/or envious. Overindulgence at this age led to fixation but with erogenous energies directed at repeating and maintaining the gratifying conditions. As an adult, such a person was overly optimistic, gullible, cockish, manipulative, and admiring.

Anal Stage

This stage of psychosexual development lasted from 18 months to 3 years of life. The erogenous zone at this stage was the buttocks or anal region. Before toilet training, the child was free to let go at any time when pressure built up on the sphincter muscles. During the socialization process, which included toilet training, the child was required to hold anal contents until a socially appropriate time and place. If the parents were too demanding at this time, the individual became fixated at this stage and developed an anal personality as an adult, characterized by holding-on tendencies such as stinginess, constrictedness, stubbornness, obsession with orderliness, meticulousness, punctuality, precision, and so on. Overindulgence at this stage led to fixation, but with a resultant personality characterized by letting-go tendencies such as overgenerosity, expansiveness, acquiescence, messiness, tendency toward dirt, tardiness, and vagueness.

Phallic Stage

This occurred between 3 and 6 years of age. The erogenous zone was the genitals. This phase was characterized by an increase in masturbatory behavior. Children were now beginning to get interested in members of the opposite gender. They examined each other as a result of sexual curiosity. Freud's conceptualization of this stage was one of the reasons his theory came into attack in the late twentieth century, because of his problematic theorization about women, at least by today's opinions.[78] According to Freud, the conflict at this stage arose from love of the parent of the opposite gender and competition with the parent of the same gender. For the boy, he named this phenomenon the "Oedipal complex," after Oedipus Rex in Greek mythology,

who unknowingly fell in love with his mother and killed his father.

According to Freud, the boy desired to have his mother sexually. However, this filled him with anxiety because the father was big and strong, and could punish him if he were to know his desires. Furthermore, the little boy could have noticed that his sister, or some other girl, did not have a penis. He hypothesized that her penis was cut off as punishment for desiring her mother sexually. He feared that the same fate would befall him. This fear filled him with castration anxiety. Due to this anxiety, he repressed his desire for the mother and his rivalry to the father. He identified with the father by copying his characteristics so that he could avoid castration but at the same time enjoy his mother sexually vicariously through the father.

The same dynamics occur in the girl, but Freud named the phenomenon the "Electra complex" in this case. His hypothesis was that after discovering that she had no penis, the girl became hostile to her mother for cheating her by not giving her a penis. She desired to have a penis (what Freud called "penis envy"). So, she turned her erotic desire to the father in the hope of sharing with him his phallus. However, for the girl, the situation was even more complicated because she had to shift her primary object of love, from the mother (every child's first object of love) to the father. She therefore had more difficulty developing her heterosexuality. Similarly, however, her erotic feelings toward her father made her anxious. To alleviate the anxiety, she repressed the erotic feelings toward her father and the hostility toward her mother, and identified with her mother in order to share the father vicariously through the mother. Obviously, in the late twentieth and early twenty-first century, Freud's insinuation that women were lacking because they did not have a penis and envied men for possessing that organ is outrageous. But considering the status of women at the time Freud was developing his theory, this suggestion made sense. It would have been similar to someone arguing that black people envied and desired to be white. No one would have thought that it would not have been so. After all, the white male held a particularly prestigious place in society.

A feeling of rejection by the parent of the opposite sex at this stage, Freud hypothesized, led to development of feelings of self-hatred, humility, plainness, shyness, isolation, and shyness as an adult. In other words, the child seemed to think that since the parent of the opposite sex did not hug or kiss him or her, he or she had to be undesirable. Therefore there was no need to flirt, dress stylishly, be outgoing, or take pride in oneself. Overindulgence by the parent of the opposite sex led to an adult who was vain, proud, stylish, flirtatious, gregarious, and brash.

Latency Stage

From 6 years through puberty, pregenital sexual desires were temporarily repressed. So much energy had been expended in repressing sexual desire at the phallic phase that at the latent stage, sexual activity was more or less banished from consciousness. Curiosity about the world, school work, and peer-related activities took precedence over sexual expression.

Genital Stage

According to Freud, this was the stage of fully developed sexuality. The individual fully outgrew the pregenital (infantile) sexual desires and began to get involved in mature heterosexual relationships. If all previous stages had been negotiated successfully, the individual would begin dating and eventually get married. Overgratification or undergratification in previous infantile stages would lead to neurotic personality at this phase, making adult relationships difficult. When this happened, the psychoanalyst could help the individual by delving into his or her childhood experiences to trace the root of neurosis and help him or her work through those experiences.

Psychoanalytic Method

Based on the hypothesis that the root of neurosis was repressed painful childhood experiences, the main goal of psychoanalysis was to make conscious the contents of the unconscious. Instincts and impulses were expressed maturely, and psychological needs were met appropriately.[30,82] The psychoanalyst began by relating to the ego (conscious experiences) and gradually delved deeper into the unconscious. Because repressed experiences were painful and threatening to the ego, the client usually unconsciously resisted examining the contents of the unconscious. To break through the resistance and access the unconscious, psychoanalysts used a variety of techniques, including free association and interpretation. Psychoanalysts still use these techniques today, with a particular focus on the dynamics of *transference* and *countertransference*.[*] These terms will be defined and explained later in the chapter.

Free Association

The client lies on a couch with the therapist sitting behind him or her and freely articulates whatever appears on his or her mind. The therapist speaks very little, if at all; he or she acts as a mirror, reflecting the client's unconscious back to him or her.

Interpretation

The therapist assigns meaning to psychological phenomena, such as dream symbols, the unconscious material explicated through free association, and transference. Freud had specific ideas about the symbolic meaning of objects exposed from the unconscious. For example, "travel symbolized death; falling symbolized giving in to sexual temptation; boxes, gardens, doors, or balconies symbolized the vagina; and cannons, snakes, trees, swords, church spires, and candles symbolized the penis" (p. 472).[37] The analyst had to be knowledgeable about these symbols in order to accurately interpret the unconscious material.

Transference

Transference refers to transfer of emotions associated with a previous object to another object in

*References 30,39,68,78,82,84.

the present. For example, a client with deep-seated repressed hostility toward his or her father during childhood may behave toward a male therapist as if the therapist were the father by demonstrating hostility in the therapeutic relationship. The therapist notes these incidences of transference and interprets them in order to give the client insight regarding the reason for the neurotic behavior and offer a chance to "work through" the hostility toward the father. Sometimes, the therapist responds to a client's transference by portraying behavior similar to the client's initial experiences. For example, an older therapist who has a client behaving toward him as if he were her grandfather (who made her feel secure and loved as a child) may respond to the client as if she were actually his granddaughter. This phenomenon is referred to as *countertransference*. Freudian analysts recommend that the therapist be aware of this dynamic, and when it occurs, make *countertransference* part of therapeutic interpretation to help the client increase insight regarding the origin of his or her neurosis.[78] Refer to Lab Manual Exercise 6-1, *A*, to learn how to apply the Freudian technique of "free association" in clinical practice.

The Neo-Freudians

In his younger years, Freud was rather rigid and unforgiving of anyone who disagreed with his theory and technique of psychoanalysis, although in his maturity he became quite humble and flexible.[18,33,42,78] Many of his close associates who did not fully agree with him broke away and developed their own systems of analysis. They came to be known as Neo-Freudians because they retained some of the basic tenets of psychoanalytic theory but modified them in significant ways. Some of the neo-Freudians included Carl Jung and Alfred Adler, among others. One of the neo-Freudians who emerged much later and who is well known in occupational therapy is Erik Erikson. In this chapter, we will discuss Carl Jung because of his significance in the development of depth/analytic psychol-

ogy. We will also discuss Erik Erikson in the "Developmental Psychology" section later in the chapter. Erickson's theory of the eight stages of humans has been used in occupational therapy primarily to provide an understanding of human development.

Carl Gustav Jung

Carl Gustav Jung was a close acquaintance of Freud who saw him as his successor as leader of the psychoanalytic movement and even referred to him as "his son."[18,33,37,42] However, as they worked together, Jung began to disagree with Freud on some important aspects of his psychoanalytic theory. For example, he disagreed with Freud's view of the unconscious and the postulation that all neurosis originated from sexual trauma. He also did not agree with Freud's interpretation of the Oedipus complex. These disagreements led to his break with Freud in 1914. Subsequently, he developed his theory and techniques of analytic psychology.

Jung's psychology may best be understood as teleological (purposeful), where the purpose of psyche development (individuation) was seen as integration of the conscious and unconscious.[34,37] He is best known for his work on the structure of the psyche, personality types, individuation, and the theory of synchronicity. We will discuss the first three aspects of Jung's analytic psychology next. We will not examine his theory of *synchronicity* (coincidence of causally unrelated events by similarity in meaning) in this text because it is more or less mystical. Therefore it is not applicable in occupational therapy or consistent with the profession's empirical orientation.

Structure of the Psyche

Jung agreed with Freud on the concept of unconscious motivation and the expansiveness of the unconscious part of the psyche. However, unlike Freud, he did not see the unconscious as the trash bin of traumatic, undesirable experiences. Rather, he saw it as storage for psychic material that he viewed as analogous in value to gold.[11]

He also viewed the psyche as a whole entity comprising the totality of psychological structure of the human. In other words, he saw it as the spirit and the soul embracing all thought, feeling, perception, and behavior, both conscious and unconscious. Furthermore, he saw the psyche as creative, bringing life and creativity to man, and creating its symbols.[45] In that sense, he postulated, the mind has godlike qualities and could be thought of as a concentrated representation of God. In other words, "As the eye is to the sun, the soul is to God" (p. 64).[45] So to Jung, instead of psychic energy being sexual, it was *creative*.

Another important argument in Jung's conceptualization of the mind was the idea of lost wholeness. In his view, a person was born with a whole psyche. In the process of socialization, the individual began to disavow parts of the psyche as unacceptable by significant others, which led to fragmentation of the psyche. To him, this was a psychic illness. The purpose of psychotherapy was to help the individual recapture the original psychic wholeness and strength, so that he or she acted as an autonomous, integrated person, rather than a split individual with multiple conflicting splinter subpsyches. To understand the concept of psychic wholeness and how it is lost, one must understand its layered structure. According to Jung, the psyche consisted of the ego (conscious) and the unconscious. However, instead of the unconscious consisting of a single layer as in Freud's theory, for Jung, it was made of two layers: the *personal* and *collective unconscious*.[34,45]

The Ego
The *ego* was the center of consciousness. It contained all the conscious perceptions, feelings, thoughts, and memories, and provided one a sense of continuity and identity through selection and censorship of the psychic material that was consciously expressed or lived out.

The Personal Unconscious
The *personal unconscious* was next to the conscious layer of the psyche and contained psychic material that was particular to the individual, such as memories that could easily be retrieved, repressed memories of traumatic experiences whose retrieval could be more resisted and forgotten, and subliminal memories. All psychic material that could be threatening to the conscious (because it was inconsistent with the identity or moral values, or it was irrelevant to one's life circumstances) was relegated to this layer of the psyche.

The Collective Unconscious
The *collective unconscious* was the most original of Jung's contribution to psychology and also the most controversial.[34,37] It was the information in the psyche that was *transpersonal* and contained traces of memory inherent in the past experiences of all humanity. Jung perceived this part of the psyche as consisting of traits comparable to genetically inherited biological characteristics. He considered these traits (e.g., fear, danger, hate, love, birth, death) to be present in our psyches before birth such that we inherited them like physical characteristics from previous generations.

These memories were in the form of what Jung called the *archetypes,* which he explained as the blueprints of reality, analogous to undeveloped photographic negatives. These "negatives," consisting of an unclear sense of psychic reality, were in time clarified and filled out by experience. For example, every newborn has a primordial idea of the ideal person of the opposite gender. However, a complete perception of erotic love is not realized until the individual has matured and experienced heterosexual relationships. According to Jung, archetypal images consisted of the *persona, shadow, anima/animus,* and the *self*.

The *persona* was the part of ourselves that we present to others. It was conceptualized as a mask that we wear, symbolically speaking, to help us adapt to our various social roles. For example, when one assumes the role of a teacher, he or she has a different persona from that assumed in the role of a parent, lover, or friend. It was postulated to be close to the ego because it reflected our identity as perceived by the ego. However, it was an archetype because it developed out of archetypal patterns of idealized self as a social person.

The *shadow* was made of content from both the personal and collective unconscious. As one experienced the process of socialization, traits that were not consistent with identity as perceived by the ego were disavowed and pushed down into the unconscious. Those traits did not develop and were not expressed consciously. For example, a person who grew up with values emphasizing being nice and generous to others repressed all urges to express disapproval of others or to say no when asked for help. In fact, criticism of other people and all traces of selfishness were disavowed. Those traits formed part of the person's shadow. However, they did not disappear. Rather, they acted like splinter personalities and were expressed inappropriately, causing incongruities in behavior, confusing other people and causing discomfort to the ego. For example, the nice, generous person may often act toward others in conniving, malicious ways, quite contrary to the nice, generous persona. The collective part of the shadow on the other hand contained imagery of polarities between bad and good, desirable and undesirable, and so on, which were inherited from experiences of good and evil, desirable and undesirable, over many generations of human existence. These images were expressed through religious rituals, fairy tales, and myths found in cultures all over the world.

It was understood that the shadow was usually projected to other people. For example, the nice, generous person in our example may see his or her mean, selfish part in other people perceived to exemplify those traits. When he or she acts like those people, he or she feels guilty and uncomfortable. Jung's recommendation was that whenever we feel dissatisfied with ourselves or feel guilty for no apparent reason, we should look for projections of our shadow to those close to us.[69] Moreover, the shadow was seen as always projected to people of the same gender.

A man projected his shadow to another man, such as a friend. The same case applied to a woman. The collective shadow was exemplified in activities such as political scapegoating.[44]

The *anima/animus* referred to the archetype of contra sexual traits in every person. Jung postulated that every man had an eternal image of a woman in his psyche, which he called the *anima*. Similarly, every woman had an eternal image of a man (the *animus*). Thus

> Every man carries within him the eternal image of the woman, not the image of this or that woman, but a definite feminine image. This image is fundamentally unconscious, an hereditary factor of primordial origin engraved in the living organic system of the man, an imprint or archetype of all the ancestral experiences of the female, a deposit, as it were, of all the impressions ever made by woman (vol. 17, pp. 101-102).[45]

Whereas the shadow was understood to be projected to the person of the same sex, contrasexual characteristics of the psyche were projected to the person of the opposite sex, "and is one of the chief reasons for passionate attractions or aversions" between people in heterosexual relationships (p. 183).[45] For example, a woman who did not recognize characteristics such as aggressiveness in herself projected them to men, and she admired and was attracted to aggressive men. Similarly, a man who was not able recognize the feeling, relational part of himself projected these characteristics to women. He was therefore attracted to women who were warm, feeling, and good at relationships.

However, similar to the shadow, contrasexual characteristics that were disavowed were postulated to be expressed negatively. For example, when a woman who saw herself as feminine and nonaggressive was faced with a challenging situation in which her ability to cope was questioned, she became *animus possessed* and was blunt, emotional, inflexible, judgmental, and so on. She expressed herself like a second-rate man, so to speak. Similarly, a man who was unable to live out his feminine, feeling, relational characteristics became *anima possessed* and was moody, peevish, angry, brutal, unfeeling, violent, and so on. That is, he behaved like a second-rate, immature woman. However, the anima/animus were not always seen as negative. They were important mediators of the unconscious and links to the deeper layers of the psyche.

The *self* in Jungian analytic psychology referred to the "true self" at the depth of one's psyche.[45] It was the central archetype, and all other parts of the psyche were constellated around it.[34] It was conceived to be the center of totality of the psyche, embracing both the conscious and unconscious, and was represented symbolically in dreams by circles (mandalas), the royal couple, a divine child, a church, or any other symbol of divinity. It was not limited by the ego structures of time and space. It transcended these structures and could get in touch with the past, the future, and could even travel to places that one had never been physically. The self strived toward integration of all parts of the psyche so as to capture original wholeness, a process that Jung referred to as *individuation*.

Personality Types

Jung's personality types referred to one's way of functioning in or relating to the world. As he put it, "The relation between subject and object, considered biologically, is always a *relation of adaptation*, since every relation between subject and object presupposes mutually modified effects from either side" (p. 414).[43] He characterized these types as consisting of two major attitudes (referring to one's orientation to the world in general) and four psychological functions (expression of the personality type or the general attitude).[34] The relationship between personality types and functions are shown in Figure 3-1.

Attitudes

The two attitudes or ways of relating to the world are *extraversion* and *introversion*.[34,43,83] Extraverted types orient themselves to the world externally, focusing on objective reality. They are open and outgoing and are energized by relating

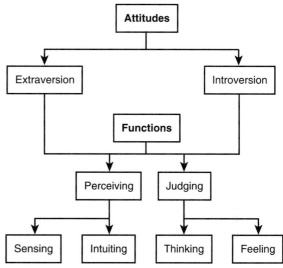

Figure 3-1. Jungian psychological types. The two attitudes defining general orientation to life are extraversion and introversion. These orientations are served by psychological functions classified in the categories of perception and judgment. The functions of perception are sensing and intuiting, and those of judgment are thinking and feeling.

to other people and to the objective world of sense data. They have numerous relationships, but not of an intensive nature. Extraverts talk as they think, without reflecting first on what they are saying. Their orientation is on interaction rather than concentration. By contrast, the source of energy for introverted types is from within. They orient their libido inside themselves. They are good listeners rather than speakers. They have few relationships but those few are intense. They think and reflect before they speak and therefore are often sure of what they say; their words are carefully measured. They have good concentration on the subject at hand. Both attitudes are in every person. However, only one of them is predominantly manifested in a person's orientation in or psychological adaptation to the world. The subordinate attitude is unconscious. Thus, for extraverted persons, their introversion is unconscious, and vice versa.

Functions

Within the two psychological attitudes are functions of the psychological types. These are generally classified into two categories, namely, *perceiving* and *judging* functions. Perceiving functions are sensing and intuiting, and judging functions are thinking and feeling. Those who perceive through sensing gather data from the environment through their senses. They attend to specific concrete facts that are verifiable through the senses. They are preoccupied with accuracy and are chronological in their thinking, always taking into account factual experiences in their past and present. At work, they are patient with routine tasks and are able to work steadily. They like to use skills already learned. Because of their orientation to the objective world, extraverted individuals are likely to use the perceiving function of sensing predominantly.

The intuiting function refers to attention to experiences in ways that transcend the senses. People using this function seek to understand the deeper meaning of events. They examine patterns and relationships between events. Their thinking is abstract, and they examine possibilities rather than what is apparent. Because of their ability to analyze patterns, relationships, possibilities, and to be abstract, people who use this function are able to formulate ideas, have profound insights, make surprising discoveries, and therefore approximate and predict future events. At work, intuitives are impatient with routine tasks. They may have outbursts of enthusiasm but dislike tasks involving precision. They like to learn new skills, but as soon as they master them, they abandon them and seek new ones. They thrive on novelty.

Thinking, the first function of judging, is an approach to events in an objective manner. Thinking types are impersonal and firm-minded. They tend to be critical and are concerned with fair play. They value facts and whether those facts are true or false. In other words, their preoccupation is with justice. Feeling types evaluate events subjectively. They are personal and sympathetic. They use persuasion rather than command to convince people of their values. In conflicts, they seek conciliation rather than right and wrong. They value the work of others and are usually not critical. Their interest is quality of human relationships rather than facts. In other words, their basis of evaluating events is whether those events are good or bad for people rather than whether the facts involved are true or false. So, their preoccupation is humanity rather than justice. According to Jung, all the psychological functions are integrated into one totality:

> Sensation establishes what is actually present, thinking enables us to recognize its meaning, feeling tells us its value, and intuition points to possibilities as to whence it came and whither it is going in a given situation. In this way we can orient ourselves with respect to the immediate world as completely as when we locate a place geographically by latitude and longitude (p. 126).[34]

Although all the previously discussed psychological functions are inherent in every human's psyche, one of the functions (referred to as the *superior function*) is the most developed and therefore dominant. The least developed function (referred to as the *inferior function*) is repressed and expressed only in dreams and fantasies, and is sometimes projected to other people. For example, for an extraverted sensist, sensing would be a superior function. Such a person would primarily orient himself or herself to the objective world of facts. If the intuitive function in such a person is inferior, he or she will be unconscious of his or her ability to infer reality beyond available facts and may project this ability to others.

Individuation/The Transcendent Function

According to Jung, the psyche was splintered with those aspects of it that were consistent with the ego identity being the most developed and expressed and those that were not consistent with identity being unconscious, undeveloped, and unexpressed.[34,37,43,71] Thus the shadow was in conflict with the consciousness, the anima with the animus, introversion with extraversion, the superior function with the inferior one, and so on. This conflict led to neurosis. The psyche's drive was to integrate the different aspects so that the original wholeness that was there at birth could be regained. The goal of this integration was "realization of selfhood" (p. 137).[34] For this integration to occur, different aspects of the psyche had to be fully developed, differentiated, and expressed in conscious life. Thus characteristics of the shadow had to be expressed consciously, so that a person who identified himself or herself as generous had to own his or her jealousy, a woman had to live out her masculine qualities (animus), the man had to live out his feminine qualities (anima), an extrovert had to develop his or her introverted reflective qualities, and so on. This process of differentiation, development, and conscious expression of different parts of the psyche was what Jung called *individuation*. This occurred throughout a person's life but was the primary task of the second half of life (this is discussed further in the "Developmental Psychology" section).

Once different parts of the psyche had been differentiated, developed, and fully expressed, they had to be integrated so that psychic wholeness was attained. Once this happened, a person had integrity, which meant that he or she acted from the center of an authentic self. This process of synthesis and integration occurred through a process that Jung called the *transcendent function*. As Hall and Lindzey state, "This function is endowed with the capacity to unite all of the opposing trends of the several systems and to work toward the ideal goal of perfect wholeness (selfhood)" (p. 138).[34]

Analytical Therapy

According to Jung, when various parts of the psyche that were underdeveloped were ready to be differentiated, expressed, and integrated, they presented themselves in dreams, projections, and fantasies.[34,37,45,71] The goal of analytic therapy was and today is to facilitate this process by making associations and interpreting symbols from dreams, fantasies, and creative works of clients (such as mandalas or magic circles, which are artistic creations within a circle). Other methods of working with clients in Jungian analytic therapy include active imagination (where the client acts out in turn each figure appearing in a dream to apprehend its message to the conscious identity). Active imagination can also be done with figures appearing in myths, stories, or rituals that have particular attraction to a person, or those appearing in fantasies. Refer to

 Lab Manual Exercise 6-1, *B*, to learn how to apply the Jungian technique of active imagination in clinical practice.

Application of Psychoanalytic and Analytic Psychology in Occupational Therapy

A review of the literature reveals documented application of the Freudian version of psychoanalysis since the 1950s, which coincides with the period when psychoanalysis was most influential[37] and occupational therapy was struggling to be accepted as a medical discipline (see Chapter 2). During this time, occupational therapy was seen as a projective means of helping clients with psychiatric diagnoses bring to consciousness their unconscious psychic conflicts.

Azima and Azima[4] outlined a dynamic theory of occupational therapy, based on the psychoanalytic view of the relationship between people and human and nonhuman objects. Azima[3] developed a battery of tests for occupational therapy evaluation, using a variety of activities that were employed as projective media on which clients could project their intrapsychic conflicts. The battery was based on the object relations theory developed by Anna Freud, Sigmund Freud's daughter. Fidler and Fidler[27] wrote a book in which they suggested that activities in occupational therapy could be used as media through which clients could communicate with therapists the contents of the unconscious. Mosey[58] outlined the analytic frame of reference based on psychoanalytic theory as one of her proposed three frames of reference. These are just a few of the ways in which occupational therapy incorporated psychoanalytic theory. Although this approach has lost momentum since the 1980s, psychoanalytic concepts are still used in occupational therapy (see Chapter 9 for a detailed discussion of the psychodynamic conceptual model of occupational therapy).

A review of the literature reveals no indication of significant use of Jung's analytic psychology in occupational therapy. This is surprising considering the emphasis on symbolism in this theory, which would come in handy in helping clients achieve wholeness and live meaningful lives. For example, activities such as painting, sculpting, dancing, and writing (which are important leisure activities for many people) may reveal important images from a client's unconscious. One could use Jungian techniques such as active imagination to help them become more integrated. In fact, I have applied Jungian techniques in the context of occupational therapy with notable success (see Chapter 9 for details).

Behavioral Psychology

Background

The origin of behaviorism is often associated with the Russian psychologist, Ivan Pavlov. However, its roots go even further back than Pavlov. Behaviorism actually originated from what was known as the Russian objective psychology, which was started by Ivan M. Sechenov.[37] Sechenov started with German structuralist principles since he had studied with well-known structuralists such as Herman von Helmholtz in Berlin. He was of the opinion that the cause of behavior was external stimulation and not internal thought processes as held by many psychological schools at the time. He regarded the idea of internal thought etiology of behavior as "the greatest of falsehoods." Rather, "the initial cause of any action always lies in external sensory stimulation, because without this thought is inconceivable" (p. 89).[76] Therefore, for him, behavior was reflexive since it originated from physiological processes of the brain. He sug-

gested that investigation in psychology needed to be pursued using methods of physiology.

Ivan Pavlov, who had studied with Karl Ludwig at the University of Leipzig, agreed with Sechenov.[37] He tried to apply Sechenov's ideas by taking a physiological approach to the study of behavior. He prepared a gastric fistula from a dog's digestive system to outside of its body and used the fistula to study gastric activities as the dog received different forms of stimulation. This research led to development of the foundational concepts of classical conditioning, and a Nobel Prize in physiology in 1904. Following is a discussion of the basic constructs of classical conditioning, the basis of behaviorism, based on Pavlov's research.[63-65]

Conditioning

In his experiments, Pavlov discovered that secretions in the dog's digestive system occurred not only when food was in the dog's mouth but also at the sight of food. He named this response the unlearned or *unconditioned response* (UCR). Pavlov figured that the response by the dog when food was placed in its mouth was learned and therefore named it a learned or *conditioned response* (CR). These observations made him curious about how these responses were formed. To satisfy his curiosity, he tried a number of experiments. He paired a variety of signals, such as light, sound, and so on, with presentation of food. Pavlov's observations led to the conclusion that stimulus-response associations could be created through this pairing process. He observed that learning to respond to these signals took place in stages.

First, Pavlov presented the signal (light or sound). He called this an *unconditioned stimulus* (UCS). In the second stage, whenever he presented the UCS, he simultaneously presented food, which stimulated digestive system secretions (UCR). After several trials, he withdrew the food and presented the signal alone. He noticed that the dog produced secretions as if food was present. He concluded that this was a *conditioned response* (CR). At this point, the signal became a *conditioned stimulus* (CS). He then noticed that as long as a CS was followed by the presentation of food, the response (CR) became stronger. He called this *reinforcement* of conditioned behavior. However, if he presented the CS several times without presenting food, the CR (secretion of the digestive system) disappeared. He called this disappearance of response due to lack of reinforcement *extinction*. He observed that after extinction, sometimes the secretions of the digestive system of the dog would spontaneously occur when the CS was presented. He called this tendency *spontaneous recovery*.

As he continued with his experiments, Pavlov also found that in time, the CR could be generalized to other signals that were similar to the CS. For example, a dog that was conditioned to produce digestive secretions at the sound of a bell could also respond to the sound of chimes of a clock produced at a certain frequency. Thus, through Pavlov's work, basic constructs of conditioning theory, namely, unconditioned stimulus, unconditioned response, conditioned stimulus, conditioned response, reinforcement, extinction, spontaneous recovery, and generalization of learning were defined.

Application of Conditioning Theory in the US: John B. Watson and Behaviorism

Pavlov's conditioning theory was the basis of the school of behaviorism in the United States. This school was founded by John Broadus Watson. Watson was somewhat influenced in his intellectual development by both functionalism and pragmatism.[32,37] However, his main interest was neurology; particularly, animal studies, which was the subject of his dissertation. His intellectual position was that the traditional methods of studying animal psychology were the only legitimate methods of scientific psychology. Thus he emphasized the study of observable behavior and rejected introspective methods and the notion of the unconscious prevalent in psychoanalytic psychology. In this emphasis, he was highly influenced by the work of Ivan Pavlov.

Consistent with Pavlov's experiments, Watson came up with the branch of psychology referred to as *behaviorism*, in which he proposed that behavior be described in terms of physiological responses of organisms. He adopted Pavlov's reflexological terminology so that it was applicable to human behavior. An example of this application was his experiment with "Little Albert" in which he conditioned a child named Albert to fear a rabbit by pairing presentation of the rabbit with the loud sound of a clanging metal bar.[85] Gradually, he was able to demonstrate that this fear generalized to all furry objects. Watson used his position as editor of the journal *Psychological Review* to influence the development of American psychology in the direction of behaviorism.

B.F. Skinner and Operant Conditioning

Burrhus Frederic Skinner was one of a group of psychologists referred to as neo-behaviorists, who were influenced by the philosophy of *logical positivism*.[37] A philosopher named Auguste Compte developed positivism; Sechenov, Pavlov, and Watson all ascribed to it. Positivism was based on the radical empiricist position that the only valid information about the world was that which could be positively, objectively observed. Metaphysical speculation was to be avoided because it could not provide any valid knowledge of the world. However, with recognition in science of phenomena such as gravity, electromagnetism, and so on, it became apparent that directly observable data as the only basis of reality was not plausible. This necessitated a search for another approach to explanation of reality. A group of philosophers in Vienna came up with what came to be known as *logical positivism*, where empiricism was used to gather objective facts, and rationalism was used to explain the observed facts. This led to development of the concept of *operationalization*, where it was proposed that abstract concepts be operationalized according to methods used to measure them. These ideas were adopted in psychology, and neo-behaviorism emerged from them. Skinner was part of this new movement in psychology.

Basic Propositions

Consistent with logical positivism, Skinner disagreed with the positivistic position that "something is meaningful or scientific (objective) only if at least two observers agree on its existence."[53] Rather, to him, even private experiences were valid data, and thinking was as much activity or behavior as walking. Instead of concentrating on mentalism as psychoanalysts did, or ruling it out altogether as classical behaviorists did, he sought, in the true logical positivistic fashion, to strike a balance between the two.[80] Another important observation in understanding his development of operant conditioning was the influence of the theory of evolution. He saw this theory as providing a means of explaining operant behavior. Thus he stated that "Important consequences of behavior which could not play a role in evolution because they were not sufficiently stable features of the environment are *made effective through operant conditioning* during the lifetime of the individual" (pp. 51-52, emphasis mine).[53] Obviously, Watson's behaviorism was also an important influence on his thought.[37,70] Based on these influences, he developed a theory of operant conditioning consisting of the propositions described below.[10,37,80]

First, Skinner observed that learning occurred as the organism operated within the environment. As it operated, it encountered a rewarding stimulus after portraying certain behaviors. He called this the *reinforcing stimulus* or *reinforcer*. When a reinforcer for a behavior was present, the tendency toward the behavior that was immediately reinforced *(operant)* increased. He named this phenomenon *operant conditioning*. Skinner made the observations that were the basis of his theory while he was experimenting with rats. He had devised a box (Skinner's box) that had a bar with a pedal attached to one wall. Pressing the pedal led to a pellet of rat food being released into the box. When Skinner

placed the rat in the box, he noticed that it bounced around in the box aimlessly until it accidentally pressed on the pedal and a pellet of food was released. After this, the behavior became more and more precise. Very soon the rat was pressing the pedal quite regularly and intentionally in order to obtain food. This led to the first proposition of operant conditioning: *rewarding behavior (presence of reinforcers for the behavior) increased the probability of the behavior being repeated.*

Skinner started wondering what would happen if food did not appear when the pedal was pressed. So he removed the food and no pellets were released when the rat pressed the pedal. After a few trials without food, the rat stopped its pedal-pressing behavior. Skinner called this phenomenon *extinction*. This led to his second proposition of operant conditioning that *if behavior was not reinforced, the probability of its recurrence decreased.*

Schedules of Reinforcement

Very soon, as Skinner continued experimenting, he discovered that certain variations of how reinforcement was presented were more effective than others in ensuring that the rat repeated the desired behavior. He called these variations *schedules of reinforcements.* In *continuous reinforcement,* every time the rat pressed the pedal, food was released into the box. However, when food was not made available, the pedal-pressing behavior went into *extinction* very quickly.

In the *fixed ratio schedule,* food was released after a certain number of pedal pressings (e.g., every second, third, fourth time). Very soon the rat learned to press the pedal the required number of times in order to obtain food. However, like the continuous schedule, when food was not released at the scheduled occurrence of the behavior, after a while the pedal-pressing behavior disappeared.

In the *variable schedule,* Skinner varied the number of times that the rat needed to press the pedal before food was released. First the food would be released after pressing the pedal two times, another time it would be after five times, another time after three times, and so on. He found that when food was withdrawn, the pedal-pressing behavior persisted longest when this type of schedule was used. He concluded that the *variable schedule* of reinforcement was the most effective when the goal was to make learned behavior permanent. This is the mechanism of addiction to gambling.[10] People continue to gamble because they do not know when they might win. It may be the next hand in a game of poker, or the next trial in a roulette table.

Shaping

In addition to establishing reinforcement schedules, Skinner experimented with complex behaviors. He found that when behaviors that successively approximated desired behavior were rewarded, beginning with the least to most complex, in time it was possible for organisms to learn fairly complex behaviors. In fact, this is the basis of all education. For example, a child is first taught to write single letters of the alphabet and is rewarded for accomplishing this task. Then, he or she is taught to join the letters with vowels to make simple sounds and is rewarded for being successful until this is mastered. Next, he or she is taught how to write whole words, and finally whole sentences. Skinner called this technique *shaping*.

Punishment and Negative Reinforcement

Continuing with his experiments, Skinner rigged the box such that every time the rat pressed the pedal, it received an electric shock. After a few trials, the rat stopped pressing the pedal altogether. His discovery led to the third proposition of operant conditioning that when *aversive stimulus* followed behavior, the likelihood of the behavior being repeated was decreased. This form of conditioning was called *punishment*.

In a separate experiment, Skinner continuously used a low electric current to shock the rat until it pressed the pedal and the current stopped.

Very soon, it pressed the pedal frequently in order to stop the discomfort of being shocked. He called this type of conditioning (where aversive stimulus is removed when desired behavior is performed) *negative reinforcement*. His observations led to his articulation of the fourth proposition of operant conditioning that *removal of aversive stimulus when behavior was performed led to an increase in the probability that the behavior would be repeated*.

Criticism of Behaviorism

Some of the criticisms of behaviorism include its insistence that most behavior is learned. Critics propose that behaviorism tends to ignore the genetic origin of behavior.[37] Furthermore, behaviorism, according to critics, ignores the importance of language in shaping behavior since behaviorists insist that thinking and language are activities just like walking. This argument ignores the fact that since language is separate from physical activity, it influences the way we think, and therefore our behavior. Furthermore the idea that we can learn something about humans by observing animal behavior has been questioned because animals are significantly different from humans. It is doubtful that animal models can be used to help us understand human behavior in any useful way.

The biggest criticism of behaviorism is that it ignores mental events as causes of behavior. This is important, considering that it has been demonstrated clearly that what we believe about ourselves (including what we believe to be our abilities) often determines what we choose to do and how well we do it. Based on the above-mentioned criticisms, some academic and clinical psychologists developed new systems of psychology (cognitive and cognitive behavioral psychologies) by modifying behavioral concepts to incorporate the idea of mental processes as causes and mediators of behavior. We will discuss these systems of psychology next. Refer to Lab Manual Exercise 6-2 to learn how to apply behavioral strategies in a clinical setting.

Cognitive and Cognitive Behavioral Psychologies

Cognitive behavioral psychologies were developed as clinical disciplines in an attempt to incorporate cognitions (e.g., thinking processes, images, beliefs), emotions evoked by those cognitions, and behavior in response to perceived shortcomings of both behaviorism and psychoanalysis. The goal of therapeutic interventions based on this psychological system was to change thought processes and through them change behavior. Cognitive behavioral psychology has replaced behaviorism as the most influential psychological movement of the twentieth and early twenty-first century. This is evidenced by the fact that in any counseling journal today you will find an article discussing some aspect of cognitive behavioral therapy, and every counseling graduate program incorporates training in that approach to therapy.[88] As Borgen states, cognitive behavioral-oriented approach to therapy "may be the most popular orientation of clinicians, aside from eclecticism" (p. 581).[12] Chief among cognitive/behavioral psychologists are Albert Ellis, Aaron Beck, and Albert Bandura. We will discuss these psychologists next.

Albert Ellis's Rational Emotive Behavior Therapy

Albert Ellis was educated and was quite successful as a psychoanalyst. However, he disliked the psychoanalytic method of trying to increase client insight and subsequently waiting for changes to occur.[37,62] He wanted to be more directive, giving authoritative information to clients and using pointed questions and remarks to help facilitate behavioral change. He tried conditioning theory during which he attempted to decondition his clients from engagement in harmful behaviors. However, he was still not satisfied because behaviorism did not attempt to give clients insight regarding why changes were necessary in the first place. This led to his development of Rational Emotive Techniques (RET) in

1955.[62,89] In 1993, the name changed to Rational Emotional Behavior Therapy (REBT).[57]

Basic Premise

The basic proposition of REBT is that humans are both rational and irrational beings.[62] When they think rationally, they are efficient in their behavior, happy, and competent. When they are irrational, they are inefficient, unhappy, and incompetent. This is the root of neurosis. At birth, humans tend to be irrational, which leads to self-defeating behaviors.[57,62] How a person subsequently develops depends on early learning as determined by his or her environment during upbringing, with particular focus on the parents. When early learning is faulty, the person develops *irrational values,* which leads to neurosis. Ellis[23] identified the following irrational values that are universal among individuals from all cultures who develop neurosis:

- *I must be loved and approved by everybody in the community*. This value is irrational because it is virtually unachievable. It does not matter how nice or integrated you are. At some point, you will meet someone who does not like you, may even hate you, or someone who does not approve a single thing you do. Striving to be loved and approved by everybody is therefore a self-defeating objective whose pursuit can lead to inevitable failure and misery.

- *I must be competent, adequate, achieving, and therefore perfect if I am to be worthwhile.* A person who thinks like that falls apart every time he or she does anything that appears to be less than perfect, which is very much most of the time. Such a person lives a very unhappy life, striving to achieve unachievable perfection.

- *Some people are bad and must be blamed and punished.* This type of thinking is based on the mistaken assumption that people are rational, intelligent, infallible human beings. Reasonable people know that this is not true. When others make mistakes, they try to understand and to forgive them. When others point their mistakes to them, they try to correct them, and if what they did was not a mistake, they ignore the criticism and try to get on with their lives without letting the criticism bring them down. They accept their mistakes and take responsibility for them without it causing them to feel worthless.

- *When things do not go my way, it is terrible. It is a catastrophe.* The self-fulfilling consequences of this type of thinking are obvious. We are not the only actors in this world. Every person that we meet has his or her individual objectives, desires, beliefs, values, and so on. Therefore once in a while, we will meet people who do things that are contrary to our desires. Also, some things are beyond our control; therefore there is no way we will always get our way. We must accept disappointments in life but not let them destroy us. The healthy way to view disappointing events is to accept that they are not catastrophes. We will survive them and live to see more of them. As Ellis states, it is not the goals that people have that are the problem. Rather, it is "what they tell themselves when those goals and values are thwarted or blocked."[57]
- *My unhappiness is caused by other people or events that are out of my control.* This is obviously not true. What other people do and outside events can be upsetting. However, they cannot make you unhappy unless you allow them to. It is not what happens that is the problem. It is how you perceive, interpret, and act on it.
- *I must continually dwell on things that are fearsome and dangerous because they are of great concern.* The irrationality of this thought process is obvious considering that worrying about things does not do anything to make them better. In fact, rational people know that worry and anxiety have exactly the opposite effect. When you are worried and anxious, your ability to evaluate dangerous events objectively and deal with them effectively is significantly diminished. The rational thing to do is to be most clearheaded during dangerous

situations so that your reactions are calculated, rational, and effective. Furthermore, some events are beyond our control. For example, we cannot do anything about whether or not a tornado strikes us. Since it is out of our control, instead of worrying about it, the rational thing to do is to have a contingency plan in the event of the situation arising, and then hope for the best.
- *It is easier for me to avoid difficult situations and responsibilities rather than face them.* Rationality and experience should tell us that it is easier in the long run to face situations that are difficult, deal with them, and be done with them. Then, they are out of our lives. Usually, when a difficult situation is avoided, it gets worse and leads to more problems.
- *I should have someone stronger than I am to take care of me and whom I can rely on.* This is irrational because dependency leads to loss of individuality, and eventually it stifles us. Furthermore, when we are dependent, we are very insecure because however reliable the other people are, we can never really be sure that they will be there when we need them. Rational people recognize this fact and strive for independence, individuality, and self-expression, even though they know that independence can be risky (because when we make autonomous decisions we also have to live with the consequences, even if undesirable). However, in the long run, autonomy is more rewarding than security in dependence.
- *Our past determines our present circumstances, and we cannot do anything to change the consequences of our past.* This is irrational because while it is true that our present difficulties can be traced back to what happened to us in the past, we have choices now. We do not have to be dependent on the vulnerabilities of our past. We can change the direction of our future by exercising responsible choices now. Besides, past solutions to past problems may not work for the problems facing us in the present.

- *I should be upset about other people's problems and disturbances*. This is irrational because other people's problems really have nothing to do with you. While others' behavior may be of concern, a rational person knows that instead of being upset, the judicious thing to do would be to do something to try to help them change their behavior. If attempts to help others change their behavior are unsuccessful, then you should just accept the situation and go on with your life. Getting upset will not do any good.
- *There is always a perfect solution to every problem and I must find it, otherwise catastrophe will befall me*. This is not correct. The truth is, there are many solutions to every problem, and none of them is really perfect. Striving for perfectionism is a recipe for a very unhappy life. Furthermore, perfectionism leads to poorer solutions because the person is not open to a variety of possible solutions. Rationality demands openness of mind so that as many possibilities as possible are considered and the best among them is chosen.

Ellis summarizes the above irrationalities, which are the basis of neuroses, as follows:

> REBT is more philosophical than other therapies because you change your basic outlook, philosophy and give up those musts, shoulds, oughts, and demands and just go back to having preferences. *'I would like to do well but I never have to; it would be great if you treat me kindly but you don't have to'* and if you do, then you would rarely make yourself neurotic (p. 310).[57]

Therapeutic Intervention

Therapeutic intervention based on Ellis's REBT involves use of the G, ABC, D formula. *G* refers to one's goals, such as *"to do well, to get along with people, to enjoy yourself"* (p. 310).[57] *A* refers to anteceding events that block or thwart achievement of conceptualized goals. They are viewed as adversities. *B* refers to what the person tells himself or herself about these events, or the belief system associated with the event, one's preferences, and one's goals, such as *"I don't like it, I wish it weren't so"* (p. 310).[57] An irrational belief system composed of *musts, shoulds,* and *oughts* is somewhat like this: *"therefore, it [the event thwarting your goal] shouldn't exist, I know the right way, you know the wrong way and you should die"* (p. 310).[57] *C* refers to the emotional and behavioral consequences of the event, such as feelings of anxiety and depression, as well as behaviors such as compulsion, procrastination, and so on. *D* refers to the therapeutic intervention that primarily consists of finding and disputing irrational beliefs so that the person changes them to preferences rather than *musts, shoulds,* and *oughts*. In addition, behavioral techniques are used "where we get people to do what they are afraid of, do public speaking, go for job interviews, approach members of the opposite sex" (p. 311).[57] The behavioral changes are used to support modified cognitions.

Aaron Beck's Cognitive Therapy

Like Ellis, Beck started out as a psychoanalyst, because, as he explains, "Once I got into psychiatry and everybody was talking about psychoanalysis, I felt I had to go through psychoanalysis to really understand things" (p. 162).[87] However, once he started working with depressed clients, he realized that the psychoanalytic model was not really supported by clinical observations. In the mid-1950s, Beck developed the cognitive model, which seemed to fit observations of his depressed clients better. His model was therefore developed initially for treatment of depression, anxiety, and other related conditions such as phobias. However, recently cognitive therapy (CT) has been used quite successfully with clients suffering from eating disorders, alcoholism, manic-depressive psychosis (bipolar disorder), and victims of incest, rape, and so on. Beck's biggest contribution is research. He has generated enormous amounts of research investigating the effectiveness of cognitive therapy,[57,87] in which he demonstrates that cognitive therapy is more effective than psychopharmacotherapy alone, and that a combination of the two is most effective in the treatment of most psychiatric conditions.[87] His research efforts led to widespread recognition of cognitive therapy. For example, Tony Blair, the British prime minister, is on record as stating in parliament that "cognitive behavior therapy is indeed as cost-effective as pharmacological treatment, and moreover; it is often preferred among patients" (p. 1).[9]

The Cognitive Theory of Psychopathology

According to Beck, people experience dysfunction in affect and behavior because of their excessive and inappropriate interpretation of experiences.[87] They distort their experiences, their images of themselves, and their circumstances. For example, consider a student who thinks/believes that it is essential to score an *A* in every course, but for some reason believes that he or she is inadequate. Such a person may become anxious or even depressed because he or she focuses on biased evidence from the environment that supports his or her image of self as inadequate. So the student focuses on the occasional *A*– or *B+*, then draws broad conclusions that go beyond the evidence, such as, "I am totally inadequate and a failure as a student. I will never make it, and I will be a failure in life." Then, the student looks back to and excavates the occasional time that he or she did less than perfectly (e.g., in school, a part-time job, dating) and uses that evidence to further support the conclusion that he or she has always been a failure. These distorted cognitions pop up in a person's mind spontaneously. Beck called them *automatic thoughts*.[8] In a way, according to Beck, we make ourselves psychologically sick, so to speak.

Therapeutic Interventions

In both depression and anxiety, cognitive interventions consist of helping the client:

> identify the kinds of interpretations and expectations that lead to the painful effects of sadness and anxiety, to avoidance and inhibition, and adjust them to realistic situation. We also identify and test the dysfunctional attitudes underlying the misin-

terpretations and catastrophic interpretations. The behavioral approaches are particularly important in inducing patients to test their catastrophic interpretations in anxiety-producing situations and in breaking through their avoidances and inhibitions. (p. 161)[87]

Therefore therapy consists of helping people change their cognitive processes, and this is expected to correspond to change in feelings and behavior. For panic disorders, cognitive therapists try to reproduce experiences interpreted by clients as catastrophic and reframe them so that they are viewed more realistically. This leads to a reinterpretation of symptoms of panic when they occur. In psychotic conditions, the cognitive therapist helps the client test the validity of strong beliefs (delusions) by comparing data that supports these beliefs with those that are contradictory to the beliefs.

Beck's CT is therefore very similar to Ellis' REBT, in that both types of therapy try to identify cognitive processes that lead to a distorted view of reality and cause emotional distress and behavioral dysfunction. They then intervene to change those cognitive processes so that interpretation of experiences is more realistic. This leads to alleviation of emotional distress with a corresponding modification of behavior. The major differences include the fact that REBT was originally broader in application than CT. CT was initially developed specifically to treat depression and anxiety, although recently it has expanded its scope to include other types of mental disorders. Furthermore, Beck has devoted much effort to development of classifications of specific characteristics associated with each condition (e.g., depression, anxiety).[8,87] He has developed a wide variety of assessment instruments, such as the Beck Depression Inventory, Cognitive Checklist, and Panic Belief Questionnaire. Beck was also instrumental in developing and carrying out numerous outcome studies establishing the clinical effectiveness of CT. Finally, he specifically disagrees with Ellis' list of irrational cognitions[23] because, according to him, "It is only according to the therapist's frame of reference that they are irrational" (p. 162).[87] The cognitions may be quite justifiable and if they are not contributing to the disorder of focus, Beck does not see why they should be dealt with

in therapy. Refer to Lab Manual Exercise 6-3 to learn about cognitive/behavioral therapeutic techniques.

Albert Bandura's Cognitive Social Learning Theory

The last cognitive psychology theorist we will discuss in this chapter is Albert Bandura, who developed the Cognitive Social Learning Theory (CSLT).

Theoretical Principles

Bandura's theory is concerned with motivational factors and self-regulatory mechanisms that contribute to acquisition of behavior.[70] He believes that behavior is acquired by observing other people and then imitating what is observed.[5,6] Based on this belief, Bandura developed his theory of cognitive social learning (CSL), or what may be referred to as observational learning. This theory is summarized below.[5,6,41,61]

Basic Assumptions

Central to CSLT is the belief that application of consequences is not necessary for learning to occur. Rather, all that is needed is observation of other people engaging in activities and experiencing consequences of their behavior. In this sense, CSLT combines cognitive and operant principles of learning.

The Building Blocks of Human Learning and Agency

Agency (human ability to produce activity) is based on *efficacy expectations,* which refer to the expectation that we are capable of doing something and doing it well. There are two types of expectations, and they can be summarized logically as follows:

- "If I do *A*, *B* will follow. I like *B*. I am confident that I can do *A* successfully. Therefore I will do *A* in order to achieve *B*."

- Alternatively, "I do not like *B*. I can resist doing *A*. Therefore I will not do *A* and I will avoid *B*."
- Or, "I like *B*, but I am not confident that I can do *A* well. Therefore I will not try *A*."
- Or, "I do not like *B* but I am not sure I can resist doing *A*. Therefore I will do *A* anyway, and live with *B*."

Therefore the probability that behavior will occur is based on a combination of efficacy, or one's confidence that the behavior can be produced effectively and adequately, and outcome expectations or consequences of the behavior. Efficacy is a cognitive process, while consequences constitute environmental response (reinforcement or punishment as a result of engaging in behavior), hence, the argument that CSLT is a combination of cognitive and operant principles.

Learning Process

For learning to take place, the following four processes have to occur: (1) *attention*—a person has to be able to notice something in the environment, (2) *retention*—the observed event has to be remembered, (3) *reproduction*—action has to be produced to imitate what was observed, and (4) *motivation*—the consequences from the environment have to be reinforcing to the behavior. Initially, reinforcement is external, such as praise by other people. Many times, it is also vicarious. The person observes other people engaging in behavior and receiving reward or punishment for their actions. This determines whether or not he or she engages in the behavior. For example, a student sees other students being praised for academic accomplishments. He or she may engage in scholarly behavior in an attempt to do well and receive similar rewards. Finally, over time, the student internalizes the reinforcement and does not need external rewards in order to produce the behavior. For instance, in time, the student in our example internalizes the value of education, and doing well academically eventually constitutes self-reinforcing behavior.

Refer to Lab Manual Exercise 6-4 to learn about Albert Bandura's CSLT therapeutic techniques.

Cognitive Learning Theories

Cognitive learning theory originated from Gestalt psychology and was given impetus by computer science and what later came to be referred to as artificial intelligence (AI).[37,86] Newell, Shaw, and Simon[60] published an article in which they argued that the human mind is similar to a computer program in terms of information processing and problem solving. This marked the formal bridge between cognitive psychology and computer science or AI. According to Newell and colleagues,[60] computer programs receive information (input), process it, keep it in memory, and produce an output. This is the same process for human cognition. Thus "By analogy, that is the most of what cognitive psychology is about. It is about how people take in information, how they recode and remember it, how they make decisions, how they transform their internal knowledge states, and how they transform these states into behavioral outputs" (p. 559).[37]

This analogy assumes that computer information input is comparable to stimuli received by humans through their senses. Computer output is analogous to human response or behavior after processing stimulus from the environment. Computer information processing is analogous to human information storage, encoding, processing, capacity, retrieval, conditional decisions, and programs. Based on this model, it is perceived that cognitive processes consist of input of information into the neural system, its organization into larger cognitive units, and its representation so that it stands for properties absent in the immediate stimulus and is based on past learning experiences.[50] In this sense, representation in cognitive processes is a synthetic process in which "Our representational mechanisms create a psychological environment or apparent reality which seems so real—so inexorably given by our objective environment—that we do not dream that *we* are producing such effects" (p. 36).[50]

Furthermore, as already suggested above, representation depends on past learning that is represented in the mind in the form of schemas. A *schema* is a framework upon which information is interpreted and the environment understood. According to Piaget, learning is an *adaptive* process.[31] This process consists of a balance between accommodation and assimilation. *Accommodation* refers to the phenomenon in which general concepts are used to adapt schema to fit reality. In other words, if cognitive schema becomes inadequate in interpreting events, it is replaced by another schema. In *assimilation,* experience is interpreted using current cognitive schema.

Application of Behavioral Psychology and Cognitive-Behavioral Psychology in Occupational Therapy

A review of the literature reveals that behavioral psychology has been systematically applied in occupational therapy since the 1970s, and probably even earlier. Sieg[79] proposed a framework for application of operant conditioning in occupational therapy, where she suggested that in treatment planning, occupational therapists identify terminal behavior and baseline data, and (using appropriate reinforcers) facilitate attainment of the terminal behavior. This is the model of goal setting and therapeutic planning in occupational therapy today.[22,74] Mosey[58] outlined the acquisitional frame of reference in occupational therapy, which is very much a behavioral conceptual model of practice since the emphasis was on acquisition of behavior through learning. Cognitive approaches have been used extensively in occupational therapy to help clients acquire adaptive behaviors.[14,22,81] We will discuss the cognitive and cognitive/behavioral conceptual model of practice in greater detail in Chapter 10.

Humanistic Psychology

Humanistic psychology, referred to as "third force" psychology, emerged in the 1960s. It was developed mostly by Abraham Maslow and

Carl Rogers.[17,38] This psychological movement emerged in reaction to the prevailing psychological systems at the time that were viewed as lacking in terms of addressing the needs of relatively healthy individuals who wanted to optimize their growth. The feeling was that clinical psychology, dominated at the time by Freudian psychoanalysis, focused exclusively on individuals who were emotionally/psychologically disturbed. Behaviorism, on the other hand, was seen as too reductionistic and therefore not really able to address human needs in any meaningful way. The third force psychology was developed primarily to help people become better, optimize their existence, and foster their emotional development. As mentioned, Maslow and Rogers were leading personalities in this psychological movement.

Abraham Maslow

Abraham Maslow's view of human development was based on his perception of happiness. He saw happiness as originating from the ability to experience "real emotions over real problems and real tasks" (p. 23).[40] He saw attainment of happiness as the primary motivation of behavior. Therefore his theory was based on human motivation and the construct of *self-actualization*.[35,38,40,45]

Motivation

According to Maslow, the motivation of humans was need fulfillment. When needs become active, they have to be satiated so that a state of homeostasis can be reestablished in the individual. When needs are satisfied, they cease to be active. These needs are arranged in a hierarchical order. At the base of the hierarchy are *basic needs,* which are physiological, such as the need for food, water, air, and so on. If these needs are not met, the individual dies. Therefore they have to be met before any other needs can become active. Once basic needs are satisfied and the organism is now assured of continued existence, attention is turned to *safety*. One has to be able to avoid predators, or any threats to existence. Once safety and security are achieved, the next

need is for *belonging*. One needs to feel that he or she belongs to an accepting community. Related to this need for acceptance by significant others is the need to be *esteemed* by others and by self. Once esteem needs have been met, then one strives for *self-actualization*.

As is apparent from the above summary, needs lower in the hierarchy are more urgent and must be met before higher needs can be activated. Thus one must have enough food, water, air to breathe, and so on, and then feel a sense of security before he or she can worry about being respected by others. Respect means nothing to someone who is struggling for survival and is threatened by death through starvation.

Self-Actualization

Self-actualization is defined as "the desire to become more and more of what one is, to become everything that one is capable of being" (p. 22).[54] This is the highest human need. Once all needs that are lower in the hierarchy have been met, this need has to be met (failure of which leads to a sense of meaninglessness, and could even lead to suicide). Maslow identified some of the characteristics of self-actualized individuals as including the following:

- *A sense of adventure and novelty:* Self-actualized individuals are not afraid to try new things, new ways of doing things, and new ideas, or to reconsider old ideas in a new way. They are energized by novelty.
- *Confidence:* Self-actualized individuals are comfortable with themselves, and they do not rely too much on approval by other people.
- *Non-prejudicial:* Self-actualized individuals are open minded and accepting of others from a variety of backgrounds. They are comfortable with ideas and viewpoints that are different from theirs.
- *Empathic:* Self-actualized individuals empathize with humanity in general.
- *Above polarities:* Self-actualized individuals are neither good nor bad, neither introvert nor extrovert, and so on. They transcend polarities.

Transcendent Actualization

Transcendent actualization refers to attainment of the spiritual aspect of self. It is "an optimal way to give spiritual meaning to one's life and live this meaning in every day life" (p. 4).[35] Maslow considered as healthiest those people who can express their eternal, sacred, spiritual self, as exemplified by values of truth, justice, and beauty.

Carl Rogers

Carl Rogers is regarded as the founder of professional counseling.[48] While practicing Freudian analysis, he found it wanting. Even with the most skilled directive questioning and interpretation, some clients were extremely resistant to therapy and did not seem to benefit. Gradually, he realized that "it is only the client who knows what hurts, what directions to go, what problems are crucial, what experiences have been deeply buried" (p. 11).[73] This epiphany was the beginning of what was later to become client-centered/person-centered therapy, which he developed for the rest of his life while he held a variety of teaching positions and did research to substantiate his ideas.

Theory of Personality

Central to Carl Rogers' client-centered therapy was his theory of personality. This was based on the core hypothesis that

> The client has within himself the capacity, latent if not evident, to understand those aspects of his life and of himself which are causing him pain, and the capacity and the tendency to reorganize himself and his relationship to life in the direction of self-actualization and maturity in such a way as to bring greater degree of internal comfort (p. 443).[72]

This vote of confidence in the potential of humans was based on his view of how selfhood emerged. According to Rogers, the theory of personality was really a theory of self-emergence.[48,68,73] As the self emerged, he postulated, socialization led to a distrust of one's feelings and sense of self. Here is how the distrust develops: according to Rogers, we are born with two inherent forces within us; an actualizing force that motivates us, and a valuing process that regulates us. If we trust these processes, they serve us well. However, if we actualize ourselves, we experience reality subjectively and not as real or pure objective reality. Other people cannot understand us unless they make an attempt to place themselves in our internal frame of reference. In other words, there is reality as shaped by our environment, and reality as shaped by our internal frame of reference.

In the process of actualization, we are able to differentiate between experiences that are part of our personal frame of reference and those that belong to others. Experiences that we accept as part of ourselves are *self-experiences*. We become conscious of those experiences by representing them in language and in other symbols. As we interact with those who are significant to us, the self-experiences become elaborated into self-concepts. Self-concept is a series of beliefs, or a view of self that forms our perception of what is characteristic of "I" or "me." As we develop, a crystallized consciousness of this self emerges and we develop a need for positive regard of ourselves, which leads to a need to be loved, prized, accepted, and regarded positively. A little child constantly looks at the face of the mother or other significant adult, scanning for signs of positive regard. The way these significant adults respond to what the child does strengthens or weakens the child's sense of self, leading to the child developing a positive or negative view of self. If the response to one's behavior is positive, one's sense of self as a loved individual is strengthened. If the response is negative, the sense of self as a loved one is weakened. The desire for positive regard by significant others becomes so strong that it overshadows the organismic self-valuing process. The person is therefore more apt to seek experiences of positive regard by others and sacrifice those that may not be regarded positively by others but are actualizing to the individual.

If the need to be loved and accepted dominates, the person guides his or her behavior by his or her judgment of the likelihood that he or she will receive love and acceptance rather than by what is best for organismic well-being. The person perceives a sense of significance in life on the basis of what other people attribute to him or her as significant, even though organismically, it may not be experienced as satisfying. For example, a little boy who grows up in a family where professionalism is emphasized as a measure of individual worth may organismically find it more fulfilling to work with his hands; for example, he may want to be a mechanic. However, because he knows that his father and mother would regard him more highly if he were a doctor, he will pursue a career as a doctor (although it may be extremely dissatisfying and meaningless to him personally). He therefore ignores or disavows his desire to work with his hands. Other behaviors that are disavowed because they do not meet other peoples' approval include sexual desires and expression of emotions such as anger, doing good for oneself (regarded by some as selfishness), and so on. A person who regularly ignores personal desires/needs is not guided by valuing of organismic experiencing. In other words, we learn very early in life to sacrifice our basic tendency toward actualization for conditional love from others and internalized conditional love of ourselves. In other words, we see ourselves as lovable only when we behave in ways that meet other peoples' approval, irrespective of our organismic needs.

This variance between our behavior, which is pegged on conditional positive regard from others and ourselves, and organismic needs is the basis of psychopathology. For instance, it is the basis of workaholism for those who think they only have self worth when they are working and being productive and will work themselves to death before taking a vacation. The result of this variance is incongruence between what is organismically fulfilling and what is symbolically perceived as part of one's self-concept. The symbolized perception of self is the ideal self, and the organismic self is the actual self toward which we naturally tend before the process of socialization. The variance between the ideal self and the actual self leads to loss of wholeness. This loss of wholeness creates anxiety and discomfort, which we try to alleviate by using perceptual distortions such as projection, rationalization, denial, and so on.

Lack of wholeness also becomes apparent in somatic symptoms that we exhibit, as well as in incongruence between our verbal and nonverbal signals when we communicate. For example, you may be the kind of person who when angry at someone is wary of expressing your anger because you have internalized the ideal self, that you are acceptable and lovable only when you are nice and do not express negative feelings such as anger. However, the impulse of your actual disavowed self is to burst out and really let the person know how you feel. You may then smile at the person and tell him that you are fine and not to worry, while at the same time clenching your teeth and fists. You are communicating two messages simultaneously. Verbally, the message is that you are fine with whatever is happening. Nonverbally, you are communicating anger. The two messages are not consistent with one another and are confusing.

Therapeutic Intervention

Rogerian client-centered therapy is nondirective and emphasizes therapeutic or helping relationship. A helping relationship, according to Rogers,[72] requires that the therapist be (1) accepting of the client as he or she is (unconditionally), (2) empathic (able to place himself or herself in the client's shoes and to experience reality as perceived through the client's personal frame of reference), and (3) congruent (able to model genuineness in verbal and nonverbal communication). Thus Rogers felt that central to the therapeutic relationship was behaving naturally which "seemed to help his clients more than acting as a scientist with specialized knowledge" (p. 79).[7]

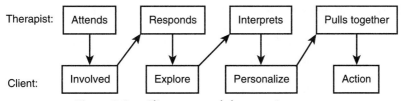

Figure 3-2.   Client-centered therapeutic process.

This relationship consists primarily of the therapist communicating empathy and acceptance to the client, then using the skills of responding, summarizing, and interpreting to help the client do in-depth self-exploration, leading to insight and action that results in expression of the actualized self.[68] The process of therapy can be summarized diagrammatically (Figure 3-2).

As shown in Figure 3-2, the initial role of the therapist is to attend to the client by communicating acceptance or unconditional positive regard through a nonjudgmental attitude, empathy, and genuineness. If this is done successfully, the client gets involved and begins talking. As the client talks, the therapist responds and demonstrates interest and understanding, encouraging the client to do self-exploration. As the client explores personal experiences more deeply, the therapist summarizes and paraphrases these experiences to provide clarification and focus (interpretation). This encourages *personalization* of these experiences, or taking of responsibility on the part of the client. Finally, the therapist pulls together all the information explicated through self-exploration giving it a sense of immediacy, and this facilitates contemplation of action by the client to resolve any issues. Refer to Lab Manual Exercise 6-5 to learn how to respond appropriately using Carl Rogers' client-centered therapeutic intervention.

Phenomenological and Existential Psychologies

This is a group of psychological approaches originating from the phenomenological philosophical orientation of Søren Kierkegaard, based on the argument that "it is the personal, subjective aspects of human life that are the most important" (p. 208)[52] because the only reality that is meaningful is individual reality. This idea was extended by Edmund Husserl in his *Doctrine of the Lived World,* in which he formulated a philosophy devoted to "examination of consciousness and its objects. It was a systematic analysis of experience, and became known as phenomenology, because it treated everything as phenomena" (p. 211).[52] In this philosophical approach, emphasis is placed on the lived world as experienced subjectively by the individual. It is validation of subjective experience as the basis or foundation of the known world of reality. The psychological systems based on this philosophical orientation include Frederick (Fritz) Perls' Gestalt psychology, and Martin Heidegger, Gabriel Marcel, and Jean-Paul Sartre's existential-phenomenological psychologies.[62]

Collectively, phenomenological/existential psychologies are based on the philosophical view exemplified in the following seven propositions:

1. Humans are responsible for their lives. This responsibility is exercised by fulfilling one's obligation or responsibility to make choices. Humans are influenced by environmental factors. However, these factors do not determine what one becomes. It is choices that are made freely and consciously that determine the quality of one's existence in this otherwise meaningless world. We are therefore largely responsible of our existence and the meaning of this existence.

2. The human is in a constant state of emergence. One emerges, becomes, or self-actualizes, by

fulfilling inner responsibilities through continual participation and interaction in the world of people and objects. Healthy humans focus on their future (emergence) rather than dwelling in the past.

3. Humans are conscious of the fact that at some point in the future, they will cease to be, or that they will die. This realization is what gives reality to life, for it is the only absolute certainty of our existence. Humans must therefore confront the reality of their death or nonexistence.

4. This threat of nonexistence or death creates *anxiety,* which is "normal" or "existential" anxiety. It is normal because it is a condition shared by all humans.

5. When we abdicate the responsibility to exercise our freedom to choose and to actualize our potentialities, we experience guilt, or *neurotic anxiety.* This is what makes people feel uncomfortable when they are not doing what they think they should be doing. For instance, if I take a break to watch television rather than continue to write this book as I think I should, I may feel anxious because writing the book is part of my self-actualization. By choosing not to engage in the task when I should, I feel that I am abdicating my responsibility and this fills me with neurotic anxiety.

6. As mentioned earlier, our past circumstances contribute to our current reality. For instance, I was born in a poor family in a poor rural community in Kenya, East Africa. This historical fact has contributed to who I am today in the sense that the circumstances of my birth determined the resources available to me, the kind of relationships I had and continue to have today, and the kind of personality I developed. However, we are responsible of who we subsequently become. Thus we are capable, and in fact are responsible of tra- scending circumstances into which we are thrown through the choices that we make in life. For example, the fact that my family was poor and material resources were

limited did not prevent me from getting the education that would help me actualize my potential.

7. Finally, modern life is such that we all experience alienation from ourselves, other people, and our communities. Thus loneliness, isolation, and detachment are conditions that are shared by all humanity. We have lost our world and have become strangers in our own homes. The biggest need in the modern world is therefore the need for belonging, connectedness, and meaning.

Therapeutic Intervention

Based on the above seven propositions, the role of the phenomenological/existential therapist is to facilitate development of insight illuminating the client's condition of his or her *being in the world.* In the therapist-client relationship, the therapist enters the client's existential world, tries to understand it, and helps him or her experience it as real. The client is then helped to develop orientation to this world, make a commitment to exercising freedom of choice, and make decisions that lead to an authentic existence, where potentialities are actualized. In this endeavor, techniques that lead to attainment of that objective are useful, including those drawn from psychoanalysis, client-centered therapy, and so on. It is not the techniques themselves that are of concern to an existential therapist; it is the therapist's attitude and objective.

Application to Occupational Therapy

Humanistic and phenomenological-existential psychologies have contributed significantly to occupational therapy practice and theory development. Client-centered occupational therapy, which was developed in Canada,[16] was a direct attempt to apply Rogerian client-centered principles in occupational therapy. This is the basis of current professional focus on collaborative, client-centered interventions.[1,16] Furthermore, occupational therapy emphasizes the need for clients to exercise choice, responsibility, and sense of agency as a means to attain meaning in life. These are the fundamental tenets of existential/phenomenological psychologies.

Developmental Psychology

Developmental constructs are also used extensively in occupational therapy. This means acquisition of increasingly complex behaviors in various domains of performance through growth (e.g., physiological bodily changes in height, strength), maturation of structures, and learning.[20] Thus development has many dimensions, including physical (physiological), cognitive, social, moral, and so on. In this book, developmental theories that are of interest are those that are related to psychosocial functioning, including cognitive, social, and moral theories. The developmental psychological theories that have contributed to the development of psychosocial occupational therapy include Freud's psychosexual stages of development, Erik Erickson's psychosocial stages of development, Robert Havighurst's developmental tasks, and Jean Piaget's cognitive development theory.

Application of Kohlberg's and Gilligan's theories of moral development is not common in occupational therapy. Therefore we will not discuss these theories in this book. We have already discussed Freud's psychosexual development,

and we will now discuss Carl Jung's analytical theory, Erikson's theory of psychosocial development, Havighurst's developmental tasks, and Piaget's theory of cognitive development in detail in this section.

Jung's View of Human Development

According to Jung,[46] the first half of life is devoted to establishment of identity. For instance, a man needs to develop his masculine characteristics. Similarly, a woman needs to develop her feminine characteristics. The second half of life (which Jung saw as from 45 years of age and up) is devoted to development of the undeveloped and unexpressed characteristics. The introvert has to develop skills of extraversion; a woman has to develop masculine characteristics of aggressiveness, use of logic, and so on; the man has to develop female characteristics of being in touch with feelings and relationship skills.

Robert Havighurst

For Havighurst,[36] development was seen as a continuous process in which the individual had to accomplish specific tasks at each stage of development. The stages of development and tasks that had to be accomplished at each stage are presented in Table 3-1.

Table 3-1. Havighurst's Stages and Developmental Tasks

Developmental Stage	Developmental Tasks
Infancy/early childhood	Learning: To walk, eat solid food, talk, manage toileting needs, sex differences and sexual modesty, concepts and language, reading, and distinguishing right from wrong (i.e., forming a conscience).
Middle childhood	Learning: Physical skills, attitudes toward oneself, how to get along with peers, masculine and feminine social roles, reading, writing and calculating, concepts, conscience, morality and values, personal independence, and attitudes toward social groups and institutions.
Adolescence	Achieving: mature relations with peers of both sexes, masculine/feminine roles, acceptance of one's body physique and effective use of body, emotional independence from parents and other adults, preparation for marriage and family life, preparation for an economic career, set of values and an ideology, and socially responsible behavior.

Data from Havighurst R: *Developmental tasks and education,* New York, 1972, McKay; and Uhlendorff U: The concept of developmental tasks and its significance for education and social work, *Social Work Soc* 2(1):54-63, 2004.

Erik Erikson's Theory of Psychosocial Development

Erikson agreed with Freud's concepts of the id, ego, and superego. However, he thought that development was related to how a person negotiated social requirements rather than solely to sexual expression as Freud postulated. Thus he developed what he called psychosocial stages of development.[24-26] Moreover, while Freud saw human psychic development as being complete in the first 5 or 6 years of life, Erikson viewed psychic development as going on through the entire lifespan. He identified eight stages of psychosocial development. In all stages, establishment of identity was central, where the individual negotiated a conflict of opposing instincts, such as trust versus mistrust. How the conflict was resolved at each stage determined how the next stage was negotiated. Thus the stages built on each other with development in lower stages determining subsequent development. Erikson's stages of psychosocial development are outlined in Table 3-2.

Jean Piaget's Stages of Cognitive Development

Jean Piaget's theory of cognitive development was based on his construct of cognitive structure.[13,66,67,75] By cognitive structure, Piaget meant patterns of physical/mental action underlying acts of intelligence. He also called these structures cognitive *schema*. The *schema* are used to interpret information in such a way that it makes sense and helps one understand the environment. He saw these structures as corresponding to stages of child development. In Piaget's view, the purpose of intelligence was to help humans *adapt* to the environment. In the process of adaptation, cognitive structures changed through the process of *assimilation* and *accommodation*.

Assimilation referred to interpretation of events according to existing cognitive structures/schema. *Accommodation* referred to change in cognitive structure to accommodate changes in the environment. Cognitive development was conceptualized to be a constant effort to adapt to the environment by continual balance between assimilation and accommodation. As this process of adaptation took place, Piaget argued, a child went through stages of cognitive development where increasingly complex cognitive processes were used at every stage to solve environmental problems. Piaget's stages of cognitive development are presented in Table 3-3.

Application in Occupational Therapy

Developmental constructs have been used extensively in occupational therapy. Mosey[58] identified the developmental frame of reference as one of the frames of reference guiding occupational therapy practice. Ayres[2] used developmental concepts in

Table 3-2.   ERIKSON'S STAGES OF PSYCHOSOCIAL DEVELOPMENT

Stage	Conflict to be Resolved	Positive Outcome	Negative Outcome
1 (birth to 24 months)	Trust vs. mistrust	A sense of trust	A sense of mistrust
2 (2 to 3 years)	Autonomy vs. shame and doubt	A sense of autonomy	A sense of shame and doubt
3 (3 to 6 years)	Initiative vs. guilt	A sense of initiative	A sense of guilt
4 (6 to 12 years)	Industry vs. inferiority	A sense of industry	A sense of inferiority
5 (12 to 18 years)	Identity vs. identity diffusion	A sense of clear identity	A sense of identity and role confusion
6 (18 to 35 years)	Intimacy vs. isolation	A sense of intimacy	A sense of isolation
7 (35 to 60 years)	Generativity vs. stagnation	A sense of generativity	A sense of stagnation
8 (60 years to death)	Integrity vs. disgust and despair	A sense of ego integrity	A sense of despair

Table 3-3. PIAGET'S STAGES OF COGNITIVE DEVELOPMENT

Stage	Label	Cognitive Skills
1 (birth to 2 years)	Sensorimotor	Activity is mostly limited to reflexive reaction to stimuli, e.g. sucking, kicking, and in the latter part of the stage acting on objects to make stimulus last longer (e.g., picking up and shaking a rattle).
2 (2 to 7 years)	Preoperational	Child is able to use signs and symbols as representation of something else, is egocentric (unable to see another person's point of view), and focuses on salient aspects of stimuli to the exclusion of others.
3 (7 to 12 years)	Concrete operations	Child is able to grasp mathematical concepts, decenter from egocentricity, has a sense of identity (objects are the same irrespective of orientation), and is able to understand relationships.
4 (12 years and over)	Formal operations	The individual is now at the highest level of cognitive development characterized by highly evolved symbolic thought and representation, and is able to perform mental operations that are highly abstract.

her conceptualization of how children develop perceptual motor abilities. Llorens[51] presented an overview of how various developmental theorists have contributed to our understanding of human occupational performance and mastery throughout the life span. In the current edition of *Willard and Spackman's Occupational Therapy,* an entire chapter is devoted to "Developmental and Neurological Perspectives."[19] Thus it is clear that developmental theories are central to occupational therapy theory and practice. Like behavioral and cognitive behavioral principles, even where it is not stated explicitly, developmental constructs are implicitly used in practice. Developmental principles are applied any time a therapist makes an assessment to determine whether a proposed intervention is consistent with a client's skills as determined by current developmental level (in order to offer the "just right challenge"[56]).

SUMMARY

In this chapter, we examined the psychological theories underlying occupational therapy practice. We also discussed each theory's contribution to the development of occupational therapy concepts/constructs used in psychosocial practice. Figure 3-3 illustrates the relationship between these theories.

As Figure 3-3 indicates, in the 1950s (around the same time that occupational therapy adopted the reductionistic, mechanistic, medical model) two psychological theories that were most influential were Freudian psychoanalysis and behaviorism. From Freudian psychoanalysis emerged neo-Freudian psychological orientations. In response to the perceived shortcomings of psychoanalysis and behaviorism, cognitive/behavioral and cognitive learning theories were developed, borrowing from both psychoanalysis and behaviorism. "Third force" (humanistic) psychology emerged, also borrowing some concepts from psychoanalytic theory. Developmental theories were developed based on Freudian, neo-Freudian, and cognitive principles. All these psychological traditions have contributed and continue to contribute to the development of psychosocial occupational therapy.

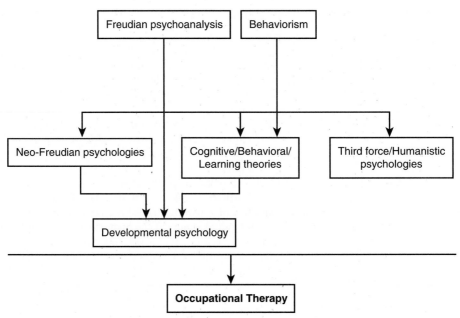

Figure 3-3. The relationship between the various psychological theories that have contributed to occupational therapy in psychosocial practice.

REFERENCES

1. American Occupational Therapy Association: Occupational therapy practice framework: domain and process, *Am J Occup Ther* 56(6):609-639, 2002.
2. Ayres JA: The development of perceptual motor abilities: a theoretical basis for treatment of dysfunction, *Am J Occup Ther* 17:221-225, 1963.
3. Azima F: *Introduction to dynamic occupational therapy: object relations and the Azima battery*, Buffalo, NY, 1967, State University of New York Press.
4. Azima H, Azima FJ: Outline of a dynamic theory of occupational therapy, *Am J Occup Ther* 13:215-221, 1959.
5. Bandura A: *Social learning theory*, New York, 1977, General Learning Press.
6. Bandura A: *Social foundations of thought and action*, Englewood Cliffs, NJ, 1986, Prentice-Hall.
7. Barresi J: On becoming a person, *Philosophical Psychology* 12(1):79-98, 1999.
8. Beck Institute: *Dr. Aaron T. Beck's Biography*, 2000. Retrieved August 2005, from http://www.beckinstitute. org/Library/InfoManage/Zoom.asp?InfoID=302&Red irectPath=Add&FolderID=196&SessionID={9F49D49 A-9AFD-42E5-AC2E-0D5F6CB8ACDF}&InfoGroup= Main&InfoType=Article.
9. Beck Institute: *Summary of a question/answer exchange related to cognitive behavior therapy between the British Prime Minister and a member of parliament*, 2000. Retrieved August 2005, from http://www.beckinstitute. org/Library/InfoManage/Zoom.asp?InfoID=350&Red irectPath=Add&FolderID=212&SessionID={9F49D49 A-9AFD-42E5-AC2E-0D5F6CB8ACDF}&InfoGroup= Main&InfoType=Article.
10. Boeree CG: BF Skinner: 1904-1990. *Personality Theories*, 1998. Retrieved August 2005, from http://www. ship.edu/'cgboeree/skinner.html.
11. Boland L: *Carl Jung's theory of personality*, Lectures presented to counseling students at Amani Counseling Center, Nairobi, Kenya, 1987.
12. Borgen FH: Counseling psychology, *Annual Review Psychol* 35:579-604, 1984.
13. Brainerd C: *Piaget's theory of intelligence*, Englewood Cliffs, NJ, 1978, Prentice Hall.
14. Bruce M, Borg B: *Psychosocial frames of reference: core for occupation-based practice*, ed 3, Thorofare, NJ, 2002, Slack.
15. Bryden P, McColl MA: The concept of occupation: 1900 to 1974. In McColl MA, Law M, Stewart D, et al., eds: *Theoretical basis of occupational therapy*, ed 2, Thorofare, NJ, 2003, Slack.
16. Canadian Association of Occupational Therapists: *Occupational therapy: guidelines for the client-centered practice*, Toronto, ON, 1983, CAOT ACE.
17. Cassel RN, Reiger RC: New third force psychology promises to reduce the growing prison population

through student-centered high schools, *Educ* 121(1):34-37, 2000.

18. Corbett L: Kohut and Jung: a comparison of theory and therapy [electronic version]. In Detrick DW, Detrick SB, eds: *Self psychology: comparisons and contrasts,* Hutsdale, NJ, 1989, The Analytic Press. Retrieved April 2006, from http://www.findingstone.com/professionals/monographs/KohutandJung.doc.

19. Crepeau EB, Cohn ES, Schell BA: *Willard and Spackman's occupational therapy,* ed 10, New York, 2003, Lippincott Williams & Wilkins.

20. Cronin A, Mandich M: *Human development and performance throughout the lifespan,* Clifton Park, NY, 2005, Thomson Delmar Learning.

21. Detweiler J, Peyton C: Defining occupations: a chronotopic study of narrative genres in a health discipline's emergence, *Written Communication* 16:412-468, 1999.

22. Early MB: *Mental health concepts and techniques for the occupational therapy assistant,* New York, 2000, Lippincott Williams & Wilkins.

23. Ellis A: *Reason and emotion in psychotherapy,* New York, 1962, Lyle Stuart.

24. Erikson EH: *Childhood and society,* New York, 1950, Norton.

25. Erikson EH: *Identity: youth crisis,* New York, 1968, Norton.

26. Erikson EH, Erikson JM: *The life cycle completed,* New York, 1987, Norton.

27. Fidler GS, Fidler JW: *Occupational therapy: a communication process in psychiatry,* New York, 1963, McMillan.

28. Freud S: A difficulty in the path of psychoanalysis. In Strachey J, ed: *The standard edition,* Vol. 17, London, 1955, Hogarth Press, pp. 136-144.

29. Freud S: *Beyond the pleasure principle,* London, 1955, Hogarth Press.

30. Goldberg A: Postmodern psychoanalysis. *Psyche Matters,* 2001. Retrieved July 2005, from http://www.psychematters.com/papers/goldberg.htm.

31. Goswami U: Cognitive development: no stages please—we're British, *Br J Psychol* 92:257-277, 2001.

32. Green CD: Introduction to "Psychology as the behaviorist views it." In Watson JB: *Classics in the history of psychology,* 2001. Retrieved August 2005, from http://psychclassics.yorku.ca/Watson/Intro.htm.

33. Hakohain YL: *The nature of the archetypes,* 2004. Retrieved April 2006, from http://www.kheper.net/topics/Jung/archetypes.htm.

34. Hall CS, Lindzey G: *Theories of personality,* New York, 1978, John Wiley & Sons.

35. Hamel S, Leclerc G, Lefrancoise R: A psychological outlook on the concept of transcendent actualization, *Internat J Psychol Religion* 13(1):3-15, 2003.

36. Havighurst R: *Developmental tasks and education,* New York, 1972, McKay.

37. Hergenhahn BR: *An introduction to the history of psychology,* ed 3, Pacific Grove, CA, 1997, Brooks/Cole.

38. Heylighen F: A cognitive-systemic reconstruction of Maslow's theory of self-actualization, *Behavioral Sci* 37(1):39-59, 1992.

39. Hinshelwood RD: Evidence-based psychoanalysis: symptoms or relationships: a comment on Jeremy Holmes', "All you need is CBT," *Psych Matters,* 2002. Retrieved July 2005, from http://www.psychematters.com/papers/hinshelwood3.htm.

40. Hoffman E, ed: *Future visions: the unpublished papers of Abraham Maslow,* Thousand Oaks, CA, 1996, Sage.

41. Huitt W: Observational (social) learning: an overview, *Educational psychology interactive,* Valdosta, GA, 2004, Valdosta State University. Retrieved August 2005, from http://chiron.valdosta.edu/whuitt/col/soccog/soclrn.html.

42. Institute of Transpersonal Psychology: *Transpersonal pioneers: Carl Jung,* 2003. Retrieved April 2006, from http://www.itp.edu/about/carl_jung.cfm.

43. Jung CG: Psychological types [Electronic version]. *Classics in the history of psychology, an Internet resource developed by Christopher D. Green.* Retrieved August 2005, from http://psychclassics.yorku.ca/Jung/types.htm.

44. Jung CG: *The unconscious self,* New York, 1958, Mentor Books.

45. Jung CG: *The collected works of C.G. Jung,* Princeton, 1953–1983, Princeton University Press.

46. Jung CG: Integrating anima and animus, *Therapy Weekly* 15, 1985.

47. Kielhofner G: *Conceptual foundations of occupational therapy,* ed 3, Philadelphia, 2004, FA Davis.

48. Kirschenbaum H: Carl Rogers's life and work: an assessment on the 100th anniversary of his birth, *J Counseling Development* 82:116-124, 2004.

49. Krupa T: The psychological-emotional determinants of occupation. In McColl MA, Law M, Stewart D, et al, eds: *Theoretical basis of occupational therapy,* ed 2, Thorofare, NJ, 2003, Slack.

50. Leeper RW: *What contributions might cognitive learning theory make to our understanding of personality?* Oregon, 2003, Ebsco.

51. Llorens LA: Performance tasks and roles throughout the lifespan. In Christiansen C, Baum C, eds: *Occupational therapy: overcoming human performance deficits,* Thorofare, NJ, 1991, Slack, pp. 45-68.

52. Magee B: *The story of thought: the essential guide to the history of Western philosophy,* New York, 1998, The Quality Paperback Book Club.

53. Malone JC, Cruchon NM: Radical behaviorism and the rest of psychology: a review/precis of Skinner's *ABOUT BEHAVIORISM, Behavior Philosophy* 29:31-57, 2001.

54. Maslow AH: *Motivation and personality,* ed 2, New York, 1970, Harper & Row.

55. Masson JM: *The assault on truth: Freud's suppression of the seduction theory,* New York, 1984, Farrar, Strauss, & Giroux.

56. McColl MA: Therapeutic processes to change occupation. In McColl MA, Law M, Stewart D, et al, eds: *Theoretical basis of occupational therapy,* ed 2, Thorofare, NJ, 2003, Slack, pp. 179-182.

57. McGinn LK: Interview: Albert Ellis on rational emotive behavior therapy, *Am J Psychother* 51:309-316, 1997.

58. Mosey AC: *Three frames of reference for mental health,* Thorofare, NJ, 1970, Slack.

59. Mosey AC: Involvement in the rehabilitation movement: 1942-1960, *Am J Occup Ther* 25:234-236, 1971.

60. Newell A, Shaw JC, Simon HA: Elements of a theory of problem solving, *Psychological Review* 65:151-166, 1958.

61. Niaura R: Human models in craving research: cognitive social learning and related perspectives on drug craving, *Addiction* 95:S155-S163, 2000.

62. Patterson CH: *Theories of counseling and psychotherapy,* New York, 1980, Harper & Row.

63. Pavlov IP: *Lectures on conditioned reflexes,* New York, 1928, Liveright.

64. Pavlov IP: *Conditioned reflexes: an investigation of the activity of the cerebral cortex,* New York, 1960, Dover.

65. Pavlov IP: *Work of the principle digestive glands,* St. Petersburg, Russia, 1987, Kushneroff.

66. Piaget J: *The origins of intelligence in children,* New York, 1963, Norton.

67. Piaget J: *The psychology of intelligence,* New York, 1963, Routledge.

68. Prochaska JO: *Systems of psychotherapy: a transtheoretical analysis,* Chicago, IL, 1984, Dorsey.

69. *Projections to persons of the opposite sex,* Princeton, 1983, Princeton University Press.

70. Psy Café: *B.F. Skinner: 1904–1990,* 2001. Retrieved August 2005, from http://www.psy.pdx.edu/PsiCafe/KeyTheorists/Skinner.htm.

71. Randall F: *Lectures in Jungian psychology,* Presented to counseling students at Amani Counseling Center, Nairobi, Kenya, 1987.

72. Rogers CR: A current formulation of client-centered therapy, *Social Service Review* 24:442-450, 1950.

73. Rogers CR: *On becoming a person,* Boston, 1961, Houghton Mifflin.

74. Sames KM: *Documenting occupational therapy practice,* Upper Saddle River, NJ, 2005, Pearson/Prentice-Hall.

75. Saxe GB, Shaheen S: Piagetian theory and the atypical case: an analysis of the developmental Gerstmann syndrome, *J Learning Disabil* 14:131-135, 1981.

76. Sechenov IM: *Reflexes of the brain,* Cambridge, Mass, 1965, MIT Press.

77. Sechenov IM: *I.M. Sechenov: biographical sketch and essays,* New York, 1973, Arno Press.

78. Sedgwick D: Freud reconsidered: the technique of analysis. *Psyche Matters,* 2005. Retrieved July 2005, from http://www.psychematters.com/papers/sedgwick2.htm.

79. Sieg KW: Applying the behavioral model to the occupational therapy model, *Am J Occup Ther* 28:421-429, 1974.

80. Skinner BF: *About behaviorism,* New York, 1974, Knopf.

81. Stein F, Cutler SK: *Psychosocial occupational therapy: a holistic approach,* ed 2, Albany, NY, 2002, Delmar Thompson Learning.

82. Strachey J: *Two short accounts of psychoanalysis, five lectures on psychoanalysis, the question of lay analysis,* London, 1957, Horgath.

83. Sullwood E: *Reconnection with resources in the psyche,* Lectures presented to counseling students at Amani Counseling Center, Nairobi, Kenya, 1989.

84. von Salis T: What exactly is psychoanalytic psychotherapy? Some remarks on research in psychotherapy. *Psyche Matters,* 2003. Retrieved July 2005, from http://www.psychematters.com/papers/vonsalis.htm.

85. Watson JB, Rayner R: Conditioned emotional responses, *J Experiment Psychol* 3:1-14, 1920.

86. Web Quest: *Cognitive learning theory,* 2005. Retrieved August 2005, from http://suedstudent.syr.edu/-eberrett/ide621/cognitive.htm.

87. Weinrach SG: Cognitive therapists: a dialogue with Aaron Beck, *J Counseling Development* 67:159-164, 1988.

88. Weinrach SG: Rational emotive behavior therapy: a tough-minded therapy for tender-minded profession, *J Counseling Development* 73:296-300, 1995.

89. Weinrach SG: Nine experts describe the essence of rational-emotive therapy while standing on one foot, *J Counseling Development* 74:326-331, 1996.

90. Wilcock AA: *An occupational perspective of health,* Thorofare, NJ, 1998, Slack.

II

Contemporary Conceptual Foundations of Psychosocial Occupational Therapy

In Chapters 1 and 2, we discussed the origins of occupational therapy and analyzed the intellectual contexts within which the profession developed. In Chapter 3, we continued to analyze the conceptual foundations of the profession, focusing on the psychological theories from which constructs used in psychosocial occupational therapy practice are derived. In Part II of this book, we will complete the discussion of the conceptual foundations of the profession.

At the end of Chapter 2, we noted that a new paradigm of occupational therapy has emerged in the last two decades, culminating in articulation of what might be viewed as a *paradigmatic consensus* in the new Occupational Therapy Practice Framework (at least in occupational therapy literature; it is recognized that some therapists in practice may not yet be aware of the paradigm).[1] In Part II of this book (Chapter 4), we will discuss this paradigm in detail. We will also examine the social/intellectual context that has influenced its emergence and the implications of the new paradigm to occupational therapy practice.

One may wonder why so much space needs to be devoted to discussion of the professional paradigm. Would it not be more convenient to present the core constructs, principles, and guidelines spelled out in the Occupational Therapy Practice Framework and provide instructions on how to apply them in practice? In response to this question, it is argued that first of all, the Framework is not a prescription for practice techniques. It offers general guidelines that need to be interpreted by the therapist in order to apply them in practice. For example, the Framework

suggests that the therapeutic process revolves around "the collaborative therapeutic relationship between the client and the occupational therapist" (pp. 613-614).[1] However, it does not give the therapist step-by-step directions about how this collaboration can be achieved. The therapist has to *interpret* this general guideline. Suppose that a clinician argues that collaborative treatment planning means that a therapist sets treatment goals, presents them for discussion with the client, and then convinces him or her that these goals should be achieved. Would such an interpretation be correct? In order to determine whether or not such an interpretation would be correct, one must understand the spirit of the Framework. One can compare it to the U.S. Constitution; an attorney has to understand the spirit of the Constitution in order to interpret it correctly for application in specific situations.

Secondly, the Framework represents a consensus in occupational therapy literature, not only in the United States but all over the world, regarding what the nature of occupational therapy ought to be (there are other documents used to guide therapy in other countries, such as the Canadian Guidelines for Client-Centred Practice.[2] The constructs on which these documents are based are similar to those underlying the Framework, such as occupation-centeredness, client-centeredness, collaboration, and so on). That is why it is argued that the Framework (along with other similar documents used in other countries) represents a distilled presentation of the new consensual professional paradigm. This consensus within the community of occupational therapists constitutes the spirit of the paradigm. In order to interpret the guidelines of the Framework correctly, a therapist needs to understand the nature of this consensus, its context, and how it came to be. When that happens, the Framework becomes a guide to insightful practice. Since information about the evolution of the new paradigm is extensive, a complete discussion is not possible in a short chapter. Therefore, in this chapter, the goal is to sensitize the reader about the proposed paradigmatic consensus, its context, and how it arose within the profession.

REFERENCES

1. American Occupational Therapy Association: Occupational therapy practice framework: domain and process, *Am J Occup Ther* 56(6):609-639, 2002.
2. Canadian Association of Occupational Therapists: *Occupational therapy guidelines for client-centred practice*, Toronto, ON, 1991, CAOT Publications ACE.

4

The Occupational Therapy Paradigm

Preview Questions

1. What is a paradigm?
2. What is the relationship between a paradigm and a theory?
3. Explain the paradigm shifts that have occurred in occupational therapy since the introduction of the formal therapeutic use of occupations during the moral treatment era.
4. Describe the core constructs, focal viewpoint, and integrating values of the newly emerged occupational therapy paradigm.
5. Demonstrate analytically how the newly emerged occupational therapy paradigm is articulated in the new *Occupational Therapy Practice Framework*.
6. Discuss the proposed philosophical foundations and the scientific framework of the new occupational therapy paradigm.
7. What are the implications of the above-mentioned framework to occupational therapy practice?

The term *paradigm* was introduced by Thomas Kuhn,[35] a philosopher of science. Kuhn started as a physicist whose appetite for the history of science was whetted after he taught a class in science for humanities at Harvard University.[6] The class involved historical analysis of scientific case studies. This experience led to his acquaintance with the scientific work of Aristotle, after which he decided to concentrate his academic efforts on the history and philosophy of science. His inquiries in this field led to the publication of his book, *The Structure of Scientific Revolutions*.[35] In the book, because of his interest in the his-

tory of science, he introduced a new method (the historical method) to the study of the philosophy of science.[6]

Kuhn's Core Argument

Before Thomas Kuhn, the most influential philosopher of science was Karl Popper.[20] Popper agreed with the positivistic position that scientific observations are those that are objective and verifiable. In other words, they are "knowable truths" that can be established through observation of facts that are publicly verifiable. However, he disagreed with the positivists' doctrine that merely observing facts and explaining them constituted science. Rather, he argued that without a targeted object of observation, it was not possible to do science. Therefore scientific observations were selective. Furthermore, he argued, what separates science from nonscience is falsifiability of explanations of observations. A useful scientific theory must make predictions that can be proved false by observations. If an explanation is *post-diction* (occurs after observations), he considered it to be nonscientific and useless. Popper also prescribed to the prevalent view that the use of scientific procedures led to progressive production of information or knowledge, such that new knowledge built on to old knowledge, and new knowledge progressively approximated objective truth.

Thomas Kuhn disagreed with this view; his approach was revolutionary.[35] First, he disputed the idea of science as an objective endeavor.

Rather, he argued that the subjectivity of the scientist is part of scientific enterprise. Furthermore, he disputed the idea that development of science is progressive and cumulative. Instead, he suggested that science develops through revolutions. First, it is guided by what he called a *paradigm* (which he initially referred to as a *matrix*[6]). A *paradigm* consists of shared theoretical beliefs, values, instruments, and techniques of scientific endeavor, to which members of the scientific discipline commit. He also used the analogy of a puzzle to explain the construct of paradigm. According to Kuhn, puzzles are presented to scientists, and the scientific methods, as guided by a paradigm, help them solve those puzzles. During what he called *normal science,* nothing much happens in the way of introducing radical new knowledge. After a while, the methods of solving scientific puzzles are more or less standard. During these times, development of science is consistent with the progressive view where knowledge accumulates gradually in small increments.

During normal science, there is usually a resistance to change. Therefore when events that do not fit the explanatory framework of the paradigm occur (what Kuhn referred to as *anomalies*), they are ignored or explained away as best as possible. However, when the anomalies accumulate to the point where they cannot be ignored, scientists begin to lose confidence in the ability of the prevailing paradigm to explain the events. When this lack of confidence becomes critical, there is a *crisis.* Normally the response to this crisis is attempting to revise the prevailing paradigm so that the most pressing anomalies are explained and outstanding puzzles are solved. This revision constitutes a scientific revolution. This revisionist period is characterized by competition between varying ideas, which are compared on the basis of their rational merits in explaining the anomalies. Eventually, the idea that has the most explanatory or problem-solving power (and retains the problem-solving power of the preceding matrix) emerges as the new paradigm.

Kuhn's Construct of Paradigm: Application to Occupational Therapy

Although Kuhn developed the paradigmatic model to explain development of knowledge in the basic sciences, it can be applied to practice disciplines such as occupational therapy to explain evolving discipline's core constructs, focus, and values.[33] Kielhofner and Burke[34] used the model to explain occupational therapy's changing identity since the moral treatment era. According to Kielhofner,[33] the formal founding of occupational therapy as a profession was preceded by a pre-paradigm (the moral treatment movement). During this era, the idea that mental illness was caused by environmental factors emerged. It was argued that effective treatment of the mentally ill was environmental modification. Furthermore, society had an obligation to help the mentally ill return into the mainstream of life.

Central to this form of milieu therapy was the therapeutic use of daily occupations including self-care, education, physical exercises, and recreation designed to "interrupt the chain of morbid thoughts," direct "the attention on more pleasant subjects," and "maintain order" (p. 20)[46] among clients. Also, therapy was based on the premise that the mentally ill retained a certain measure of rationality. This residual intellectual capacity could be appealed by use of intellectually challenging occupations, resulting in a return to rationality through the individual patient's actions.[55] Thus the responsibility of healing was on the patient, and the therapist was a facilitator. Although Kielhofner does not state it, it may be argued that the arts and crafts movement was also part of the pre-paradigm. As discussed in Chapter 1, this movement introduced the idea that alienation in the industrial society caused mental illness, and engagement in arts and crafts helped decrease this sense of alienation, leading to better mental health.[46] Thus arts and crafts became a media of therapy and would remain so after occupational therapy was founded, perhaps even until the 1970s.

At the turn of the twentieth century, a variety of ideas from the moral treatment movement and the arts and crafts movement coalesced into the formal founding of the profession of occupational therapy. Principles of the new profession were articulated, constituting the first paradigm for the profession—the paradigm of occupation. In this paradigm, the founders of the profession saw their task as convincing the public "of the important relationship between creative work and health" (p. 32).[46] However, beginning in the era of the Great Depression, and exacerbated by the rise of the rehabilitation movement, an anomaly arose in which the medical profession challenged occupational therapists to explain what they were doing scientifically. This anomaly/challenge led to a loss of confidence in the ability of the paradigm of occupation to offer scientific justification of the existence of the profession.[13,33] Occupational therapists responded to this crisis by revising the paradigm and adopting the reductionistic, mechanistic medical model. Normal practice within this paradigm included a focus on the internal intrapsychic, kinesiological, and neurological systems in therapeutic interventions.

Very soon, however, the reductionistic medical model proved inadequate as a guide for occupational therapy. The profession began to look more and more like physical therapy with predominant use of exercises as therapeutic media or like social work with extensive use of talk therapy.[19,31] Thus there was role blurring.[18] Furthermore, this paradigm did not address the problems of chronically ill patients. Also, it was inadequate in helping therapists address the full spectrum of occupational problems of humans as they interacted with the environment.[33] This led to a loss of confidence in the paradigm and the rise of another crisis. The response to this crisis was a call to return to the roots of occupational therapy in the moral treatment movement and the principles articulated by the founders of the profession at the turn of the twentieth century (see Chapter 2). This call led to concerted activity among scholars in the professional commu-

nity, leading to articulation of a new paradigm in the early twenty-first century. Since the paradigm is client-centered,[1,33] we will refer to recipients of occupational therapy services as *clients* and not *patients*.

Articulation of the Paradigm in the *Occupational Therapy Practice Framework*: An Analysis

The role of the occupational therapist is primarily facilitation of occupational performance by providing opportunities for engagement in occupation, assistive devices, education/counseling, and modifying the environment. This role is well articulated in the new practice framework (see "The New Occupational Therapy Paradigm" in Chapter 2 for a detailed discussion).

Similar to the occupational therapy paradigm articulated by Kielhofner,[33] the primary focus of the AOTA in the *Occupational Therapy Practice Framework* (OTPF) is client "engagement in occupation for participation in life" (p. 609).[1] Similarly, the role of the occupational therapist is conceptualized in the OTPF as follows:

- The use of self, or use of what is known as the therapeutic relationship
- Use of occupations/activities (i.e., occupation-based practice)
- Consultation and education, which corresponds to counseling/education in the paradigm as presented by Kielhofner[33]

Similar to the expressed values of the paradigm outlined by Kielhofner,[33] the OTPF emphasizes client-centered, collaborative therapeutic interventions. In other words, therapy revolves around "the collaborative therapeutic relationship between the client and the occupational therapist" (pp. 613-614).[1] This collaboration is based on clients engaging in occupations by self-choice and motivation, which makes those occupations meaningful to them. One can see from the above analysis that the shared opinion about the nature of occupational therapy in the new paradigm is that the profession's existence is necessitated by its mission to use client-centered, occupation-based, collaborative, therapeutic interventions, with the goal of facilitating engagement in meaningful occupations for effective participation in life. This opinion is expressed both in the professional paradigm as articulated by Kielhofner[33] and in the AOTA OTPF.[1]

The Context of the New Paradigm

The new professional paradigm did not originate in a vacuum. Therefore in order to understand its spirit and therefore the spirit of the OTPF, one needs to understand the context within which it emerged. As mentioned earlier, the paradigm emerged mostly as a response to a call to return to the roots of occupational therapy following a crisis due to lack of confidence in the reductionistic, mechanistic paradigm of the medical model. However, this response occurred in context. For example, in mental health, there was the influence of the community mental support movement.[54] The movement emphasizes the view that, with adequate support by making available resources and opportunities such as vocational opportunities and housing, disabled individuals, including the mentally ill, can be helped to reintegrate into the mainstream of society and become fully functioning community citizens. Thus the movement advocates recovery of clients in the community.

From the community support movement has emerged a new discipline of psychiatric rehabilitation (PsyR).[45] Professionals subscribing to this new discipline share certain principles and values. These include individualized interventions so that "The uniqueness of each person's rehabilitation has a direct bearing on PsyR services" (p. 91).[45] In this individualized intervention, clients are encouraged to examine their life aspirations and if necessary, formulate new personal world views, dreams, and aspirations. This principle seems consistent with the objective to conduct client-centered, collaborative interventions in occupational therapy, where

the client is seen as an active agent in his or her own therapy. Individualization of therapy has also been popularized by humanistic psychologies,[37,48] with their emphasis on the dignity of the individual and the need to facilitate individual growth.

Other themes that are found in PsyR that are also prevalent in occupational therapy include integration of clients into the community, focus on their quality of life, and consideration of their contextual (environmental and social) circumstances. From the ensuing discussion, it is clear that emergence of the new occupational therapy paradigm has been influenced significantly by the humanistic psychology, community support movement, and the call by the profession's leaders to return to the roots of the profession.

Philosophical Basis of the Paradigm: Pragmatism as a Philosophy of Occupational Therapy

There seems to be a converging consensus in occupational therapy that the philosophical foundations of occupational therapy are to be found in the philosophy of pragmatism.* Evidence that pragmatism is the philosophy of occupational therapy is provided by the extensive historical relationships between the founders of occupational therapy and the leading pragmatic philosophers, particularly William James, John Dewey, and George Herbert Mead. (See discussion of these historical connections in Chapter 2. See also Breines,[8] who gives an in-depth discussion of these historical links.) Therefore it is imperative that the occupational therapist understand prevailing themes in the philosophical principles, assumptions, and values of pragmatism and how these themes are consistent with those of occupational therapy.

Breines[8] provides an analysis indicating that the principles of occupational therapy are clearly consistent with those of pragmatism. Both disciplines focus on individual experiences as

---

*References 8,11,22-25,29,47,60.

humans act on their environment. Both emphasize mind/body unity as individuals interact adaptively with their environment. This consistency led Breines to conclude that: "Pragmatic principles were placed in the medical arena as occupational therapy" (p. 92).[8] Further analysis of the philosophical writings of four leading pragmatic philosophers (Charles Sanders Peirce, William James, John Dewey, and George Herbert Mead) and the literature of occupational therapy revealed that the themes underlying the principles, assumptions, and values of the two disciplines are consistent.[22,29] Figure 4-1 shows a logistic mapping of themes illustrating this consistency.

Following is a discussion of the themes in Figure 4-1. The contemporary consensual definition of occupation may be understood to be as presented in the *Occupational Therapy Practice Framework:*

activities...of every day life, named, organized, and given value and meaning by individuals and a culture. Occupation is everything people do to

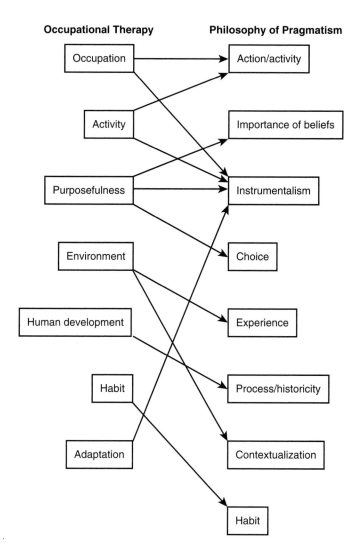

Occupational Therapy   **Philosophy of Pragmatism**

Occupation — Action/activity

Activity — Importance of beliefs

Purposefulness — Instrumentalism

Environment — Choice

Human development — Experience

Habit — Process/historicity

Adaptation — Contextualization

Habit

Figure 4-1.   Logistic mapping illustrating the consistency between themes underlying the assumptions, principles, and values of occupational therapy *(left column)* and those of the philosophy of pragmatism *(right column).* Occupational therapy themes in the left column were derived from analysis of occupational therapy literature and Slagle lectures delivered between 1955 and 1995. Pragmatic themes in the right column were derived from analysis of the literature from the writings of the four leading American pragmatic philosophers. Adapted from Ikiugu MN, Schultz S: An argument for pragmatism as a foundational philosophy of occupational therapy, *Canad J Occup Ther* 73(2):86-97, 2006.

occupy themselves, including looking after themselves...enjoying life...and contributing to the social and economic fabric of their communities (p. 610).[1]

The above definition identifies occupations as *activities*. Activity is a popular theme in occupational therapy as identified in the analysis of occupational therapy literature and Slagle lectures (see Figure 4-1). This theme is consistent with the emphasis on *action/activity* in the philosophy of pragmatism. Pragmatism is primarily a philosophy of doing (action) because, as Dewey states, it is "The theory that the processes and the materials of knowledge are determined by practical or purposive considerations—that there is no such thing as knowledge determined by exclusively theoretical, speculative, or abstract intellectual considerations" (p. 27).[17] *Practical* or *purposive* considerations referred to by Dewey are only achievable through action, or as Peirce stated,

It is certainly best for us that our beliefs should be such as may truly guide our actions so as to satisfy our desires; and this reflection will make us reject every belief which does not seem to have been so formed as to insure this result (p. 10).[43]

Also, the purpose of occupation is identified in the definition as including humans' use of their capacity and need for action through occupation to contribute *to the social and economic fabric of* communities. This purpose of occupation is consistent with Dewey's instrumental view of the mind, where the purpose of the mind is seen as to produce actions that enable us to perform occupations that make it possible to take care of ourselves and contribute to our communities. To this end, Dewey saw all the products of the mind in its role as a guide for action as instrumental. By *instrumental* he meant using the mind to create social institutions and solve problems to make it possible for humans to adapt to their environment. Thus he stated that when belief, as a function of the mind, is apprehended "as a tool and only a tool, an *instrumentality* of direction, the same scrupulous attention will go to its formation as now goes into the making of

instruments of precision in technical fields" (p. 375, emphasis mine).[16]

Purposefulness, which is identified in Figure 4-1 as a common theme in occupational therapy, is one of the characteristics of occupation that makes it therapeutically valuable. AOTA defines engagement in occupation in part as participation in "objective and subjective aspects of carrying out occupations and activities that are meaningful and *purposeful* to the person" (p. 618, emphasis mine).[1] A purposeful activity is further defined as one that "Allows the client to engage in goal-directed behavior or activities within a therapeutically designed context that lead to an occupation or occupations" (p. 628).[1] This definition implies *use of the mind* as may be understood from Dewey's instrumental perspective, since goal-directedness implies use of the mind to formulate goals for action. In that sense, purposefulness is consistent with the emphasis on the importance of *beliefs* (products of the mind in its use as a tool) in pragmatism where it is postulated that "Our beliefs guide our desires and shape our actions" (pp. 9-10).[43] Therefore by virtue of consistence of purposefulness with the importance of beliefs, it is also consistent with the pragmatic construct of instrumentalism.

Purposefulness also implies *choice,* since being goal oriented means that one makes action-oriented choices. The concept of choice is an important theme in pragmatism, particularly in the philosophy of John Dewey, who saw all human endeavors, including politics, as

the struggle to construct an optimum environment for the realizing and sanctioning of the aesthetic processes of living. Finally, the entire human endeavor should be an effort to apply the method of creative intelligence in order to achieve optimum possibilities in the never-ending moral struggle to harmonize the means-end relationship for the purpose of enhancing human life and achieving growth (pp. xxv–xxvi).[39]

Application of creative intelligence is a matter of choice for all humans, which defines their *agency* as they act on the environment.

It is by now clear that the environment is an important theme in occupational therapy.[1,38,60] McColl observes that "the theoretical literature in occupational therapy most commonly identifies occupation as a function of the person on one hand and the environment on the other" (p. 2).[38] Furthermore, the environment is conceived to consist of "both the physical and the social environments" (p. 3).[38] This emphasis on the importance of the environment is consistent with the value placed on experience in the philosophy of pragmatism. As McDermott observes, the entire corpus of Dewey's philosophy, for example, may be seen as a philosophy of "experience which is 'had'–that is, undergone, lived" (p. xxiv).[39] Emphasis on experience in pragmatism speaks to perceived supremacy of mundane facts gathered from sensations emanating from the environment. Combined with the logic of science, this perceived supremacy of environmental experiences allows humans to look at the facts of experience without despising them as imperfect evils or inferior to transcendent superior knowledge of some final cause (as had been the case in philosophy for centuries).[14] Since the environment is a context for experience, the construct of *contextualization* is very important in pragmatism. Indeed, because of Hegelian influence, Dewey saw a philosophy that is removed from context as useless in addressing human needs. Thus he saw pragmatism as a contextual philosophy[15] that addresses real, contemporary human problems. Thus the theme of *environment* in occupational therapy is consistent with the pragmatic theme of *contextualization*.

Human development is another important theme in occupational therapy. As McColl states, the view in occupational therapy is that "*Developmental changes* in occupation occur when an external or internal demand sets in motion an intrinsically programmed change that is sequential and predictable" (p. 4).[38] Sequential and predictable change implies taking into account past, present, and future events. This developmental view is consistent with the construct of *process/historicity* in pragmatism. In this context, *historicity* means that as humans we

may, by appealing to dynamic laws, "and earlier states or events, explain later states or events" (p. 75).[59] Thus historicity, like development, appeals to continuity of life through sequencing of events that connect the past, present, and future into one continuum.

Habit is another theme present in both the philosophy of pragmatism and occupational therapy literature. In the early 1900s, when the profession of occupational therapy was still in its infancy, Slagle developed habit-training programs to treat the mentally ill (see Chapter 2).[50,60] These programs consisted of a structured 24-hour regimen of activities. They were based on the rationale that "Occupation usually remedially serves to overcome some habits, to modify others, and to construct new ones to the end that habit reactions will be favorable to the restoration and maintenance of health" (p. 178).[60] As discussed in Chapter 2, this rationale for habit training seems remarkably similar to William James' admonition that

> The hell to be endured hereafter, of which theology tells us, is no worse than the hell we make for ourselves in this world by habitually fashioning our characters in the wrong way. Could the young but realize how soon they will become mere walking bundles of habits, they would give more heed to their conduct while in the plastic state (p. 20).[30]

Thus Slagle and other occupational therapists of her time seem to have developed their therapeutic interventions based on James' notion of the importance of habits in the formation of humans. Today, habits still play a big part in occupational therapy practice (see Kielhofner's *Model of Human Occupation* [MOHO][32]), indicating that the pragmatic notion of habit is still influential in occupational therapy practice.

Finally, *adaptation* is one of the core constructs in occupational therapy. Occupation is seen as a means by which humans attain mastery and adapt to their environment.[51,52] In recent years, with the advent of occupational science, investigation of "a common evolutionary view of human history in which occupational development is considered in conjunction with the biological and cultural development of the human species" (p. 71)[60] is already under way. This supports the argument that the concept of adaptation in occupational therapy is based on Darwin's theory of evolution with its doctrine that organisms adapt as they interact with the environment and change in order to survive.[12] In this case, occupation is seen as the means by which the human organism interacts with the environment and in the process changes itself and the environment in order to survive. The construct of adaptation is also prevalent in the philosophy of pragmatism (as has already been argued in Chapter 2) through which it infiltrated occupational therapy.

The central role played by evolutionism in the formulation of the philosophy of pragmatism is not only apparent in Peirce's[43] professed respect for Darwin and his theory, but also in a reiteration of this sentiment by Dewey in his statement that "The influence of Darwin upon philosophy resides in his having conquered the phenomenon of life for the principle of transition, and thereby freed the new logic for application to mind and morals and life" (p. 35).[12] Thus one can conclude that the theme of adaptation, drawn from Darwin's evolutionism, is a central construct in both occupational therapy and pragmatism.

The above discussion leads to the conclusion, as proposed by Ikiugu[22] and Ikiugu and Schultz,[29] that indeed, as Breines[8] argued, the philosophy of pragmatism is a likely philosophical foundation of occupational therapy. Therefore the principles, assumptions, and values of pragmatism can be used to provide a philosophical foundational framework for occupational therapy theory and practice. Propositions, such as the importance of beliefs as a basis for actions and human agency in choosing and initiating action, can be operationalized for application both in clinical practice and occupational therapy research. They can be used as a foundation for a framework to provide the rationale

for core constructs, focal viewpoint, and integrating values[33] shared by occupational therapists as defined in the new professional paradigm. Those constructs and propositions have already been used in practice (see the $OTPF^1$), but their pragmatic basis has not been made explicit. Such explicit awareness of the philosophical framework is essential for a shared definition of professional identity.[8] Already, the construct of instrumentalism has been operationalized to develop a conceptual practice model.[23-25] This model is an example of direct application of pragmatic principles in occupational therapy practice.

Complexity/Chaos Theory: A Scientific Framework for Occupational Therapy Theory and Practice

In her Slagle lecture, Royeen[49] proposed that complexity/chaos theory is more suited as a scientific framework than linear science for the study of human occupation both in occupational science and occupational therapy. She argued that a shift from linearity to chaos perspective is necessary because occupations are complex, nonlinear phenomena that cannot be adequately understood using linear scientific methods. Other authors have proposed similar sentiments and indeed, chaos theory is now used to provide concepts to describe and study occupations and related phenomena.[26,28,36,44]

This chapter proposes that complexity/chaos theory be integrated explicitly in the new occupational therapy paradigm as a scientific framework to inform an understanding of the role of human occupation in facilitating adaptation. In this sense, the philosophical foundation of the paradigm is conceptualized to be pragmatism, while its scientific framework is the complexity/chaos theory, and the theoretical content comes from the literature of occupational therapy and related scientific disciplines such as psychology, anatomy, developmental studies, disability studies, social work, and so on. In this section, we will discuss complexity/chaos/dynamic systems theory, its place as a scientific framework for the occupational therapy paradigm, and practice implications of using it.

Introduction

Complexity theory, also known as *chaos theory*[53] or *dynamics systems theory,*[36] has a history similar to that of occupational therapy or occupational science. Similar to the founding of occupational therapy, and recently occupational science, renowned researchers from a variety of backgrounds (e.g., Murray Gell-Mann, a physicist; John Holland, a biologist; W. Brian Arthur, an economist; Christopher Langton, a researcher in artificial life) came together to found the new scientific discipline. Their interest was to create a science of non-*linear dynamics,* or as Prigogine[45a] asserted, a scientific discipline to replace the Newtonian paradigm focusing on stability, order, uniformity, equilibrium, and linear relationships within and between systems. But, what do we mean by complexity and linearity? Following are some definitions.

Dynamic Systems

A *dynamic system* is one that changes over time[58]; such a system may be simple or complex. An example of a simple dynamic system is a pendulum. It has a simple path (trajectory) that is in the shape of an arc. Complex dynamic systems, on the other hand, consist of multiple agents acting and interacting dynamically within an environment.[53] It is an interaction between systems coupled with flux.[58] Complexity/chaos theory is a science of such complex, dynamic systems.

Complex, Dynamic, Adaptive Systems

According to Waldrop, complex, dynamic, adaptive systems interact adaptively with the environment.[57] Living organisms are such systems. Researchers in complexity propose that life emerges at the edge of chaos and order, which means that the creativity associated with a living organism emerges at the point where the system is beginning to be chaotic but there is still structure to give its activity order. Thus one may argue that life is bounded by order (often associated with stagnation) on one side and chaos (associated with lack of focus or structure) on the other.[2]

The science of complex, dynamic, adaptive systems seems to be a hybrid of the older systems theory characterized by the view of multiple systems that influence each other (in the older systems theory, the systems were conceptualized to be hierarchical)[56] and Darwin's theory of evolution as indicated by the construct of adaptation to the environment through organismic change.[12] Complexity theory may therefore be seen as a superior theory in terms of its explanatory power to both the older systems theory and the theory of evolution. We have already seen that the theory of evolution, through pragmatism, has been a part of occupational therapy conceptual foundations since the formal founding of the profession. Hence it is logical that complexity/chaos theory would be adopted by the profession as its scientific framework. Complex, dynamic, adaptive systems are characterized by nonlinearity, dependence on initial conditions, disproportion between input and outcome(s), deterministic chaos, self-similarity, self organization, and emergence.[5,7,42,57,58]

Nonlinearity, Disproportion Between Input and Output, and Dependence on Initial Conditions

For those who are analytically inclined and would like to explore complexity theory in depth, the mathematical analogies used in this section may offer an interesting and stimulating approach that is different from other discussions of application of complexity in occupational therapy to date. However, it is recognized that some individuals are not mathematically oriented and may be discouraged by the dryness of the algorithmic discourse presented here. Since this section is not extremely crucial to an understanding of the applicability of the constructs from complexity theory to psychosocial occupational therapy, those who prefer to skip the mathematical discourse may move on to the "Implications to Clinical Practice" section.

Newtonian science is characterized by linear relationships between events such that event A causes event B. For example, in the typical medical model, drug A (for example, a diuretic), will cause reaction B in the human body (removal of excessive accumulation of fluids in the extremities). This relationship is predictable. It can be characterized by a linear mathematical function, such as $2x$, and the output is proportional to the input. In complex, dynamic, adaptive systems, there is no linear causal relationship between events because of the complex multiple interactions between subsystems involved.[36] Rather, there is dependence on initial conditions such that "In complex adaptive systems, cause and effect relationships are bidirectional and nonlinear, meaning a small change can have large effects" (p. 35).[42]

In other words, the output is not proportional to the input. This happens, for instance, in marital relationships in which a simple, seemingly inconsequential statement may lead to a big argument and possibly even a threat to the ensuing relationship. This phenomenon occurs in therapy as well. For example, an off-hand statement by the therapist during therapy may cause far-reaching life changes in a client. The disproportion between cause and effect may be expressed mathematically by a nonlinear function such as x^2, such that $1^2 = 1$, $2^2 = 4$, $3^2 = 9$, and so on.[58] It is evident that the output is significantly disproportional to the input. This property of nonlinearity is referred to as *dependence on initial conditions*. The function of x^2 also introduces another characteristic of nonlinearity. It "implies the possibility of very rapid change" (p. 359).[58]

This possibility of sudden, rapid change is even more noticeable if you take the outcome of x^2 and feed it back as input. Thus the iteration becomes: $2^2 = 4$, $4^2 = 16$, $16^2 = 256$, and so on. In such iterations, the output very quickly becomes extremely large compared to the original input. Dependence on initial conditions

happens because systems are sensitive to environmental input (known as *noise* or *perturbation*). A small perturbation reverberates within the system because of the multiple interactions between subsystems within the system, leading to multiplicity of effects. This reverberation, where the input is magnified by reactions from the agents in the system, is known as *recursive effect*.[58] It is postulated that this causes escalation in relationships (such as the marital relationship discussed earlier), leading to a possible breakdown of the relationship due to a small initial disagreement. The effects are also unpredictable,[7] or at least, "long-term predictions are limited if not impossible" (p. 348).[36] In the relationship example for instance, it is impossible to predict the specific outcome of saying something seemingly insignificant. One can guess that generally, insensitivity to another person's feelings could lead to deterioration of a relationship, but no one can predict with precision the direction of deterioration because of the recursive feedback reverberating between the two subsystems (the two individuals) in the relationship system.

This unpredictability of the effects of input to a system means that complex, dynamic, adaptive systems can be nudged to move in a certain direction,[58] for example, by giving timely feedback to a student or client to facilitate change in a desired direction, but they "cannot be controlled in the usual sense of the term" (p. 2). In other words, therapists have to use what Lazzarini calls "windows of opportunity"[36] to make well-timed interventions in therapy to push the system toward increased adaptive functioning.

Deterministic Chaos

It has been found that determinism and chaos can coexist in the same system.[41,58] Within complex dynamic systems, events occur at random without repeating themselves, but they stay within certain defining parameters. For example, an adolescent with behavioral and emotional difficulties engages in activities such as truancy, drug use, and violence, and does poorly in school. If we were to keep a record

Table 4-1.   ITERATED CALCULATED VALUES
USING THE LOGISTIC EQUATION
$X_{t+1} = RX_t(1 - X_t)$ WITH R = 3.8
AND X = 0.6

x_t	$Rx_t(1 - x_t)$
X_1	0.9120000
X_2	0.3049728
X_3	0.8054646
X_4	0.5954272
X_5	0.9153958
X_6	0.294296
X_7	0.7892062
X_8	0.6321671
X_9	0.883621
X_{10}	0.3907727
X_{11}	0.9046636
X_{12}	0.32774
X_{13}	0.8372406
X_{14}	0.5178213
X_{15}	0.9487931

$$x_{t+1} = Rx_t(1 - x_t),$$

where t = time (0, 1, 2...), R = rate of change (1 to 4), and x is a variable (0 to 1).

Table 4-1 shows iterated values calculated using the logistic equation $x_{t+1} = Rx_t(1 - x_t)$, where R = 3.8 and x = 0.6 (randomly chosen values). Figure 4-2 shows a graph of x at time t plotted against the values of $Rx_t(1 - x_t)$.

As shown in Figure 4-2, iterations of the values of x_{t+1} are confined between 0 and 1, and they are random iterations with no value repeated. In other words, the values are chaotic but are bounded within certain parameters. This is deterministic chaos. It is a mathematical analogy of an adolescent whose scores on tests are random but remain within a region defined as the fail score region, consistent with his general poor performance pattern. This pattern has been found to characterize peoples' occupational performance. In a study by Ikiugu and Rosso,[28] study participants completed daily occupational inventories where they logged occupations in which they engaged on an hourly basis for 21 days. The occupations were grouped into seven categories as defined in the Practice Framework developed by the AOTA[1]: activities of daily living, instrumental activities of daily living, education, work, play, leisure, and social participation.

Daily frequencies of engagement in categorized occupations as determined from the completed daily occupational inventories were

of his scores in a test or a variety of tests, we would have scores that are random, where most often no two scores are similar. However, because he is in a constraining pattern defined as "poor performance" in school-related work, we would expect that the scores would fall within a certain region (in the category of fail scores). Such behavior of complex dynamic systems may be described by a generic equation known as a *logistic equation,* which is often used in chaos theory of the type:

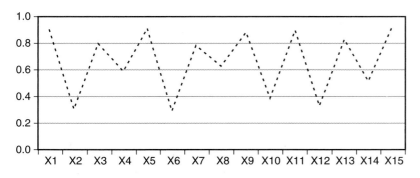

Figure 4-2.   A graph of x at time t (*x-axis*), plotted against $Rx_t(1 - x_t)$ (*y-axis*).

tallied. Occupational performance scores were calculated as a function of the frequency of engagement in the top five occupations (as ranked by participants on the basis of their perceived importance in the participants' lives) using the following algorithm:

$$P_t = \Sigma(P_i) = \Sigma(F \times PI),$$

where P_t = total performance score for the day, P_i = performance score for each of the occupations, F = frequency of engagement in the occupation as determined from the daily occupational inventory entries, and PI = performance index of each activity according to rank (I = 5 for the occupation ranked number 1, 4 for number 2, 3 for number 3, 2 for number 4, and 1 for number 5). Refer to the Occupational Performance Calculation Guide (OPCG) by Ikiugu and Rosso[28] in Chapter 8 of the Lab Manual.

When each of the participant's daily performance scores were plotted, the graphs, without exception, revealed patterns that were similar to the graph in Figure 4-2. This pattern suggested that the study participants' occupational performance fell within bounded chaos (deterministic chaos) as described above. Now, suppose we plot iterations of x_{t+1} in Table 4-1 against subsequent iterations (Figure 4-3).

As is apparent in Figure 4-3, when each iteration of x_{t+1} is plotted against the next iteration, a graph in the shape of a parabola results. Thus the seemingly chaotic iterations have a deterministic form. Derivatives of the logistic equation must

fall somewhere along this parabola. The region defined by the parabola is known as a *strange attractor*,[58] and it determines the otherwise chaotic trajectory of a complex, dynamic, adaptive system. An *attractor* is a point that determines the trajectory or path of the system or the point to which the behavior of a system is attracted or at which it settles.[4,9,10] For simple systems, such as a pendulum, the attractor is a single point (the point of equilibrium). For complex systems, the attractor consists of multiple points that form a basin of attraction.[26,28] Such a basin is known as a *strange attractor*.

Therefore deterministic chaos is a function of boundaries of chaotic behavior determined by systemic attractors. In our earlier example of a poorly performing student, such a basin of attraction may be formed by multiple points in the basin of attraction such as lack of discipline, impulsive behavior, inability to delay gratification, exposure to pernicious environmental factors, and so on. Notice also that the parabola (basin of attraction) resulted from iterations in which values from the operations of the logistic equation were fed back as input for the calculation of the next value, and then the former value was plotted against the latter value. This suggests that in complex, dynamic systems, the basin of attraction itself is an emergent phenomenon, emerging from the recursive feedback resulting from interactions between the multiple subsystems within the system. This conclusion would have far-reaching implications in education, parenting, and therapy, in explaining the value of modifying the environment to produce

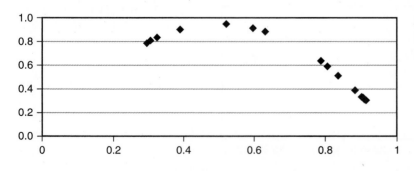

Figure 4-3.   A scatter diagram of iterations of x_{t+1} plotted against subsequent iterations.

desirable perturbations on the one hand, and creating opportunities for positive communication between subsystems on the other, so that attractors that structure the trajectory so that it moves toward a general positive direction emerge. This concept is discussed further in the "Implications to Clinical Practice" section.

Self-Similarity

System trajectories in complex dynamic systems are characterized by patterns that, when examined, reveal properties at small scales that are replications of the properties of the entire system. Such patterns are referred to as *self-similarity,* and a self-similar system is known as a *fractal.*[5] Again, we'll illustrate this property of complex, dynamic, adaptive systems using the logistic equation of the type

$$x_{t+1} = Rx_t(1 - x_t)$$

where t = time (0, 1, 2, 3...), R = rate of change (3.3), and x is a variable (.2).

Table 4-2 shows fifteen iterations of the values of x_{t+1}. When the value of R is greater than 3.0,

Table 4-2. Illustration of Periodicity (Self-Similarity) of Fractal Systems

x_t	x_{t+1}
0.2	0.528
0.528	0.8224128
0.8224128	0.4819644
0.4819644	0.8239265
0.8239265	0.4787363
0.4787363	0.8235078
0.8235078	0.4796309
0.4796309	0.8236307
0.8236307	0.4794328
0.4794328	0.823604
0.823604	0.4794254
0.4794254	0.823603
0.823603	0.4794276
0.4794276	0.8236033
0.8236033	0.4794269

the values of x_{t+1} will cycle, or portray a mathematical characteristic known as *periodicity.* This is true even though the values of x_{t+1} vary. When the value of R is less than 3.0, the system is in a "stable, steady state" (p. 19.)[41] Therefore one may assume that it is closest to the point of equilibrium and therefore least amenable to change. When R = 3.3, the system has two cycles, alternating between 0.823…and 0.479…. Such a system is self-similar and is known as a *period 2 system,* with 0.823… and 0.479…being "periodic attractors for the system" (p. 193).[41]

In real life, such self-similarity is indicated by the general patterns of one's life. For instance, in our earlier example of an adolescent who has emotional and behavioral problems and performs poorly in school, we can expect a life pattern consistent with that characterization. For instance, instead of going to school and studying regularly as required, he may cut school, drink or engage in drug consumption with friends, and so on. Although we cannot predict precisely what he will do at a specific point in time, we can, based on the pattern of his life, guess that on Saturdays he will go to the mall to meet his buddies and then drink until after midnight. Then on Sundays he will probably sleep until after midday, and so on. His life pattern is therefore characterized by a stable, steady state with periodic frequency of certain activities within the week, although this pattern can only be predicted in general terms and not specifically. We can also hypothesize that if we want him to develop a more adaptive approach to life, we have to push him out of this "stable, steady state" and help him change his entire life pattern rather than trying to change specific activities piecemeal. This brings us to the question of how change occurs in complex, dynamic systems.

Change in Complex, Dynamic Systems

If we gradually increase the value of R in the above discussion, we will reach a point where the values of x_{t+1} form a periodic pattern with oscillations between 4 points. After another increase in R, the pattern will oscillate between 8 points, and so on. This phenomenon is known as *period doubling* (p. 193).[41] This suggests that as long as the rate of change is within a certain range, the values of x_{t+1} stay within certain parameters and the system is in a stable, steady state. Once the threshold of the rate of change is reached, there is a sudden rapid change and the system goes into a new stable, steady state. Therefore change in a complex, dynamic system occurs when the system is farthest from equilibrium (where proximity to equilibrium is represented by a stable, steady state). Many small changes in the system in the desired general direction propel the system further and further away from equilibrium until finally the system is tipped over, resulting in rapid changes and reestablishment of a new, stable, steady state.[42]

As an illustration of this dynamic, let us consider a student who is embarking on a new area of study. In the beginning, everything is new, and it is a struggle for the student to master the basics of what is being studied. However, once a certain threshold is reached, the ability to learn new concepts in that area of study increases rapidly and the student suddenly finds it easy to get through the various courses, until a completely new level of learning is introduced. Then the student starts struggling again, *ad infinitum*.

Self-Organization and Emergence

The above-described dynamic, where the system moves into a new stable, steady state once the rate of change reaches a certain threshold, indicates another important property of complex, dynamic, adaptive systems: they are self-organizing.[36,40] Each stable steady state described above is a new level of self-organization of the system. At each of these levels, new properties emerge that are specific to that level and that transcend the sum of individual parts of the subsystems involved.[5] These emergent properties enable the system to adapt to its environment. In the earlier example of a troubled adolescent, if environmental perturbations were introduced that pushed his entire life performance system into a more adaptive direction, then eventually a

threshold might be reached, and the young man may decide to get his act together. Such a decision may lead to a restructuring of his entire life such that his life patterns are quantitatively and qualitatively different from his previous life, and conducive to more adaptive functioning. In other words, self-organization would have occurred leading to new personality properties that make him more adaptive.

Implications to Clinical Practice

Adopting the complexity/chaos theory as a scientific framework for occupational therapy has far-reaching implications for practice and research. First, we would need to regard the occupational human as a complex, dynamic, adaptive system, with characteristics such as dependence on initial conditions, disproportion between input and output, self-organization, and emergence.[24,26,28] Such a framework would enable us to appreciate underlying order in seemingly chaotic client performance.[7] As therapists, we must bear in mind that once the rate of change reaches a certain threshold, sudden, rapid change may occur; thus we would focus on introducing small, well-timed perturbations to nudge the system in the general desired direction, without trying to control it.[7,58] Such perturbations may be in the form of occupations designed "to elicit change" by providing experiences that "lead to the development of new habits, beliefs and value systems" (p. 349).[36]

The nudges may also be in form of timely information given to the client to create insight of the need to change, or offering occupations that pose the right challenge to force the client to develop increasingly organized adaptive capabilities (emergence), and so on. Following is a mathematical illustration of how the nudges would be timed. In this illustration, we will borrow constructs from Bandura's Cognitive Social Learning Theory (CSLT).[3] The reader should remember that these mathematical illustrations are not literal but are mere analogies.

In Bandura's theory (discussed in more detail in Chapter 3), it is proposed that performance (which we may regard as occupational performance for the purpose of this illustration) depends on the meaningfulness *(M)* (for our purposes of an occupation), drive *(D)* [to engage in an occupation], and sense of efficacy *(E)*. Based on that proposition, and assuming that drive is a function of meaningfulness, we can develop a method of measuring meaningfulness and sense of efficacy. If we let drive *(D)* to perform an occupation *(P)* equal the meaningfulness score *(M)* multiplied by the efficacy score *(E)*, we can visualize facilitation of change as follows:

$$D = M \times E$$

If we calculate and document D over time, we can observe a change in D over time (ΔD) that corresponds to a change in P over time (ΔP). Let us suppose that ΔD and ΔP have hypothetical values of 3.3 each, and the values D_t and P_t are 0.2 each. Using the logistic quadratic equation for complex, dynamic systems [$D_{t+1} = \Delta D_t(1 - D_t)$] and [$P_{t+1} = \Delta P_t(1 - P_t)$], respectively, we can iterate values of D and P. The iterations would lead to values similar to the ones shown in Table 4-2 with both drive D_{t+1} and occupational performance P_{t+1} forming self-similar stable, steady state systems of period 2, each oscillating between 0.823…and 0.479…We can hypothesize that as ΔD and ΔP increase, the values would eventually reach a threshold, leading to new patterns of D and P values, respectively.

Since we can measure performance *(P)* (e.g., by documenting frequency of engagement in occupations (refer to Ikiugu and Rosso[28] Chapter 8 of the Laboratory Manual) and Drive *(D)* [by multiplying Meaningfulness score *(M)* with Efficacy score *(E)* as measured for instance using Likert-type scales], we can theoretically identify the critical values of ΔD and ΔP that result in sudden, rapid change, and higher levels of self-organization. Such ability would be useful in helping clients to develop increasing adaptive capabilities as required. Helping clients develop adaptive capabilities would in turn be consistent

 with the construct of instrumentalism that we saw might be a useful philosophical construct in occupational therapy.

Following is a summary of how complexity/chaos theory may be used to understand and guide occupational therapy clinical practice[36] (see also Okes'[42] discussion of how similar principles would be applied in business):

1. In order to facilitate change of the client from a maladaptive to a complex, dynamical, adaptive system, the therapist should strive to create attractor conditions. One way to do this may be by helping the client clarify what is important in his or her life, or what is worth doing or pursuing.[25,27] This sense of purpose in life would create meaningfulness of chosen occupations, thus serving as a basin of attraction that would structure the client's occupational life trajectory so that it moves generally toward a more adaptive direction.

2. The therapist should avoid trying to control the client. Instead, provide rules to help the system move toward a desired general direction. Such rules may include that the client will commit to engaging in at least two occupations per week that are meaningful to him or her and that will help him or her move closer to achievement of a visualized future life.

3. The therapist should offer and create opportunities for the environment to provide timely feedback (perturbations) to the client. This may be achieved by creating what Lazzarini calls "occupational crisis and dynamic instabilities" (p. 349),[36] which means pushing the client away from the steady, stable state, or in common language, the comfort zone. For instance, if you are working with a student who is about to graduate high school, providing opportunities for the student to obtain information regarding career opportunities would provide the necessary small nudges that may lead to the student eventually deciding to choose and commit to a career path.

4. Number 3 above also indicates the need for the therapist to rely on small, timely, perturbations

as a means of creating a chance for sudden, rapid, systemic change, due to recursive feedback. Thus discussing career issues of concern with a group of students who are about to graduate high school would make it possible to input little pieces of information at strategic times, and allow the information to reverberate within the group, thus magnifying the effect (in this case, motivation to commit to a career path).

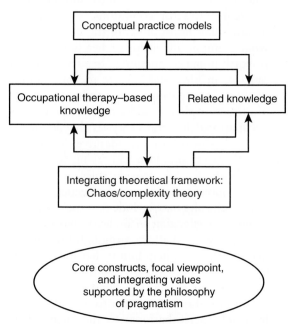

Figure 4-4. Proposed anatomy (structure) of the new occupational therapy paradigm. At the base of the paradigm, forming the foundation of the profession, are the core constructs, focal viewpoint, and integrating values derived from the philosophy of pragmatism. Next to the foundation is the complexity/chaos theory, which forms the integrating theoretical framework to help explain, operationalize, and apply the philosophical constructs. This theoretical framework is strengthened by knowledge from occupational therapy literature and related disciplines, such as anatomy, psychology, and so on. Conceptual practice models are the tools for application of occupational therapy knowledge in clinical practice.

In general, practice based on complexity/chaos theoretical framework would aim at facilitating emergence of the client's adaptive capability by presenting occupations that challenge problem-solving skills. This overarching goal is consistent with pragmatic philosophical principles that emphasize active participation (agency), doing, and using the mind as a tool to help one adapt to the environment (instrumentalism).

SUMMARY

In this chapter, we discussed the contemporary paradigm of occupational therapy, the structure of the paradigm, and its articulation in the new AOTA Practice Framework. The new paradigm focuses primarily on an occupation-based, client-centered, collaborative intervention process, where the overarching goal is to facilitate engagement in meaningful occupation to enable participation in life. The role of the therapist in the new paradigm is fourfold: (1) providing opportunities for engagement in meaningful occupations, (2) providing environmental modification, (3) providing assistive devices, and (4) providing education and counseling in order to facilitate occupational performance. Pragmatism has been identified and discussed as the philosophical foundation of the new paradigm, and it has been argued that complexity/chaos theory may be the most appropriate scientific framework for the paradigm. The paradigm of occupational therapy is illustrated in Figure 4-4.

REFERENCES

1. American Occupational Therapy Association: Occupational therapy practice framework: domain and process, *Am J Occup Ther* 56(6):609-639, 2002.
2. Arndt M, Bigelow B: The potential of chaos theory and complexity theory for health services management [Electronic version], *Health Care Management Review* 25:35-41, 2000. Retrieved July 2002, from the Proquest database.
3. Bandura A: *Social learning theory,* New York, 1977, General Learning Press.
4. Bassingthwaighte JB, Liebovich LS, West BJ: *Fractal physiology,* New York, 1994, Oxford University Press.

5. Bell IR, Baldwin CM, Schwartz GE: Alternative therapies in health and medicine [Electronic version], *Aliso Viejo* 8:58-66, 2002. Retrieved July 2002, from the Proquest database.
6. Bird A: Thomas Kuhn [electronic version]. In Zalta EN, ed: *The Stanford encyclopedia of philosophy, 2005.* Retrieved August 2005, from http://plato.stanford.edu/archives/spr2005/entries/thomas-kuhn/.
7. Brack CJ, Brack G: How chaos and complexity theory can help counselors to be more effective, *Counseling and Values* 39:1-7, 1995.
8. Breines E: *Origins and adaptations: a philosophy of practice,* Lebanon, NJ, 1986, Geri-Rehab.
9. Buell M, Cassidy D: The complex and dynamic nature of quality in early care and educational programs: a case for chaos [Electronic version], *J Res Childhood Educ* 15:209-219, 2001.
10. Crutchfield J, Farmer J, Parkard N, et al: There is order in chaos: randomness has an underlying geometric form. Chaos imposes fundamental limits on prediction, but it also suggests causal relationships where none were previously suspected. In Russell R, Murphy N, Peacocke S, eds: *Chaos and complexity: scientific perspectives on divine action,* Berkeley, CA, 1995, The Center for Theology and the Natural Sciences, pp. 35-48.
11. Cutchin MP: Using Deweyan philosophy to rename and reframe adaptation-to-environment, *Am J Occup Ther* 58:303-312, 2004.
12. Darwin C: *The origin of species by means of natural selection,* New York, 1985, Penguin Books.
13. Detweiler J, Peyton C: Defining occupations: a chronotopic study of narrative genres in a health discipline's emergence, *Written Communication* 16(4):412-468, 1999.
14. Dewey J: *Reconstruction in philosophy,* Boston, 1957, Beacon Press.
15. Dewey J: The influence of Darwinism on philosophy. In McDermott JJ, ed: *The philosophy of John Dewey: two volumes in one,* Chicago, 1981, University of Chicago Press, pp. 31-41.
16. Dewey J: The construction of good. In Fisch MH, ed: *Classic American philosophers,* New York, 1996, Fordham University Press, pp. 360-381.
17. Fisch MH, ed: *Classic American philosophers,* New York, 1996, Fordham University Press.
18. Gritzer G, Arluke A: *The making of rehabilitation: a political economy of medical specialization—1890-1980,* Los Angeles, 1985, University of California Press.
19. Haase B: Clinical interpretation of occupationally embedded exercise versus rote exercise: a choice between occupational forms by elderly nursing home residents, *Am J Occup Ther* 49:403-404, 1995.
20. Hergenhahn BR: *An introduction to the history of psychology,* ed 3, Albany, NY, 1997, Brooks/Cole.
21. Hooper B, Wood W: Pragmatism and structuralism in occupational therapy: the long conversation, *Am J Occup Ther* 56:40-49, 2002.
22. Ikiugu MN: *The philosophy and culture of occupational therapy, doctoral dissertation, 2001,* Texas Woman's University, Dissertation Abstracts International 62(12B):5678, 2001.
23. Ikiugu MN: Instrumentalism in occupational therapy: an argument for a pragmatic conceptual model of practice, *Internat J Psychosocial Rehabil* 8:108-117, 2004.
24. Ikiugu MN: Instrumentalism in occupational therapy: a theoretical core for the pragmatic conceptual model of practice, *Internat J Psychosocial Rehabil* 8:150-162, 2004.
25. Ikiugu MN: Instrumentalism in occupational therapy: guidelines for practice, *Internat J Psychosocial Rehabil* 8:164-177, 2004.
26. Ikiugu MN: Meaningfulness of occupations as an occupational-life-trajectory attractor, *J Occup Sci* 12:102-109, 2005.
27. Ikiugu MN, Ciaravino AE: Assisting adolescents with emotional and behavioral difficulties (EBD) transition to adulthood, Manuscript submitted for publication, 2006.
28. Ikiugu MN, Rosso HM: Understanding the occupational human being as a complex, dynamical, adaptive system, *Occup Ther in Health Care* 19(4):43-65, 2005.
29. Ikiugu MN, Schultz S: An argument for pragmatism as a foundational philosophy of occupational therapy, *Canad J Occup Ther* 73(2):86-97, 2006.
30. James W: Habit: its importance for psychology. In McDermott JJ, ed: *The writings of William James: a comprehensive edition,* Chicago, 1977, University of Chicago Press, pp. 9-21.
31. Joe BE: 50 years an occupational therapist and still going strong: Gail Fidler, *OT Week* 22-23, 1995.
32. Kielhofner G: *Model of human occupation: theory and application,* ed 3, Philadelphia, 2002, Lippincott Williams & Wilkins.
33. Kielhofner G: *Conceptual foundations of occupational therapy,* ed 3, Philadelphia, 2004, FA Davis.
34. Kielhofner G, Burke JP: Occupational therapy after 60 years: an account of changing identity and knowledge, *Am J Occup Ther* 31:675-689, 1977.
35. Kuhn T: *The structure of scientific revolutions,* ed 2, Chicago, 1973, University of Chicago Press.
36. Lazzarini I: Neuro-occupation: the nonlinear dynamics of intention, meaning and perception, *Br J Occup Ther* 67(8):342-352, 2004.
37. Maslow AH: *Motivation and personality,* ed 2, New York, 1970, Harper & Row.
38. McColl MA: Introduction: a basis for theory in occupational therapy. In McColl MA, Law M, Stewart D, et al,

ed: *Theoretical basis of occupational therapy,* Thorofare, NJ, 2003, Slack, pp. 1-6.

39. McDermott JJ, ed: *The philosophy of John Dewey: two volumes in one,* Chicago, 1981, University of Chicago Press.

40. Mendenhall M, Macomber J, Curtright M: Mary Parker Follet: prophet of chaos and complexity [Electronic version], *J Management History* 6:191-207, 2000.

41. Mouck T: Capital markets research and real world complexity: the emerging challenge of chaos theory, *Accounting Organization Soc* 23:189-215, 1998.

42. Okes D: Complexity theory simplifies choices, *Quality Progress* 36(7):35-37, 2003.

43. Peirce CS: The fixation of belief. In Buchler J, ed: *Philosophical writings of Peirce,* New York, 1955, Dover Publications, pp. 5-22.

44. Persson D, Erlandsson L, Eklund M, et al: Value dimensions, meaning, and complexity in human occupation—a tentative structure for analysis, *Scand J Occup Ther* 8:7-18, 2001.

45. Pratt CW, Gill KJ, Barrett NM, et al: *Psychiatric rehabilitation,* New York, 2002, Academic Press.

45a. Prigogine I: *The end of certainty,* New York, 1997, Simon & Schuster

46. Quiroga VA: *Occupational therapy: the first 30 years—1900 to 1930,* Bethesda, MD, 1995, AOTA.

47. Reed K, Sanderson SN: *Concepts of occupational therapy,* ed 4, New York, 1999, Lippincott Williams & Wilkins.

48. Rogers CR: A current formulation of client-centered therapy, *Social Service Review* 24:442-450, 1950.

49. Royeen CB: Chaotic occupational therapy: collective wisdom for a complex profession, *Am J Occup Ther* 57:609-624, 2003.

50. Sabonis-Chafee B, Hussey S: *Introduction to occupational therapy,* St Louis, 1998, Mosby.

51. Schkade J, Schultz S: Occupational adaptation: toward a holistic approach for contemporary practice, part 1, *Am J Occup Ther* 46:829-837, 1992.

52. Schultz S, Schkade J: Occupational adaptation: toward a holistic approach for contemporary practice, part 2, *Am J Occup Ther* 46:917-925, 1992.

53. Underwood M: *Introductory models and basic concepts: complexity,* 2005. Retrieved from http://www.cultsock.ndirect.co.uk/MUHome/cshtml/introductory/complex.html.

54. United States Surgeon General: *Mental health: a report of the Surgeon General,* 2005. Retrieved May 2005, from http://www.surgeongeneral.gov/library/mentalhealth/home.html.

55. van Atta K, Roby DS, Roby R: *Friends hospital: an account of the events surrounding the origin of Friends hospital and a brief description of the early years of Friends asylum 1817–1829,* 1988. Retrieved June 2005 from http://www.friendshospitalonline.org/eventsaccount.htm

56. von Bertalanffy L: General systems theory and psychiatry. In Arieti S, ed: *American handbook of psychiatry,* vol. 3, New York, 1966, Basic Books, pp. 705-721.

57. Waldrop MM: *Complexity: the emerging science at the edge of order and chaos,* New York, 1992, Simon & Schuster.

58. Warren K, Franklin C, Streeter CL: New directions in systems theory: chaos and complexity, *Social Work* 43:357-372, 1998.

59. White M: *Pragmatism and the American mind: essays and reviews in philosophy and intellectual history,* New York, 1973, Oxford University Press.

60. Wilcock AA: *An occupational perspective of health,* Thorofare, NJ, 1998, Slack.

PART III

General Practice Considerations in Psychosocial Occupational Therapy

In Parts I and II of this book, the proposed conceptual foundation of psychosocial occupational therapy was established. In Part III, we will discuss general practice skills and techniques used by occupational therapists. By general practice skills we mean intervention techniques that are the basis of practice and that every occupational therapist uses, irrespective of the chosen conceptual practice model. We will discuss intervention using specific conceptual practice models in Part IV. In Part III, we will discuss general practice skills and techniques, including client assessment, clinical reasoning and treatment planning, and general intervention techniques. The reader should refer to Chapters 6 to 9 of the Laboratory Manual for specific exercises to help him or her practice and master the skills and techniques discussed in this part of the book.

Chapter 5

Client Evaluation

Preview Questions

1. What is the difference between evaluation and assessment?
2. How is medical chart review used in the process of client evaluation in psychosocial occupational therapy?
3. Why is it important that occupational therapists understand the DSM-IV-TR diagnostic categories?
4. Discuss the importance of the initial interview in setting the foundation for a good therapeutic relationship.
5. Discuss the difference between standardized and nonstandardized assessment instruments.
6. Should occupational therapists use nonstandardized instruments in assessing clients? Explain.
7. Discuss how the occupational therapy paradigm guides the process of client evaluation.

According to the American Occupational Therapy Association (AOTA), *evaluation* refers to the process of gathering information about occupations or activities of daily living that are problematic to the client.[3] It is a more broad process of information gathering; *assessment* refers to the use of specific strategies and tools to gather this information.[8,9,27] The evaluation process includes use of interviews, observation, and standardized and nonstandardized instru-ments to gather information so that problem areas in occupational functioning are identified and a treatment plan established.

This process is crucial to appropriate therapy because it is difficult to institute meaningful interventions without accurate information about the client's interests, desires, aspirations, and functional status. It is also important to remember that the evaluation process is driven by the profession's paradigm, as discussed in Chapter 4. The paradigm defines the core constructs, focal viewpoint, and integrating values shared by members of the profession[13]; therefore, it is used in the evaluation process. For example, in the current occupational therapy paradigm, core constructs include the view of therapy as occupation-based, client-centered, and collaborative.[4,13] Meaningful occupation is seen as an integral part of good quality of life. Therefore, the client's engagement in occupation to enhance participation in life is valued. The evaluation process driven by the new professional paradigm should involve use of assessment instruments and techniques that are occupation-based, address occupational performance needs, and encourage collaboration with the client. In this chapter, we will discuss the various aspects of this evaluation process briefly and in general terms. Later, we will explore specific applications when the conceptual models of practice are expounded.

Gathering Information from the Client's Chart

Not all occupational therapy clients have a medical chart. Charts are relevant in the rehabilitation of clients within the medical model (those seen in institutional medical care facilities). For those seen in the community, school system, work settings, and so on, the medical model is not applicable.[6] For such clients, there are no charts to review. For clients in medical institutions, once a referral to treat is received, the first task is to review the chart and gather pertinent information related to the referral.[9,25] The therapist notes the documented diagnosis and any necessary precautions, as well as details of the history of the illness. In order to read and interpret information in the chart accurately, the therapist needs to be familiar with the *Diagnostic and Statistical Manual of Mental Disorders—Text Revision* (DSM-IV-TR),[5] which psychiatrists use to make the diagnoses.

The Diagnostic and Statistical Manual of Mental Disorders

Attempts to develop a *nosological* system of classifying diseases date back to 1891, when the International Statistical Institute developed *Classification of Causes of Death*.[32] In 1948, after several revisions, the document became the *International Classification of Diseases, Injuries, and Causes of Death*. In 1965, WHO experts met in Geneva and revised the manual. The product was the seventh edition of the *International Classification of Diseases* (ICD). The ICD-9 was published in 1975, and the current edition, the ICD-10, was published in 1992.

The first edition of the *Diagnostic and Statistical Manual of Mental Disorders* (DSM) was published by the American Psychiatric Association in 1952.[6] The second edition was published in 1968, coinciding with the eighth edition of the ICD. These two initial editions were highly influenced by the psychodynamic approach to mental health, with the cause of mental illness seen as originating from environmental experiences, especially in the early years of life. Classification in these editions simply placed mental illnesses into two categories: psychosis (characterized by loss of touch with reality) and neurosis (where reality is distorted but the individual is not completely severed from it). In the 1980s, the DSM-III was published, coinciding with the ICD-9. This edition was based on a biomedical model and clearly distinguished between normal and abnormal behavior. However, it was atheoretical because it offered no theory of etiology but simply provided taxonomy of clinical conditions and their features.[6] Clinical features in this edition were hierarchical, based on the assumption that symptoms higher in the hierarchy were found in the lower hierarchies but not vice-versa.

Research challenged the assumption of hierarchical arrangement of symptoms. This resulted in the publication of subsequent editions (the DSM-III-R and DSM-IV) in 1987 and 1994, respectively. The later editions (DSM-III to IV) were originally intended for research in mental health. However, they became tools for diagnosis of mental illness. In the 1990s, there was strong consensus that the diagnostic system used in the United States should be compatible with the *International Classification of Diseases*, tenth edition (ICD-10), which was used in Europe and much of the rest of the world.[24] Thus the DSM-IV-TR was published to achieve this objective.[5,6]

Characteristics

The DSM is not a textbook of psychiatry. Rather, it is a system of classification of psychiatric disorders into nosological categories, according to described clinical features. It does not offer a theory of etiology or explain the pathological processes involved in mental illness.[6] Diagnostic criteria are listed along with clinical features necessary for a diagnosis. In other words, it offers the minimum criteria required for diagnosis of each mental disorder. It also offers a systematic description of epidemiological factors associated with a condition such as age, gender, prevalence, incidence, and other related factors.[5] In the DSM, a multi-axial system of diagnosis is used, where diagnostic categories are classified into five axes.[5,24]

Axis I diagnoses consist of clinical psychiatric disorders or other conditions that may be of clinical focus such as schizophrenia, eating disorders, dissociative disorders, impulse-control disorders, and so on. Axis II diagnoses are personality disorders and mental retardation. They include paranoid personality disorder, schizoid personality disorder, borderline personality disorder, mental retardation, and so on. Axis III diagnoses consist of physical disorders and general medical conditions that a client may have in addition to the mental disorder(s), such as diabetes mellitus, CAD, COPD, and so on. Axis IV diagnoses consist of psychosocial and environmental factors that cause stress and exacerbate the mental disorder, such as divorce or other relationship problems, loss of a job, death in the family,

relocation to a new place, and so on. Axis V diagnosis is referred to as the Global Assessment of Function (GAF).

Psychiatrists' acknowledged that psychiatric diagnoses were not well-linked to function, so Axis V diagnosis was established to provide this link.[6] For Axis V diagnosis to be made, the client's overall level of functioning, including danger to self and others, relationship issues, prediction of remission (based on the number of rehospitalizations), employment history and current employability, and ability to take care of self are assessed. This assessment might be used by occupational therapists as a starting point for further evaluation, leading to subsequent treatment planning.

Occupational Therapy Implications

The following case description will be used to demonstrate how understanding of the DSM-IV-TR diagnosis would help a therapist form a hypothesis of possible functional limitations of the client.

CASE STUDY: FRANCINE

Francine is a 17-year-old female who lives at home with her biological parents. She is the oldest of five children. Her mother is a recovering alcoholic who has been sober for 10 years and regularly attends Alcoholic Anonymous (AA) meetings. Francine's father goes on drinking binges, especially when he is unemployed. During such times, he tends to become violent. Francine's mother then takes Francine and her two brothers and two sisters to a shelter for battered women. When her father gets another job, Francine's mother and the children usually move back home. This cycle of events has been occurring for as long as Francine can remember.

Recently, Francine's father lost his job, which led to increased tension in the family as usually happens during such times. Francine's mother has threatened to leave him if he starts drinking again.

In recent weeks, Francine has become increasingly irritable with her brothers and sisters and has lost interest in her usual activities such as going to the movies, visiting the mall, and hanging out with her friends. She states that she feels worthless and often stays up late, sometimes up to 3:00 A.M. watching television. When she's not in school, Francine watches television and does nothing else. Her dog died four years ago. On the latest anniversary of her dog's death, Francine attempted to commit suicide by ingesting a bottle of sleeping pills. She was hospitalized with a diagnosis of depression with suicidal tendencies.

Normally, Francine is an average student both in academics and sports. She has poor problem-solving skills and tends to blame other people for all her problems. Just before her suicide attempt and subsequent hospitalization, her boyfriend

CASE STUDY: FRANCINE—CONT'D

ended a relationship with her and started dating her best friend. She verbalizes that she feels rejected by both her friend and her boyfriend. Neither of them talks to her any more.

Upon reviewing Francine's chart, the therapist notices the following information from the admitting note.

Diagnoses:

Axis I—Depression with suicidal tendencies.

Axis IV—Increased tension in the family, recent breakup with her boyfriend, loss of her best friend, anniversary of her dog's death.

Axis V—Lacks skills to cope with family and other stressors, loss of interest in usual activities, poor problem-solving skills, inability to take responsibility for her life, may injure herself.

From this diagnostic information, it is apparent that precautions are needed while working with Francine in the occupational therapy department because of the possibility of Francine using tools

in the department to attempt to commit suicide. It is also clear that she needs to learn coping skills, which indicates that she may benefit from social skills and assertiveness training groups. The therapist needs to help her modify her thinking processes that lead to self-depreciation and sense of worthlessness. This can be done using challenging occupations that she can complete successfully, with esthetically pleasing outcomes. Engagement in such occupations can be combined with disputing those thought processes that lead to negative feelings. Her success in producing esthetically pleasing occupational products can be used as evidence for the need to question the validity of her self-denigrating thoughts. Therefore, from the diagnoses, especially Axis I, III, IV, and V diagnoses, the therapist can form a fairly good hypothesis of the nature of indicated therapeutic intervention for the client. However, the therapist must bear in mind that this is only a hypothesis.

It is important for a therapist to maintain an open mind when meeting a client, so that he or she can objectively assess the client's problems firsthand. Information gathered from the client's chart, however, helps focus this assessment.

Other Important Information from the Client's Chart

The client's psychiatric history is also found in the admission note. In the psychiatric evaluation, a detailed history is usually taken, covering the areas listed in Box 5-1.[12,24]

From this history, the therapist is primarily interested in the chief complaint and, particularly, what the client views as the reason for hospitalization. This information can help the therapist make preliminary prediction of a possible outcome of therapy. For instance, the outcome of therapy for a client who states that he was hospitalized because his wife wanted to

get rid of him, and he has no problem, is more guarded than one who states that he is hospitalized because he failed to take his medications

Box 5-1	Areas Covered in a Detailed History

- Identifying data such as name, age, marital status, gender, and occupation
- Chief complaint or primary reason for hospitalization
- History of present illness from onset to hospitalization
- Past illnesses and hospitalizations, how long hospitalized, and the outcome of each hospitalization
- Family history
- Personal history including past experiences, relationships, and so on, and how they relate to the present illness
- Regimen of medications, both past and current

and has difficulty controlling his anxiety. The first client has no insight and sees no need for therapy; if he does not develop insight, the outcome will not be successful. This does not mean that he cannot be treated. It is possible that the therapist can help him develop insight and invest himself in the therapeutic process. However, it will be an uphill task. The second client already sees the need for change; therefore it will be easier to treat him.

Information about past history of an illness is also important because it indicates to the therapist the client's pattern of coping, the coping skills that have been used in the past and how successful they have been, and the coping abilities that the client needs to develop. Finally, information about the client's educational background and occupational and work history can be gleaned from the social worker's note. Nurses' notes can offer clues regarding how the client is coping in the hospital, and thus indicate what needs to be addressed in therapy.

Client's Initial Interview

Once the therapist has reviewed the chart and gathered preliminary information, it is time to contact the client for screening.[17,18,25] The initial contact is crucial because it is the beginning of a therapeutic relationship. It is the time when the therapist begins establishing rapport by communicating to the client understanding, empathy, and respect.[23] Therefore the therapist needs to be conscious of how this first introduction is conducted. The session usually takes place in the client's room, although it may also be at the occupational therapy clinic (or office in case of community-based interventions). Irrespective of where the interview is conducted, the therapist needs to be respectful to the client. This respect, as mentioned above, is communicated by being sincere, empathetic, understanding, supportive, and nonjudgmental.[7,10,22]

Before the interview begins, the therapist should make sure that the environment is conducive to the interview. For example, the client should be com-

fortable. If the interview is conducted in the client's room, the therapist should be seated on a chair (not the client's bed) in a location where he or she can easily be seen and heard.[7] Other factors to consider when planning an interview environment include the possibility of interruption by the phone ringing, noise from outside the interview room, the possibility of the conversation being overheard by unauthorized individuals, and so on.[23]

Also, the interview should be conducted at a time that is conducive to the client. Some clients perform better in the morning rather than in the afternoon. It may be necessary to visit the client several times before completing the initial interview in order to determine the time when you can obtain the most accurate representation of his or her mood, performance, and so on. During the first contact with the client, the therapist should begin by introducing himself or herself and stating his or her role in the treatment of the client.[7,9] To illustrate with Francine's case described above, a brief initial screening interview may go as follows:

Therapist: Good evening, Ms. Daniels. My name is Mary. Your doctor has ordered occupational therapy for you, and I will be your therapist. Would you prefer that I call you Francine or Ms. Daniels?

Client: Francine is fine.

Therapist: Okay, Francine. I'd like to talk to you for a few minutes to find out how occupational therapy may be of help to you. This won't take more than 15 minutes. Okay?

Client: Fine.

Therapist: By the way, I would like to commend you on your taste in fashion. I like the way you have chosen a sweater to match your top and jeans in such a subtle way. Very stylish.

Client: Thank you.

Therapist: Now, have you had occupational therapy before?

Client: No. I haven't met an occupational therapist before. What is occupational therapy?

Therapist: Occupational therapists help people who may have lost the ability to do daily things they enjoy doing, or need to be able to do, so that they are able to do those things again. People lose the ability to do things they enjoy doing or need to do every day because they have either been injured, are ill, or have lost the desire and feel that they do not have energy to do those things. Have you ever felt that way?

Client: I feel that way right now. I used to go to the movies, visit with friends, talk to my friends over the phone…I don't feel like doing any of those things anymore. My best friend recently stole my boyfriend…the slut. I used to do a lot of things with both of them. Now, I don't have anybody to do anything with. I'm so terrible and people can't stand me.

Therapist: You feel sad because you think that you are a horrible person and people can't stand you?

Client: Yes. Even dad can't stand me. That's why he is so mean to mom. It's because of me.

Therapist: I understand that you are saying people can't stand you because you are a horrible person, and that makes you feel sad. But I don't feel that you are a horrible person. I actually have a feeling that you are a very nice person, and the nurses seem to think so as well. Ms. Green at the nursing station was just telling me how you are such a sweet young woman.

Client: Well, I don't know.

Therapist: Would you like to be able to go to the movies and do other things with your friends again?

Client: Yes, but I know it won't happen.

Therapist: How about we give it a shot? Occupational therapists such as I help people just like you be able to do just what you say you would like to be able to do. What do you think? Shall we try and see how it works?

Client: Okay.

Therapist: Francine, I'm glad to hear that. I look forward to working with you to see what we can do together. I'll meet you tomorrow morning at the occupational therapy department. Ms. Green will bring you over. At that time, I'll complete an evaluation to help us find out what your needs are, and what skills you have to help you do the things you want to be able to do. The evaluation will take about one hour. Together, we will make goals. On Friday, we'll start working to help you achieve those goals. Do you have any questions?

Client: (After a few seconds) No. No questions.

Therapist: All right then, Francine. See you tomorrow morning. It's been really nice talking to you.

Client: Bye.

Notice how the therapist introduced herself in the above dialogue. She asked the client, right from the beginning, how she would like to be addressed. This is a sign of respect. The therapist then explained who she was and why she was there. She explained what occupational therapy was and how it could help the client (what Peloquin[19] calls developing a *therapy set*). The therapist communicated with sincerity, was genuinely attentive to the client's concerns, and was not judgmental. Consistent with the client-centered collaborative approach advocated in the new occupational therapy paradigm, she followed the client's process rather than trying to establish an agenda. She allowed the client to state, in her own words, what she perceived to be her problems. She demonstrated understanding by responding both to the content of what the client said as well as to the feeling associated with that content. She also paraphrased the client's statements to bring clarity to them. She gave the client a chance to ask questions or to seek clarification. When the interview was over, she explained what was going to happen next (that evaluation was going to be completed next day, and therapy would begin soon after that). Her communication skills, therefore, helped her gain Francine's trust, which is a big step in establishing a therapeutic relationship.

Other Suggestions for Conducting a Successful Initial Interview

Sometimes it is not easy for a client to talk about personal details, especially if they involve information that he or she perceives to be embarrassing.[7,9,17] It is important that the therapist makes the client feel as comfortable as possible, including conducting the interview in a place where it will not be overheard. As mentioned above, the therapist should also make sure that he or she can be heard clearly and seen by the client. Another important clue is that the therapist should be attentive to how he or she feels during interaction with the client. Sometimes the therapist's feelings, especially if unexpectedly strong, may be an indication of what the client is feeling. For instance, when the therapist feels as if he or she is on edge for no good reason, this may be an indication that the client is probably feeling anxious. Noticing such clues is helpful in conducting the interview in such a way that the client feels understood and respected, leading to a sense of trust.

Many times the therapist needs to take notes because it is not possible to accurately remember all the details of an interview. It is important to explain to the client beforehand that notes will be taken during the interview and the reason for taking those notes. Note taking should not interfere with the interview process. Only key words should be jotted down to help the therapist remember what transpires in the interview. The content of the session should then be transcribed as soon as the interview is over, before the therapist forgets important details. The same interview process should be used during the client's evaluation and reassessment.

Observation

During the initial interview and throughout the therapeutic process, the therapist observes both the content and process of interaction.[21] Observation of content means noting what is said, the client's tone of voice, language used, compulsive talking, attention-seeking self-expression, expression of interest, avoidance of issues, and self-disclosure. For example, if you are talking to a client about the events that led to admission (e.g., loss of a loved one, violence) and the client keeps changing the subject and talking about the nice people in the hospital, this may indicate that he or she is avoiding the topic at hand. Avoidance usually indicates that the issue being discussed is either uncomfortable or too painful. Similarly, a client who continually describes himself or herself as helpless or constantly apologizes may be seeking the therapist's attention by playing a helpless person. The client's tone of voice may indicate anger or anxiety irrespective of whether he or she states the opposite of those feelings.

Content observation may be enhanced by the therapist using a sensory grounded structural framework to increase efficiency of observation. The framework may include auditory, visual, affective, relationship, and attitudinal cues, among other things. Auditory cues include what is said, tone of voice, and so on, as discussed above. Visual cues include noting the client's facial expression, posture, gestures, and so on. For example, slouching may indicate tiredness or depression, while wringing of hands may be an indication of anxiety. Sitting on the edge of the chair may suggest that the client is uncomfortable. The affective component of observation includes noting the ability of the client to share emotions and the appropriateness of both verbal and nonverbal expression. Relationship cues include how comfortable or close you feel to the client. If you feel apprehensive, it may mean that trust has not been established, and both you and the client are guarded. This would suggest that you still need to think of ways to bring down the walls between you and the client. Attitudinal cues include a general appraisal of the client's view of world issues and concerns. Some people tend to be generally optimistic, while others are invariably pessimistic. Determine the category in which your client falls.

Throughout the evaluation process, the therapist also observes the client and notes important clues that may indicate functional problems and possible indications for therapeutic interventions. As mentioned above, some of the cues to be noted are nonverbal signals such as body posture, movement, gestures, facial expression, type of clothes worn, and grooming.[7,9,17] Other behaviors that can be observed include the client's interaction with other clients, values, interests, skills, patterns, routines, strengths, and limitations. These clues are deduced from the client's choice of activities, performance, and interaction with others in the occupational therapy department.[17,20]

Assessment

Apart from interview and observation, the therapist completes the occupational therapy evaluation using specific assessments. Part of client observation is done using assessment tools to guide what is being observed. The interview is also part of assessment since an assessment is defined as a "Critical appraisal of client's functional abilities in every day tasks. [It] includes clinical observations, tests, facility-generated procedures, and client interviews" (p. 244).[27] Some assessments are standardized, and others are nonstandardized.[9,17,27] A standardized assessment has an established procedure for administration, and research has been conducted to establish its validity and reliability. Examples of standardized instruments include the Kohlman Evaluation of Living Skills (KELS),[29] the Canadian Occupational Performance Measure (COPM),[15] the Bay Area Functional Performance Evaluation (BFPE),[14] and the Stress Management Questionnaire,[26] among others.

According to Mosey, the choice of assessment instrument depends on the frame(s) of reference (called *conceptual practice models* in this book) chosen to guide therapy for a particular client.[17] For example, a client who has intact cognitive skills but feels a general sense of meaninglessness

may be treated using the Canadian Client-Centered Occupational Performance Model, in which case the COPM would be used to complete the assessment. Similarly, a client with cognitive deficits may benefit from intervention guided primarily using Allen's Cognitive Disabilities Model, which would necessitate the use of the Allen Cognitive Level Screening tool (ACLS) and/or the Allen Diagnostic Module (ADM) as data-gathering instruments.[1,2]

We will discuss these assessments in detail in subsequent chapters in which the corresponding conceptual practice models will be expounded. It is important to point out that a single conceptual practice model does not often address all the client's problems (see Chapter 17 for a discussion of how conceptual practice models are integrated in practice). Therefore it is necessary to use a combination of conceptual practice models as indicated by the needs of a specific client. A therapist will often use as many assessment instruments as the conceptual models chosen to address the client's problems.

Nonstandardized instruments include unstructured clinical observations with no developed protocols of administration, or instruments whose reliability and validity has not been established through research. Facility-specific assessments are often nonstandardized instruments. Therapists are encouraged to use standardized assessment tools as much as possible in order to ensure accuracy and validity of client evaluation.[17,27] However, this does not mean that nonstandardized instruments are not useful. A therapist can still gather important information that may prove useful in guiding treatment planning using these tools. Furthermore, there are good assessment tools that have not been rigorously standardized through research or are in the initial stages of the process (for example, the Assessment and Intervention Instrument for Instrumentalism in Occupational Therapy[11]). Although these instruments are useful even though they have not been standardized, the therapist needs to corroborate the data gathered using them with standardized tools in order to establish their concurrent validity.

Finally, as mentioned earlier, the process of evaluation and assessment must be completed in such a way that it is consistent with the profession's prevailing paradigm. This means that from the initial contact and throughout the evaluation process, the client must be involved collaboratively as an equal partner in the process. In this regard, the AOTA unequivocally states that "the evaluation process is focused on finding out what the client wants and needs to do and on identifying those factors that act as supports or barriers to performance." Further, "During the evaluation, a collaborative relationship with the client is established that continues throughout the entire occupational therapy process" (p. 616).[4] During evaluation, the therapist must bear in mind that the whole purpose of the process is to facilitate the client's engagement in meaningful occupations for satisfactory participation in life. That is why AOTA suggests that evaluation begin with an appraisal of the client's occupational profile. The occupational profile is a person's occupational history, interests, values, needs, and experiences. For example, an occupational profile for a recently retired teacher might include a history of 30 years teaching, participation in a teacher association's political action committee, participation in car racing activities as part of his leisure pursuits, and so on. The therapist would be aware that this client values education and is interested in car racing and politics. All this information would be very useful when planning therapeutic interventions and choosing meaningful therapeutic occupations for this individual.

As the AOTA states in the practice framework, "During the process of collecting this information, the client's priorities and desired targeted outcomes that will lead to engagement in occupation to support participation in life are also identified" (p. 616).[4] Therefore, the entire evaluation process, as it is with therapy, is guided by the client-centered, collaborative, occupation-based approach to information gathering.

Also, consistent with the complexity/chaos theory perspective, the therapist should pay attention to the client's maladaptive self-similar patterns. These are the patterns that will need to be changed in therapy. For example, in Francine's case, one can already see a pattern that primarily consists of introjection of negative qualities so that she "nullifies or negates" her loss "by taking on characteristics of" (p. 60)[28] those who hurt her, such as her boyfriend, her best friend, and her father. As a result, she blames and denigrates herself for what these individuals do to her. Consequently, she loses her self-esteem and confidence and is unable to manage her life in such a way that she is able to meet her needs adequately. The therapist may surmise that Francine is stuck in a maladaptive pattern characterized by a basic need to be esteemed and accepted by others, and to esteem herself according to Maslow's hierarchy of human needs.[16] This pattern will probably need to be changed in therapy using choice meaningful occupations that pose just the right challenge to Francine coupled with timely feedback about her performance. This may help challenge her self-denigrating thoughts[30,31] so that change can occur and her response pattern can reorganize at a higher, more adaptive level.

SUMMARY

The occupational therapy evaluation process consists of reviewing the client's chart and making initial contact with the client after receiving the psychiatrist's referral to treat. We have discussed important aspects of reviewing the chart, including understanding psychiatric diagnoses based on the DSM-IV-TR criteria. Initial contact with the client is crucial because it is the beginning of a therapeutic relationship. We also covered the fundamentals of a good initial interview, including self-introduction to the client, demonstrating respect and understanding, and eliciting the client's collaboration. We also emphasized the importance of observation as part of the evaluation process. Finally, we discussed the use of both standardized and nonstandardized assessment instruments. This chapter provided a general overview in an attempt to give the occupational therapist/occupational therapy student a sense of the evaluation process. In subsequent chapters, we will discuss in detail the specific evaluation protocols associated with each conceptual practice model.

REFERENCES

1. Allen CK: *Allen cognitive level screen (ACLS): test manual,* Colchester, CT, 1998, S&S Worldwide.
2. Allen CK, Earhart CA, Blue T: *Allen diagnostic module: instruction manual,* Colchester, CT, 1993, S&S Worldwide.
3. American Occupational Therapy Association: The association: clarification for the use of the terms assessment and evaluation, *Am J Occup Ther* 49:1072-1073, 1995.
4. American Occupational Therapy Association: Occupational therapy practice framework: domain and process, *Am J Occup Ther* 56(6):609-639, 2002.
5. American Psychiatric Association: *Diagnostic and statistical manual of mental disorders—text revision,* ed 4, Washington, D.C., 2000, APA.
6. Bonder BR: *Psychopathology and function,* ed 3, Thorofare, NJ, 2004, Slack.
7. Bongiovi ME, Cournos F: Introduction to medical interviewing. In Kay J, Tasman A, Lieberman JA, eds: *Psychiatry behavioral science and clinical essentials: a companion to Tasman, Kay, Lieberman: psychiatry,* pp. 24-40, Philadelphia, 2000, Saunders.
8. Cohn ES, Schell BA, Neistadt ME: Introduction to evaluation and interviewing. In Crepeau EB, E Cohn ES, Schell BA, eds: *Willard and Spackman's occupational therapy,* ed 10, New York, 2003, Lippincott Williams & Wilkins, pp. 279-297.
9. Early MB: *Mental health concepts and techniques for the occupational therapy assistant,* ed 3, New York, 2000, Lippincott Williams & Wilkins.
10. Flaskas C: Thinking about the therapeutic relationship: emerging themes in family therapy, *New Zealand J Fam Ther* 25(1):13-20, 2004.
11. Ikiugu MN: Instrumentalism in occupational therapy: guidelines for practice, *Internat J Psychosocial Rehabil* 8:164-177, 2004.
12. Kay J, Tasman A, Lieberman JA, eds: *Psychiatry behavioral science and clinical essentials: a companion to Tasman, Kay, Lieberman: psychiatry,* Philadelphia, 2000, Saunders.
13. Kielhofner G: *Conceptual foundations of occupational therapy,* ed 3, Philadelphia, 2004, FA Davis.
14. Klyczek JP: The bay area functional performance evaluation. In Hemphill-Pearson BJ, ed: *Assessments in occupational therapy mental health: an integrative approach,* Thorofare, NJ, 1999, Slack, pp. 87-107.
15. Law M, Baptiste S, Carswell A, et al: *Canadian occupational performance measure,* Toronto, ON, 2000, CAOT Publications ACE.
16. Maslow AH: *Motivation and personality,* ed 2, New York, 1970, Harper & Row.
17. Mosey AC: *Psychosocial components of occupational therapy,* New York, 1996, Lippincott Williams & Wilkins.
18. Page M: Interviewing as an assessment tool in occupational therapy. In Hemphill-Pearson BJ, ed: *Assessments in occupational therapy mental health: an integrative approach,* Thorofare, NJ, 1999, Slack, pp. 19-39.
19. Peloquin SM: The development of an occupational therapy interview/therapy set procedure, *Am J Occup Ther* 37:457-461, 1983.
20. Pitts DB: Evaluation and assessment. In Cara E, MacRae A, eds: *Psychosocial occupational therapy: a clinical practice,* Clifton Park, NY, 2005, Thomson Delmar Learning, pp. 477-507.
21. Posthuma BW: *Small groups in counseling and therapy: process and leadership,* ed 4, Boston, 2002, Allyn & Bacon.
22. Roberts AR: Assessment, crisis intervention, and trauma treatment: the integrative ACT intervention model, *Brief Treatment Crisis Intervention* 2:1-21, 2002.
23. Sadock BJ, Sadock VA: *Kaplan and Sadock's synopsis of psychiatry: behavioral sciences/clinical psychiatry,* ed 9, New York, 2003, Lippincott Williams & Wilkins.
24. Sadock BJ, Sadock VA: *Concise textbook of clinical psychiatry,* ed 2, New York, 2004, Lippincott Williams & Wilkins.
25. Sames KM: *Documenting occupational therapy practice,* Upper Saddle River, NJ, 2005, Pearson/Prentice-Hall.
26. Stein F, Bentley DE, Natz M: Computerized assessment: the stress management questionnaire. In Hemphill-Pearson BJ, ed: *Assessments in occupational therapy mental health: an integrative approach,* Thorofare, NJ, 1999, Slack.
27. Stein F, Cutler SK: *Psychosocial occupational therapy: a holistic approach,* ed 2, Albany, NY, 2002, Delmar.
28. Stubbe DE: Psychological theories of human development and behavior. In Kay J, Tasman A, Lieberman JA, eds: *Psychiatry behavioral science and clinical essentials: a companion to Tasman, Kay, Lieberman: psychiatry,* pp. 43-85, Philadelphia, 2000, Saunders.
29. Thomson LK: The Kohlman evaluation of living skills. In Hemphill-Pearson BJ, ed: *Assessments in occupational therapy mental health: an integrative approach,* Thorofare, NJ, 1999, Slack.
30. Weinrach SG: Cognitive therapists: a dialogue with Aaron Beck, *J Couns Dev* 67:159-164, 1988.
31. Weinrach SG: Rational emotive behavior therapy: a tough-minded therapy for tender-minded profession, *J Couns Dev* 73:296-300, 1995.
32. World Health Organization: *History of the development of the ICD* [electronic version], 2005. Retrieved August 2005, from http://www.who.int/classifications/icd/historyoficd.pdf.

Chapter

6

Clinical Reasoning: Goal Setting and Treatment Planning

Preview Questions

1. What is clinical reasoning?
2. Explain how cognitive psychology may be used to explain the clinical reasoning process.
3. Discuss the following six types of clinical reasoning skills used by occupational therapists in clinical practice:
   a. Procedural/scientific
   b. Interactive
   c. Narrative
   d. Conditional
   e. Pragmatic
   f. Ethical
4. Explain the M-A-P-P model of teaching students clinical reasoning. Explain how the different types of clinical reasoning skills can be taught using this model.

Clinical reasoning refers to the process used by clinicians in medical disciplines to collect client data and use it to make decisions about treatment.[9,15] It is the process of planning, directing, performing, and reflecting on client care by the therapist.[24] More specifically, it is "the thinking, decision-making and 'know-how' that therapists use in the conduct of their work, including the way they seek information, how they interpret the client's overall situation and how they derive a 'best' course of action with a particular client" (p. 15).[16]

Clinical reasoning has been studied extensively in medicine[5,6,11]; however, these studies have focused mostly on the process of making medical diagnoses. Occupational therapy is remarkably different from medicine. The diagnostic clinical reasoning process used in medicine may not be adequate to identify occupational problems that occupational therapists try to address. This is why a study sponsored by the American Occupational Therapy Association (AOTA) and the American Occupational Therapy Foundation (AOTF) was designed "to identify the reasoning strategy that occupational therapists used to guide their practice" (p. 1007).[6]

Significance of Clinical Reasoning in Occupational Therapy

Clinical reasoning is crucial in occupational therapy because it is the means by which therapists identify clients' problems accurately and determine effective treatment protocols. The extent to which a therapist is able to use clinical reasoning skills effectively determines the quality of care given to a client.[21] Furthermore, clinical reasoning is the means by which therapists are able to translate theory into practice (and therefore conduct theory-based therapy). Therefore, it determines the difference between a professional therapist and a layperson, such as a therapists' aide.[11,17,22] It is important that occupational therapy students be equipped with clinical reasoning skills before they go out into the field as therapists.

It has been noted that clinical reasoning is difficult to teach; questions have been raised regarding whether it can even be taught at all.[25] A literature search reveals that attempts have been made to develop programs to teach medical students clinical reasoning skills. The impact of these programs has been investigated through research.[23,27] There is continuing research exploring the clinical reasoning processes of occupational therapists in a variety of settings, including the relationship between the pre-theoretical world views held by therapists and the clinical reasoning processes they use in practice,[11] the clinical reasoning of occupational therapists treating patients with spinal cord injuries,[3] and the clinical reasoning of community health occupational therapists (CHOTs) during home visit assessments.

Hinojosa and Blount[10] present thoughtful ways of facilitating learning of skills needed to apply occupations in clinical practice through creative use of case studies and a variety of exercises. They use language from the new *Occupational Therapy Practice Framework*[1] and the World Health Organization's *International Classification of Functioning, Disability, and Health*[28] to demonstrate how activities can be linked to clinical interventions through activity analysis, synthesis, and reasoning. However, few systematic approaches to teaching clinical reasoning skills per se to occupational therapy students were revealed in the literature search. Certainly, none were found that were similar to the approach suggested in this book.

In this book, it is proposed that clinical reasoning skills can be taught and should be taught in a systematic manner. A protocol for teaching occupational therapy students such skills is suggested. In this chapter, we will explore the proposed protocol as follows: we will discuss different types of clinical reasoning skills and present a model for teaching occupational therapy students clinical reasoning skills using a case study to illustrate the model. Refer to Lab Manual Exercise 7-1 to learn how to apply these skills in practice.

Clinical Reasoning Skills Used in Occupational Therapy

In studies conducted by Fleming,[6] Gillette and Mattingly,[7] and Mattingly,[14] it was found that occupational therapists primarily used four types of clinical reasoning: *procedural, interactive, narrative,* and *conditional reasoning*. These four types of clinical reasoning were used to address clients' problems at three levels: (1) physical ailment, (2) personal experiences and concerns, and (3) the client's familial, environmental, and cultural context. In later studies, procedural reasoning was renamed *scientific reasoning*,[24] and *pragmatic* and *ethical reasoning* were added.[16,20,24,26] We will discuss the six types of clinical reasoning (procedural/scientific, interactive, narrative, conditional, pragmatic, and ethical) later in this chapter.

Consider the idea that clinical reasoning is a cognitive process, which may be understood using the cognitive psychology framework.[24,25] In Chapter 3, we mentioned that Piaget,[18,19] one of the leading theorists in cognitive psychology, suggested that there were cognitive structures called *cognitive schema* underlying acts of intelligence. He proposed that an individual uses the schema to interpret information so that it makes sense and the environment is understandable. He suggested that new information is either *assimilated* to the current schema (which consists of past experiences and existing knowledge) or if the information is not compatible with the current structure, the schema is modified so that it accommodates the new knowledge. He called the later process *accommodation*. By balancing *assimilation* and *accommodation*, one is able to adapt to the environment.

Piaget's theory of cognitive structure can be applied to the clinical reasoning process. The therapist observes cues from the client's performance or context (new information) and organizes these cues into patterns. Then the therapist assimilates the patterns into the existing cognitive schema consisting of his or her theoretical knowledge and experience.[24,25] According to Hooper,[11] the therapist's clinical reasoning process is influenced in part by his or her pre-theoretical world view. We may argue that this pre-theoretical world view consists of assumptions, principles, and values that are obtained from a philosophical orientation adopted by the therapist. The philosophical framework is part of what forms the cognitive structure (schema) that the therapist uses to interpret observed clinical cues and thus understand the client's condition. Based on the discussion in Chapter 4, it can be argued that pragmatism, along with the complexity/chaos theory, should be part of the philosophical and scientific frameworks forming the therapists' clinical cognitive schema. In any case, the cognitive protocol of clinical reasoning may be conceptualized to proceed as shown in Figure 6-1.

In Figure 6-1, the therapist identifies cues through observation, which includes listening to what the client or others say. The therapist identifies patterns from these cues (e.g., Do symptoms tend to occur or get worse at certain times? Does there seem to be a sequence of presentation, such as some of them invariably occurring before others? Do they tend to occur in certain clusters?). The therapist then compares the observed pattern to the frameworks available in his or her cognitive schema. For example, a group of symptoms such as sadness, loss of interest, agitation, being tearful, guilt, and so on may remind the therapist of a cluster constituting a clinical condition labeled "depression."

The process of making sense of symptom patterns by comparing them to a conceptual framework in the cognitive schema constitutes

a reflective process, which Dewey suggested was the essence of thinking: "The material of thinking is not thoughts, but actions, facts, events, and the relations of things" (p. 156).[4] This type of thinking is what has been termed by education theorists as *thinking in action*.[8,12] It is comparable to what educationists call *dialogic reflection* in that it is essentially a process of discourse or internal dialogue with the self.[8,12,13] However, unlike the common education practice of dialogic reflection, use of reflective journaling is not mandated or commonly used in clinical reasoning, although it probably could be helpful in focusing the therapist's awareness. We will now discuss the six types of clinical reasoning.

Procedural/Scientific Reasoning

Procedural/scientific reasoning is the process by which the therapist identifies the problem by observing cues, determining patterns, and comparing to type.[6,14,16] Once the problem is identified, the therapist sets goals and establishes a treatment plan. In other words, through scientific/procedural reasoning, therapists are able to match the ensuing clinical conditions or problems with treatment procedures to address those problems.[24] The therapist answers the following questions: What is the problem and what activities or procedures can be used to address the problems resulting from the condition? The medical problem-solving process, whose focus is mainly diagnosis, utilizes this type of clinical reasoning.[2,24,25,27]

Interactive Clinical Reasoning

Through interactive clinical reasoning, the therapist is able to relate to and understand the client as a person[6,14] and thus individualize therapy

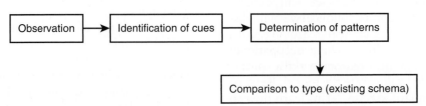

Figure 6-1. Cognitive protocol of the clinical reasoning process.

according to the needs of the client.[16] This type of clinical reasoning occurs through a dialogue with the client[20] and observation of verbal and nonverbal cues and subsequent recognition of patterns based on those cues, leading to a deeper understanding of the client as a person.

Narrative Clinical Reasoning

Narrative reasoning is based on the view of the person as a life, which denotes an attempt to understand the meaning of the condition of the individual client.[24] Stories are used in an attempt to understand the person as a unique individual. Through these stories, the therapist gets a sense of a client who has a life with continuity (a past, present, and projected future).[20] By understanding the client's story, the therapist can help him or her establish therapeutic goals that are meaningful to his or her life circumstances. Occupational performance is viewed as part of story making, contributing to the shared life stories of both the client and the therapist. Narrative reasoning is also used to help both the therapist and client project to the future and anticipate activities for the next therapy session, thus ensuring a sense of continuity of the therapeutic process. For example, in a study by Creighton and colleagues, it was found that therapists "often spent the last few minutes of each session reviewing with the patient what was accomplished and discussing follow-up activities or plans for the next day's therapy" (pp. 315-316).[3] They concluded that this event constituted therapists' use of narrative reasoning.

Conditional Reasoning

Conditional reasoning is used when the therapist thinks about "the whole condition and about the patient's possible future" (p. 313).[3] The therapist constantly pays attention to the client's current and possible future contexts.[26] In other words, the client's current status is used to conceptualize a detailed image of him or her and project this image to the future, taking into account his or her expected progress in therapy and living context. Conditional reasoning may therefore

be understood simply as "the ability of skilled occupational therapy practitioners to 'form an image of future life possibilities for the person' " (p. 138).[24]

Pragmatic Reasoning

Therapists use pragmatic reasoning to guide their decisions and choices of actions during therapy. This type of reasoning refers to the nuts and bolts of moment-to-moment decision making. In the study by Creighton and colleagues,[3] it was found that therapists used this type of reasoning when making decisions regarding activities to be used in therapy, and the grading and modification of those activities given the environmental context. When a therapist was asked to give a reason for making a certain decision, he or she "gave a pragmatic reason for modifying an activity" that was "often prefaced...with the word *realistically* (e.g., 'realistically, the nursing staff won't be able to provide the structure she would need to feed herself upstairs')" (p. 315).[3] In other words, pragmatic reasoning enables therapists to make clinical decisions about practical actions on the basis of "what is realistically achievable given their own and the client's world" (p. 12).[20]

Ethical Reasoning

Ethical reasoning is "the thought process involved in making economic, moral, and political decisions" (p. 9)[20] while balancing the ethical requirement of beneficence and the need to allow the client autonomy to make decisions and thus be an agent of change in his or her life. This type of clinical reasoning leads to "an ethical decision, rather than a scientific one" (p. 137).[24] It allows the therapist to answer the question: What ought to be done given contextual limitations? Ethical principles guiding therapists in ethical decision making will be discussed in detail in Chapter 7.

Teaching Clinical Reasoning Skills

In medicine, clinical reasoning skills are challenging to teach.[25] This challenge is also apparent in occupational therapy. For example, in a study by Creighton and colleagues,[3] therapists found it difficult to teach students didactically how to modify activities. One therapist observed: "I can tell a student how to do the treatment, but I don't know if you can verbally instruct somebody in why, and how you know, and what to look for" (p. 316).[3] However, attempts have been made to develop methods for teaching medical students the clinical reasoning skills that would enable them to become better diagnosticians.

Bleakley and colleagues,[2] for example, describe a program in which medical students are taught to be more astute in observing and noticing cues through training in observation, description, and judgment of esthetic qualities in the visual arts. Similarly, van Gessel and colleagues[27] developed a program at the University of Geneva, School of Medicine, where a 12-week unit of introduction to clinical reasoning was introduced as part of problem-based learning for fourth-year medical students. After going through the unit, students' feedback indicated that their level of confidence in gathering, interpreting, and weighting relevant patient data increased. They concluded that the unit was useful in easing the "students' transition from the preclinical to clinical years" by giving them an "opportunity to train their clinical reasoning processes on standardized and prototypical problems, before encountering real patients with more ill-structured problems during clerkships" (p. 966).[27]

Ryan, Dolling, and Barnet developed a tutorial guide "to promote effective clinical reasoning" that was "based on iterative information gathering as" hypothesis were "framed, tested, and modified or discarded" (p. 639).[23] The web-based guide consisted of case information triggers followed by prompt questions to facilitate the student's clinical reasoning process. When the student's response was submitted, a clinician's response became available. Thus, the student was able to compare his or her response to prompt questions with the clinician's responses. They found the guide to be "an effective tool for augmenting the PBL (Problem Based Learning)

process in clinical settings and promoting the development of clinical reasoning" (p. 638).[23]

It is evident that a similar guide would be useful in helping occupational therapy students develop clinical reasoning skills. However, a review of the literature revealed that no such guide is systematically used by occupational therapy educators. That is why it is proposed in this book that there is a need to develop a model for use in the profession to help educators systematically facilitate occupational therapy students' development of clinical reasoning skills. The M-A-P-P is proposed to be one possible model, and is presented below.

Manifestations, Assessment, Priorities, Plan (M-A-P-P)

M-A-P-P[*] is an acronym for Manifestations, Assessment, Priorities, and Plan. Manifestations (M) refer to the presentation of the clinical condition through the signs and symptoms (cues) observed by the therapist. Assessment (A) refers to the therapist's clinical interpretation of those cues and the patterns they present. In addition to the Manifestation and Assessment, a section for comments about the reasons for suggested assessments was added to the original M-A-P-P. This section is similar to the "clarifying comments" (p. 640)[23] component in Ryan and colleagues' web-based clinical reasoning guide. By completing this section, the student is encouraged to think of the conceptual schema guiding his or her pattern recognition and subsequent interpretation of the pattern. Priorities (P) are the therapist's analysis of the client's strengths and limitations based on the assessments. The Plan (P) refers to the therapist's conclusions drawn

*I am grateful to Neil Penny, Assistant Professor of Occupational Therapy at Alvernia College, for introducing me to the M-A-P-P (see Figure 6-2). Neil used this instrument as a tool for teaching students client assessment in psychosocial rehabilitation when he was at the University of Scranton. I found the instrument to be suitable for teaching clinical reasoning skills and adapted it for this book. Professor Penny was unsure of the instrument's origin, and I was unable to find its author in my search.

CASE STUDY: DRAKE

Drake is a 46-year-old Caucasian male living in rural east North Carolina. He was diagnosed with bipolar disorder 13 years ago. Currently, Drake is being treated at a mental health facility. He was born in North Carolina and grew up in northern Georgia. He served in the U.S. Marines for 14 years but has been unemployed for the last 4 years. Drake still has a strong interest in being a church minister.

Drake is the second of six children. He has two surviving brothers and another brother who committed suicide at age 15. Drake has been married for 27 years; he and his wife have two children, a daughter and a son. His wife is 45 years old and is employed by the state. Drake reports that the relationship with his wife has been increasingly strained over the years because of his illness. At one time, he and his wife were temporarily separated. His son, who is 20 years old and was diagnosed with depression at age 14, is currently in the U.S. Navy. Drake and his 26-year-old daughter have a strong relationship. She shows understanding of her father's illness while his son is in denial about the illness. Drake's daughter attends the state university in the area and visits him frequently at home or at the mental hospital.

Drake enjoys walks, working out with weights, and riding his motorcycle. He reports that he often eats only one meal a day and sometimes may go for 7 or 8 days without food. His sleep pattern is highly irregular and disruptive to his wife's sleep. He often sleeps for less than 4 hours a night. He reports that he has abused substances such as PCP, LSD, marijuana, downers, black beauties, and powder cocaine in the 1960s and 1970s. Currently he abuses alcohol. Recently, his driver's license was suspended for a DUI. He also smokes about one pack of cigarettes per day. Drake has never been treated for substance abuse, although he quit all other substances except alcohol and cigarettes.

This is Drake's ninth admission to the mental health facility in 2½ years. Prior to the first admission, he had attempted to commit suicide. He has received electroconvulsive therapy, among other types of treatment, after which he reports noticing improvement in mood. Drake also has a diagnosis of Wolff-Parkinson-White Syndrome and coronary artery disease (CAD).

Drake's M-A-P-P Assessment is shown in Figure 6-2.

Concise Statement of Treatment Goals for Drake

Short-Term Goals (STGs)

1. By the end of 3 weeks, Drake will demonstrate improved performance of his role as a husband as indicated by spontaneously making a romantic gesture such as making a romantic card two times a week in the OT department and giving it to his wife during her regular hospital visits.
2. By the end of 3 weeks, Drake will demonstrate increased initiative toward resumption of his worker role as indicated by updating his resume and mailing applications for a job as a minister to at least three churches.
3. By the end of 3 weeks, Drake will demonstrate the ability to follow an adaptive routine as indicated by engaging in a regimen of personally meaningful productive and leisure occupations, and sleeping at least 6 hours per night for at least 3 days of the week.
4. By the end of 4 weeks, Drake will demonstrate improved ability to care for himself as indicated by his ability to plan three meals for a typical day, shop for groceries, and make meals independently in the OT kitchen.

Long-Term Goals (LTGs)

1. By the end of 6 weeks, Drake will successfully resume his roles as a husband and worker.
2. By the end of 6 weeks, Drake will be able to care for himself, including making and eating healthy meals three times per day, pursuing healthy and meaningful leisure occupations, and having adequate sleep and rest.

The M-A-P-P Process of Assessment

MANIFESTATION (What is Observed)	ASSESSMENT (Clinical Interpretations of Observations)	REASONS FOR SUGGESTED ASSESSMENT	PRIORITY (Importance to Client's Treatment)
1. Bipolar disorder	Has oscillations of mood between manic and depressive episodes	Interpretation based on therapist's education about the clinical features of psychiatric conditions	**Strengths/Assets** 1. Has leisure interests 2. History of ability to sustain employment 3. Maintains father role: strong relationship with his daughter 4. Motivated to resume his role as a church minister 5. Has educational and experiential background to resume his worker role
2. Heart problems (CAD)	Physical condition may be a trigger for the bipolar disorder	There is evidence in literature suggesting that physical illness triggers and exacerbates an existing mental condition	
3. Religious minister for 13 years	History of ability to sustain employment	Sustaining employment for 13 years is a big accomplishment	
4. Unemployed	Loss of worker role		
5. Irregular sleep pattern	Disrupted roles, routines, and habits	Based on chaos theory, irregular sleep pattern seems to be an indicator of a larger problem, including disruption of roles and routines in general	**Limitations** 1. Decreased IADL performance 2. Strained marital relationship 3. Suicidal 4. Loss of roles 5. Disrupted roles, routines, and habits 6. Loss of control, impulsiveness 7. Physical illness: heart condition
6. History of drug abuse; currently abuses alcohol	Loss of control, impulsiveness	Drug abuse is usually an expression of feelings of loss of control	
7. History of attempted suicide	Suicidal	This is inferred from his own attempt to commit suicide and his brother's suicide (genetic component)	
8. Strained relationship with wife	Relationship stress may be exacerbating the mental illness	It is documented in literature that relationship problems trigger mental illness	

Figure 6-2.   The M-A-P-P is an instrument to help teach students the clinical reasoning skills necessary for effective observation of cues, interpretation of the cues, and arrival at clinical decisions. *ADLs*, Activities of Daily Living; *IADLs*, instrumental activities of daily living; *wk(s)*, week(s); *OT*, occupational therapy.

9. Eats one meal a day and sometimes does not eat for up to 7 days	Decreased IADL performance	Being able to make and eat healthy meals is IADL performance
10. Smokes		
11. Enjoys walking, working out with weights, and riding his motorcycle	Has leisure occupational interests	Taking walks, working out, riding a motorcyle, etc., are leisure activities
12. Has children	One of his central roles is that of a father	
13. Served in the military	Has self-discipline to achieve goals if he decides to focus	He could not have lasted in the Marines for 6 years if he had no discipline

Continued

Figure 6-2.   Cont'd.

PLAN
Proposed Treatment Plan to Facilitate Change by Building on Existing Strengths

CONCLUSIONS (What are your conclusions given the manifestations, assessments, and priorities?)	GOALS (What, Where, When, Why)	METHODS (Who, How)
Drake is a 45-year-old Caucasian male with an axis I diagnosis of bipolar disorder, who presents to the psychiatric hospital for the ninth time in 2 years. He has a history of drug abuse and attempted suicide. He presents to the occupational therapist with c/o:	What 1. Help Drake resume satisfactory performance of his roles as husband and worker 2. Help Drake re-establish an adaptive routine consisting of balance between work, rest, sleep, and leisure 3. Help Drake develop healthy eating and sleeping habits	Who 1. Occupational therapist 2. Occupational therapist and nursing staff 3. Occupational therapist and dietician
1. Loss of roles 2. Disrupted roles, routines, and habits 3. Decreased IADL functioning	Where 1. Occupational therapy clinic 2. Occupational therapy clinic and other places in the hospital as indicated 3. Occupational therapy clinic	How 1. By helping Drake and his wife find ways of sharing chores, finding interesting activities they can engage in together etc., and updating his resume and sending out applications for a job 2. By helping Drake develop and follow an individualized daily routine consisting of balanced performance in productive activities, ADLs, leisure, and rest
He has a history of ability to sustain employment and has a very supportive daughter. He also has a variety of leisure interests including walking, working out, and riding his motorcycle.	When 1. Wednesdays at 3 PM 2. Every day from waking up to going to sleep 3. Wednesdays at 3 PM	3. Meal planning and cooking activities, and relaxation exercises
	Why 1. To increase his participation and sense of meaning in life 2. To increase his adaptive capabilities and his quality of life 3. To improve his health status	

Figure 6-2.   Cont'd.

PLAN
Summary of Intervention Plan

Problem	Goals	Interventions	Frequency	Target Date
Loss of husband role	Drake will demonstrate improved performance of his role as husband as indicated by spontaneously making a romantic gesture, such as making a romantic card in the OT department and giving it to his wife during her regular hospital visits	Making available opportunities, materials, and instructions to help Drake learn relevant skills	Once a week	9/21/2005
Loss of worker role	Drake will demonstrate increased initiative toward resumption of his role as a worker as indicated by updating his resume and mailing an application for a job as a minister to at least three churches	Using activites to help Drake develop resume writing, job searching, job application, and job interview skills	3 times a week	9/21/2005
Disrupted roles, routines, and habits	Drake will demonstrate ability to follow an adaptive routine as indicated by engaging in a regimen of productive and leisure occupations with minimal cuing from the therapist and nurses, and sleeping at least 6 hours every night, 3 days/wk	Collaboratively working with Drake to make a schedule of daily activities that are meaningful to him; teaching him relaxation exercises	One day during the first week of therapy	9/7/2005
Decreased IADL performance	Drake will demonstrate improved ability to take care of himself as indicated by ability to plan three balanced meals (breakfast, lunch, and dinner), shop for groceries, and make the meals in the OT kitchen	Grocery shopping, meal planning and meal preparation activities, and education regarding the value of good nutrition	2 times a week	9/21/2005

Figure 6-2.   Cont'd.

from the analysis of manifestations, assessments, and priorities, leading to establishment of goals and a treatment plan. Use of the M-A-P-P is illustrated using the case study of Drake.

Analysis of Drake's M-A-P-P Assessment

Manifestation consists of facts resulting from the client's condition, such as the diagnosis, employment history, relationships, and so on, as gleaned from the case description without interpretation. They include what is observed about Drake and what is reported by family members, nurses, or other therapists, as well as by Drake himself. This part of the tool educates the student to develop close noticing skills, which have been suggested to be crucial to good clinical reasoning skills.[2] In other words, there is a need to educate the student's attention because "informational images must first be accurately discriminated (attention to form)" (p. 545)[2] before they can be interpreted. Without accurate observation of cues, correct problem identification is not possible.

Once the therapist accurately identifies the cues, he or she organizes them into patterns (what Schuwirth referred to as *chunking*[25]) and compares the patterns to an existing cognitive structure (schema) consisting of past experiences, education, the profession's paradigm, and so on. In the example of Drake, the fact that he is unemployed, his sleep pattern is irregular, and he does not eat three meals a day leads the therapist to conclude that Drake has developed a self-similar trajectory of maladaptive occupational behavior patterns that have disrupted his roles, routines, and habits. This conclusion is based on past occupational therapy education and informed by the professional paradigm with its emphasis on occupational behavior, as viewed within the framework of pragmatic constructs of "doing" and "agency," and the complexity/chaos theoretical constructs of "fractality" and "recursive feedback" within a system. The inference that Drake has a self-similar trajectory consisting of maladaptive patterns leading to disrupted

roles, routines, and habits is a clinical *assessment* of the manifestations (he is unemployed; has an irregular sleep pattern; goes sometimes for days without meals).

Once manifestations have been identified and clinical assessments inferred, the therapist sorts the manifestations into strengths/assets and limitations. This part of clinical reasoning is informed by a holistic outlook that is a central tenet of the new occupational therapy paradigm. A holistic approach means that the therapist is not only interested in the client's problems but also in his or her strengths, since good therapy focuses on building on strengths to address the problems.

The conclusions help the therapist distill identified manifestations and their assessments into specific problems that are relevant to occupational therapy intervention. The goal setting and delineation of methods of intervention encourages the therapist to think of the client's condition, now and in the future. For instance, Drake's condition is a married client with bipolar disorder, whose marriage is strained because of the manifestations of the disorder, and the therapist projects him to the future and visualizes him as someone who has a satisfactory relationship with his wife, is healthy, and is gainfully employed in something he loves to do. This is *conditional* reasoning.[3,6,20,24] The conclusion also prompts the therapist to think about the client's life as continuous, where past experiences, employment, and relationships are examined in relationship to current circumstances and expected outcome of therapy. For example, in the case of Drake, his story consists of a past as a church minister and a marine, as well as a drug abuser. This helps the therapist to infer that Drake can sustain employment, has the potential to be disciplined enough to pursue desired goals successfully, and so on. This is *narrative* reasoning.

Also, the *what*, *where*, *when*, *who*, and *how* parts of the M-A-P-P force the therapist to think of the practical aspects of therapy, such as what kinds of activities are available in the department to help work on the client's goals, what staff members (e.g., the nurses) need to be involved in the client's interventions, and so on. This constitutes *pragmatic* reasoning.[11,20] Thus, the M-A-P-P may be a useful instrument to teach the student procedural/scientific, narrative, conditional, and pragmatic clinical reasoning skills. Interactive skills can be taught as students learn therapeutic use of self (refer to Lab Manual Exercise 7-1 to learn how to apply these skills in practice). Ethical clinical reasoning skills can be taught when ethical decision making is discussed. Based on the above illustration, it is evident that the M-A-P-P can be an effective tool to help teach students clinical reasoning skills (at least the skills required to identify the clients' problems) and appropriate occupational therapy interventions consistent with the clients' past, present, and projected future contexts. It is recommended that research be conducted to investigate the effectiveness of the tool as a clinical reasoning teaching instrument.

SUMMARY

In this chapter, we discussed clinical reasoning. We can understand the clinical reasoning process within the framework of cognitive psychology. As discussed in Chapter 5, the interview and observation of a client leads to identification of cues that are then organized into patterns. The therapist interprets the patterns through assimilation to available cognitive structure (schema) consisting of the therapist's education, experience, and professional paradigm (as discussed in Chapter 4). We explored the different types of clinical reasoning skills, namely, procedural/scientific, interactive, narrative, conditional, pragmatic, and ethical. Contrary to arguments in some areas of literature, clinical reasoning skills can be taught and learned, and a model for teaching occupational therapy students clinical reasoning skills (the M-A-P-P) was proposed. However, research is needed to test the effectiveness of the proposed model as a clinical reasoning teaching tool.

REFERENCES

1. American Occupational Therapy Association: Occupational therapy practice framework: domain and process, *Am J Occup Ther* 56(6):609-639, 2002.
2. Bleakley A, Farrow R, Gould D, et al: Making sense of clinical reasoning: judgment and the evidence of the senses, *Med Educ* 37:544-552, 2003.
3. Creighton C, Dijkers M, Bennett N, et al: Reasoning and the art of therapy for spinal cord injury, *Am J Occup Ther* 49:311-317, 1995.
4. Dewey J: *Democracy and education*, New York, 1916, MacMillan.
5. Elstein A, Schulman LS, Sprafka SA: *Problem solving: an analysis of clinical reasoning*, Cambridge, MA, 1978, Harvard University Press.
6. Fleming MH: The therapist with the three-track mind, *Am J Occup Ther* 45:1007-1014, 1991.
7. Gillette NP, Mattingly C: The foundation—clinical reasoning in occupational therapy, *Am J Occup Ther* 41:399-400, 1987.
8. Herrington J, Oliver R: Designing for reflection in online courses (Electronic version), 2002. *HERDSA*. Retrieved March 2006, from http://elrond.Scam.ecu.edu.au/oliver/2002/HerringtonJ.Pdf#Search='dialogic%20reflection'.
9. Higgs J, Jones M: Clinical reasoning in the health professions. In Higgs J, Jones M, eds: *Clinical reasoning in the health professions*, pp. 3-14, Melbourne, 2000, Butterworth Heinemann.
10. Hinojosa J, Blount M, eds: *The texture of life: purposeful activities in occupational therapy*, ed 2, Bethesda, MD, 2004, AOTA.
11. Hooper B: The relationship between pretheoretical assumptions and clinical reasoning, *Am J Occup Ther* 51:328-338, 1997.
12. Hughes HW: *Dialogic reflection: a new face on an old pedagogy*. Retrieved March 2006, from http://gsep.pepperdine.edu/_whughes/Journaling.html.
13. Irvin LL: *Reflecting on reflections—the central role reflection plays in teaching writing in a computer networked environment*, 2002. Retrieved March 2006, from http://www.accd.edu/sac/english/lirvin/cw2002paper.htm.
14. Mattingly C: What is clinical reasoning? *Am J Occup Ther* 45:979-986, 1991.
15. Mattingly C, Fleming MH: *Clinical reasoning: forms of inquiry in a therapeutic practice*, Philadelphia, 1994, FA Davis.
16. Mitchell R, Unsworth CA: Role perceptions and clinical reasoning of community health occupational therapists undertaking home visits, *Austr J Occup Ther* 51:13-24, 2004.
17. Parham D: Nationally speaking—Toward professionalism: the reflective therapist, *Am J Occup Ther* 41: 555-561, 1987.

18. Piaget J: *The origins of intelligence in children,* New York, 1963, W.W. Norton.
19. Piaget J: *The psychology of intelligence,* New York, 1963, Routledge.
20. Precin P: *Client-centered reasoning: narratives of people with mental illness,* Boston, 2002, Butterworth-Heinemann.
21. Rogers JC: 1983 Eleanor Clarke Slagle lecture—clinical reasoning: the ethics, science, and art, *Am J Occup Ther* 37:601-616, 1983.
22. Rogers JC: Clinical judgment: the bridge between theory and practice. In *Target 2000: occupational therapy education,* Rockville, MD, 1986, AOTA.
23. Ryan G, Dolling T, Barnet S: Supporting the problem-based learning process in the clinical years: evaluation of an online clinical reasoning guide, *Med Educ* 38:638-645, 2004.
24. Schell BA: Clinical reasoning: the basis of practice. In Crepeau EB, Cohn ES, Schell BA, eds: *Willard and Spackman's occupational therapy,* ed 10, New York, 2003, Lippincott Williams & Wilkins, pp. 131-139.
25. Schuwirth L: Can clinical reasoning be taught or can it be learned? *Med Educ* 36:695-696, 2002.
26. Schwartzberg SL: *Interactive reasoning in the practice of occupational therapy,* Upper Saddle River, NJ, 2002, Prentice Hall.
27. van Gessel E, Nendaz MR, Vermeulen B, et al: Development of clinical reasoning from the basic sciences to the clerkships: a longitudinal assessment of medical students' needs and self-perception after a transitional learning unit, *Med Educ* 37:966-974, 2003.
28. World Health Organization: *International classification of functioning, disability and health,* Geneva, 2001, WHO.

Chapter 7

Intervention

Preview Questions

1. What is ethical reasoning?
2. Explain the concept of ethical cognitive schema and the sources of its content.
3. Distinguish between the deontological and teleological perspectives in ethics.
4. Discuss with examples the six steps of the ethical decision making model.
5. Why is it important for occupational therapists to understand the therapeutic relationship?
6. Discuss at least four components of a therapeutic relationship.
7. What is the difference between a purposeful activity and a meaningful occupation?
8. Explain with examples how meaningful occupations are used as a tool in occupational therapy.
9. Discuss and illustrate with examples how Cole's seven-step group therapy format is used in occupational therapy.
10. Explain how culture may shape the therapeutic relationship and subsequent outcome of occupational therapy intervention.

In Chapters 5 and 6, we discussed the general process of client assessment and the clinical reasoning skills used to interpret gathered data and establish a treatment plan. In this chapter, we will explore occupational therapy intervention. We will also explain the ethical clinical reasoning process in psychosocial occupational therapy intervention. We will broach the intervention process by examining the following topics: (1) use of therapeutic relationship, use of meaningful occupations and activities, and use of groups

and group processes. Finally, we will examine the cross-cultural issues affecting intervention.

The Ethical Clinical Reasoning Process in Psychosocial Occupational Therapy Intervention

In Chapter 6, we noted that ethical decision making is one of the clinical reasoning skills in occupational therapy.[69,76,77] According to Rogers, it is the process by which a therapist arrives at "an ethical decision rather than a scientific one" (p. 602).[74] Thus ethical decision making is not a passive process. It occurs in the course of interaction with the world where the professional encounters ethically challenging situations in the process of conducting his or her business in an endeavor to meet professional responsibilities. By intelligently reasoning, guided by principles of ethics, he or she arrives at ethical decisions to resolve obtaining situations. Therapists need to learn this decision-making process because it is an acquired skill.

Ethics: A Definition

Many definitions seem to equate ethics with morality. For example, Bailey and Schwartzberg believe it is "a branch of applied philosophy and is a careful and systematic study of the nature of morality" (p. 3).[6] Kornblau and Starling adopt the view that ethics is "The study of the general nature of morals and of specific moral choices" (pp. 3-4).[53] It may be useful to make a clear distinction between *ethics* and *morality*.

Morality pertains to social norms. What is moral is defined by social institutions such as the church. However, *what is moral may not always be ethical.* For instance, in the Middle Ages, the Catholic Church participated in events such as burning of witches at stake.[84] Similarly, at one time in the United States and other parts of the world, owning and trading in slaves were morally and socially widely-tolerated practices. It took a while even for the Church to start revising its position and declaring slavery an unacceptable practice. In these instances, what might have been accepted morally was unethical.

Therefore a definition of ethics that makes this distinction clear could be useful. An example of such a definition is provided by the Josephson Institute of Ethics: "Ethics refers to principles that define behavior as right, good and proper. Such principles do not always dictate a single 'moral' course of action, but provide a means of evaluating and deciding among competing options" (p. 1).[49] Sibley concurs with this view by asserting that "Ethics denotes a valuational process where all rules, regulations, and/or mores are critically examined rationally" (p. 2).[81] Thus it seems that morality consists of a list of socially agreed-upon rules by which members of a community are required to abide, while ethics is a process of evaluation of the goodness or otherwise of those rules. Thus ethical decision making is an intelligent, rational process, whereas moral decision making calls for simple adherence to moral rules. With this distinction made, we will examine the process of evaluating these rules.

Ethical Decision Making

As the above-discussed definition infers, like other clinical reasoning skills, ethical decision making is a cognitive process. It is proposed here that the therapist uses *ethical cognitive structure (schema)* to interpret ethically-oriented data and arrive at a decision about action. Thus it is essential that therapists explore the content of their cognitive structures so that they have insight regarding how they go about making ethical decisions. Refer to Lab Manual Exercise 8-1, *A,* to learn how to facilitate this reflective self-exploration.

Ethical Cognitive Structure

The ethical cognitive structure (schema) is a framework consisting of information derived from one's social experiences (including upbringing, education, religious experiences, and so on). Thus part of the ethical cognitive schema consists of internalized moral rules derived from one's social context. Other information in the ethical cognitive schema is derived from professional education, including education in models of ethical decision making. We will discuss each of the above-proposed aspects of the ethical cognitive schema.

Social Context as a Source of Ethical Cognitive Schema

According to social constructivists, reality is socially constructed through consensus.[18,53,58] By extension, it can be argued that this socially constructed reality defines concepts of what "is good," "is bad," "ought to be done," "ought not to be done," and so on, for those who share in it. These values are instilled in a person through upbringing (including religious education and other forms of education subscribed to by the community) and other socialization processes. As a student is assisted to make the transition from a novice to an expert in occupational therapy, professional socialization through education about the beliefs, values, and domains of concern agreed upon by consensus in the professional community provides experiences that contribute toward the formation of this cognitive schema. For instance, learning about the professional paradigm discussed in Chapter 4 socializes the practitioner about what should be the overarching goal of the profession (to promote engagement in meaningful occupations to facilitate participation in life). Socialization through education about this paradigm significantly influences a therapist's decision making regarding what should be legitimate therapeutic media and interaction processes in the process of planning interventions and providing what are ethically considered to be adequate occupational therapy services.

A personal example is provided here to illustrate what is meant by development of ethical cognitive schema through the process of socialization. I was brought up in a society in which children were revered. I was taught that they always come first. Through example, the adults demonstrated that sacrifices must always be made for children. Because of that experience, if I am working as a therapist and encounter a situation in which the best interests of an adult are in conflict with those of a child, my decision regarding how to act will likely be in favor of the child. In this case, it happens that the ethical principles of my profession (occupational therapy) are consistent with the values instilled in me by upbringing. My ethical cognitive schema in this regard consists of the concept that the welfare of children comes first, and this concept guides me in my interpretation of client data in the process of making an ethical decision.

In addition to past experiences, it has been found that the current social context affects ethical decision making. Cottone, Tarvydas, and House concluded in part from a study that "relationships seem to influence ethical decision making linearly and cumulatively" (p. 63).[20] It can be argued that the social context, including social relationships, contribute to the formation of the ethical cognitive schema. To give another personal example, many of my current friends share my belief in the autonomy of other people, and in the value of respect and being nonjudgmental. These values are therefore strengthened by my current relationships. Interaction with my friends helps strengthen that part of my ethical cognitive schema.

Professional Education as a Source of Ethical Cognitive Schema

In considering how professional education contributes toward formation of the ethical cognitive schema, it is important to understand how education in ethical decision making is implemented. Ethics fall under one of the branches of applied philosophy.[5] Traditionally, philosophers assumed that universal truths could be defined, and individual cases of sense data simply needed to be subsumed under these universally defined principles.[25,81] Although early Greeks attempted to arrive at ethical decisions through rational, logical inquiry, they followed the framework of their time. They assumed that through rational inquiry, they could arrive at universal truths about the good and end of humankind. Some philosophers, like St. Augustine, argued that the end of ethical inquiry should be to discover the divine will. Others such as John Stuart Mill saw maximization of pleasurable consequences as the end of philosophical inquiry. Still others such as Immanuel Kant appealed to a sense of duty that they assumed was innate in every human.

 Refer to Lab Manual Exercise 8-1, *A* to learn how to develop insight into the origin of your ethical cognitive schema.

Today, there are probably many ethical conceptual frameworks. In the model presented here, ethicists may be considered to fall in a continuum between two positions: those like Kant,[50] who see the end of ethics as adherence to a sense of duty to uphold universal principles (deontological perspective), and those who emphasize maximization of "good" consequences, or aim at achieving "the greatest good for the greatest number of people" in the fashion of John Stuart Mill[61] (teleological perspective).[18,36,53] The teleological approach is also known as *utilitarianism* because it emphasizes decision making aimed at arriving at what is the most useful in terms of producing the greatest good for the greatest number of people.[19,61] Because of their belief in existence of irrefutable universal ethical principles, deontologists tend to be absolutists. In other words, they do not allow exception to adherence to established principles. It is argued here that deontologists tend to be more moralistic because of their strict conformity to moral rules that they see as the universal principles of right and wrong.

While recognizing that there could be many other ethical conceptual frameworks, professionals who would like to consider the one proposed here as a guide for their ethical decision-making process may want to reflect on their ethical cognitive schema so that they understand where they fall in the continuum (between the deontological and teleological positions). This would give them insight regarding how to go about making ethical decisions. Each perspective has its own shortcomings. For instance, the absolutism of the deontological perspective may not be workable at times. One of the dilemmas often posed to illustrate this shortcoming is about Immanuel Kant's insistence that it is wrong to tell a lie irrespective of circumstances (adherence to the moral principle of complete honesty at all times).[82]

The scenario is that in Nazi Germany Kant is hiding a friend sought by the Gestapo. While the friend hides in the basement, Kant and his colleagues engage in a discussion upstairs. The Gestapo asks Kant whether he has seen the friend. If he says no, he will have lied. If he tells the truth, his friend will be killed. What is he to do? In this case, adherence to a moral principle would seem to bring about worse consequences. One may argue that it would be better to tell a lie and save a person's life. This is the greatest shortcoming of the deontological perspective: There is no consideration of the consequences of acting or not acting on principles.

On the other hand, the teleological approach does not seem to provide a method of deciding what would be considered to be the greatest good for the greatest number of people. For example, during the World War II, the Nazis performed horrible medical experiments on individuals who were incarcerated in concentration camps. This abuse led to the famous Nuremberg War Crime Trials and subsequent drafting of a code specifying standards for judging physicians and scientists who had conducted experiments on concentration camp prisoners.[87] This code became a prototype for the Belmont report published on April 18, 1979, and updated in 1998. One may argue that the abuses uncovered in the Nuremberg Trials (and other abuses that occurred later in the United States) were beneficial because medical discoveries were made

that benefited all humanity (e.g., the discovery of the natural course of syphilis, thus enhancing its treatment). According to the logic of utilitarianism, such experiments may be judged to be ethically right since they resulted in the greatest good for the greatest number of people. Is it, however, right to hurt even one individual so that the rest of humanity can benefit? Would such a conclusion in any way be justifiable? This is an important limitation of the teleological perspective. There are no guidelines to determine when action that benefits people in the long run is justifiable.

As is usually the case, a hybrid of the two perspectives may be the most appropriate. One can refer to socially accepted rules of conduct and moral principles, examine the consequences of acting on their basis, and then make a judgment regarding whether the consequences are acceptable. This still leaves the question of how the judgment is to be made. We will discuss that later. At this point, it is important to mention that within the deontological-teleological continuum there are a variety of models of ethics.[32] These are the *virtuous, social constructivism, collaborative, rational,* and *integrative models.*

The *virtuous model* is based on individual character or virtues that include "integrity, prudence, discretion, perseverance, courage, benevolence, humility, and hope" (p. 270).[32] The *social constructivism model* assumes that ethical decisions are externally influenced because "what is real evolves through personal interaction and agreement as to what is fact" by members of society (p. 270).[32] The *collaborative model* is based on the idea that a group-derived perspective is superior to an individual one. Therefore ethical decision making should be based on cooperation and inclusion where all members of a group contribute, and it leads to emergence of a group perspective regarding what is an ethical decision. The *rational model* advocates consideration of all the different ethical principles bearing on a situation and where those principles are in conflict, choosing the best course of action. Finally, the *integrative model* is a kind of hybrid of the rational and virtue models. In this model, which seems to be more consistent with the notion of ethical cognitive schema discussed earlier, the individual making the decision analyzes his or her morals, beliefs, and experiences and then the principles underlying different competing courses of action, finally arriving at the best course of action.

It is imperative that therapists examine their ethical cognitive schema and decide whether they are deontological or teleological and whether they subscribe to the virtuous, social constructivism, collaborative, rational, or integrative models. Such awareness has significant implications regarding how decisions are made. Hadjistavropoulos and colleagues,[36] for example, completed a study in which they compared the behavioral intentions of psychologists and doctors as these intentions were influenced by ethical ideologies. They found that psychologists tended to be more absolutist in adherence to the professional code while physicians tended to be more relativistic. Thus physicians tended to be influenced more by their own personal beliefs and family values and less by their professional code of ethics (they were more integrationist), and vice versa for psychologists. The desirability of consequences obtaining from one trend or the other depends on the ethical situation in question. However, this book proposes that neither extreme is desirable and that the middle ground is always the safest place.

The Ethical Decision-Making Process

Having discussed the philosophical/theoretical basis of ethics, we will now examine the process of professional ethical decision making. There seems to be a consensus in literature that ethical decision making involves a number of steps that do not necessarily constitute a linear process[19,32,88]:

1. *Identifying the ethical problem and defining it as clearly as possible, taking into account its personal, interpersonal, social, and environmental implications.* In other words, who and/or what are affected by the situation? Is it only an ethical issue, or is it a legal or institutional one as well? What would be the consequences of not acting on the situation?

2. *Gathering information.* What are the facts involved? What is at stake? Who has something at stake in relation to the issue? What options for action are available?

3. *Consulting legal and ethical guidelines to find out how it is proposed that you act in relation to the situation.* In the case of occupational therapy, this means consulting legal guidelines as well as the professional principles of ethics.

4. *Evaluating different options for action generated in #2 above on the basis of legal and ethical guidelines.* If your perspective is deontological, you will probably focus on trying to do what is consistent with the established moral/ethical guidelines. If you are teleological in perspective, you will examine what option will produce the most good for the greatest number of people and result in the least harm. As mentioned earlier, many people fall somewhere in the middle within the deontological-teleological continuum. Whatever your perspective, you have to examine outcomes very closely before making an ethical decision.

5. *Making a decision and implementing the chosen option.*

6. *Monitoring the action and evaluating its outcome.* If indicated, make modifications accordingly.

To make the decision-making model more complete, it is proposed that a step based on social constructivism be added between numbers 4 and 5. In this step, the therapist should "identify the levels of consensus that operate around" (p. 41)[18] the chosen action (Box 7-1). This is because it is important to be cognizant of what is agreed upon among colleagues regarding the appropriate course of action, whether it is defined in the written principles of ethics or

---

<table>
<tr><td>

Box 7-1   Seven Steps to Ethical Decision Making

1. Identify the ethical problem.
2. Gather information.
3. Consult legal and ethical guidelines.
4. Evaluate options.
5. Identify levels of consensus that operate around the chosen action.
6. Make a decision and implement it.
7. Monitor the action and evaluate its outcome.

</td></tr>
</table>

not. This does not mean that decisions should be made on the basis of peers' opinions. It means that if there is a need to disagree with those opinions, one needs to be clear about them, and why they are not appropriate given the circumstances of the ethical situation at hand.

 Refer to Lab Manual Exercise 8-1, *B* to learn how to develop your ethical decision-making skills.

Principles of Ethics in Occupational Therapy

The principles of ethics that occupational therapists use to guide them as they make ethical decisions were largely derived from Beauchamp and Childress's *Principles of Biomedical Ethics*.[8] In this work, Beauchamp and Childress suggest four principles *(nonmaleficence, beneficence, justice,* and *autonomy)* and four supplementary rules *(veracity, privacy, confidentiality,* and *fidelity)*.[1,8,9] Occupational therapy adopted these four principles as well as the four supplementary rules, as can be seen in the discussion below.[3]

Principle 1: Nonmaleficence

This is the principle directing a therapist, above all, to do no harm. In other words, the therapist should not inflict evil on others, such as causing death, harm, or suffering.[5,9,53] The AOTA words this principle as follows: "Occupational therapy personnel shall take measures to ensure a recipient's safety and avoid imposing or inflicting harm" (p. 640).[3]

Principle 2: Beneficence

This principle is closely related to the principle of nonmaleficence. It directs the therapist to do good and to prevent or remove harm from happening to those for whom he or she is placed in charge.[9] In this principle, the therapist has an obligation to act to prevent injury or harm to others, except in situations in which an attempt to rescue another from harm would cause personal injury.[53] According to Kornblau and Starling, simply stated, this principle denotes the ethical obligation to look out for the well-being of his or her clients or to act for the client's good.[53] The AOTA states this principle as follows: "Occupational therapy personnel shall demonstrate a concern for the safety and well-being of the recipients of their services" (p. 639).[3]

Principle 3: Justice

This is the principle of fairness. It mandates that resources be distributed fairly, appropriately, and equitably according to prevailing social contract.[9] This takes the form of either comparative justice, where equal cases are treated in the same way, or noncomparative justice, where each person receives what he or she needs.[5,53] This principle denotes that all people requiring a service should have equal access to that service. Of course, it is also recognized in the notion of noncomparative justice that treating some people the same may actually be unjust. For instance, treating a person with a bruise first because he or she came to the emergency room first while a person with life-threatening multiple injuries waits may hardly be called justice. Obviously, even if the person with serious injuries came later, he or she deserves to be attended to before those with less serious injuries. On the other hand, if all injuries are of equal seriousness, then justice demands that individuals be treated on first-come, first-served basis.

The AOTA calls this principle "procedural justice" and states it as follows: "Occupational therapy personnel shall comply with laws and Association policies guiding the profession of occupational therapy" (p. 640).[3] In this statement, the AOTA speaks of adherence to laws but does not address the need for therapists to advocate for equitable and just distribution of resources to facilitate equal accessibility of therapeutic services. There may be an oversight as far as the spirit of this principle is concerned, and there is a need to address this anomaly.

Principle 4: Autonomy

This principle refers to the need to respect the ability of clients to govern themselves and make reasonable choices and decisions.[5,8,53] In the principle, the right to self-determination by individuals through action based on individual choice and decision making, free from any undue coercion or influence, is recognized. The goal of occupational therapy is generally acknowledged as to facilitate client autonomy,[2] which is consistent with this principle. Thus the AOTA states that "Occupational therapy personnel shall respect recipients to assure their rights" (p. 640).[3]

In addition to the four principles, Beauchamp and Childress identified four supplementary rules.[8,9] The AOTA presents these rules as principles or incorporates them into one of the four principles.[3] Following is a discussion of the four rules as proposed by Beauchamp and Childress and as they are presented by the AOTA. According to Beauchamp and Childress, the rules of veracity, privacy, and confidentiality may be understood to be supplementary to the principle of autonomy, or the right of the client to govern him or herself or make personal decisions.[8,9]

Rule 1: Veracity

This is the rule of truthfulness, which is part of informed consent.[1,8,9] In other words, the therapist needs to be honest with clients about his or her intentions so that they can make informed decisions regarding whether or not to be involved in the therapist's therapeutic plans.[53] This obligation is based on the realization that without accurate information truthfully conveyed by the therapist, he or she cannot make truly informed, autonomous decisions about therapy. The AOTA presents this as an independent principle, although according to Beauchamp and Childress, it is a rule supplementing the principle of autonomy. The association presents it as follows: "Occupational therapy personnel shall provide accurate information when representing the profession" (p. 640).[3]

Rule 2: Privacy

The client has a right to privacy. This means that he or she has freedom to share or not to share pertinent information with the therapist or anyone else.[1,8,9] This rule clearly supplements the principle of autonomy. In the latest edition of the professional code of ethics, the AOTA does not clearly identify this rule; however in Principle 3D, it is stated that one of the occupational therapist's professional obligations is to "Protect all privileged confidential forms of written, verbal, and electronic communication gained from educational, practice, research, and investigational activities unless otherwise mandated by local, state, or federal regulations" (p. 640).[3] This emphasis on protection of client information may be understood to indirectly address the client's right to privacy.

Rule 3: Confidentiality

The client has a right to expect that information shared with the therapist in the course of therapy is kept confidential and not divulged to unauthorized individuals without his or her consent.[1,8,9] This rule is particularly important in therapy because it is the basis of trust that makes a therapeutic relationship possible.[68] Furthermore, confidentiality "has become increasingly the focus of legal battles" (p. 146).[68] This denotes the need for occupational therapists to pay even more attention to the rule. It is important to recognize that there are exemptions to the requirement to maintain confidentiality.[53] If risk of injury or child abuse is involved, for example, the therapist may be obligated not only by personal conscience but also by law to report the issue to relevant authorities. The therapist may consider disclosing these limitations to confidentiality before the client actually reveals any information that may need to be reported. This disclosure will allow the client to maintain individual autonomy by deciding whether or not to reveal the information. Again, this rule speaks to the principle of client autonomy and is correctly incorporated into that principle by the AOTA.[3]

Rule 4: Fidelity

Fidelity refers to faithful adherence by the therapist to the duty to care for the client.[1,8,9] This includes the therapist's duty to keep any explicit or implicit promises made to the client, including the promise to maintain confidentiality unless the law or someone's safety requires disclosing the information shared in therapy. Clearly, this rule supplements the principles of nonmaleficence (not to cause harm to clients) and beneficence (the need to do good and prevent harm to clients). However, as it is presented in the AOTA, the rule is a separate principle (Principle 7) and seems indistinguishable, to a certain extent, from the rules of veracity and confidentiality. It is

stated as follows: "Occupational therapy personnel shall treat colleagues and other professionals with respect, fairness, discretion, and integrity" (p. 641).[3] It is not clear how the rule, as stated above, relates to the duty to be faithful to client care.

We will now illustrate the process of ethical clinical reasoning using a personal example that was typical in the profession a few years ago. Although this example does not pertain directly to client care and may be removed from the experience of many occupational therapists, it is an illustration of how a therapist's ethical decision making can affect not only an individual client but can also have implications for broader social systems and the well-being of humans in general. Besides, it is possible that in the current status of the medical care system where medical care has become a business in many parts of the world, many therapists may continue to experience demands from employers to increase economic productivity, placing them in ethical binds similar to my experiences as described in this example.

CASE STUDY: AN ILLUSTRATION OF ETHICAL DECISION MAKING

I was recruited from abroad by a rehabilitation company to work in the United States as an occupational therapist in long-term care. As I migrated to the United States, I had two main objectives: to earn enough money to support my family back home and to complete my doctoral education. As such, I was very focused in my pursuits. The company I worked for sponsored my doctoral education by paying full tuition. At the same time, they held my visa, which meant that if they terminated my employment and I could not get another employer willing to apply for a visa on my behalf, I would have to go back home and terminate my studies, not to mention go back to a situation where my pay as a therapist was not nearly enough to take care of my family.

Aware of this hold, the company was putting pressure on me to increase productivity in terms of billable units of therapy that I generated. The physicians at the facility where I worked were not cooperative in referring clients to me. The company was not supportive in helping a foreigner (who was still acclimatizing to methods of therapy in the country) build necessary relationships with the physicians. Instead, they suggested that I increase my productivity by placing the few Medicare Part B clients on therapy five times a week and Medicare Part A clients two times a day, five times a week.

Being an ethically conscious therapist, I argued with my supervisors that I could not justify giving clients more therapy than was indicated by my professional evaluation; in fact, giving some clients

CASE STUDY: AN ILLUSTRATION OF ETHICAL DECISION MAKING—CONT'D

more therapy than needed may be harmful. My supervisors responded by mandating that I had 30 days to implement their recommendations or in some other way increase productivity to 75% of a workday, or I would have to leave the company. What would you have done in my position? How would you have drawn from your ethical cognitive schema in your reasoning process so that you were able to arrive at an ethical decision?

One may argue that the decision is simple. My supervisors were asking me to be dishonest and therefore I needed to stand up to them and stick to the truth. That is the kind of stance a person with a deontological perspective would take since that perspective requires adherence to one's duty to universal principles (in this case the principle of honesty above all else). That would make sense in my case considering that my upbringing, which consisted of a large dose of religious instruction, instilled in my ethical cognitive schema the value that one has to be truthful and honest at all times. It is true that ideas about honesty and truth are a large part of my ethical cognitive structure, and the idea of being less than completely truthful makes me uncomfortable. However, as mentioned earlier, adherence to a principle such as honesty is not always enough criteria for ethical decision making. Sometimes it may even be undesirable to be truthful because it may be more hurtful than beneficial to people. Suffice to say that for this reason, I do not subscribe to the deontological perspective. So, in order to make the decision, I had to appeal to other criteria, specifically, the consequences, actual or potential, of my conformity with my supervisors' demands.

While examining the consequences, I had to be cognizant of the larger picture, including the professional principles of ethics as well as the social consequences of my decision. For instance, if I submitted clients who were physically weak to strenuous therapeutic activities that they did not need, I could hurt them. This would contravene the professional ethical principle of *nonmaleficence*. Similarly, my behavior would be contrary to the principle of *beneficence* since what I would be doing would not be consistent with doing what is good and preventing what is harmful to my clients. I would also be cheating my clients by convincing them to receive therapy which they really did not need, which would be contrary to the principle of *autonomy*.

In addition, my behavior would be harmful on an even larger scale. In Chapter 4, we saw that in complex systems such as the world economy, outcomes are disproportional to the input. Thus, if every therapist billed a few units of unnecessary therapy, eventually the entire medical system would be overwhelmed with unnecessary costs. This would have dire economic consequences, not only for the United States but for the entire world. This assertion has already been proven by skyrocketing medical costs and medical insurance in the United States. These consequences directly relate to the principle of *justice* because when resources are misused, many people who actually need them in order to live go lacking. Based on careful consideration of all the above discussed consequences, I had to stand up for what was right. I left the company. Fortunately, I was able to get a job with another company, maintain my immigration status, and go on to complete my doctoral studies.

 Refer to Lab Manual Exercise 8-1, *B*, for an exercise in ethical clinical reasoning.

The Intervention Process

For some time now, it has been recognized that there are generally three legitimate tools of intervention in occupational therapy: use of self as a therapeutic tool, use of groups and group processes, and use of purposeful activities.[24,30,63,92] In this book, we will use terminology in the new proposed professional paradigm (see Chapter 4) as articulated in the *Occupational Therapy Practice Framework*[2] and explicated in current interdisciplinary therapeutic literature.[31] Thus the term *therapeutic relationship* will be substituted for the term *self* as a therapeutic tool; the term *meaningful occupations* will be substituted for the term *purposeful activities*.

The Therapeutic Relationship

Therapeutic use of relationship has been a part of psychotherapy for a long time. For example, psychoanalysts considered issues of transference and countertransference to be central to therapeutic practice.[31,34,40,78,89] These phenomena involve transfer of emotions and objects associated with earlier experiences to the therapist. This transfer can only happen in the context of a relationship, which in current psychotherapy literature is being defined as a *therapeutic relationship* because it occurs in the context of therapy. Of course transference and countertransference are strictly psychodynamic constructs. Therapeutic relationship on the other hand is a central construct in many varieties of psychotherapy (client-centeredness, cognitive approaches, existential psychotherapies, and so on). Nevertheless, it can be argued that the very idea of therapeutic relationship has its roots in the psychodynamic constructs of transference and countertransference because they represent initial attempts by therapists to take into account the effects of interpersonal dynamics in therapy.

It is only recently, however, that research has demonstrated the importance of the therapeutic relationship as a tool of therapy. Researchers have found that the outcome of therapy depends to a large extent on three factors: client factors (including the client's outlook and attitude), therapeutic relationship, and therapeutic techniques.[16,31,95] Of the three factors, it has been found that irrespective of techniques, the therapeutic relationship accounts for most of the variance in therapeutic outcome, second to client factors.[31,83]

Client factors account for 40% of the variance in therapeutic outcome, therapeutic relationship for 30%, and therapeutic techniques

for only 15%.[31] These statistics imply that the client's attitude and therapeutic relationship are the most important factors in therapy, and therapeutic techniques do not really matter as much. However, one must bear in mind that the therapeutic relationship is related to therapeutic techniques. If a therapist is confident in the techniques he or she is using, he or she is likely to be more effective in establishing a strong therapeutic relationship because of enhanced ability to instill confidence in the client. Thus the three factors should not be considered in isolation. The above-cited research indicates, without doubt, that it is very important that occupational therapists pay close attention to factors related to developing skills necessary for establishment of strong therapeutic relationships, also known as *therapeutic alliances,* with clients.[31] It is necessary to delineate components of this therapeutic relationship or alliance.

Components of the Therapeutic Relationship/Alliance

Mosey defined conscious use of self in therapy as "the use of oneself in such a way that one becomes an effective tool in the evaluation and intervention process" (p. 199).[63] Continuing, she said that

> Conscious use of self, as previously defined, involves a planned interaction with another person in order to alleviate fear or anxiety, provide reassurance, obtain necessary information, provide information, give advice, and assist the individual to gain more appreciation of, more expression of, and more functional use of his or her latent inner resources (p. 199).[63]

Crepeau referred to this process as attention to other people's experiences or what she termed establishment of "*intersubjectivity,* or entering the life-world of another person" (p. 1016).[22] The above descriptions of conscious use of self are consistent with the construct of use of therapeutic relationship in current therapeutic literature,[31,83] which Peloquin refers to as part of the art of occupational therapy practice.[66]

According to Flaskas,[31] some of the emerging themes in the construct of therapeutic relationship include the following:

- Collaboration and an attempt by therapists to be fully present to their clients
- The need for therapists to be neutral and non-judgmental and to approach the client with an attitude of curiosity, seeking to know more about the client rather than making assumptions
- Listening to the client and striving to be a witness to his or her experiences
- Transparency
- Growing attention to issues of transference and countertransference.

One may add to this list establishment of rapport, which is the beginning of a therapeutic relationship.[12]

Establishing Rapport

Establishment of rapport, defined as "a relationship of mutual trust," (p. 25),[12] is an important step in beginning to develop a therapeutic relationship. By creating trust, the therapist is able to reach out to clients and engage them in the therapeutic process.[7,66] However, what is meant by creating a relationship of trust? It means being authentic in the process of interaction with the client, communicating respect and caring, and being *empathetic*.[65,66,93] Being authentic means "being true and real" (p. 615),[66] or "the therapist allowing himself to feel real emotion as he enters into mutual relation with the client" (p. 8).[94] Empathy, as defined by Rogers, means making an effort to enter another person's subjective experience and see the world from that person's eyes (see discussion of Rogerian psychotherapy in Chapter 3), or as Eklund and Hallberg call it, "tuning one's interactions to another's needs" (p. 2).[29] It is "a way of seeing with the eyes of others to appreciate nuances in their visions of the world" (p. 26).[65] This is what makes what Crepeau[22] referred to as *intersubjectivity* between the therapist and client (see above)

possible. This intersubjectivity creates a sense of understanding and trust in the relationship.

However, how is creating a relationship of mutual trust accomplished in practice? The therapist accomplishes this from the beginning of a therapeutic relationship by communicating respect to the client through the following: self-introduction, stating his or her role in helping resolve the client's issues, and ensuring privacy.[12] Specifically, the process outlined by Rogers[72] (see discussion of the four-step client-centered process on Figure 3-2 in Chapter 3) may be helpful.

Refer to Lab Manual Exercise 8-2, *A*, to learn how to develop skills to establish rapport with clients. Also, Lab Manual Exercise 4-1 will help you practice the art of establishing rapport quickly and conducting an initial interview. The process begins with attending, where the therapist attends to the physical comfort of the client. This includes paying attention to the sitting arrangement. It is recommended that the therapist sit at a place where he or she is in full view of the client without staring. There should be no physical barriers (e.g., a desk) between the therapist and client. The therapist should also note nonverbal cues such as how the client is dressed, posture, facial expression, and so on. All these cues help the therapist to formulate a hypothesis about the client's feeling state. Reflecting to the client this feeling state through verbal and nonverbal responses conveys to him or her that he or she is understood.

The therapist's posture and demeanor should also convey warmth and unconditional acceptance of the client. For example, sitting with legs and arms crossed may communicate to the client that the therapist is not really open. This perceived lack of openness reduces the chances of developing a trusting relationship. Once the therapist has been effective in attending, the client will likely become comfortable and begin communicating openly (the communication could be verbal, nonverbal, or both). Once the client begins to get involved (through open communication), the therapist now has to listen actively. Active listening means listening not only to what is being said but also to the underlying feeling.

For example, a client says "I can't do this. It's hopeless! I've never been good at this kind of activity." The two parts of this statement include a perception by the client that he or she is inadequate in the kind of activity in question (content), and the associated feeling of hopelessness (as implied in the statement, "I can't do this. It's hopeless!"). The therapist responds to both the content and the associated feeling of what is said. In this example, the response might be "You feel helpless because you do not think you can adequately complete the task?" Such responses convey to the client the sense of being accurately understood. This is part of communicating empathy and contributes to establishment of trust, since the client feels that the therapist can be depended upon to understand what he or she is going through. This communication of understanding encourages the client to explore his or her experiences even more deeply, leading to action as required to change his or her circumstances.

Refer to Lab Manual Exercise 8-2, *B,* for an exercise to facilitate development of active listening, which is the basis of establishment of a therapeutic relationship.

Collaboration

Flaskas states that "The single most important shift in emphasis has been to collaborative (sic) descriptions of the therapeutic relationship" (p. 15).[31] This collaborative stance challenges therapists to give up the idea of being experts and requiring that clients simply go along with their prescriptions. It is consistent with the new occupational therapy paradigm,[2] which places collaboration at the center of the therapeutic process. It is also consistent with the earlier definition of the conscious use of self, which provides in part that the therapist assist the client "to gain more appreciation of, more expression of, and more functional use of his or her latent inner resources" (p. 199).[63]

Collaboration requires that the therapist genuinely seek to understand issues that are of primary concern to the client rather than attempting to impose an agenda. Successful application of this skill requires that the therapist have adequate "other-enhancing" skills,[13,84] which denotes the need to be able to truly place the client's interests first and above all else. Incidentally, this aspect of use of therapeutic relationship is consistent with the ethical principle of autonomy (discussed earlier), since the client is encouraged to make personal decisions and the therapist merely assumes the role of facilitator.

Neutrality and a Nonjudgmental Attitude

Mosey identified *empathy, compassion,* and *unconditional positive regard* as some of the qualities or characteristics that facilitate therapeutic use of self by the therapist.[63] We have discussed empathy and examined its role in the development of a therapeutic relationship consisting of mutual trust. *Compassion* refers to profound sympathy for another person's suffering and a desire to alleviate it. *Unconditional positive regard* refers to acceptance of another person as he or she is, as a valuable and dignified individual, irrespective of disagreement with the person's perspective and behavior. All the above characteristics seem to be part of the emerging theme of the need to be neutral, nonjudgmental, and curious about the client's experiences in helping disciplines.[31] This theme implies the idea of "therapist as open to the meaning and the sense of the struggle in which" (p. 16)[31] the client is engaged. The perspective of the theme, more specifically, is that "Used carefully and well, curiosity and not-knowingness should promote empathic connection with clients through demonstration of the therapist's desire to understand the client's experience" (p. 16).[31]

As mentioned earlier, it is also evident that the themes of empathy, neutrality, and nonjudgmental attitude, as is the case with most of the other themes of the therapeutic relationship, are derived from Rogerian client-centered therapy, which is defined as a process of carefully listening to the client, accepting the client for who he or she is—no matter how confused or antisocial that might be at the moment—and skillfully reflecting back the client's feelings. The acceptance and reflection of feelings would create a level of safety for deeper exploration and a mirror in which to further understand and reflect on the client's own experience, which would lead the individual to further insight and positive action (p. 118).[52]

This characteristic is also a necessary part of a collaborative relationship.

Listening to the Client and Striving to be a Witness

Closely related to the theme of neutrality and curiosity about the client's experiences is an emphasis on the therapist's quality of listening[31] (see earlier discussion of active listening). In current helping professions' literature, it is referred to as *radical listening,* which is defined as including "a deliberate listening for the context" of the client's experience (p. 17).[31] When one listens carefully, taking into account the context of the relationship within which the client's experiences are occurring (as discussed earlier), one becomes a witness to these experiences, which is very valuable for clients. The ability to listen well is similarly a necessary condition for collaborative relationships with clients.

 Refer to Lab Manual Exercise 8-2, *B,* for an exercise to help you develop responding skills in the context of active listening.

Transparency

Mosey identified self-awareness as "the ability to recognize, with a reasonable degree of accuracy, how one reacts to the outside world and how the outside world reacts to oneself" (p. 202).[63] She asserted that this self-awareness is a crucial characteristic of successful therapeutic use of self. This suggests continuous vigilance and self-auditing by the therapist, achieved through constant reflection on personal experiences. This allows the therapist to be authentic, or to demonstrate what Rogers referred to as *genuineness.*[73] This characteristic is emerging

as a theme in current therapeutic relationship literature. It emphasizes that "it is important to listen to your own thoughts in the same way that you listen to" the client's ideas, "staying curious about your own process" (p. 18).[31] This means "reflectiveness in the therapeutic use of self" (p. 18).[31] When you are reflective and are conscious of your own psychic processes as a therapist, you are likely to collaborate more effectively with your clients.

Growing Attention to Issues of Transference and Countertransference

Flaskas observes that there is a clear gravitation toward psychoanalytic concepts in current psychotherapeutic literature, particularly the constructs of "Transference, countertransference, and projective identification" as "ways of understanding unconscious communication" (p. 18).[31] It is perceived that effective handling of those processes has the potential to enrich "empathic connection through reflection on these processes" (p. 19),[31] which would subsequently strengthen the therapeutic relationship.

The above six themes define a therapeutic relationship as it is conceived in current helping professions' literature. Application of the propositions in those themes allows establishment of rapport, which is primarily a therapeutic relationship, through communication of respect and acceptance, neutrality and a nonjudgmental attitude, and restraint from imposing personal opinions or values of the therapist to the client.[71] Other benefits of adherence to the principles underlying the above themes include establishment of a therapeutic relationship that makes it possible to communicate caring and create a sense of safety for the client.[13] This leads to trust, in turn facilitating open communication, comfort with the inevitable ambiguity of the therapeutic process, and openness to change by the client.

For more practice in the use of a therapeutic relationship, refer to Lab Manual Exercise 8-2, *C,* for an exercise using client-centered therapeutic interventions.

Therapeutic Use of Meaningful Occupations

As noted in Chapters 1 and 2, occupations were always part of occupational therapy, and have indeed justified the profession's existence since its inception. However, at some point in the profession's history, the term *occupation* was dropped from the professional literature and *purposeful activity* was adopted. Mosey argued that purposeful activities are considered to be a major legitimate tool in occupational therapy. She defined purposeful activities as,

> doing processes that require the use of thought and energy and are directed toward an intended or desired end result. Purposeful activities may be contrasted with random activities, which are undirected and without a predetermined goal. They also may be contrasted with 'busy work' or mindless repetitive tasks designed primarily to keep one physically occupied and out of mischief. An activity is usually not considered purposeful unless the reason for engaging in the activity is apparent to the doer (p. 227).[63]

As is evident from the above definition, the construct of purposeful activity emphasizes goal-directedness and does not seem to take into account meaningfulness of the activity to the client, which has been proposed to be a major therapeutic ingredient of use of occupations as a therapeutic tool.*

Beginning with Reilly's call for occupational therapists to return to the roots of their profession,[70] there has been an effort to move away from the concept of "purposeful activities" in favor of resumption of the idea of "meaningful occupations," culminating in the latter being a central construct in the newly emerged professional paradigm.[2,51] In the new paradigm, there seems to be a consensus that "Occupational therapy is about providing meaningful and purposeful experiences for people within occupations" (p. 53)[15] as can be discerned from the profession's literature.† It has also been suggested that since meaningfulness is idiosyncratic,

the meaning of an occupation is specific to the individual client.[46,56] This meaningfulness may be related to the extent to which an occupation is perceived to provide one with a sense of identity, well-being, and perception of life as a continuous whole, among other factors.

Essentially, a therapeutic occupation has meaning for the client and is used by the therapist to frame therapy, communicate the value of occupations, and bridge the psychiatric institution and community.[13] Hasselkus found in a study that occupations were used not only to provide "some meaningful purpose throughout the day" for clients with dementia, but also to help clients "establish a positive self-image and sense of identity" (pp. 203-204).[37] Meaningful occupations utilize the client's abilities (by providing just the right challenge[15]), to help him or her fulfill life roles and achieve personal goals. They help increase clients' feelings of competence and mastery in self-care, work, and leisure; are congruent with their level of development; are recognized by the clients' cultures as meaningful; and involve investigating, trying out, and accumulating evidence of their skills and capacities.

Use of meaningful occupations to frame therapy means using them to facilitate change in the client.[13] Change occurs as a result of the client gaining knowledge, acquiring new skills, learning or relearning how to use capabilities, being able to identify abilities and limitations, developing new interests, learning how to use time effectively, broadening recreational and work opportunities, and increasing the network of people in his or her life as a result of engaging in the occupation. Hasselkus also found the use of meaningful occupations to be a means by which clients with dementia continued to relate to others and to the world, reconnected with their long-held identities, demonstrated a sense of independence, and experienced a sense of control over their environment.[38]

Finally, it is important to point out that use of meaningful occupations as a tool of therapy is made possible by the therapist's effective use of

---

*References 15,37-39,46,64,86.

†References 23,27,48,67,75,86,90.

therapeutic relationships. Through such relationships, the therapist effectively communicates the value of occupations, provides emotional and physical safety so that the client can confidently engage in occupations of choice, and helps the client learn how what is learned during engagement in occupation is applicable in life outside the occupational therapy clinic.[13]

Illustration

Refer to Drake's case presented in Chapter 6. Drake's short-term goals included helping him resume his roles as husband and worker, establish a balanced routine consisting of a repertoire of meaningful occupations, and take better care of himself. We know from the case description that he is interested in performing his role as husband and resuming work as a church minister. The occupations of making greetings cards, writing a resume, and applying for a job were meaningful to him; therefore they were chosen as tools for intervention in his therapy. Similarly, time was taken to develop a schedule of meaningful occupations to fill out his daily routine. Grocery shopping and cooking activities were also meaningful because he recognized that they addressed his need to be able to take better care of himself. By assisting him to engage in these occupations during therapeutic intervention, the therapist was able to help him acquire new skills to enable him to better relate to his wife, relearn job application and self-care capabilities, and learn to use time effectively so as to participate in a balanced routine of occupations.

Refer to Lab Manual Exercises 4-1 and 5-1 to learn how to identify meaningful occupations that can be used as therapeutic media.

Therapeutic Use of Groups and Group Processes

The use of groups as a tool in therapy was borrowed from group techniques in general psychological theory. The prototype of group psychotherapy in occupational therapy can be traced back to the opening of Jane Addams' Hull House in Chicago in 1889.[80] In this setting, a social work group model was used to provide intervention to assist people served by the settlement to transition to the American culture. The first group to be assembled under the aegis of medicine was by Boston internist Joseph Hersey Pratt. He formed a group whose participants were patients from impoverished environments suffering from tuberculosis. His goal was to help participants share so that they did not feel alone in their experiences (principle of universality). He recognized that recovering patients can have significant positive influence on other patients by instilling hope in them.

According to Shaffer and Galinsky,[80] group therapy was extended to patients suffering from psychological illnesses by Edward W. Lazell, a psychiatrist, in 1918 when he was working with war veterans diagnosed with schizophrenia. Gradually, group work was adopted by psychoanalysts such as Trigant Burrow who referred to group therapy in psychoanalysis as *group analysis*. Other psychoanalysts such as Louis Wender recognized transference phenomena in groups, similar to individual psychoanalysis. Paul Schilder attempted to incorporate the Freudian technique of free association by asking group members to discuss anything that came to their minds. Samuel Slavson developed activity group therapy whose objective was to enable children to express their conflicts and pent-up feelings. Slavson's model may be seen as the prototype of a modern day occupational therapy group.

The pioneers of latter-day group work in occupational therapy were Fidler and Fidler, and Mosey. These authors borrowed techniques from psychoanalytic group models and applied them to occupational therapy. Fidler and Fidler developed what they referred to as a *task group model*.[30] The purpose of the task group was to stimulate interpersonal awareness. Their rationale was that interpersonal, intrapsychic, and environmental factors influence affect, learning, and behavior. They saw occupational therapy as a learning laboratory in which skills for life could be developed. As such, occupational therapy task groups were meant to facilitate (using activities) self-exploration in the here and now to help identify clients' stress, conflicts, and problems, and elicit interaction leading to learning and change. Their emphasis was group process emphasizing the relationship between feeling, thinking, and behavior, and the effect of these factors on other people and on task performance.

Fidler and Fidler prescribed that the occupational therapy task group consist of eight clients and meet four times per week for 1.5 hours each session. During those meetings, participants were to work on a task requiring common effort and consensus of all group members. They defined a group task as an activity or process whose objective was to create an end product or a demonstrable service for group members or for other people outside the group. Examples of such tasks included publishing a hospital newsletter, cooking, gardening, participating in patient's councils, and so on.

Mosey,[62] on the other hand, saw groups as venues for evaluation and development of client social interaction skills. Thus she termed them *developmental groups*. She conceived them to be hierarchical and identified five types of groups corresponding to five levels of social-skill development. The lowest in the hierarchy was the *parallel group*. Participants in this type of group had to be able to function in the presence of other people, but were not expected to be able to share roles. This type of group had no common goal. There might be verbal and nonverbal interaction between group members. The only expectation was that group members be able to observe common social manners, such as saying "please," "thank you," and so on.

In the second type of group in the hierarchy *(project group)*, there was a shared *short-term* task. Members of this type of group should be able to share and compete with each other. To participate in a group at this level, clients had to be able to interact with other group members competitively and seek assistance when needed.

The third type of group was the *ego-centric cooperative group*. Tasks in this type of group were relatively *long-term*. Group members were still preoccupied with self interest. However, it was now *enlightened self-interest*. Members realized that their need fulfillment was dependent on other peoples' needs being met. Members of this level of group should be able to engage in cooperative as well as competitive tasks, and recognize and adhere to group norms.

At the fourth level in the hierarchy was the *cooperative group*. This type of group was homogenous, and its sole purpose was mutual need satisfaction. Members of the group shared similar views and feelings. The task was not as important as need satisfaction of group members. To participate in this type of group, clients had to be able to perceive others' needs and try to meet them. Mosey considered the *mature group* to be at the top of the hierarchy. This type of group was conceived to be heterogeneous in its composition. The leader and follower roles were clearly delineated. To participate in this type of group, clients had to be able to share group leadership roles and to distinguish between task-oriented and socio-emotional roles.

Mosey suggested that for a client to benefit from group therapy, he or she needed to be placed in a group immediately next in the hierarchy to his or her level of social-skill development. For example, a client who was able to function in the presence of others (parallel group) needed to be placed in a project group.[62] This would ensure an opportunity to learn social interaction skills at the next developmental level but not to be overwhelmed as to be discouraged. More recently, Mosey[63] has expanded her conceptualization of therapy groups to include a discussion of group stages, roles, goals, and norms, and other types of activity groups such as evaluation and task-oriented groups in addition to developmental groups.

Apart from Fidler and Fidler's and Mosey's groups, other models are currently being used in occupational therapy. For example, Yalom's[93] focus on the group process as opposed to group content is used as a guide to the developmental phase of occupational therapy groups. Other models used include client-centered group leadership based on

Rogerian theory and drawing from existentialism.[17] Also, task groups have become increasingly a part of occupational therapy since the late 1990s, during what Howe and Schwartzberg call "the Wellness Era," during which

the focus of group work has shifted from diagnosis or pathology to an emphasis on the health of the individual, on the inborn capacity for wholeness and well-being that exists in every person and can be supported and developed through the use of groups engaged in occupations (p. 74).[43]

In a survey by Duncombe and Howe,[28] ten types of task groups commonly used by therapists were identified: cooking, activities of daily living, arts and crafts, special task, self-expression, exercise, discussion, sensorimotor and sensory integration, and educational groups.

Cara[14] identifies five types of groups that are commonly used by occupational therapists: (1) task groups (group members try new behaviors and adaptive modes through problem solving in an attempt to complete a task collaboratively), (2) developmental groups (see Mosey's developmental groups discussed above), (3) directive groups (most useful for the more severely affected or acutely mentally ill where the therapist needs to provide more structure and control for group members), (4) neurodevelopmental groups (based on the sensory integration theory and utilizing movement), and (5) other types of groups, such as the psychoeducational group (where the educational format is used to facilitate acquisition of information and techniques by clients).

All group models, however, present a format that generally can be summarized as consisting of three phases: *preparation, development,* and *closure.*[13] In the preparation phase, introductions are made, group goals are stated, and group norms (dos and don'ts) are reviewed. In the development phase, there is discussion of the experiences of group members. During group activity, the therapist notes patterns of group participation including nonverbal expressions of group members. Participation in group activity is facilitated by minimization of cliques in the group. In the closure phase, the therapist summarizes group experiences by restating the group purpose, clarifying outcomes of the group process, and helping group members connect their experiences in the group to their life outside the treatment setting.

A commonly used group intervention approach in occupational therapy is the seven-step format by Marilyn Cole,[17] which consists of *introduction, presentation of the activity, sharing experiences, processing, generalizing, application,* and *summary.* During introduction, the purpose of the group is explained, and group goals are clearly stated. The activity is explained, including supplies needed and the step-by-step procedure to complete it. During the activity phase, group members participate in the activity. Choice of the activity is based on goals of the group members. During the sharing phase, group members present their feedback regarding how the activity was facilitated. This feedback is directed toward the therapist's group leadership skills and how effective group members feel the therapist was in facilitating activity performance.

In the processing phase, group members share their experiences and try to help each other. In the generalizing phase, group members try to find commonalities and differences between their experiences. In the application phase, the therapist uses concreteness (examples) to help group members develop "greater self-awareness, new learning, skill development, greater self-understanding, new choices, or new solutions or strategies for stated problems" (p. 74).[17] During the summary phase, the therapist encourages group members to summarize group proceedings. This format is similar to the group protocol outline suggested by Cara,[14] consisting of group purpose, goals, content, structure, logistics, and methods. However, in Cara's protocol, processing after the group activity is not emphasized. Establishment of a group protocol using Cole's seven-step group therapy format is illustrated in Figure 7-1.

The clients in Figure 7-1 were part of a group of participants in a research study completed

Group Participant Goals	Group Protocol
Participant A 1. By the end of 3 weeks, I will demonstrate improved ability to pay attention in church as indicated by remembering content of the sermon and writing it down immediately after church service. **Participant B** 1. By the end of 3 weeks, I will improve my ability to listen to other people as indicated by consciously listening to at least three friends without interruption, 3 times a week. 2. By the end of 3 weeks, my study habits will improve as indicated by studying for at least 1 hour a night, 3 times a week. **Participant C** 1. By the end of 3 weeks, my participation in family chores will improve as indicated by helping out with cleaning in the kitchen after dinner 3 times a week and vacuuming the house once a week. 2. By the end of 3 weeks, I will demonstrate increased seriousness about church as indicated by attending church service every Sunday.	**Title of the Group** Cultivating good study habits needed to be successful in school. **Purpose of the Groups** To assist group members identify their level of motivation for success in school and use that awareness to develop strategies to complete school-related occupations more satisfactorily. **Description of the Group Activity** Participants will complete a motivation checklist inquiring about their perceptions of why they are attending school, what they hope to achieve, and what hinders their ability to achieve their goals. The relationship between success in school and achievement of life goals will be discussed. Each participant will then read a newspaper article and summarize in writing his or her understanding of the article. Another article will be read aloud by the therapist to the group. Participants will be asked to take notes while listening to the reader. Then they will be requested to summarize in writing what they understood the gist of the article to be. A discussion and other related activities will be facilitated to help participants identify what might have interfered with their ability to understand what they read or listened to. Finally, the group members will be encouraged to formulate a plan for time budget so that enough time is allowed to complete school-related occupations successfully using skills learned from the group activities. **Supplies Needed to Complete Activity** 1. Enough copies of two newspaper articles 2. Instrument to assess and facilitate discussion of study skills (see Texas A & M University's suggestions[85])

Figure 7-1. The application of Cole's seven-step format of occupational therapy group process.

Goals of the Group

By the end of the group session, each group member will demonstrate an understanding of the following as expressed in group discussion:

1. His or her source of motivation to succeed in school.
2. Sources of hindrance to successful completion of academically related occupations.
3. Strategies to minimize the effect of those hindrances so as to be more successful in academic occupations.
4. The importance of being successful in school as a means of achieving life goals.

Questions to Guide Discussion

Processing:

1. How did you feel about today's group activities?
2. How did you feel about how the activity was presented and facilitated?
3. What do you feel was the significance of today's activities to you personally?

Generalization:

1. How do you feel that the problems you experience when you try to study are the same or different from those of the other group members as expressed today?
2. How were your experiences in today's activities in general similar or different from those of the other group members?

Application:

Explain how what you learned in today's group activities may be helpful to you in the future, not only in school but in your life in general.

Summary

Please summarize for me today's group proceedings as you understand them.

Participant D

1. By the end of 3 weeks, my participation in the family will improve as indicated by engagement in family-oriented activities such as playing card games or outdoor games 3 times a week.

Participant E

1. By the end of 3 weeks, my initiative will lead to increased family closeness as indicated by sitting at table for dinner with mom 2 times a week.
2. By the end of 3 weeks, my study habits will improve to enable me to be successful at school as indicated by studying for at least 2 hours once a week.

Participant F

1. By the end of 3 weeks, I will demonstrate increased communication and closeness with my family as indicated by participation in a family board game or some other family leisure activity at least 2 times a week.
2. By the end of 3 weeks, I will demonstrate increased sense of responsibility as indicated by decreased disruptive behavior in class to no more than once a week.

Figure 7-1. Cont'd.

by the author. Their therapy goals were established in collaboration with each client and were therefore stated in first person, using the client's words. The reader will notice that the majority of participant's goals identified development of school-related occupational skills, such as good study habits and being less disruptive in class (three out of the six clients stated this as one of their goals). Thus development of study habits and being successful in school were chosen as themes for the first group session for this group of participants, and group goals were generated accordingly.

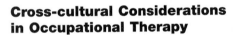 Refer to Lab Manual Exercise 8-3 for experiential learning of how to prepare and use a group protocol to run a therapeutic occupational therapy group.

Cross-cultural Considerations in Occupational Therapy

In this section, we will examine the cultural issues affecting occupational therapists' effectiveness in delivery of services. As Crabtree, Royeen, and Benton state,

> The most critical issue in culturally proficient rehabilitation is to recognize that individuals receiving rehabilitation services are part of a multifaceted system of shared beliefs, meanings, values, and the like, that are expressed through those individuals' beliefs about things like independence, health, and function (p. 4).[21]

In order for occupational therapists to deliver services to clients from varying backgrounds guided by a client-centered model, they need to develop cultural proficiency so that they can be truly collaborative with clients irrespective of disparities in beliefs.

The need for cultural proficiency by members of helping professions is well-recognized in the literature. Culture is a decisive factor in counseling theory and practice, so it is important to know how it limits the effectiveness of any therapy.[44] Similarly, Lawless, Gale, and Bacigalupe observed that "The family therapy supervision literature clearly states that issues of REC (Race, Ethnicity,

and Culture) should be part of the discourse in clinical supervision" (p. 191).[57] In occupational therapy, it is being increasingly recognized that due to increasing numbers of minorities and individuals with a variety of cultural experiences,[10] there is need "to examine how culturally relevant occupational therapy really is for both its colleagues and its clients" (p. 1).[47]

The discussion in this section is meant to provide a general awareness of cultural issues in therapy with the hope that the therapist will be inspired to seek more education to develop cultural proficiency.

Culture: A Definition

A review of the literature indicates that a clear definition of culture is elusive.[11,26,47] Sometimes it is defined in terms of cultural esthetic products such as arts, music, theater, and so on, while in other instances it is defined in terms of ethnicity (e.g., Italian culture, Irish culture). However, culture is more than just cultural artifacts or ethnicity. For instance, there is increasing recognition that cultural differences exist, even within the same ethnic or racial groups in terms of age (e.g., youth versus traditional cultures), sexual orientation (gay/lesbian versus heterosexual cultures), geographical locality (Eastern, Midwestern, Western, and Southern cultural factors within the United States), and so on.[10] It has even been suggested that gender constitutes a cultural difference (genderlects)[68] because women perceive reality and communicate differently from men. Men tend to value logic over emotion, while women tend to prioritize relationships and affect over logic.

One way of understanding culture broadly is as a determinant of "individual's actions, and their attributions of meaning and value to those actions" (p. 160).[11] Dickie suggests that culture may be seen "as a central part of daily life for most people" (p. 169).[26] Iwama sees culture "as shared spheres of experience and the means through which meaning is ascribed to objects and phenomena around us" (p. 1).[47]

Bonder and colleagues propose three ways of defining culture that may be of interest to occupational therapists. The first is a descriptive definition emphasizing "the technological, economic, political, kinship, and religious characteristics of a people" (p. 160).[11] An example of such a definition is culture as "knowledge, beliefs, art, morals, laws, customs, and any other capabilities and habits acquired by members of a society" (p. 12).[44] In such a definition, culture consists of beliefs and values that shape the way we think, perceive, feel, and behave/act. It encompasses behavior as well as products of labor and industry for a society at a given place and time. The danger with this type of definition is the possibility of stereotyping individuals on the basis of superficial group characteristics, which describe groups generally but do not explain individual choices and behavior.

The second approach is the rule-based definition. These types of definitions tend to focus on rules that guide behavior and interactions between individuals, for example, determining the appropriate roles of men, women, boys, and girls (e.g., in some cultures, women cook and take care of the home and children, while men work out in the fields and perform jobs in towns) and how women and men should interact with each other (e.g., in fundamentalist Muslim communities, the woman's face is not supposed to be seen by any man other than the husband). These types of definitions help us understand generally how individuals from a certain culture interact and make decisions, and how to interact with clients from such cultures during therapy. This understanding is crucial in establishing rapport with the client, which in the previous chapter was found to be extremely important in the development of a therapeutic relationship. However, the rule-based definitions are also limited. They describe general rules guiding interactions in a group of individuals but do not provide an understanding of how we should interact with a specific client.

Bonder and colleagues propose a third approach to defining culture: the pragmatic approach.[11] In this type of definition, culture is perceived to emerge from the interaction between individuals. In this view, individual behavior is seen as emerging from an interaction between cultural and individual factors (this is close to what are referred to below as *culturals* and *individuals*). In other words, "each person's contact with and interpretation of the culture is unique" (p. 5).[54] Culture provides behavioral guidelines, but the individual ultimately makes choices and acts.

It is also important to point out that culture is primarily a creation of humans, for the service of those in a specific community. In that sense, culture is a social institution. As Dewey pointed out, social institutions are creations that help humans adapt to their environment.[60] Similarly, Grady proposed that humans organize themselves and their environment (other people, objects, space, and relationships) in the process of adaptation.[35] The need for organization of others and the environment in order to adapt is further indication that culture is a tool for adaptation, since relationships denote the socio-cultural aspect of the environment. It can therefore be safely concluded that culture is a human creation, designed specifically to make interaction possible, which then facilitates collective community adaptation to the environment.

Characteristics of Culture

According to Bonder and Gurley, "culture is learned, localized, patterned, and evaluative" (p. CE-1).[10] The first characteristic is that culture is a *learned* phenomenon. In this sense, "some cultural belief structures and behavior patterns are laid down in early childhood through learning and experience within the family and community" (p. 162).[11] This learning occurs primarily through observation and discourse. This implies that certain aspects of culture are acquired through upbringing. However, some cultural characteristics are acquired through education and other life experiences as well. For example, occupational therapists are enculturated through education and modeling by professionals.

Because culture is learned, it means that it is also not static. It evolves and changes, both for the community and the individual.

The second characteristic is that culture is a *localized* phenomenon. This means that cultural perspectives are shared and therefore are meaningful to individuals within a certain locale, who share in those perspectives. The fact that culture is localized also means that one may have more than one set of cultural identities. For instance, as an occupational therapist, you share a certain perspective with the occupational therapy community regarding the value and meaning of occupation, client-centeredness, and so on. However, once you leave the professional setting and go back to your community, you share in your community's cultural values and beliefs. This means that each person has a variety of cultural perspectives that are expressed in different settings as indicated.

The third characteristic is that behaviors are *patterned* by cultural perspectives that make individual actions meaningful. This meaning is expressed through routines, habits, and rituals. The third characteristic is that culture provides a group of people shared *values* that guide their choices and interactions. However, cultural values are not always agreed upon by individuals in a group. Like culture, values also evolve and change over time, both for the group collectively, as well as for the individual.

Finally, culture provides *stability* of perspective in life, even as it evolves and changes. Some cultural values remain the same through time but may be expressed differently. For example, an immigrant from Africa may not abandon the value for strong family ties. However, being several thousand miles away from home, it may be difficult to visit family members regularly, which would be typical if he was living at home. He may adopt cell phone and e-mail technology as a way of keeping in touch with family members regularly. In this case, the value for strong family ties remains constant, while the means of keeping in contact with family members over long distances changes because of technology.

The characteristics of culture notwithstanding, people's knowledge, beliefs, art, morals, laws, customs, and other habits defined by culture differ because they depend on the geographical, religious, educational, social, and political context within which they are cultivated.[44] The environment to which a community is trying to adapt determines how those aspects of a culture develop. For instance, the African's largely agrarian environment characterized mostly by subsistence farming facilitates greater awareness of the need for a strong social support system in order to survive, given the uncertainty associated with dependence on environmental factors such as whether or not it rains. This leads to development of a culture in which social relationships are prioritized and ownership of property in the Western sense of individual ownership is deemphasized.[79] On the other hand, individualism is encouraged in Western industrialized cultures based on competition for industrial trappings, since personal strength and ability to compete effectively is perceived to be a way to ensure community survival. Thus individuals from these two cultures have different perspectives on life. That being the case, how can there be any understanding between them? This necessitates a conceptualization of what happens when different cultures meet.

In this conceptualization, the reader should bear in mind that as discussed earlier in the chapter, ethnicity is not the only factor that constitutes cultural differences. Other factors include age, geographical locality, and sexual orientation. However, ethnically-based differences are particularly important for occupational therapists because they have been found to have a significant effect on health factors such as life expectancy, incidence of certain types of diseases, practices that have a bearing on health such as use of tobacco or alcohol and exercising, access to health care, and so on.[10] That is why ethnicity will be emphasized in the following discussion, rather than other forms of cultural differences.

What Happens when Two Disparate Cultures Meet

Figure 7-2 shows a hypothetical illustration of three possible outcomes that can take place when two cultures meet.

The scenarios illustrated in Figure 7-2 are based on the assumption of cultural advantage derived from each culture's strength. The strength of a culture is assumed to obtain from many factors including its military, technological, or material wealth. In Scenario 1, Culture A is stronger than Culture B. A possible outcome of the two cultures meeting is annihilation of Culture B. Attempts to annihilate other cultures abound. For example, Nazi Germany attempted to annihilate the Jewish culture in Europe through genocide. The same case occurred in Africa when the Hutu attempted to eliminate the Tutsi in Rwanda. Crabtree, Royeen, and Benton call this the "overt *cultural destructive behavior,*" which they see as including "intentional and militant actions to destroy and eradicate a particular culture or group and the values it represents" (p. 5).[21]

In Scenario 2, Cultures A and B are equal in strength. When the two meet, sharing occurs, resulting in mutual enrichment where each culture adopts the other's positive aspects. This is the ideal situation where a hybrid culture emerges. The dominant U.S. culture may to a certain extent be seen as representing this ideal situation, where different European cultures have interacted, leading to an emergence of a distinctly American culture (see discussion of the values of this culture by Crabtree, Royeen, and Benton[21]).

Finally, in Scenario 3, Cultures A and B, which are of equal strength, do not interact. Each culture stays independent, and there is no sharing. An example of this outcome can be found among the Maasai peoples of Kenya and Tanzania. All attempts by the British to conquer the Maasai and bring them under British rule along with the rest of the Kenyan and Ugandan peoples (Tanzania was then a German protectorate) failed. Consequently, the Maasai people of East Africa are the only group of African people who have never been colonized and therefore have never experienced forceful loss of culture. Their culture has been maintained very much in its original form to this day, in the midst of rapid Westernization of the rest of Africa.

It is important to emphasize that the above-discussed possible outcomes are hypothetical. In real life, interaction between cultures is complex and does not in reality result in such neat, well-delineated outcomes. For example, even a dominant culture that somehow manages to subdue a weaker culture borrows some characteristics from that culture. Thus no culture really remains pure after an encounter with another one.

Implications of Cultural Factors to Therapeutic Discourse

It is important for occupational therapists to realize that culture provides an explanatory model of disease, health, disability, and performance—not only for the client but also for the therapist.[10] This means that a client's choice of occupations perceived to be appropriate and meaningful and the patterning of his or her performance depends on his or her cultural perspective. If the therapist's view, based on his or her culture, is different from that of the client, there is a likelihood of differences in valuation of the meaning of behaviors in therapy and subsequent miscommunication. For example, a client who perceives an occupation to be culturally meaningless may resist involvement in it, which may be interpreted by the therapist as

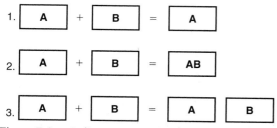

Figure 7-2.   A diagrammatical illustration of three possible outcomes when two cultures meet.

laziness. Also, culture affects communication between the client and therapist. If a therapist is not sensitive to cultural nuances in a therapeutic relationship, he or she may miss what is truly meaningful to a client and may offend the client by statements and behaviors perceived to be inappropriate.

It is also argued in this book that when a therapist meets a client from a different cultural background, it is important to remember that it is a meeting of two cultures. Therefore the same dynamics that occur when two cultural groups meet are experienced in the therapist-client relationship. Similar cultural struggles ensue. In this case, since the therapist holds a position of power bestowed by the profession, most probably he or she will be representing the cultural perspective perceived to have the upper hand. The result of the therapist-client interaction may be an attempt by the therapist to change the client's views (subduing the client's perspective), an effort to understand the client's perspective so that there is mutual enrichment, or remaining aloof so that neither of them is affected by the other.

Another thing to remember is that when two people meet, it is not just the two of them in communication. The entire history of their respective cultural experiences is present in their interaction. This will be illustrated with Drake's case introduced in Chapter 6. Suppose that I were Drake's therapist. From the first moment of our meeting, the fact that I represent a cultural heritage of a people who have been abused for hundreds of years through slavery, colonization, and economic unfairness is a significant potential influence on my communication with him. On the other hand, he represents the heritage of the abuser (a Caucasian white male). Because of this history, certain dynamics may occur between us, which may have nothing to do with us as individuals. For example, I might be thinking that he is looking down upon me. After all, there is a historical indication (which in all likelihood is wrong given that social views have changed drastically since the slavery and colonial eras)

that people of his ethnic persuasion do not think favorably of people from my ethnic background. For instance, David Hume, one of the greatest Western philosophers of all time, once expressed the opinion that: "The Negro is naturally inferior to the whites. There scarcely ever was a civilized nation of that complexion, nor even any individual, eminent either in action or speculation. No ingenious manufacturers among them, no arts, no science" (p. 14).[91]

Drake, a modern Caucasian American, may not share Hume's sentiments. However, the fact that I may unconsciously be thinking that he does, based on our cultural histories, is likely to affect how I interact with him, unless I am able to maintain a reflective stance and with awareness decide not to let prejudices based on historical events interfere with our relationship. This suggests the need for the therapist to maintain cultural competence, which Crabtree and colleagues define as "self-exploration in relation to one's own culture, values, beliefs, and experiences of people from different ethnic groups and cultures" and "to apply those relevant cultural concepts in every day practice to patients of different cultural backgrounds" (p. 5).[21] The recommendation calls for vigilance, as suggested by Flaskas,[31] where the therapist consistently dwells in self-exploration so as to effectively distinguish factors of the therapeutic relationship that pertain to the client and those that pertain to the therapist. Dickie,[26] Bonder and colleagues,[11] and Bonder and Gurley[10] similarly emphasize the importance of this self-reflection through which the therapist should aspire to understand how his or her own cultural perspective as well as the client's perspective affects the therapeutic discourse.

Through such self-reflection, I would be able to realize that although Drake is a Caucasian American, it does not mean that he shares in the negative stereotypes about Africans propagated over history. I would be able to come to a conscious awareness of the dynamics of our relationship, allowing it to progress without prejudice. To develop vigilance, a model for understanding

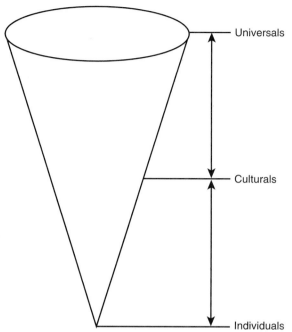

Figure 7-3. An illustration of culture as a filter of experiences that influence interaction in a therapeutic relationship. *Universals* refer to experiences that are common to all humans irrespective of cultural background. *Culturals* refer to experiences acquired in the process of socialization in a particular culture. *Individuals* refer to individual characteristics that set one apart from all other humans.

how cultural issues filter into the therapeutic relationship is suggested in Figure 7-3.

Figure 7-3 is presented as a funnel because it is meant to demonstrate the filtering process that occurs in a therapeutic relationship. This is consistent with the idea of culture as "a filter or veil through which people perceive life's experiences" or the view that: "Talk and action are 'processed through the filter of interpretation'" (p. 108).[55] When a therapist meets a client, he or she is able to relate to that client because of an understanding of certain experiences that are common to all humans. For instance, irrespective of cultural background, we all experience pain when hurt, love when we meet someone who really connects to how we feel, hate when we meet someone who intentionally wants to hurt us, and so on. We can relate to these experiences in another person because we have experienced them in our lives at one time or another. They are universal experiences, common to all humanity. This shared common humanity is what makes empathy, which has been repeatedly emphasized in this book, possible. Because we can relate to experiences of others, we can place ourselves in their shoes, so to speak, and see the world from their frame of reference.

As discussed earlier, cultural experiences, values, beliefs, and customs are instilled in us through education, which includes verbal instruction, modeling, and interaction with other people. The culture in which we grow up initially determines our interpretation of experiences and therefore our world outlook. For example, Crabtree and colleagues[21] point out that there is a set of values specific to mainstream America that includes acceptance of a scientific orientation to the world, an attempt or desire to control the environment, materialism, individualism, strict adherence to prescribed time use, and so on. People from other parts of the world view these values differently. For instance, in Africa, keeping time is not as important as socializing.[45,59] Individualism is deemphasized in favor of the clan, and property is seen as communal rather than individual.[79]

Thus, although all humans have a concept of property, time, community, and individual worth, how these universal human characteristics are interpreted, understood, and prioritized depends on the culture in which one is socialized. Dickie refers to this as knowledge of what is typical for a certain culture.[26] As discussed earlier, the cultural perspectives that structure the meaning of these universal characteristics evolve and change over time as individuals acquire new experiences. However, there are also some cultural factors that remain stable and therefore contribute to a person's enduring identity.[10,11]

Finally, even in the same culture, individuals have idiosyncratic characteristics that set them apart from all other individuals. In the final analysis, it is the individual who is the cultural actor.[11] As Krefting states, "each person's contact with and interpretation of culture is unique" (p. 5).[54] For instance, American culture may emphasize individualism and materialism. However, how individuals exercise the autonomy associated with this individualism, or use property accumulated from their work, is unique. One person may use his or her property to help others, while another may use it to seek more luxury. One may choose to use the latitude allowed for self-determination by the cultural value of individualism to spend discretionary time volunteering to serve the less-advantaged members of the world community, while another may decide to spend the same discretionary time traveling to see the world. These individual differences result in part from the values that one learns from his or her family and in part from one's constitution.

It is these individual characteristics that a therapist seeks to uncover in the therapeutic process. However, in order to uncover these traits, he or she has to be able to relate to the client. Relating to the client is possible in a sound therapeutic relationship. To establish this relationship, the therapist needs to be able to communicate effectively with the client. This necessitates that he or she be able to identify characteristics shared with the client as a member of the human race, and how expression of those characteristics is shaped by cultural experiences.

Suggested Outline for Culturally Sensitive Therapeutic Discourse

Bonder and colleagues[11] and Bonder and Gurley[10] suggest a three-step process of conducting culturally sensitive occupational therapy interaction:

1. If you are scheduled to meet a client from a culture that is different from yours, educate yourself about at least the basic characteristics of his or her culture. This will help you develop the cultural sensitivity necessary for communication with the client in such a way that rapport may be established quickly.

Self-education may be achieved by attending "workshops, courses, or reading about specified cultures" in order to gain "helpful insights and strategies for working with people of those cultures" (p. 172).[26] An addition to this list could be searching for information on the Internet or interviewing people who may know about the culture in question.

2. Make a hypothesis about how the client's occupational performance issues may be framed based on an understanding of his or her culture. At the same time, reflect on how your own view of the clues you are picking up in the therapeutic discourse may be influenced by your own cultural perspective, and how this cultural interpretation may color your hypothesis about the client.

3. Finally, test your hypothesis by questioning the client about whether or not your interpretation of cues and attribution of meanings to them is accurate.

The above three steps infer that, as a therapist, you need to maintain vigilance by paying attention at every moment to the client's "word choice, facial expression, body posture, voice tone, gestures, and other clues to the feelings and attitudes of the individual" (p. 166).[11] This is the same kind of vigilance needed for therapeutic communication in general (see section on the therapeutic relationship above).

Illustration

To illustrate the cultural influence in a therapeutic relationship, when working with Drake in the case example in Chapter 6, the therapist would need to understand that Drake probably experiences anxiety related to the strained relationship with his wife. We know from experience that when valued relationships do not go well, there is psychological pain. It is an experience common to all humanity (referred to as *universals* in Figure 7-3). We also can guess that he might be feeling good (joyous, uplifted, and so on) because of his closeness with his daughter. These are other universal feelings. However, being a

Caucasian American, we can guess that Drake probably values punctuality, the ability to make personal decisions, privacy, and so on, because these are characteristics shared in the dominant American culture (referred to in Figure 7-3 as *culturals*). We also know that he has interests that are particular to him apart from his culture, such as taking walks, working out, riding his bike, and so on *(individuals)*. These individual interests define his autonomy (a cultural value) by helping him express it in a very individual manner. For example, he might choose to deal with his psychological pain associated with the strained relationship with his wife (universal experience) by working out vigorously (an autonomous way of relieving stress through a personally meaningful occupation). A culturally competent therapist would be able to maintain awareness of all these different levels of Drake's processing of experiences in order to relate to him in such a way as to conduct therapy in true collaboration with him.

However, as Crabtree and colleagues[21] aptly point out, it is important to realize that cultural competence is not something that a therapist achieves once and for all. As Bonder and colleagues argue: "It is impossible to know all there is to know about every labeled cultural group, Hispanics, for example, or Blacks" (p. 166).[11] Cultural competency is a process. It is more about relating to clients with the understanding that their world views may be significantly different from yours, respecting those views, and demonstrating the respect by genuinely seeking to understand the unique world view without trying to impose your own values on the client. As mentioned earlier, if as a therapist you know you will be treating a client from a culture that is different from yours, you may want to find more information about the culture before the initial meeting. In today's technological age, you can find such information easily from the Internet.

For instance, imagine that you were meeting a client from Meru (an ethnic group in Kenya). A Google search would inform you that there is a strict adherence to "age-sets," in that community, where people are expected to socialize mostly within their own age groups.[42] You would also learn that among the Meru people, interdependence is emphasized over independence, and the extended family is a very important component of life. You would therefore conclude that important decisions are made by the family rather than the individual. Such knowledge would be crucial to help you relate to a client from that community.

For another example, imagine that you are meeting a client from India. A search would reveal that some people from that country prefer their culture to be identified as *Indian* rather than *Hindu,* because they believe that the term *Hindu* has religious connotations.[41] You would also realize that Indian practices such as poetry, astrology, yoga, and so on derive from Hindu religious teachings. Thus religion to a large extent permeates the whole of Indian culture.[4] This influences the Indian view of the world, which holds that there is the divine immanent in all forms of life. Also, you would find that traditionally, women were venerated in the Indian culture. However, in the contemporary Indian society, you would learn that there are concerns about dowry-related murders of women, problems with the caste system, and so on. All of these factors may be significant in your interaction with a client from that culture. However, the final source of information is ultimately the client. To increase your sensitivity, you can use the information obtained from other sources (workshops, classes, or the Internet), but ultimately the client is the authority on how he or she prefers to be addressed and treated.

Refer to Lab Manual Exercise 8-4 for experiential learning to help you begin developing cultural competency in clinical practice.

SUMMARY

In this chapter, we reviewed general occupational therapy intervention skills. These skills include ethical clinical reasoning, use of a therapeutic relationship, use of meaningful occupations, and use of groups and group processes. We emphasized that ethical clinical reasoning is a cognitive process. We introduced the concept of an *ethical cognitive schema* (ideas, experiences, knowledge, and so on that form a framework to help the therapist interpret ethical data) as a way of offering occupational therapists a tool to analyze ideas that they use in their ethical decision-making process. We also discussed a six-step model of ethical decision making consisting of identification of the ethical problem, gathering pertinent information, consulting legal and ethical guidelines, evaluating options, making a decision and acting, and evaluating the course of action.

We then outlined the importance of a therapeutic relationship and its components in occupational therapy intervention, and examined their application in occupational therapy practice. We then explored the use of meaningful occupations in occupational therapy intervention. We discussed the use of groups and group processes with an emphasis on Cole's seven-step group therapy format. Finally, we briefly expounded cultural factors affecting occupational therapy intervention, and advanced a model for developing cultural awareness and competency in clinical practice.

REFERENCES

1. Adams J: *Prescribing: the ethical dimension*, 2004. Retrieved September 2005, from http://www.nurse-prescriber.co.uk/Articles/Ethical_prescribing.htm.
2. American Occupational Therapy Association: Occupational therapy practice framework: domain and process, *Am J Occup Ther* 56:609-639, 2002.
3. American Occupational Therapy Association: Occupational therapy code of ethics (2005), *Am J Occup Ther* 59:639-642, 2005.
4. A Tribute to Hinduism: *Hindu culture part I*, 2006. Retrieved April 2006, from http://www.atributetohinduism.com/Hindu_Culture1.htm.
5. Bailey DM, Schwartzberg SL: *Ethical and legal dilemmas in occupational therapy*, Philadelphia, 1995, FA Davis.
6. Bailey DM, Schwartzberg SL: *Ethical and legal dilemmas in occupational therapy*, ed 2, Philadelphia, 2003, FA Davis.
7. Baum CM: 1980 Eleanor Clarke Slagle lecture—Occupational therapists put care in the health system, *Am J Occup Ther* 34:505-516, 1980.
8. Beauchamp TL, Childress JF: *Principles of biomedical ethics,* ed 4, New York, 1994, Oxford University Press.
9. Beauchamp TL, Childress JF: *Principles of biomedical ethics,* ed 5, New York, 2001, Oxford University Press.
10. Bonder B, Gurley D: Culture and aging: working with older adults from diverse backgrounds, *OT Practice* 10(3):CE1-CE7, 2005.
11. Bonder BR, Martin L, Miracle AW: Culture emergent in occupation, *Am J Occup Ther* 58:159-168, 2004.
12. Bongiovi ME, Cournos F: Introduction to medical interviewing. In Kay J, Tasman A, Lieberman JA, eds: *Psychiatry: behavioral science and clinical essentials: a companion to Tasman, Kay, Lieberman: psychiatry,* pp. 24-40, Philadelphia, 2000, WB Saunders.
13. Bruce MA, Borg B: *Psychosocial frames of reference: core for occupation-based practice,* Thorofare, NJ, 2002, Slack.
14. Cara E: Groups. In Cara E, MacRae A, eds: *Psychosocial occupational therapy: a clinical practice,* ed 2, Clifton Park, NY, 2005, Thomson Delmar Learning.
15. Christie A: A meaningful occupation: the just right challenge, *Austr Occup Ther J* 46:52-68, 1999.
16. Coady NF: The association between client and therapist interpersonal processes and outcomes in psychodynamic psychotherapy, *Res Social Work Practice* 1:122-138, 1991.
17. Cole MB: *Group dynamics in occupational therapy: the theoretical basis and practice application of group intervention,* ed 3, Thorofare, NJ, 2005, Slack.
18. Cottone RR: A social constructivism model of ethical decision-making in counseling, *J Couns Dev* 79:39-45, 2001.
19. Cottone RR, Claus RE: Ethical decision-making models: a review of the literature, *J Couns Dev* 78:275-283, 2000.
20. Cottone RR, Tarvydas V, House G: The effect of number and type of consulted relationships on the ethical decision making of graduate students in counseling, *Couns Values* 39:56-68, 1994.
21. Crabtree JL, Royeen M, Benton J: Cultural proficiency in rehabilitation: an introduction. In Royeen M, Crabtree JL, ed: *Culture in rehabilitation: from competency to proficiency,* Upper Saddle River, NJ, 2006, Pearson/Prentice Hall, pp. 1-16.
22. Crepeau EB: Achieving intersubjective understanding: examples from an occupational therapy treatment session, *Am J Occup Ther* 45:1016-1025, 1991.
23. Csikszentmihalyi M: *Creativity: flow and the psychology of discovery and invention,* New York, 1996, HarperCollins.
24. Cynkin S: *Occupational therapy: toward health through activities,* Boston, 1979, Little Brown.

25. Dewey J: *Reconstruction in philosophy,* Boston, 1957, Beacon Press.
26. Dickie VA: Culture is tricky: a commentary on culture emergent in occupation, *Am J Occup Ther* 58:169-173, 2004.
27. do Rozario L: Ritual, meaning and transcendence: the role of occupation in modern life, *J Occup Sci* 1:46-53, 1994.
28. Duncombe L, Howe MC: Group work in occupational therapy: a survey of practice, *Am J Occup Ther* 39:163-170, 1985.
29. Eklund M, Hallberg IR: Psychiatric occupational therapists' verbal interaction with their clients, *Occup Ther Internat* 8(1):1-16, 2001.
30. Fidler G, Fidler J: *Occupational therapy: a communication process in psychiatry,* New York, 1963, McMillan.
31. Flaskas C: Thinking about the therapeutic relationship: emerging themes in family therapy, *Austr New Zealand J Family Ther* 25(1):13-20, 2004.
32. Garcia JG, Cartwrite B, Winston SM, et al: A transcultural integrative model for ethical decision making in counseling, *J Couns Dev* 81:268-277, 2003.
33. Gazda GM: *Group counseling: a developmental approach,* ed 4, Boston, 1989, Allyn & Bacon.
34. Goldberg A: Postmodern psychoanalysis, *Psyche Matters,* October 11, 2001. Retrieved July 2005, from http://www.psychematters.com/papers/goldberg.htm.
35. Grady AP: 1994 Eleanor Clarke Slagle lecture—Building inclusive community: a challenge for occupational therapy. In Cottrell RP, ed: *Purposeful activity: foundation and future of occupational therapy,* Bethesda, MD, 1996, AOTA, pp. 229-240.
36. Hadjistavropoulos T, Malloy DC, Sharpe D, et al: The ethical ideologies of psychologists and physicians: a preliminary comparison, *Ethics Behavior* 13:97-104, 2003.
37. Hasselkus BR: The meaning of activity: day care for persons with Alzheimer's disease, *Am J Occup Ther* 46:199-206, 1992.
38. Hasselkus BR: Occupation and well-being in dementia: the experience of day-care staff, *Am J Occup Ther* 52:423-434, 1998.
39. Hasselkus BR: *"Everyday ethics" and "everyday occupations and well-being,"* 2006. Retrieved March 2006, from http://faculty.arts.ubc.ca/graham/hasselk2.htm.
40. Hergenhahn BR: *An introduction to the history of psychology,* ed 3, Pacific Grove, CA, 1997, Brooks/Cole.
41. Hindunet: *The value of the Hindu culture for the world,* 2006. Retrieved April 2006, from http://www.hindunet.org/alt_hindu/1995_June_2/msg00010.html.
42. *History of churches of Christ in Meru: the setting and history of the Meru mission,* 2005. Retrieved September 2005, from http://www.faulkner.edu/admin/websites/rtrull/mfc/kenya/history_churches_meru.htm.
43. Howe MC, Schwartzberg SL: *A functional approach to group work in occupational therapy,* ed 3, Baltimore, MD, 2001, Lippincott Williams & Wilkins.
44. Ikiugu MN: Process-oriented psychology and African culture, *J Process Oriented Psychol* 4(1):11-22, 1992.
45. Ikiugu MN: African thought and spiritualism, *J Process Oriented Psychol* 5(2):73-79, 1993.
46. Ikiugu MN: Meaningfulness of occupations as an occupational-life-trajectory attractor, *J Occup Sci* 12:102-109, 2005.
47. Iwama MK: Guest editorial—Meaning and inclusion: revisiting culture in occupational therapy, *Austr Occup Ther J* 51:1-2, 2004.
48. Johnson JA: Occupational science and occupational therapy: an emphasis on meaning—applications in occupational therapy. In Zemke R, Clark F, eds: *Occupational science: the evolving discipline,* Philadelphia, 1996, FA Davis, pp. 393-397.
49. Josephson Institute of Ethics: Making sense of ethics. *Resources: Making ethical decisions,* 2002. Retrieved September 2005, from http://www.josephsoninstitute.org/MED/MED-1makingsense.htm.
50. Kant I: *Grounding for the metaphysics of morals,* Cambridge, England, 1981, Hackett.
51. Kielhofner G: *Conceptual foundations of occupational therapy,* ed 3, Philadelphia, 2004, FA Davis.
52. Kirschenbaum H: Carl Roger's life and work: an assessment on the 100th anniversary of his birth, *J Couns Dev* 82:116-124, 2004.
53. Kornblau BL, Starling SP: *Ethics in rehabilitation: a clinical perspective,* Thorofare, NJ, 2000, Slack.
54. Krefting LH: The culture concept in the everyday practice of occupational and physical therapy, *Occup Phys Ther Pediatr* 11(4):1-16, 1991.
55. Krefting LH, Krefting DV: Cultural influences on performance. In Christiansen C, Baum C, eds: *Occupational therapy: overcoming human performance deficits,* pp. 102-122, Thorofare, NJ, 1991, Slack.
56. Law M, Baptiste S, Carswell A, et al: *Canadian occupational performance measure,* ed 3, Ottawa, ON, 2000, CAOT Publications ACE.
57. Lawless JJ, Gale JE, Bacigalupe G: The discourse of race and culture in family therapy supervision: a conversation analysis, *Contemporary Fam Ther* 23:181-197, 2001.
58. Maturana HR: Biology of language: the epistemology of reality. In Miller GA, Lenneberg F, eds: *Psychology and biology of language and thought,* pp. 27-63, New York, 1978, Academic Press.
59. Mbiti JS: *African religions and philosophy,* Nairobi, Kenya, 1972, Heinemann Educational Books.
60. McDermott JJ, ed: *The philosophy of John Dewey,* Chicago, 1981, The University of Chicago Press.
61. Mill JS: *Utilitarianism,* New York, 1957, Bobbs-Merrill.

62. Mosey AC: *Three frames of reference for mental health,* Thorofare, NJ, 1970, Slack.

63. Mosey AC: *Psychosocial components of occupational therapy,* New York, 1996, Lippincott Williams & Wilkins.

64. Nelson DL: Therapeutic occupation: a definition, *Am J Occup Ther* 50:775-782, 1995.

65. Peloquin SM: The fullness of empathy: reflections and illustrations, *Am J Occup Ther* 49:24-31, 1995.

66. Peloquin SM: 2005 Eleanor Clarke Slagle lecture—Embracing our ethos, and reclaiming our heart, *Am J Occup Ther* 59:611-625, 2005.

67. Persson D, Erlandsson L, Eklund M, et al: Value dimensions, meaning, and complexity in human occupation—a tentative structure for analysis, *Scand J Occup Ther* 8:7-18, 2001.

68. Posthuma BW: *Small groups in counseling and therapy: process and leadership,* ed 4, Boston, 2002, Allyn & Bacon.

69. Precin P: *Client-centered reasoning: narratives of people with mental illness,* Boston, 2002, Butterworth-Heinemann.

70. Reilly M: 1961 Eleanor Clarke Slagle lecture—Occupational therapy can be one of the great ideas of 20th century medicine, *Am J Occup Ther* 16:1-9, 1962.

71. Roberts AR: Assessment, crisis intervention, and trauma treatment: the integrative ACT intervention model, *Brief Treatment Crisis Intervention* 2:1-21, 2002.

72. Rogers CR: A current formulation of client-centered therapy, *Social Service Rev* 24:442-450, 1950.

73. Rogers CR: *On becoming a person: a therapist's view of psychotherapy,* Boston, 1961, Houghton Mifflin.

74. Rogers JC: 1983 Eleanor Clarke Slagle lecture—Clinical reasoning: the ethics, science, and art, *Am J Occup Ther* 37:601-616, 1983.

75. Scheerer CR, Cahill LG, Kirby K, et al: Cake decorating as occupation: meaning and motivation, *J Occup Sci* 11:68-74, 2004.

76. Schell BA: Clinical reasoning: the basis of practice. In Crepeau EB, Cohn ES, Schell BA, eds: *Willard and Spackman's occupational therapy,* ed 10, pp. 131-139, Philadelphia, 2003, Lippincott Williams & Wilkins.

77. Schwartzberg SL: *Interactive reasoning in the practice of occupational therapy,* Upper Saddle River, NJ, 2002, Prentice Hall.

78. Sedgwick D: Freud reconsidered: the technique of analysis, *San Francisco Jung Institute Library J* 16(1):5-25, 1997. Retrieved July 2005, from http://www.psychematters.com/papers/sedgwick2.htm.

79. Senghor LS: *De la negritude psychologie du negro-Africain,* Nairobi, Kenya, 1962, Heinemann Educational Books.

80. Shaffer J, Galinsky M: *Models of group therapy and sensitivity training,* Upper Saddle River, NJ, 1974, Prentice Hall.

81. Sibley J: *Classical ethics for contemporary times: a heuristic approach,* unpublished manuscript, Denton, Texas, Texas Woman's University.

82. Sibley J: Personal communication, 1997.

83. Smith SA, Thomas SA, Jackson AC: An exploration of the therapeutic relationship and counseling outcomes in a problem gambling counseling service, *J Social Work Pract* 18:99-112, 2004.

84. Stein F, Cutler SK: *Psychosocial occupational therapy: a holistic approach,* ed 2, Albany, NY, 2002, Delmar Thompson Learning.

85. Texas A&M University: Basic study techniques, *Texas A&M University student counseling service,* 2005. Retrieved September 2005, from http://www.scs.tamu.edu/selfhelp/elibrary/basic_study_techniques.asp.

86. Trombly CA: 1995 Eleanor Clarke Slagle lecture—Occupation: purposefulness and meaningfulness as therapeutic mechanisms, *Am J Occup Ther* 49:960-972, 1995.

87. U.S. Food and Drug Administration: The Belmont report: ethical principles and guidelines for the protection of human subjects of research, *Information Sheets: Guidance for Institutional Review Boards and Clinical Investigators,* 1998. Retrieved September 2005, from http://www.fda.gov/oc/ohrt/irbs/belmont.html.

88. Velasquez M, Andre C, Meyer TM: *A framework for thinking ethically,* Markkula Center for Applied Ethics, Santa Clara University, 2005. Retrieved September 2005, from http://www.scu.edu/ethics/practicing/decision/framework.html.

89. von Salis T: What exactly is psychoanalytic psychotherapy? Some remarks on research in psychotherapy, *Psyche Matters,* September 10, 2003. Retrieved July 2005, from http://www.psychematters.com/papers/vonsalis.htm.

90. Vrkljan B, Miller-Polgar J: Meaning of occupational engagement in life-threatening illness: a qualitative pilot project, *Canad J Occup Ther* 68:237-246, 2001.

91. wa Thiong'o N: *Writers in politics,* Nairobi, Kenya, 1981, Heinemann Educational Books.

92. Yalom ID: *Theory and practice of group psychotherapy,* ed 2, New York, 1975, Basic Books.

93. Yalom ID: *Theory and practice of group psychotherapy,* ed 4, New York, 1995, Basic Books.

94. Yerxa EJ: 1966 Eleanor Clarke Slagle lecture—Every one counts, *Am J Occup Ther* 12:1-9, 1967.

96. Young TM, Poulin JE: The helping relationship inventory: a clinical appraisal, *Fam Soc* 79(2):123-133, 1998.

PART IV

Specific Interventions: Application of Conceptual Models of Practice in Occupational Therapy

In Parts I, II, and III of this book the foundation for occupation-based practice was laid. In Part I, the historical origins of occupational therapy and the constructs that inform professional practice were explained. Psychological theories that have contributed to the development of psychosocial occupational therapy were also discussed. In Part II, the occupational therapy paradigm, which is suggested to be the conceptual foundation of the profession, was presented. In Part III, general occupational therapy practice skills, including clinical reasoning, use of therapeutic relationship, use of meaningful occupations, use of groups and group processes, and cultural influences on practice were explained. The reader may now recognize a pattern in this book: occupational therapy practice is presented deductively, beginning with general professional issues, and gradually progressing toward specific application.

Continuing in this pattern, in Part IV we will discuss specific interventions. The objective of this part is to provide the reader with a bridging framework that connects theory and practice. The conceptual foundations of the profession explicated in Parts I to III will be operationalized through specific conceptual models of practice used in the profession. However, before presenting these guidelines for application of theory, we will discuss the meaning of a conceptual model of practice.

Authors have viewed theoretical models differently. For example, Mosey[3] sees the construct *model* as overused in health professions, basic and applied sciences, and philosophy, and poorly defined. Thus she refrains from using it, instead preferring the construct *frame of reference* to refer to organized sets of guidelines for application of theory in practice professions such as occupational therapy. Mosey sees frames of reference as consisting of a theoretical base, a description of the function/dysfunction continuum, postulates regarding change, and technology for application including evaluation and intervention guidelines. Kielhofner, on the other hand, sees the means of application of theory as a conceptual model of practice that he defines as "a way of thinking about and doing practice that is constantly refined and improved" (p. 74).[1] In his view, models both explain phenomena and provide guidelines for practice that are based on the explanation of those phenomena. His definition of a model seems clearer and more complete than Mosey's definition of a frame of reference. Therefore we will adopt Kielhofner's idea of a conceptual model of practice in this book.

Similar to Mosey's view of a frame of reference, Kielhofner sees a conceptual model of practice as consisting of an interdisciplinary theoretical base consisting of constructs and propositions. However, unlike Mosey, who sees the constructs and propositions of the frame of reference as being derived wholly from disciplines outside occupational therapy, Kielhofner sees the constructs and propositions of a conceptual model of practice as derived from both within and outside the profession. He also views models as consisting of technology for application, which includes assessment and intervention tools and guidelines.

Other occupational therapy theorists and occupational scientists seem to fall somewhere in between Kielhofner's idea of conceptual models of practice and Mosey's idea of a frame of reference. McColl adopts the construct of *theory* to refer to "conceptual tools that help to explain or predict a central construct or that promote the understanding of a central phenomenon—in our case, occupation" (pp. 21-22).[2] Thus her interest here is purely theoretical, and her definition reflects this focus. Reed and Sanderson[4] on the other hand distinguish between *conceptual models* and *practice models*. They see conceptual models as providing explanations regarding *why*, while practice models explain *how*. Their definition of practice models seems to be closer to Kielhofner's,[1] where assessment instruments are viewed as a means of measuring concepts proposed by the model.

As mentioned earlier in this book, a conceptual model of practice will be understood as defined by Kielhofner. However, analysis of conceptual models of practice will follow the guidelines proposed by Mosey,[3] which in my view are well-defined and therefore useful for such analysis. Thus for each model, we will identify the interdisciplinary conceptual base;

articulate postulations about function, dysfunction, and change; and explain the guidelines for client evaluation and therapeutic intervention. In addition, we will evaluate the model in terms of the extent to which it is consistent with the new professional paradigm proposed in Chapter 4. In this regard, we will evaluate the model in terms of its consistency with the philosophy of pragmatism, and the complexity/chaos theoretical framework, which are both proposed as constituting part of the conceptual foundations of the new occupational therapy paradigm. Also, consistent with the emphasis on evidence-based practice in contemporary practice, we will discuss research demonstrating clinical efficacy of the conceptual model to provide the reader with research evidence supporting it.

REFERENCES

1. Kielhofner G: *Conceptual foundations of occupational therapy,* ed 3, Philadelphia, 2004, FA Davis.
2. McColl MA: Using the taxonomy to classify occupational conceptual models. In McColl MA, Law M, Stewart D, et al., eds: *Theoretical basis of occupational therapy,* Thorofare, NJ, 2003, Slack, pp. 21-26.
3. Mosey AC: *Applied scientific inquiry in the health professions: an epistemological orientation,* ed 2, Bethesda, MD, 1996, AOTA.
4. Reed KL, Sanderson SN: *Concepts of occupational therapy,* ed 4, New York, 1999, Lippincott Williams & Wilkins.

Chapter 8

Instrumentalism in Occupational Therapy

Preview Questions

1. Discuss the interdisciplinary conceptual basis of Instrumentalism in Occupational Therapy (IOT).
2. Concisely state the theoretical core of IOT.
3. Explain the postulations of IOT about the following:
   a. Function
   b. Dysfunction
   c. Change
4. Describe the assessment and intervention process as outlined in IOT and guided using the Assessment and Intervention Instrument for Instrumentalism in Occupational Therapy (AIIIOT).
5. Explain the consistency of IOT with the following:
   a. The occupational therapy paradigm
   b. The philosophy of pragmatism
   c. The chaos/complexity theoretical framework
6. Discuss available empirical evidence supporting clinical effectiveness of IOT as a guide to intervention in occupational therapy practice.

Instrumentalism in Occupational Therapy (IOT) is not a mainstream model of practice in occupational therapy. It is newly developed, and its validity has not been established. However, it is presented here because it is based on the new proposed professional paradigm (see Chapter 4) and therefore presents a yardstick with which to judge other models regarding their consistency with the paradigm. In that sense, it is one among many ways of helping the reader shape his or her thinking about theory and philosophy-based occupational therapy practice.

The IOT was developed as a philosophically based model meant to guide practice in a way that was perceived to be unique to the identity of occupational therapy.[12-14] It was based on the proposition that the themes underlying the assumptions, principles, and values of the philosophy of pragmatism are consistent with those of occupational therapy,[11,18] and therefore pragmatism is most probably the foundational philosophy of the profession[3,10,33] (see Chapters 2 and 4 for a detailed discussion of the influence of pragmatism in occupational therapy).

Using the extrapolation method[6] as presented by Mosey,[24] the model was developed through six steps: identification and analysis of the problem, identification of constructs that would form the theoretical core of the model, selection and synthesis of postulations to establish the theoretical core, deduction of guidelines for problem identification and intervention, and assessment of completeness and internal consistency of the model. We will discuss the model in detail as follows: We will present the interdisciplinary conceptual base and highlight its postulations about function, dysfunction, and change. We will provide guidelines for client evaluation and intervention with an illustration using a case study. Then we will explore the consistency of the model with the new occupational therapy paradigm, the philosophy of pragmatism, and the chaos/complexity theory. We will also discuss pilot studies providing preliminary evidence of model construct validity and clinical applicability.

Interdisciplinary Conceptual Base

Constructs used to formulate the IOT conceptual practice model were derived from the occupational therapy literature, the philosophy of pragmatism (particularly the philosophical writings of Peirce, James, and Dewey), chaos/complexity theory, and various psychological theories (particularly cognitive behavioral therapy literature). Client-centered practice constructs were derived from the occupational therapy literature.[4,5,22,23] The AIIIOT, which is the primary tool for IOT, was based in part on the Canadian Occupational Performance Measure (COPM).[22] Constructs derived from the above-mentioned sources included the mind, occupation, environment, belief as a rule for action, activity or "doing," consequences, instrumentalism, contextualization, disproportion between initial conditions and outcomes, emergence, the fractal nature of human occupational behavior, and attractor conditions.

Postulations About Function, Dysfunction, and Change

The IOT model postulates that the human is a complex, dynamic, adaptive system engaged in interaction with the physical and social environment.[13] This interaction is perceived to occur through occupational performance for the purpose of changing self and the environment so as to adapt and survive both physically and psychologically. As one interacts dynamically with the environment, there is self-organization leading to increasingly more adaptive behavior. In this interaction, the mind is used as a tool for shaping, through occupational performance, the environment so that it is suitable for human survival.[8,9,25,29,32]

Consistent with the philosophy of pragmatism,[19-21,26,27] instrumental use of the mind is conceived to occur through formation of beliefs, acting on the basis of those beliefs, and using the consequences emanating from action either to alter behavior or modify beliefs. The constel-lation of factors under which beliefs about self, others, and the world are formed is particularly important because it determines an individual's typical patterns of behavior. This is because of dependence on initial conditions where small differences in a combination of factors may result in radically big differences in beliefs and subsequent behavioral patterns.[1] For instance, a little comment by a teacher in the fifth grade about how bright someone is may lead to a general lifelong self perception of intellectual adequacy leading to a choice of occupations requiring intellectual challenge.

We will illustrate the construct of dependence on initial conditions with a personal example. A specific combination of factors resulted in my beliefs about me and the world that affect my life every day. For example, during my childhood, my mother consistently emphasized to my sisters and me that what is important in life is not to get rich but to work hard and make sure that we live by the product of our labor. My mother, sisters, and many people around me also believed in my abilities and made it clear to me that there were great expectations of me. The family and community in which I was brought up instilled in me the value of a good education as a way to a good life. I particularly learned the value of education from the example of my sisters, who I saw working very hard in school. When I worked similarly hard, I was at the top of my class, received much praise from my family and teachers, and was afforded prestige by my peers.

All the above experiences constelled to form in me a firm belief in the value of education and my ability to achieve anything to which I aspired. As a result, throughout my life, my occupational life trajectory has consisted of engaging increasingly in challenging intellectual occupations, such as doing research and writing, leading to increasing levels of self-organization and emergence of greater ability to process and present ideas. If my family had not been as supportive of me as it was, or my community had not communicated a value for education, and so on, my life might have turned out significantly differently than it is today.

Function

In the IOT model, a person's occupational life is conceptualized to consist of a repertoire of occupations forming a trajectory consisting of self-similar patterns.[15,17] The self-similar patterns of the trajectory may be either adaptive or maladaptive.[13] Perception of meaningfulness forms attractor conditions for one's occupational life trajectory, with various factors that make occupations meaningful constituting a basin of attraction.[15,17] Function is conceptualized to consist of adaptive occupational patterns that lead to adaptation to the environment, and a meaningful, satisfying life, in which one is living according to perceived mission in life.

Dysfunction

Dysfunction is seen as constituting an occupational life trajectory consisting of a repertoire of occupations forming maladaptive self-similar patterns that lead to decreased ability to adapt. Such occupational patterns result from belief systems that are inconsistent with adaptive behavior. For example, a person who believes that he or she is incapable of accomplishing anything useful may engage in a pattern of giving up every time when faced with a challenge, which then reinforces and amplifies the belief of inefficacy. When such a person is observed over a period of time, it may be observed that he or she avoids initiating or engaging in occupations where a possibility of failure is perceived. Even when there is belief that engagement in an occupation may result in fairly successful outcomes, if unexpected difficulties are encountered, the task is abandoned. The individual ends up sustaining a pattern of failure in most of the attempted occupations.

Change

The objective of occupational therapy is seen as to facilitate change of a client's occupational life from a maladaptive to an adaptive system.[13] This is achieved by helping the client identify beliefs that lead to maladaptive occupational patterns and substituting them with those that support adaptive patterns. Occupations are used to challenge faulty beliefs about self, others, and the world, similar to Albert Ellis' idea of "disputing."[31] For example, a woman who believes that she is incapable of succeeding in occupations requiring leadership may be given tasks in a group activity in which she is skilled and that involve organizing other people. Success in such tasks is used to challenge or dispute her belief that she cannot be a leader. Thus, intervention in this model is perceived to consist of a *belief establishment phase,* in which current beliefs that lead to maladaptive occupational patterns are challenged and those supporting adaptive patterns are established; the *action phase* in which the client is engaged in specific occupations designed to support newly established beliefs; and the *consequence appraisal phase* in which consequences of actions resulting from newly established beliefs are evaluated and, if not desirable, either changed or the beliefs modified accordingly (Figure 8-1).

Guidelines for Client Evaluation and Therapeutic Intervention

Intervention using the IOT conceptual practice model comprises ten steps.[14] The belief establishment phase consists of introduction, articulation of a personal mission statement, choice of occupations to help one achieve the stated mission, clarifying beliefs supporting action geared toward the mission, and challenging beliefs that do not support the mission. The process begins with the therapist introducing himself or herself to the client and explaining what occupational therapy is and what will transpire in therapy. Through a visualization exercise (Figure 8-2), the client creates a personal mission statement that includes an envisioned desired life in four different areas: family, socialization, school/work, and church/community participation. According to chaos/complexity theory terminology,[15,17] creating a personal mission statement may be seen

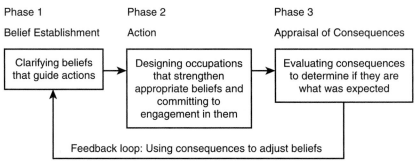

Figure 8-1. Instrumentalism in occupational therapy: a pragmatic conceptual model of practice. (Adapted from Ikiugu MN: Instrumentalism in occupational therapy: a theoretical core for the pragmatic conceptual model of practice, *Internat J Psychosocial Rehabil* 8:151, 2004.)

as establishment of attractor conditions that will organize occupational performance patterns. It is predicted that the client will regularly choose occupations that are consistent with the articulated mission and that are therefore more adaptive.

The next step is to list two occupations under each of the four areas of the mission statement (family, socialization, work/professional life, and religious/community organizations) in whose regular satisfactory engagement would lead to achievement of the mission. The client is requested to rate himself or herself on four Likert-type scales regarding his or her perception of frequency and adequacy of engagement, satisfaction with engagement, and belief about ability to engage in each of the eight occupations with desired frequency and adequacy. In chaos theory terminology, by facilitating identification of occupations and having the client rate himself or herself regarding frequency and adequacy, satisfaction, and belief about ability to engage in those occupations, the therapist is introducing perturbations in order to nudge the client's occupational life trajectory into a more adaptive direction.[2,30] This nudging continues into the action phase.

Once the client has rated himself or herself regarding frequency and adequacy, satisfaction, and ability to engage in each of the listed occupations, short-term and long-term goals are established in collaboration with the client to address each of the occupations whose rating on satisfaction is less than 4. In the action phase, the client commits to regular engagement in each of the listed occupations so as to create a new routine or pattern of occupational performance that is consistent with the conceived mission in life. Reassessment is conducted every week to track changes in perceived frequency and adequacy, satisfaction, and belief about ability to engage in each of the occupations. Progress is indicated by a positive change in aggregated self ratings in each of the four scales. If significant progress is not observed (consequence appraisal phase), the therapist and client discuss and either change the occupations or modify the mission as indicated.

Revisions

The AIIIOT presented in Figure 8-2 is a revised version of the instrument developed by Ikiugu.[14] The language of the new paradigm, as discussed in Chapter 4, has been incorporated in the version in this chapter. Therefore reference to *activities* has been changed to *occupations*, and *performance* to *engagement*. Also, based on the findings from a pilot study completed by Ikiugu and Ciaravino,[16] the client's perception of occupations crucial to attaining the articulated mission in life may change after intervention. Therefore, it is recommended that during reassessment, the client be asked to reexamine the

Assessment and Intervention Instrument for Instrumentalism in Occupational Therapy (AIIIOT)

When using this instrument, the therapist should find a quiet place where the client can concentrate and respond in detail to all items without interruption. The client should be given as much time as necessary to respond to all the items in this instrument exhaustively. The instrument consists of four sections. Section I is designed to lead the client to formulate a personal mission statement to create a purpose toward which to strive. Section II involves identification of some of the occupations in which to engage so as to attain the stated mission. Section III provides scales for evaluation of the frequency and perceived adequacy of engagement in the occupations, satisfaction with that engagement, and the beliefs about ability to engage in the occupations adequately. Finally, in section IV, ratings are added together to give an index of frequency, adequacy, satisfaction, and beliefs about ability to engage in the listed occupations.

I.   Personal Mission Statement

The therapist should read the following directions loudly and guide the client to complete the exercise (see Covey[7]).

Imagine that you are attending your own funeral. It is now time to read the eulogy. Write down in detail what you would like each of the following to say about you:
- Family (father, mother, spouse, son/daughter, sister/brother, cousin, any other family member that you feel close to)
- Friends (one or two close friends)
- Work/professional associate
- A member of the church, temple, or other community organization to which you are affiliated.

Now go over what you have written and take a few moments to think about what you imagine each of the people is saying about you. These statements represent the kind of person that you would like to be and that you can be. Summarize the statements in a few sentences, stating what you consider to be your personal mission statement. Your mission statement will provide direction toward which you will strive from now on. The statement should consist of four aspects as identified in the eulogy: family, friends, work/professional life, and engagement in religious/community organizations.

II.   Identification of Occupations

For each of the four areas, identify two concrete occupations in which you will need to engage on a regular basis in order to achieve your mission in life.

A. Family

1.
2.

Figure 8-2.   Assessment and Intervention Instrument for Instrumentalism in Occupational Therapy (AIIIOT). (Adapted from Ikiugu MN: Instrumentalism in occupational therapy: guidelines for practice, *Internat J Psychosocial Rehabil* 8:176–177, 2004.)

Continued

list of occupations in whose regular engagement would lead to achievement of the stated mission, and change the list if so indicated.

Reassessment of frequency, adequacy, satisfaction, and belief in ability to engage in occupations would be based on the new list. This will help take into account changes in perception regarding what occupations are important as a result of intervention. The reader should also note that, as mentioned earlier, this instrument was based in part on the COPM[22]; therefore it is similar to other client-centered instruments such as the Occupational Circumstances Assessment Interview and Rating Scale (OCAIRS), the Role

B. Social (Friendship)

1.
2.

C. Work/Profession

1.
2.

D. Affiliation to Religious/Community Organizations

1.
2.

III.   Evaluation

For each of the identified occupations, rate yourself on a scale of one (1) to four (4) regarding the (a) frequency, (b) adequacy, (c) satisfaction, and (d) beliefs regarding your ability to engage in the occupation.

Descriptors

Frequency

1 = does not engage in the occupation; 2 = rarely engages in the occupation; 3 = regularly engages in the occupation; 4 = frequently engages in the occupation.

Adequacy

1 = I am not able to engage in the occupation; 2 = I engage in the occupation with difficulty and the outcome is inadequate; 3 = I engage in the occupation with difficulty but the outcome is good if I complete it; 4 = I engage in the occupation easily, am always able to complete it, and the outcome is always adequate.

Satisfaction

1 = I am disappointed with my engagement in the occupation; 2 = I am somewhat satisfied with my engagement; 3 = I am satisfied with my engagement but would like to improve; 4 = I am happy with my engagement as it is.

Figure 8-2.   Cont'd.

Checklist (RC), and so on (see discussion of these instruments in Chapters 12 and 16).

A Word of Caution

The eulogy exercise in part I of the original version of the AIIIOT was designed for highly functioning adult clients with insight and good verbal skills, whose occupational participation is maladaptive for some reason. It is not suitable for clients who are likely to experience decompensation (impaired ability to maintain appropriate functional coping behaviors due to decreased touch with reality[28]) due to severe emotional disturbances or impaired reality testing. It could particularly be contraindicated for clients who have hallucinations or delusions, or those who are homicidal, depressed/suicidal, or terminally ill. For such clients, guide their visualization using the following exercise*: Imagine that one day, you come home unexpectedly to

---

* I want to acknowledge my colleague Dr. Elizabeth Ciaravino for suggesting this exercise as an alternative to guided eulogy visualization.

Belief

1 = I do not believe that I am capable of engaging in the occupation; 2 = I believe that I can engage in the occupation but with much help; 3 = I believe I can engage in the occupation with some help; 4 = I believe I can engage in the occupation adequately and independently.

	Frequency 1 2 3 4	Adequacy 1 2 3 4	Satisfaction 1 2 3 4	Belief 1 2 3 4
A. Family				
1.	— — — —	— — — —	— — — —	— — — —
2.	— — — —	— — — —	— — — —	— — — —
B. Social (Friendship)				
1.	— — — —	— — — —	— — — —	— — — —
2.	— — — —	— — — —	— — — —	— — — —
C. Work/profession				
1.	— — — —	— — — —	— — — —	— — — —
2.	— — — —	— — — —	— — — —	— — — —
D. Affiliation to religious/community organization				
1.	— — — —	— — — —	— — — —	— — — —
2.	— — — —	— — — —	— — — —	— — — —

Scores (x_{11}, x_{12}, x_{13}, x_{14})

— — — —	— — — —	— — — —	— — — —
Frequency	Adequacy	Satisfaction	Belief

Scores (x_{21}, x_{22}, x_{23}, x_{24})

— — — —	— — — —	— — — —	— — — —

To obtain total scores, add the ratings for each column and place the aggregate score at the bottom of the column. These scores are denoted x_{11}, x_{12}, x_{13}, and x_{14} for frequency, adequacy, satisfaction, and beliefs respectively.

To obtain the scores at the end of the therapy week, have the client rate himself or herself again and add the scores under each column. Denote the scores x_{21}, x_{22}, x_{23}, and x_{24}. Progress made in therapy during the week is indicated by $x_{21}-x_{11}$, $x_{22}-x_{12}$, $x_{23}-x_{13}$, and $x_{24}-x_{14}$ respectively.

Comments:

Figure 8-2.   Cont'd.

find a large group of people talking about you. They do not know you are there, so you decide to listen to what they are saying. Write down in detail what you would like to hear each of the following say about you: (a) a family member (father, mother, spouse, son/daughter, sister/brother, cousin, any other family member that you feel close to); (b) one or two close friends; (c) a co-worker/professional colleague/associate; (d) a member of the church or some other community organization to which you are affiliated. Now, go over what you have written and take a few moments to think about what you imagine each of those people is saying about you. These statements represent the kind of person you would like to be and that you can be. Summarize the statements in a few

sentences, stating what you consider to be your personal mission statement. This mission statement will provide the direction toward which you will strive from now on. The statement should consist of four components corresponding to the four areas of the overheard conversations: family, friends, work/professional life, and engagement in church/community organization(s).

The IOT conceptual model is also not suitable for use with children who may not have the maturity necessary to think about an overview of their life extending far into the future.

Refer to Lab Manual Exercise 10-1 to learn how to articulate your personal mission statement and identify occupations to help you achieve the mission.

CASE STUDY: HENRY

Henry, a 38-year-old African-American male, was referred to the occupational therapist by a friend who was a social worker. He suffered mild reactive depression as a result of a difficult divorce process. Henry was an architect who worked with a construction company that was contracted to erect a new building at the hospital where the social worker was employed. The social worker and Henry were old friends from college. So when Henry told her what was going on in his life, she suggested that he see the occupational therapist who had informed her of a new conceptual practice model that he was testing for clinical application.

Henry had been married and divorced from a first marriage and was in the process of divorce from a second marriage. He had two sons, 8 and 10 years old, and a daughter, 6 years old, from the first marriage. He had been married to his second wife for 3½ years. The marital relationship started deteriorating after the second year of marriage. They fought about everything. They attended marital therapy for 18 months. However, the ten-

sion between them continued to increase; in the last 3 months, Henry found the situation intolerable, and he filed for divorce. His wife's behavior became openly hostile. She started bringing men home and sleeping with them even when Henry was there. Henry got extremely depressed, started drinking heavily, and even contemplated suicide. It was at this time that he had talked to the social worker who suggested that he see the occupational therapist.

During the first meeting with Henry, the therapist introduced himself and explained what occupational therapy was. He observed that Henry's occupational routine had been disrupted by the difficult relationship between him and his wife and the hostile living conditions at home. He suggested that establishment of a new occupational performance routine might get Henry out of the maladaptive, self-destructive pattern in which he seemed to be at the present time. Henry responded and stated that he was ready to try anything at this point. The therapist led him through the eulogy visualization

CASE STUDY: HENRY—CONT'D

exercise and articulation of the personal mission statement. He imagined different people stating the following about him:

Family

Wife: *Henry was easy to live with. He was generous, kind, loving, and caring. He nurtured me and the children. He taught me so much. I feel that I grew so much just being around him. He was my friend, my lover, my source of support, my everything.*

Sons: *Our dad was a great man. He was loving and gentle, yet firm. Even when he disapproved of our actions, he always made us feel special and loved.*

Daughter: *In my dad, I had a teacher and friend. He made me feel that I can do and accomplish anything I set my heart to do. I feel lucky to have been his daughter.*

Mother: *My son was a very special person. He was hardworking and very generous. He never complained about his many responsibilities. He took care of me and made sure that I wanted for nothing. I was very proud of him.*

Church

Priest: *Henry was a very good member of the church. He was very giving of both his time and money. He touched everyone with whom he became acquainted in a very special way. He was gentle, caring, and a true embodiment of Christ.*

Work

Colleague: *Henry was so easy to get along with and so much pleasure as a colleague. Even in his very busy schedule, he always found time to help his colleagues whenever they needed his assistance. His work was a huge contribution to making life better for so many people. Even though he was recognized for his success in his chosen career, he was still a very humble man. He was truly a great human and will be missed so much. His legacy will live forever through the many innovations he made in the profession of architecture, and the many philanthropic projects that he began.*

Socialization

Friend: *Henry was attentive to his friends' needs and tried very hard to help a friend in need. He never said an unkind word to anyone. He was a valued friend and will be missed very much.*

Following the above visualization, Henry generated the following list of things to be included in his mission statement:

- Finding a compatible person to share his life with as a lifelong partner/spouse
- Providing generosity, kindness, love, care, and nurturance to his spouse and family
- Bringing up his children to be strong, decent, hardworking, caring, and righteous citizens
- Helping members of his family
- Taking care of his mother to the best of his ability
- Being more integrated in church and contributing to the best of his ability to the work of the church, especially in helping improve the conditions of those who are disadvantaged in society
- Doing his best to maintain good relationships with his colleagues at work
- Utilizing his talents to contribute to making life better for all humankind
- Being a good friend

He stated his mission as follows:
I am committed to living a virtuous life. Informed by values rooted in the traditions of my family, culture, and religion, I will achieve the virtue of excellence in my life by being in union with a spouse who supports my mission, nurturing her and the entire family, striving to focus on the positive side of every human that I meet, and doing my work with the greater good of humankind in my

Continued

CASE STUDY: HENRY—CONT'D

mind. In this value-filled and virtuous life, I will be a source of encouragement and growth for all people that I come to know in my journey through this life.

Henry then identified the following as the occupations in whose regular engagement would lead to achievement of the stated mission:

Family-related occupations
- Making a list of places to visit regularly where he could meet a possible future spouse
- Initiating conversation and socializing with people who could be future spouses
- Spending more time doing various activities with his children

Work
- Finding time to talk to each colleague regularly
- Publishing the innovations he made in his work in recognized professional journals

Socialization
- Calling and talking to his friends regularly on the phone

Participation in a religious/community organization
- Finding out what activities take place regularly in the church and how he could help.

He rated his engagement in the above occupations as follows:

Occupation	Frequency	Adequacy	Satisfaction	Belief
1. Engaging in social activities	2	2	1	4
2. Initiating conversation	2	2	1	4
3. Spending time with children	1	1	1	4
4. Talking to colleagues	2	1	1	4
5. Publishing	1	1	1	4
6. Talking to friends on the phone	4	4	4	4
7. Participating in church activities	2	2	2	4
Total	14	13	11	28

As can be seen in the above self rating, Henry had a high sense of belief in his ability to engage in all the occupations necessary to achieve his life mission with desired frequency and adequacy. He was however not satisfied with his engagement in six of the seven occupations identified. Therefore, in collaboration with the therapist, he set five short-term goals to address the six occupations as follows: By the end of 3 months, I will:

1. Demonstrate progress toward establishing a long-term relationship and possibly even marriage as indicated by going out on a date with a woman at least three times a week.

2. Demonstrate improved parenting skills as indicated by engaging in suitable leisure activities with my children for at least 2 hours, four times a week.

3. Demonstrate increased initiative toward establishing a better relationship with my colleagues as indicated by sparing at least 30 minutes every day to talk to a colleague.

4. Write and submit a paper about one of my innovations to a leading architecture journal for publication.

5. Demonstrate increased participation in church activities as indicated by volunteering in one church activity at least once a week.

CASE STUDY: HENRY—CONT'D

His long-term goals were as follows:
By the end of 5 years, I will:

1. Be happily married and satisfactorily perform my spousal and parental responsibilities as indicated by spending adequate time with my wife and children.
2. Have a good relationship with all my colleagues characterized by trust and mutual respect.
3. Be an active member of my church.
4. Be recognized professionally due to my contributions to the development of architecture through my publications.

Henry made a commitment to engage in the identified occupations regularly. Reassessments were completed every week. He made rapid progress toward his goals. By the end of four months, his depression had lifted. He was involved in a steady relationship with a woman with whom he was very happy. He was having a good time with his colleagues at work, and was spending a lot of time with his children. However, soon after he started dating, he moved to a new location where he had to find a new church. Therefore, he was not able to achieve his goal of being more active in church. However he was committed to continued work toward this goal.

Consistency of IOT with the Occupational Therapy Paradigm

Intervention using IOT is occupation-based. The focus of evaluation and intervention is on occupations that are meaningful to the client, because they help him or her achieve the conceptualized mission in life. The client and therapist collaborate in the process of evaluation, goal setting, and intervention. Thus, intervention based on the conceptual model is client-centered and collaborative. The role of the therapist in this model is to help the client identify and engage in occupations that would lead to a meaningful life. In that sense, the therapist provides education and counseling to facilitate engagement in meaningful occupations for participation in life. Finally, evaluation and facilitation of engagement in meaningful occupations are framed using the chaos/complexity theoretical framework. Since the conceptual model facilitates occupation-based, client-centered intervention and employs the chaos/complexity theoretical perspective, and the role of the therapist is to provide counseling and education to facilitate occupational performance, it is consistent with the new occupational therapy paradigm as discussed in Chapter 4.

Consistency with the Philosophy of Pragmatism

The formulation of IOT was based on John Dewey's philosophical construct of instrumentalism.[8,9] The idea of belief as a rule for action[26,27] was also central in the model. Other constructs derived from the philosophy of pragmatism included the value of human agency in interaction with the environment, contextualization of human experience, and so on.[18] The model's conceptual framework is therefore largely based on the philosophy of pragmatism.

Consistency with the Chaos/Complexity Theoretical Framework

Constructs borrowed from the chaos/complexity theory are used to frame and provide an understanding of the occupational human and the therapeutic process. For example, the occupational human is seen as a complex, dynamic, adaptive system interacting with the environment through occupational performance. This interaction is understood to lead to increased self-organization resulting in emergence of increasingly adaptive occupational behavior. The occupational life is viewed as constituting a trajectory consisting of a repertoire of occupations forming a self-similar pattern of performance. Therapeutic intervention begins with creation of attractor conditions that are hypothesized to organize subsequent patterns of occupational choices and behavior. Intervention is seen as introduction of perturbations that nudge the occupational life trajectory toward a more adaptive direction. Thus, in the model, chaos/complexity theory is used as a tool for understanding and explaining occupational behavior and therapeutic intervention. It can be said that while pragmatism is the philosophy of IOT, chaos/complexity theory forms its scientific framework.

Evidence-Based Practice Using IOT

Two pilot studies have so far been completed to test various aspects of IOT. Ikiugu and Rosso[17] completed a pilot study to test the hypothesis advanced in the theoretical core of IOT[13] that the occupational human may be understood as a complex, dynamic, adaptive system with characteristics of fractality, sensitivity to initial conditions, and attractor conditions. It was found that indeed performance of occupations constituting the occupational life trajectory is dependent on initial conditions until a significant event in a person's life occurs (onset of new conditions) leading to a change of trajectory. It was also concluded that the trajectory has self-similar characteristics. Finally, it was found that meaningfulness functions as an attractor for the trajectory with the various factors that make occupations meaningful, constituting a basin of attraction.[15,17] Therefore, although the sample in the pilot study was small (consisting of only nine college students), there is an indication that the occupational human may be understood as a complex, dynamic, adaptive system with characteristics of fractality, dependence on initial conditions, and attractor conditions.

Recently, Ikiugu and Ciaravino[16] completed another pilot study involving 15 adolescents with emotional and behavioral difficulties

(EBD) using a mixed quantitative and qualitative research design. They concluded that IOT may be useful in guiding intervention to assist individuals in this category transition to adulthood by encouraging them to think about their future, and to examine how current actions could affect realization of the visualized future. Many participants in the research study perceived therapeutic activities based on the model to be fun. This indicated that intervention guided by the model has the potential to encourage compliance with therapeutic activities among adolescents.

Recommendations for Future Development

Based on the two research projects, two modifications to the model are indicated. First, the instruments developed by Ikiugu and Rosso[17] seem appropriate as assessment tools if used in combination with the AIIIOT. The Daily Occupational Inventory (DOI), along with the Occupational Performance Calculation Guide (OPCG) developed by Ikiugu and Rosso for their research would be useful performance-based additions to the battery of assessments associated with IOT (refer to Chapter 10 of the Laboratory Manual for the battery of assessments in the revised IOT). The DOI requires that the client log occupations in which he or she is engaged on an hourly basis for four consecutive days. The frequency of engagement in various occupations and the client's rating of their importance in helping him or her achieve the articulated mission in life are used to calculate a performance score using an algorithm provided in the OPCG. The battery of assessments in Chapter 10 of the Laboratory Manual was used in the pilot study by Ikiugu and Ciaravino[16] with remarkable success.

Also, the findings by Ikiugu and Ciaravino indicated that following intervention, clients' insight increased and their perceptions of occupations important for achievement of mission in life changed. This suggests that new occupations perceived as important for achievement of mission in life need to be identified during reassessment as indicated (see discussion of revisions to the AIIIOT covered earlier in this chapter). After intervention, ratings on the four scales *(frequency, adequacy, satisfaction, and belief)* can still be compared with ratings before intervention because they do not pertain to occupations per se, but to the client's self-rating of engagement in occupations perceived to be important. It does not matter that there are changes in the perception of occupations that are important. Following intervention, if there is a positive change in self-perception of frequency, adequacy, satisfaction, and belief in ability to engage in occupations perceived to be important, therapy is working.

Other recommendations include the following:

- Completing research involving adequate numbers of participants, both with and without mental health issues, in order to validate the newly created assessment instruments
- Computerization of the assessment instruments (DOI, OPCG, and the AIIIOT [see Lab Manual, Chapter 10]) to make them clinically easy to use

Refer to Lab Manual Exercises 10-2 and 10-3 to help you identify your occupational performance patterns and calculate your occupational performance score.

SUMMARY

In this chapter, we presented IOT, a philosophically-based conceptual model of practice. Although IOT is not a mainstream model, it is an example of a theoretical practice framework that is consistent with the new occupational therapy paradigm, the philosophy of pragmatism, and the chaos/complexity theoretical framework. We discussed the interdisciplinary conceptual base of the model and how constructs used to develop IOT were drawn from the philosophy of pragmatism (particularly John Dewey's notion of *instrumentalism*), occupational therapy literature, psychology, and complexity/chaos theory. We also expounded the model's postulations about function, dysfunction, and change. Then we presented guidelines for evaluation and intervention using the model as a guide. We discussed pilot studies that have been completed to test the theoretical constructs and clinical usefulness of the model. Finally, we suggested modifications to the model's assessment instruments as indicated by the findings from the two pilot studies.

REFERENCES

1. Bassingthwaighte JB, Liebovich LS, West BJ: *Fractal physiology,* New York, 1994, Oxford University Press.
2. Brack CJ, Brack G: How chaos and complexity theory can help counselors to be more effective [Electronic version], *Counseling Values* 39:1-7, 1995.
3. Breines E: *Origins and adaptations: a philosophy of practice,* Lebanon, NJ, 1986, Geri-Rehab.
4. Canadian Association of Occupational Therapists: *Occupational therapy guidelines for client-centered practice,* Toronto, ON, 1991, CAOT Publications ACE.
5. Canadian Association of Occupational Therapists: *Enabling occupation: an occupational therapy perspective,* Ottawa, ON, 1997, CAOT Publications ACE.
6. Cole MB: *Group dynamics in occupational therapy: the theoretical basis and practice application of group intervention,* ed 3, Thorofare, NJ, 2005, Slack.
7. Covey SR: *The seven habits of highly effective people,* New York, 1970, Simon & Schuster.
8. Dewey J: The supremacy of method. In Fisch MH, ed: *Classic American philosophers,* New York, 1996, Fordham University Press, pp. 344-360.
9. Dewey J: The construction of good. In Fisch MH, ed: *Classic American philosophers,* New York, 1996, Fordham University Press, pp. 360-381.
10. Hooper B, Wood W: Pragmatism and structuralism in occupational therapy: the long conversation, *Am J Occup Ther* 56:40-49, 2002.
11. Ikiugu MN: The philosophy and culture of occupational therapy, doctoral dissertation, 2001, Texas Woman's University, *Dissertation Abstracts International* 62(12B):5678, 2001.
12. Ikiugu MN: Instrumentalism in occupational therapy: an argument for a pragmatic conceptual model of practice, *Internat J Psychosocial Rehabil* 8:109-117, 2004.
13. Ikiugu MN: Instrumentalism in occupational therapy: a theoretical core for the pragmatic conceptual model of practice, *Internat J Psychosocial Rehabil* 8:151-163, 2004.

14. Ikiugu MN: Instrumentalism in occupational therapy: guidelines for practice, *Internat J Psychosocial Rehabil* 8:165-179, 2004.

15. Ikiugu MN: Meaningfulness of occupations as an occupational-life-trajectory attractor, *J Occup Sci* 12:102-109, 2005.

16. Ikiugu MN, Ciaravino AE: Assisting adolescents experiencing emotional and behavioral difficulties (EBD) transition to adulthood, *Internat J Psychosocial Rehabil* 10(2):57-78, 2006.

17. Ikiugu MN, Rosso HM: Understanding the occupational human being as a complex, dynamical, adaptive system, *Occup Ther Health Care* 19(4):43-65, 2005.

18. Ikiugu MN, Schultz S: An argument for pragmatism as a foundational philosophy of occupational therapy, *Canad J Occup Ther* 73(2):86-97, 2006.

19. James W: Habit: its importance in psychology. In McDermott JJ, ed: *The writings of William James: a comprehensive edition,* Chicago, 1977, The University of Chicago Press, pp. 9-21.

20. James W: *Pragmatism,* Indianapolis, 1981, Hackett.

21. James W: The will to believe. In Fisch MH, ed: *Classic American philosophers,* New York, 1996, Fordham University Press, pp. 136-148.

22. Law M, Baptiste S, Carswell A, et al: *Canadian occupational performance measure,* Ottawa, ON, 2000, CAOT Publications ACE.

23. Law M, Baum CM, Baptiste S: *Occupation-based practice: fostering performance and participation,* Thorofare, NJ, 2002, Slack.

24. Mosey AC: *Applied scientific inquiry in the health professions: an epistemological orientation,* ed 2, Bethesda, MD, 1996, AOTA.

25. Muelder WG, Sears L, Schlabach AV, eds: *The development of American philosophy: a book of readings,* Boston, 1990, Houghton Mifflin.

26. Peirce CS: The fixation of belief. In Buchler J, ed: *Philosophical writings of Peirce,* New York, 1955, Dover Publications, pp. 5-22.

27. Peirce CS: How to make our ideas clear. In Buchler J, ed: *Philosophical writings of Peirce,* New York, 1955, Dover Publications, pp. 23-41.

28. Roth S, McCune CC: The client and family experience of mental illness. In Cara E, MacRae A, eds: *Psychosocial occupational therapy: a clinical practice,* Clifton Park, NY, 2005, Thomson Delmar Learning, pp. 3-25.

29. Sibley J: *Classical ethics for contemporary times: a heuristic approach,* unpublished manuscript, Texas Woman's University, no date, Denton, Texas.

30. Warren K, Franklin C, Streeter CL: New directions in systems theory: chaos and complexity, *Social Work* 43:357-372, 1998.

31. Weinrach SG: Cognitive therapists: a dialogue with Aaron Beck, *J Couns Dev* 67:159-164, 1988.

32. Whittemore RC: *Makers of the American mind: three centuries of American thought and thinkers,* New York, 1964, William Morrow.

33. Wilcock AA: *An occupational perspective of health,* Thorofare, NJ, 1998, Slack.

Chapter 9

The Psychodynamic Conceptual Model

Preview Questions

1. Discuss the interdisciplinary conceptual basis of the psychodynamic conceptual model of practice in occupational therapy.
2. Concisely state the theoretical core of the psychodynamic model.
3. Explain the postulations of the psychodynamic model about the following:
   a. Function
   b. Dysfunction
   c. Change
4. Describe the assessment and intervention process as outlined in the psychodynamic model.
5. Explain the consistency of the psychodynamic model with the following:
   a. The occupational therapy paradigm
   b. The philosophy of pragmatism
   c. The chaos/complexity theoretical framework
6. Discuss available empirical evidence supporting clinical effectiveness of the psychodynamic conceptual practice model as a guide to therapeutic intervention in occupational therapy.

The psychodynamic conceptual model of practice is one of the earliest theoretical frameworks to be developed in occupational therapy. It was an attempt to apply Freudian and neo-Freudian psychoanalytic constructs. Azima and Wittkower,[3] who were psychiatrists from McGill University in Canada, completed a survey involving psychiatric occupational therapists, psychiatrists, and patients in 15 occupational therapy departments in Canada and the United States. Although they

called it a survey, it was really a qualitative inquiry. To collect data, the authors used an interview guide consisting of open-ended questions such as: "What does occupational therapy mean to you?" and "What is the function of occupational therapy?" (p. 7).[3] Because of this apparent confusion about the research methodology, and especially lack of clarity about data analysis methods, their conclusions may be taken with a grain of salt. Nevertheless, their findings were instrumental in the development of the psychodynamic perspective in occupational therapy.

Based on their study, Azima and Wittkower concluded that there was too much emphasis on diversional and occupational aspects of activities, and psychodynamic problems of patients were not adequately addressed. Specifically, they asserted, there was "no fundamental conceptual framework which includes the present knowledge of dynamic psychopathology and encompasses comprehensively the field of psychiatric occupational therapy" (p. 6).[3] Further, they suggested that

The relative lack of occupational therapist–psychiatrist relationship is partly due to the anxiety aroused in the occupational therapist because of the weakness of her position in a theoretical field, and partly due to the anxiety of some psychiatrists because of their difficulty in performing the role of authority expected of them (p. 6).[3]

Thus they seemed to suggest that occupational therapists were unable to articulate a theoretical framework guiding their work. As a result, they felt somewhat inferior and uncomfortable as professionals. Some psychiatrists, on the other hand, were uncomfortable with assuming authority and giving occupational therapists the theoretical guidance that they presumably needed. These conclusions led Azima and Wittkower to recommend, "if it is thought feasible to construct a relatively autonomous psychiatric theory of occupational therapy, this should have as its *point of emphasis* the dynamics of object-relationships" (p. 6).[3]

Based on the recommendations by Azima and Wittkower,[3] Azima and Azima[2] outlined a dynamic theory of occupational therapy based on psychoanalytic and particularly object-relations concepts. In this theory, they saw the functions of occupational therapy in psychiatry as encompassing "diagnostic evaluation, change detection and therapeutic manipulation" (p. 216)[2] of psychiatric clients. Fidler and Fidler expanded this object-relations theory,[14] describing an eclectic approach in occupational therapy combining techniques from Freudian, Jungian, and humanistic psychological orientations. A review of the literature reveals that the late 1950s through the 1970s were characterized by a concerted exploration of this model by occupational therapists, because it was seen as a means of making occupational therapy more "scientific" and acceptable in the medical profession.

Apart from Azima and Wittkower[3] and Azima and Azima,[2] Llorens and Johnson[26] described a therapeutic community model used by the psychiatric rehabilitation team at Lafayette Clinic in which Freudian concepts were used by occupational therapists to explain their programs. Another example is a study conducted by Rothaus, Hanson, and Cleveland[32] to test the effectiveness of a group dynamics intervention in occupational therapy based on Bion's psychoanalytic group model. They concluded from their research that

> It is possible, reasonable and appropriate for occupational therapists to conduct such therapeutic programs to enrich the service they offer the patients and staff of a hospital and to deepen and broaden the impact and use they make of themselves and their materials (p. 187).[32]

They went on to suggest that such group interventions would improve occupational therapy because, they argued, seemingly in agreement with Azima and Wittkower,[3] that "Too much of what is required of occupational therapists seems like busy work for keeping psychiatric patients occupied during the day" (p. 187).[32] Diasio[10] explored in part the implication of Fidler and Fidler's[14] psychodynamic theory to understanding unconscious motivation in the occupational therapy process.

The above activities led to articulation of an analytic model as one of the tripartite frames of reference suggested by Mosey.[28] Mosey saw this frame of reference as focusing on the "concepts of need fulfillment, expression of primitive impulses, and control of inherent drives" (p. 47).[27] In formulating the theoretical framework, she drew constructs from Freud's psychoanalytic psychology, Anna Freud's object-relations theory, Maslow's theory of motivation, Erikson's psychosocial stages of development, and Jung's analytical psychology. Although this conceptual practice model has changed significantly over the years, some of its constructs have remained the same and are still used in occupational therapy to guide not only psychosocial but also other areas of occupational therapy practice.[9] We will now discuss these constructs in detail.

Interdisciplinary Conceptual Basis

Many occupational therapy authors suggest that the psychodynamic conceptual model of practice, as it is used today, is based on an integration of constructs from Freudian psychoanalysis and its later derivatives such as the ego psychology and the object relations theory,[9,30,34] Maslow's theory of motivation, and Rogerian client-centered therapy.[30,34] In later writings of the original founders of this conceptual framework, an anthropological perspective has been integrated to provide enhanced understanding of the symbolic meaning of objects with which clients interact in occupational therapy.[13,15] Constructs derived from the above sources include unconscious motivation, conscious awareness and cognitive processing, objects as means of need fulfillment, appropriate expression of unconscious needs and conflicts, symbolic importance of objects, need fulfillment, and self-actualization.

Postulations About Function, Dysfunction, and Change

To understand the psychodynamic conceptual model of practice, it is necessary that one have a good grasp of Freudian psychoanalytic theory (see Chapter 3 for a detailed discussion of the theory). According to Freud, the psyche consists of the id, the ego, and the superego.[20] The id (pleasure principle) seeks fulfillment of organismic needs (e.g., satiation of hunger, gratification of sexual needs, expression of hostile feelings). However, it may not be appropriate to gratify certain needs at certain times because of social convections (represented by the superego). The role of the ego (reality principle) is to find, through cognitive, logical appraisal of circumstances and processing of data, ways of gratifying needs of the id while not violating social values represented by the superego. When id drives that are inconsistent with the superego are perceived, the ego feels threatened. Therefore such drives are relegated to the unconscious. This suppression of instinctual impulses leads to disowning of aspects of self so that one has no conscious awareness of them. As a result, there is lack of balance between the conscious and unconscious aspects of self and consequent conflict between the two.[30] This conflict prevents appropriate fulfillment of needs and self-actualization.

Function

Mosey[30] suggests that the function-dysfunction continuum of this conceptual model of practice is not well-defined. However, there seems to be a consensus that function is indicated by a strong, well-functioning ego, enabling one to make a realistic appraisal of the environment leading to adaptation.[6,14,29] Cole postulates that reality testing is the most important function of the ego

and therefore a central focus of occupational therapy intervention: "It is the ego's ability to use perception and judgment to differentiate between internal needs and external demands," (p. 114)[9] she suggests, that is central to this conceptual model. She states that it is this ability of the ego to differentiate internal from external factors that "involves the use of interaction with the environment and with others in shaping and reshaping one's views of self and the world. It is precisely this process that is responsible for adaptation to the environment" (p. 114).[9] The ability to evaluate the self and the environment realistically leads to a sense of control. This enables one to defer gratification; use insight, intellect, and judgment to solve problems; and to meet needs in a socially acceptable manner without infringing on the need fulfillment of others.

Dysfunction

Based on the above definition of function, dysfunction is characterized by an unrealistic view of self, others, and the environment, lack of accurate awareness of personal feelings and how they shape one's decision-making process, lack of skills or talent development, making of choices that are in conflict with one's values, and an ultimate inability to seek and gratify needs satisfactorily and/or appropriately.[9,14,28,30] This leads to an inability to function adequately in the areas of activities of daily living (ADLs), work, social relationships, and leisure or pursuit of personal interests.

Change

The goal of occupational therapy as perceived from the perspective of this model is to access unconscious conflicts and fixations; gain insight into behavior, beliefs, and values; and integrate these insights into consciousness.[2,9,30] Psychic energy previously used to suppress content causing unconscious conflicts is released so that it is available for satisfaction of needs. Interpretation of symbols associated with the unconscious content reveals information that can be used for appropriate choice or, when necessary, substitution of objects with those that are appropriate for need fulfillment. Change therefore is achieved through accessing unconscious information; gaining insights into one's behavior, beliefs, and values; reality testing to increase the ability to distinguish internal needs from the external environment; strengthening the ego so that there is a more secure identity; and ability to exercise judgment, self-control, and autonomy.[2,6,9,10,26]

Guidelines for Client Evaluation and Therapeutic Intervention

Some of the earliest evaluation instruments in psychiatric occupational therapy were developed based on the psychodynamic conceptual model of practice. They included batteries of tests such as the Fiddler battery (*Stencil Cut-Out and Crayon, Finger Painting, Collage, Obstacle Course, Circle Ball Tag*),[11] and the *Azima battery*.[17,18,25] Collectively, these assessments are referred to as *projective techniques*,[5] or *expressive media*.[11] The most known among these early assessments are the Magazine Picture Collage and the Azima battery.

The Magazine Picture Collage

The Magazine Picture Collage was developed as a projective technique to be used for the purpose of "assessing some of the symptomatology operating in the dynamic structure of the patient's personality" (p. 36).[5] It is an unstructured activity to which "patients can and often do project their symptomatology" (p. 38).[5] The materials used include a variety of magazines with glossy pictures (e.g., *Life, Playboy, Outdoor Life, Sports Illustrated*), 12-by-18-inch sheets of colored construction paper, glue, scissors, and pens. This assessment can be completed in a group setting. Before clients arrive, all the materials are prepared. Clients are instructed to choose one or more pictures from the magazines, cut them out, and glue them onto a colored sheet of construction paper of choice. They are given 30 minutes to complete the collage. They are then asked to sign their name on the back of the collage and

answer the following two questions: "Why did you select these pictures? What meaning do these pictures have for you?" (p. 36).[5]

As the client completes the collage, the therapist observes the following[22]:

1. How he or she begins the activity (e.g., how much time is taken to select the construction paper and to scan or look through the various materials) and how the materials are assessed
2. The variety of materials and objects chosen to complete the activity
3. The client's experimentation with objects (e.g., by arranging and rearranging orientation of pictures)
4. How the client tries alternative ways of using space
5. The client's contact with other clients or the therapist and the nature of the contact
6. The client's ability to respond to the question about what he or she liked or disliked about the activity during group discussion
7. Whether or not the client has a title for the collage that denotes a specific theme

Through these observations, the therapist is able to assess the client's "attitudes and feelings about himself and the pictures he has chosen, as well as his ability to abstract ideas and clearly express his own thoughts" (p. 37).[5] Also, the client's "performance, work habits, behavior, and ability to relate" (p. 37)[5] become apparent.

Other psychodynamics that are revealed through the client's performance in this activity include control; compulsiveness; attention to detail; disorganization of the mind (as indicated by mutilation and fragmentation of pictures, pictures overlapping each other, and so on, which seem to be characteristic of schizophrenic clients); and amount of psychic energy available for investment in external objects as indicated by the number of pictures used, self image, tendency to escape from reality, and so on. The narrative on the back of the collage gives extra information about the client's psychodynamics. The current version of this tool is the Lerner Magazine Picture Collage (LMPC).[23] This assessment instrument is used frequently in both acute care and long-term psychiatric treatment because

> It is thought that patients are easily persuaded to do this assessment because the materials are familiar and it does not require use of techniques that can be interpreted as artistic or difficult. It is also inexpensive, using old magazines, construction paper, and glue—materials that are available in almost any clinic (p. 133).[11]

The Azima Battery

This assessment battery was developed by Azima[1] as part of the dynamic theory of occupational therapy outlined by Azima and Azima,[2] following recommendations by Azima and Wittkower[3] based on conclusions drawn from their research. The following materials are needed and set up before the client comes in for assessment[22]:

- Finger paints arranged in standard order (yellow, red, green, blue, brown, and black)
- Container of water
- Moistened clay or plasticine
- Pencil
- Drawing paper

Setup

The therapist places the finger paints on a small table, with the container of water on the right side and moistened clay/plasticine in a plastic container on the left side. Paper towels are also placed on the left side. Once the client comes into the room, the therapist makes an introduction as follows:

> As part of the evaluation routine of our department, I would like to carry out a set of tests with you. I am going to ask you to make some different things with various materials on this table. This is another way of finding out more about your problems. I may repeat the procedure at various intervals and at discharge to assess your progress (p. 40).[22]

Procedure

Once introduction is completed, the therapist instructs the client to (1) draw anything with a pencil, (2) draw a person and then another one of the opposite sex, (3) make anything he or she wishes with clay or plasticine, and (4) do a finger paint. After giving instructions, the therapist stands slightly behind the client so as to be out of the line of sight. This is because the assessment is projective and the therapist does not want the client to project internal psychic dynamics to him or her but rather to the creations. The therapist then records the time taken to complete each task on the record form and observes and notes the client's behavior while engaging in the activities.

Interpretation

Once the tasks are completed, the therapist asks the client to say what he or she has created. Then the therapist asks the client to describe what is in the creations and what he or she had in mind, as well as any insights realized after examining the creations further. Information obtained from observations of the client (including his or her orientation to reality, relationship with other people, ego control and ability to cope, expression of mood, and clarity of communication) and interpretation of the symbolism in the creations is used to determine the client's intrapsychic content.

Other Assessments

Other occupational therapy assessments based on the psychodynamic model include the Goodman battery, the BH battery, and the Comprehensive Assessment Process.[11] The Goodman battery assessment consists of a tile task. The client is requested to complete a tile craft, spontaneous drawing, figure drawing, and a clay task. The BH battery is another common psychodynamic assessment used in occupational therapy along with the LMPC and the Azima battery.

The BH battery assessment consists of two activities: a mosaic tile, and finger painting.[11,19] Materials and supplies for this task include:

- 6-inch masonite board
- Glue
- 7/8-inch mosaic tiles in red, green, yellow, blue, black, and white
- Mosaic tiling record form
- Liquid finger paint in red, blue, yellow, and black
- 16-by-22-inch finger painting paper
- Pan of water
- Paper towels
- Newspaper
- 6-inch ruler
- Stopwatch
- 16-by-22-inch template of plastic sheet marked into 16 squares
- Finger painting record form

The first task to be completed is the tiling task. Instructions are given to the client as follows: "Glue the tile on the board in any way, shape, or fashion, and take your time. Please, tell me when you are finished. Do not begin until I tell you" (p. 141).[19] The therapist then takes his or her position at an assigned table, obtains a record form, and states "You may begin." The therapist immediately starts the stopwatch and records the time taken to complete the task on the form. The therapist then asks the client: "If you had a use for your tile, what would it be?" (p. 141).[19] The answer is recorded on the record form.

For the finger painting task, the therapist arranges the finger painting materials (paint, paper, water, and so on) on the table. The arrangement is somewhat similar to the Azima battery (finger paints placed immediately to the client's right, water container to the upper-right corner of the table, and paper towels to the left). The finger painting paper is placed under running water or in a container of water. The therapist asks the client to place the paper on top of the newspaper, shiny side up, and open the finger painting jars. The following instructions are then given: "Do a finger painting in any way, shape, or fashion and take your time. Tell me when you are finished. Do not begin until I tell you to" (p. 142).[19] The stopwatch is set, the record form

obtained, and instructions are given as follows: "You may begin." The therapist immediately starts the stopwatch and records the time and client's behavior on the record form. After the task is completed, the client is asked to explain the painting and its contents. The answer is recorded on the record form.

Observations recorded in relation to the mosaic task include the client's posture, attitude, order, direction of movement, verbalizations about the tile and feelings about performance of the task, and time. Other observations that are recorded include the choice of tile colors, texture (in terms of the amount of glue used), how the mosaic surface is covered, whether tiles overlap, how tiles are distributed, designs, how space is used, and symmetry. Similar observations are made and recorded for the finger painting activity (posture, attitude, where the first daub of paint is made, parts of the hand used, motion, order, whether paint is placed in spaces where other paint had been placed previously [overlapping], nature of the strokes made, verbalizations, the story associated with the painting, and time taken to complete the activity). Also noted are the colors chosen; format; surface coverage; line size, texture, and quality; pressure used; detail; shape; size of objects painted; distribution of objects painted; symmetry; and content. These observations are analyzed and a hypothesis about the client's "ability to conceptualize a whole, and form a mental image" (p. 140)[19] is generated.

Another commonly used assessment is the *Build a City* task.[7] Materials and supplies for this task include:

- Two pairs of scissors
- Blunt table knife
- Clay fettling tool
- Two sheets of 36-by-24-by-2-inch Styrofoam
- Twelve sheets of construction paper (assorted colors)
- Small ball of string (12 feet)
- 50 ¾-inch or 1-inch finishing nails
- 12 ounces of clay
- 2 dozen neutral-colored pipe cleaners

This assessment is administered in a group setting. Clients are instructed as follows: "I would like all of you as a group to build your ideal city. You may use only the tools and materials provided on the table. You have 30 minutes in which to complete your ideal city. Are there any questions?" (p. 159).[7] The therapist then observes and evaluates clients as they complete the task. Each client's performance is rated on the basis of his or her positive, problem-solving, and emotionally negative responses.

Positive responses include helping others, expressing satisfaction, agreeing with others, and so on. Problem-solving responses include giving suggestions, opinions, information, clarification, and so on. Other problem-solving responses observed include asking for directions, expression of feelings, and asking for information. Negative responses include disagreement with others, withdrawal, and antagonistic behavior. The Build a City task is used for diagnostic purposes because it can be instrumental in identifying the client's communication and work skills, and symbolic content of the task.

In addition to standardized assessments, informal observation of the client while interacting with others or engaging in various activities may reveal crucial information about intrapsychic dynamics pertinent to adaptive functioning of the client. For example, giving the client a task during a group session and observing whether or not, or how he or she completes the task may give the therapist insight regarding "the client's effectiveness in approaching and following through with task behavior" (p. 95).[6] Therefore client evaluation under the aegis of the psychodynamic conceptual model of practice takes the form of both standardized and nonstandardized assessments.

Intervention

The hypothesis advanced in the psychodynamic conceptual model of practice is that unconscious intrapsychic conflicts lead to inappropriate expression of instincts and impulses and subsequent inability to meet psychological needs appropriately. Therefore the occupational therapist, similar to the psychoanalyst,[16,21,31,33,35] aims at bringing into consciousness the unconscious psychic content so that it can be examined. The difference between the psychoanalyst and the occupational therapist is that the former primarily uses talk therapy while the latter engages the client in various activities designed to be projective media into which he or she can project contents of the unconscious.

The unconscious intrapsychic drives and impulses can be accessed through dream interpretation, unstructured activities such as art into which the client can project unconscious content (a concept similar to free association) so that associated symbols are interpreted, and attendance to the phenomena of transference and countertransference while engaging in an activity either in a one-on-one session or a group context. Thus insight about the effect of these unconscious conflicts on behavior is gained. Once unconscious conflicts are brought into awareness, the client "works through" them by experiencing and re-experiencing them over and over until they are disinvested of strong affective associations. This allows conscious decision making about change without being influenced by strong emotions.[6,9,30,34]

Therefore, as Stein and Cutler state, "The psychodynamic occupational therapist uses activities to (a) uncover unconscious processes, (b) gratify psychosocial needs, (c) 'strengthen ego defenses and provide routes for sublimation of aggressive and libidinal impulses'" (p. 128).[34] The following paragraphs explain the therapeutic process using this conceptual model.[30]

First, the client is engaged in unstructured activities that allow projection of psychic content onto them. Next, communication with the therapist about the activities is facilitated, so that the client is allowed to "free associate" to the activity (verbalize freely about the personal meaning and characteristics of the activity). Symbols contained in these associations are interpreted. Ideas and emotions that are expressed are tested and validated through feedback from the therapist as well as from other clients in case of a group setting (reality testing). Issues of transference and countertransference that become apparent as the symbolism expressed in the activity is interpreted are also examined. For example, when a young woman draws a picture of the therapist, questions about who in her earlier life she associates the therapist with and why may be explored.

Another example is where admiration of an object produced by a client may challenge the validity of his or her expressed feelings of worthlessness. Through this communication process, insights about the effect of unconscious conflicts on functioning are gained, leading to an understanding of the meaning and purpose of behavior. Through activities, the unconscious conflicts are worked through and integrated into consciousness. For example, a client whose feelings of worthlessness are aroused by making a drawing of his family is encouraged to keep drawing similar pictures until it is possible to examine the facts associated with early experiences in the family without the influence of overwhelming feelings. Finally, once the unconscious intrapsychic content is understood, the client makes a conscious choice to make changes regarding how to approach life more adaptively.

Examples of activities used by occupational therapists using this conceptual model of practice include baking, pet care, cooking,[9] different types of games, gardening, relaxation exercises, sewing, and arranging flowers,[22] as well as listening to music; watching movies; taking walks; playing sports; dancing; doing expressive activities such as clay work, finger painting, and working with water colors; writing poetry; writing a diary; building models; and using a computer.[34] The choice of activity depends on the intention of therapy.[30] If the objective is to help the client work through painful psychic experiences such as issues of trust, participation in activities that require minimal trust of another person but slowly progress toward demands for more trust would be encouraged. If the purpose of therapy is reality testing, activities requiring judgment of what is real are used. Activities involving care of plants and animals are used for clients who need to develop intimacy skills, and so on.

Group therapy based on this model involves facilitation of identification and calling to the group's attention any client behavior that is disturbing to others and counterproductive to group task completion, promotion of increased feelings of adequacy and independent functioning, development of interaction skills, and learning of various adaptive skills needed to function adequately as one seeks to satisfy needs in the world.[9] Group intervention may be guided by Cole's seven-step format (see Chapter 7) using activities such as baking, cooking, publishing a group newspaper, and so on, as therapeutic media.

CASE STUDY: KARANJA

Karanja, a 14-year-old Kenyan boy, was referred to me by the psychological counselor following a head injury sustained after falling from a tree harvesting mangoes. On his first appointment, he was brought by his father to the counseling center where I worked. The presenting complaint was forgetfulness, which affected his performance in school. Karanja was distressed about this because he had been regarded as "the golden boy" in the family and was expected to do very well in school and in his life. He felt that by not doing well, he was letting down his family. He wanted to be helped in therapy to improve his memory. This would enable him to do well in school and pass the Kenya Certificate of Primary Education (KCPE) examination so that he could be admitted to a good secondary school and realize his dreams of being successful in education (which were also his family's dreams).

During the first therapy session, consistent with the psychoanalytic notion of relating to the consciousness as a way of accessing the unconscious intrapsychic content, I decided to address Karanja's conscious desire to improve his memory by teaching him cognitive strategies that he could use to improve his efficiency in accessing and processing information. However, I was also aware that he had to accept any cognitive limitations resulting from his injury so that he could establish realistic goals for himself. In order to accept these limitations, Karanja had to gain insight regarding how unconscious drives were interfering with his ability to appraise his situation realistically.

Karanja's therapy sessions were held once a week for 1 hour. At the end of each session, I gave him an assignment for the week. For the first week's assignment, in order to access unconscious drives, I requested that he start keeping a diary, taking time every evening before going to bed to record all activities completed that day. This activity would simultaneously give Karanja a feeling that he was working toward his goal to improve his memory while at the same time providing information that would allow us to explore his unconscious drives and impulses.

When he came in for the next session a week later, he had entered his daily activities neatly and in impressive detail in the diary. However, he still continued to complain that his memory was very bad. I pointed out that it could not be that bad since he was able to remember so much detail of what he had done during the day (reality testing). During this session, he also expressed a desire to go back to school (he had not been attending classes since his injury 6 months earlier). After consultation with his family, it was decided that he would begin his studies again under a private tutor.

As I continued working with Karanja and monitoring his progress, I noticed that he liked drawing and had a very active imagination. I decided to incorporate these strengths in therapeutic interventions. For the week's assignment, I asked him to draw or paint anything he wanted and bring it with him the next week. In the next session, he brought a painting of a man. The painting was large, filling the entire page. Green and blue colors were notably predominantly used. The face looked strong, and the man in the painting was slightly frowning. I was curious about the size of the painting, the use of colors, and the facial features. To explore what these symbols meant, I asked Karanja to paint a picture that was exactly the opposite of the man in his painting. After completing the activity, I asked him to tell me the difference between the two. The conversation progressed as follows:

Karanja: Oh, he is so small. He looks like a child.

Therapist: Like a child. Yeah, I see it too. He is so small. Not like the other man who is so big.

Karanja: Yes. The other man is big. He's a grown-up with children and a beard like yours (referring the therapist's facial hair).

Therapist: Yes. A beard like mine. I wonder though, what could this man do, being so big, like me?

Karanja: He could probably be an elder.

Therapist: An elder. That's wonderful. What does an elder do? If you can, show me by demonstrating what he does.

Karanja: (Assumes a wise demeanor and talks sternly the way a Kikuyu elder would talk when advising a young person)

Therapist: I like the wisdom of the elder. What do elders advise young people about?

Karanja: About not doing bad things like smoking opium, smoking cigarettes, drinking beer, fighting, and name calling.

Therapist: Those are bad things. Now, let's imagine for a moment that you could allow yourself to be really bad. Be a bad person and call me one little bad name.

Continued

CASE STUDY: KARANJA—CONT'D

Karanja: I would call you something like a "dog." But I cannot because you are older. If a young person my age annoyed me, I would probably call him that (he makes some gestures with his right hand as he talks).

Therapist: I noticed that you are doing something with your right hand. Could you do that again?

Karanja: (Starts moving his hand). It is like the movement of blood through the veins to and from the head.

Therapist: Let us follow the movement of blood. How exactly does it move?

Karanja: (Quiet for a while). The blood is entering my body to give it strength.

Therapist: Wonderful. We all need strength for... (blank access to encourage him to project intrapsychic content).

Karanja: To work.

Therapist: Yeah. That is true. We need the strength to work. What kind of work do we need to do?

Karanja: Studies, painting and drawing, and gardening.

Therapist: Okay. Bloo d has entered your body to give you the strength you need. So, for this week, I want you to do more studies, draw and paint some more, and start doing some gardening. Bring your drawings and paintings and a report of how your studies and gardening are going next week.

Consistent with the guidelines for the psychodynamic conceptual model, I started by relating to the conscious concerns of the client. This gave me a chance to establish rapport and trust so that the client could let his guard down to allow me to pass the ego defenses and delve into his unconscious. His conscious concern was memory. He also had strengths such as a strong imagination, which he used effectively in expressive activities such as painting. In the session, this strength was used to engage the client in an occupational task that he enjoyed and in which he felt competent, which was also unstructured and allowed projection of his intrapsychic content.

As can be seen in the above interaction, this client's conscious sense of self was that of a forgetful, weak person who was incapable of performing adequately in school. He did not feel that he was capable of achieving his life goals. Through the painting activity and subsequent verbal expression of the meaning of the activity, it is seen how the unconscious sense of strength was brought into consciousness, leading to a beginning attempt to integrate this strength so that it could be used adaptively. This effort at integration of the unconscious strength continued over many sessions. In one session, Karanja made a clay model of a crouching lion. Verbal processing of the symbolism associated with his model went as follows:

Karanja: (After prompts by the therapist, pretends to become the lion and starts pouncing at the therapist and trying to scratch him the way a lion would do). That's it. You are now devoured.

Therapist: Yeah. It's over. Now let's start again, and this time I will play the lion. (The intention here was to give him a visual demonstration of what he was doing in hope of helping him gain insight as to his unconscious impulses. However, in retrospect, I should have followed his lead and asked him to talk about his need and experience of "devouring" somebody. Instead, I became the lion, pounced on him and pinned him down.)

Karanja: (Lying down on the floor quietly). It is finished. I am devoured and dead.[*]

Therapist: How is it there in the other world?

Karanja: Oh. There are people singing. I can see the sky.

---

[*] Note that when a client talks about death, the therapist should be very careful, in case he or she is really suicidal or homicidal. Delving into the unconscious at this depth may not be appropriate for novice therapists. Techniques used at this level require great tact and skill, which may be accessible with experience, although thorough education may prepare an entry-level therapist to apply the techniques under supervision by an experienced therapist.

CASE STUDY: KARANJA—CONT'D

Therapist: How do you like it there? (I should have asked him to look at the sky more closely and describe it in detail.)
Karanja: I like it. But I do not want to join the skies.
Therapist: What do you want to do?
Karanja: I want to come back to earth and help people, for example my parents and my sisters. This was a very important transition for Karanja. He was integrating his unconscious strength and trying to find a meaningful outlet for it. So, we discussed how he could help people. He said he could be helpful by taking a leadership role among his peers in his neighborhood. For exam-

ple, he could facilitate engagement of other boys his age in constructive activities instead of hanging around shopping malls aimlessly or engaging in destructive behaviors such as drinking, smoking cigarettes, and so on. In subsequent weeks, Karanja went on to put together a boys' soccer team. He also redoubled his efforts in his studies. Eventually, his confidence increased and he enrolled to take the KCPE examination. Therapy was discontinued at this point. We did not stay in touch, and I do not know the outcome of his examination. However, it is evident that Karanja made significant gains in therapy that were likely to be sustained.

Refer to Lab Manual Exercises 11-1 and 11-2 to facilitate your beginning mastery of skills in administering psychodynamic assessments and planning treatment based on the conceptual model's guidelines.

Consistency of the Psychodynamic Model with the Occupational Therapy Paradigm

As discussed earlier, consistency of any model with the newly emerged occupational therapy paradigm is determined by the extent to which it is client-centered, collaborative, and occupation-based. It is also determined by the extent to which the model subscribes to the complexity theory perspective. Based on the above criteria, it is evident that the psychodynamic model, as articulated, is less consistent with the professional paradigm than some of the other models, such as the Model of Human Occupation and Occupational Adaptation. However, depending on the therapist's general perspective, it can be consistent with the paradigm to varying degrees.

For example, in Karanja's case, consistent with the occupational therapy paradigm, ther-

apy was clearly client-centered since the client's issues determined the direction of therapy. Issues that were of conscious concern to Karanja were used as a point of departure to go beyond the resistance and delve into the unconscious. Therapy was also occupation-based since occupations that were meaningful to Karanja, such as painting and clay modeling, studying, gardening, and engaging in sports, were used as media of therapy as well as the outcome toward which therapy was aimed. Therefore occupation was the means and desired outcome of therapy. However, there are no clear guidelines in the model that would ensure that all therapists using it are client-centered and occupation-based. Therefore whether or not the client is given an opportunity to engage in meaningful occupations depends on the initiative of the therapist, because the guidelines of the model do not clearly and categorically address this issue.

Also, in the model, complexity theory is not clearly identified as its scientific framework. The client is not conceptualized as a complex, dynamic, adaptive system in interaction with the environment, leading to self-organization and emergence of adaptive behavior. Rather, it seems that he or she is viewed in a deterministic perspective where unconscious instincts and impulses are understood to influence conscious behavior. Therapy seems to be conceived as a mechanistic process in which manipulation of the unconscious content is expected to change behavior. To that extent, the model may not be consistent with the occupational therapy paradigm. However, the role of the therapist in the model is seen as that of providing counseling and education to facilitate adaptive occupational functioning. To that extent, the model's view of the role of the therapist is clearly consistent with that of the professional paradigm. Therefore it can be concluded that the model is consistent with the new professional paradigm in some ways, although this consistency can be strengthened.

Consistency with the Philosophy of Pragmatism

The psychodynamic model views integration of the unconscious psychic content into consciousness as the way to adaptive behavior. This denotes use of the mind as a tool for adaptation. To that extent, the model is consistent with the postulations of the philosophy of pragmatism. It also emphasizes "doing," although it is not clear whether the model views "learning by doing" as the goal of therapy in accordance with the propositions of pragmatism. It seems that activities in this model are simply a means of providing unstructured media onto which psychic content can be projected. The real agent of change, according to the psychodynamic model, seems to be the verbal analysis of the client's psychic symbolism presented in the activities. The goal of the model is to facilitate development of psychic adaptive behaviors so that the client can meet his or her needs within his or her environment. This is consistent with the pragmatic valuing of the environment. It can therefore be concluded that inadvertently, the model is consistent with pragmatism in certain aspects and inconsistent in others.

Consistency with the Chaos/ Complexity Theoretical Scientific Framework

As mentioned earlier, the chaos/complexity theoretical framework is not explicitly incorporated in this model.

Recommendations for Reinterpretation of the Model

There is no doubt that there is a popular consensus, even among ardent critics of psychoanalytic approaches, that unconscious motivation influences behavior. The psychodynamic conceptual practice model is therefore very useful in helping therapists facilitate client awareness (insight) of how intrapsychic impulses affect behavior. However, it is easy to lose track and overuse verbal interventions to achieve this goal. This would lead to occupational therapists functioning more or less like psychologists or social workers, causing role blurring. Therefore it is imperative that the model's guidelines for practice be updated to explicitly and categorically emphasize an occupation-based, client-centered, collaborative approach to therapy, thus preserving the unique perspective of occupational therapy. Therapists using this model should focus on affording clients opportunities to participate in occupations, both as a means of intervention and as a desired outcome of therapy. The case of Karanja discussed in this chapter offers a good example of how this can be achieved.

It might also be useful for the theoretical core of this conceptual model to be updated to articulate the view of the client as a complex, dynamic, adaptive system in interaction with the environment. In this modified view, the goal of therapy would be seen as to provide *perturbations* by increasing client insight to intrapsychic processes leading to increased *self-organization* and subsequent *emergence* of more adaptive behaviors. This could be a potent conceptual framework for explaining the outcome of therapy.

Evidence-based Practice Using the Psychodynamic Conceptual Model

A search of the literature indicates that not much empirical research has been completed in connection with this conceptual model. In one study, Buck and Provancher[5] found that the LMPC (then known only as MPC) could reveal psychodynamic characteristics such as extreme overcontrol, compulsiveness, and attention to detail. They also found that certain psychic characteristics portrayed in the LMPC could be indicative of specific psychiatric conditions. For example, mutilation or fragmentation and overlapping of pictures could be indicative of schizophrenic psychic disorganization. Lack of psychic energy as is characteristic of depression could be identified by the number of pictures that a client used. Also, choice of pictures could indicate issues associated with self-image.

In another study, Lerner and Ross[24] confirmed that the LMPC was able to discriminate between patients and normal controls. For example, compared to normal controls, clients with psychiatric conditions tended to have fewer pictures, chose more animal than human pictures, their collages had no balance (symmetry), and there was no central theme. Also, their collages were more subdued in terms of colors of pictures chosen, and the few humans in their collages tended to be inactive. They also took significantly more time to complete their collages (invariably 1 hour or more compared with 30 minutes or less for normal controls).

Another study examining the characteristics of the H-T-P (House Tree Person) test[4] indicated that in their house, tree, and person drawings, compared to normal children, abused children tended to have smoke coming from chimneys, their house drawings had no windows on the ground floor, and people's feet were omitted. They also tended to have more clouds in their drawings, they drew genitalia on their person drawings, and the hands were oversized while the eyes were small or even omitted.

Apart from the above three studies, a search of the literature using *OT Search* revealed only two other studies between 1956 and 2001 related to this model. Cole[8] investigated how interaction in small groups and psychopathology of clients affected self and social perceptions of clients. She found that there was no interaction between those variables, but instead both psychotic and borderline clients preferred task-oriented occupational therapy groups to unstructured psychotherapy groups.

In the most recent study found in the search, Eklund and Hallberg[12] conducted a survey investigating how psychiatric occupational therapists in Sweden used verbal interaction in their therapeutic interventions. They found that in part, participants used verbal interaction to establish a therapeutic relationship and address clients' issues of self-image and ego strengthening among others. They also found that therapists who used the psychodynamic conceptual model of practice tended to use verbal interventions more often than those who used other models. They concluded that therapists need to "study and develop the verbal ingredient" (p. 14)[12] of their therapeutic interventions in order to provide more effective therapy. It is evident from the above review that clearly more research is needed to help validate the use of this conceptual model. This is crucial if the model continues to be used in this age of accountability (evidence-based practice).

SUMMARY

In this chapter, we presented the psychodynamic conceptual model of practice in occupational therapy and noted that it is one of the earliest conceptual practice models to be established in the profession. Based on Freud's psychoanalytic psychology, the model views psychic dysfunction as resulting from conflict between the conscious intentions and unconscious instincts and impulses. This conflict results in difficulty with meeting needs in one's environment appropriately. The purpose of therapy is therefore to bring these unconscious intrapsychic dynamics into consciousness and integrate them, allowing the client to pursue and meet needs effectively and appropriately.

In this perspective, the purpose of activities used in occupational therapy is to provide unstructured media onto which intrapsychic content may be projected, facilitating increased insight regarding how unconscious instincts and impulses affect conscious behavior, integrating unconscious content into consciousness, and strengthening the ego through reality testing. The ultimate outcome of therapy is an enhanced ability to adapt as signified by the ability to use intelligence, judgment, and logic to appraise environmental factors in order to make appropriate choices of objects needed to meet personal needs.

REFERENCES

1. Azima F: *Introduction to dynamic occupational therapy: object relations and the Azima battery,* Buffalo, NY, 1967, State University of New York Press.
2. Azima H, Azima FJ: Outline of a dynamic theory of occupational therapy, *Am J Occup Ther* 13:215-221, 1959.
3. Azima H, Wittkower ED: Partial field survey of psychiatric occupational therapy, *Am J Occup Ther* 13:1-12, 1957.
4. Buck J: *House-tree-person projective technique,* Los Angeles, CA, 1992, Western Psychological Services.
5. Buck RE, Provancher MA: Magazine Picture Collages as an evaluative technique, *Am J Occup Ther* 26:36-39, 1972.
6. Bruce M, Borg B: *Psychosocial frames of reference: core for occupation-based practice,* ed 3, Thorofare, NJ, 2002, Slack.
7. Clark EN: Build a city: A projective task concept. In Hemphill-Pearson BJ, ed: *Assessments in occupational therapy mental health: an integrative approach,* Thorofare, NJ, 1999, Slack, pp. 155-172.
8. Cole MB: A preference for activity: a comparative study of psychosocial groups vs. occupational therapy groups for psychotic and borderline inpatients, *Occup Ther Mental Health* 8(3):53-67, 1988.
9. Cole MB: *Group dynamics in occupational therapy,* ed 3, Thorofare, NJ, 2005, Slack.
10. Diasio K: Psychiatric occupational therapy: search for a conceptual framework in light of psychoanalytic ego psychology and learning theory, *Am J Occup Ther* 22:400-407, 1968.
11. Drake M: The use of expressive media as an assessment tool in mental health. In Hemphill-Pearson BJ, ed: *Assessments in occupational therapy mental health: an integrative approach,* Thorofare, NJ, 1999, Slack, pp. 129-137.
12. Eklund M, Hallberg IR: Psychiatric occupational therapists' verbal interaction with their clients, *Occup Ther Internat* 8(1):1-16, 2001.
13. Fidler GS: Introductory overview. In Fidler GS, Velde BP, eds: *Activities: reality and symbol,* Thorofare, NJ, 1999, Slack, pp. 1-8.
14. Fidler GS, Fidler JW: *Occupational therapy: a communication process in psychiatry,* New York, 1963, McMillan.
15. Fine SB: Symbolization: Making meaning for self and society. In Fidler GS, Velde BP, eds: *Activities: reality and symbol,* Thorofare, NJ, 1999, Slack, pp. 12-25.
16. Goldberg A: Postmodern psychoanalysis, *Psyche Matters,* 2001. Retrieved July 2005, from http://www.psychematters.com/papers/goldberg.htm.
17. Hemphill BJ: Mental health evaluations used in occupational therapy, *Am J Occup Ther* 34:721-726, 1980.
18. Hemphill BJ: *The evaluation process in psychiatric occupational therapy,* Thorofare, NJ, 1982, Slack.
19. Hemphill-Pearson BJ: How to use the BH battery. In Hemphill-Pearson BJ, ed: *Assessments in occupational therapy mental health: an integrative approach,* Thorofare, NJ, 1999, Slack, pp. 139-152.
20. Hergenhahn BR: *An introduction to the history of psychology,* ed 3, Pacific Grove, CA, 1997, Brooks/Cole.
21. Hinshelwood RD: Evidence-based psychoanalysis: symptoms or relationships: a comment on Jeremy Holmes' "All you need is CBT," *Psyche Matters,* 2002. Retrieved July 2005, from http://www.psychematters.com/papers/hinshelwood3.htm.
22. Kivanguli G, Kaberere J: *Role of psychiatric occupational therapy in rehabilitation,* Nairobi, Kenya, Ministry of Health.
23. Lerner CJ: Magazine Picture Collage. In Hemphill B, ed: *The evaluative process in psychiatric occupational therapy,* Thorofare, NJ, 1982, Slack, pp. 139-154, 361-362.
24. Lerner CJ, Ross G: The Magazine Picture Collage: development of an objective scoring system, *Am J Occup Ther* 31:156-161, 1977.
25. Llorens LA: Psychological tests in planning treatment goals, *Am J Occup Ther* 14:243-246, 1970.
26. Llorens LA, Johnson PA: Occupational therapy in an ego-oriented milieu, *Am J Occup Ther* 20:178-181, 1966.
27. Miller RJ, Walker KF, eds: *Perspectives on theory for the practice of occupational therapy,* Gaithersberg, MD, 1993, Aspen.

28. Mosey AC: *Three frames of reference for mental health,* Thorofare, NJ, 1970, Slack.
29. Mosey AC: *Activities therapy,* New York, 1973, Raven.
30. Mosey AC: *Psychosocial components of occupational therapy,* New York, 1996, Lippincott Williams & Wilkins.
31. Prochaska JO: *Systems of psychotherapy: a transtheoretical analysis,* Chicago, 1984, Dorsey Press.
32. Rothaus P, Hanson PG, Cleveland SE: Art and group dynamics, *Am J Occup Ther* 20:182-187, 1966.
33. Sedgwick D: Freud reconsidered: the technique of analysis. *Psyche Matters,* 2005. Retrieved July 2005, from http://www.psychematters.com/papers/sedgwick2.htm.
34. Stein F, Cutler SK: *Psychosocial occupational therapy: a holistic approach,* ed 2, Albany, NY, 2002, Delmar Thompson Learning.
35. Strachey J: *Two short accounts of psychoanalysis, five lectures on psychoanalysis, the question of lay analysis,* London, 1957, Horgath Press.

10
Behavioral/Cognitive-Behavioral
Conceptual Model of Practice

Preview Questions

1. Discuss the interdisciplinary conceptual basis of the Behavioral/Cognitive-Behavioral conceptual model of practice.
2. Explain the rationale for combining behavioral, cognitive, and information-processing techniques and constructs in one conceptual model.
3. Concisely state the theoretical core of the Behavioral/Cognitive-Behavioral conceptual model.
4. Explain the postulations of the Behavioral/Cognitive-Behavioral conceptual model about the following:
   a. Function
   b. Dysfunction
   c. Change
5. Describe the model's guidelines for clinical assessment and intervention.
6. Discuss the consistency of the Behavioral/Cognitive-Behavioral conceptual model with each of the following:
   a. The occupational therapy paradigm
   b. The philosophy of pragmatism
   c. The complexity/chaos theoretical framework
7. Discuss available empirical evidence supporting clinical effectiveness of the Behavioral/Cognitive-Behavioral conceptual model as a guide to intervention in occupational therapy practice.

As mentioned in Chapter 3, behaviorism came of age as a major psychological influence in society

in the 1950s and 1960s, around the same time that use of psychoanalysis became prevalent. It was also noted that behaviorists criticized psychoanalysts for their emphasis on the unconscious processes that were not scientifically verifiable, proposing that the scientific approaches of biology be used to study human behavior.[21] Therefore, it is logical that behaviorism should have been incorporated in occupational therapy practice around the same time that psychoanalysis did.

A review of the literature reveals that this was the case. Records of systematic use of behavioral techniques started appearing in occupational therapy literature in the 1960s. Furthermore, these records reflected the conflicts between behaviorism and psychoanalysis that were prevalent in psychology at the time. For example, Smith and Tempone wrote that "Historically, psychiatric occupational therapy has moved from the simple straightforward assumption that work is healthy, and working would have therapeutic effects on patients, through the murky conceptual framework of dynamically oriented theories in which the causes of behavioral disorders lay in the recesses of the unconscious, to the emerging emphasis upon the behavioral sciences and the effects of environmental factors upon behavioral disturbances"; it is a shift "from the former emphasis on the medical sciences to the behavioral sciences, a shift from a disease focus to a recovery focus...a shift from the therapy theoretical frame of reference to the occupational behavior frame of reference" (p. 415).[46]

The authors suggested that behavioral principles would be the way to focus on environmental causes of behavioral problems in occupational therapy. This suggestion seemed to be oblivious of the fact that right from the beginning, during the moral treatment movement, the profession's concern was always the environmental influences on human behavior and health. Furthermore, it is not clear what was meant by "a shift from the therapy theoretical frame of reference to the occupational behavior frame of reference." The main point here, however, is that these authors saw their work as a pioneering attempt at introducing behavioral principles in occupational therapy. A literature search revealed no evidence to the contrary.

Based on what can be gleaned from the publications that were available in the professional literature at the time, it seems that many occupational therapists adopted B.F. Skinner's operant conditioning principles. For instance, Smith and Tempone described the operant technique of *shaping* as a way of facilitating client behavioral change in therapy.[46] Ellsworth and Colman developed a program to motivate "psychiatric patients to participate in therapeutic work activities" at Walter Reed Army Hospital using operant conditioning principles such as "a point economy" (p. 562)[11] for reinforcement. The point economy system may be viewed as an antecedent to the currently used token economy.[4,51] Rugel and colleagues used the operant conditioning method of reinforcement to teach a child with quadriplegic cerebral palsy (mixed type) to abandon a maladaptive behavior of slumping forward on his arms while up on his walker, which prevented him from using his upper extremities for productive activities.[43]

The above are only a few examples of the early use of operant conditioning behavioral principles in occupational therapy. However, even at the time, consistent with the proponents of cognitive approaches in psychology, there was recognition of the limitations of behavioral psychology because of its tendency to ignore mental events as significant factors in the causation of behavior.[21,59] Ellsworth and Colman presented an example of recognition of this limitation in occupational therapy and the need to incorporate inner cognitive processes in order to facilitate self-motivation of clients at Walter Reed Army Hospital. They stated that

> One source of the morale problem was the men's lack of involvement in planning their own work tasks or in wage distribution. They had and felt little responsibility for the work they did and were either apathetic or openly belligerent (p. 563).[11]

To address the issue of self-motivation by clients, integration of behavioral and cognitive principles was suggested. Diasio pointed out that although principles for intervention in issues of motivation and the environment in learning theory were originally founded on behavior therapy:

> Over the years, however, there has been an evolution in learning theory toward recognition that central processes, or "intervening variables" as Tolman called them, mediate between stimulus and response in order to explain many goal-directed behaviors. A growing group of neo-behaviorists, including Berlyne, Hebb, and others, have been increasingly absorbed in what goes on in the "black box" between stimulus and response in the form of cognitive processes (p. 402).[8]

Intervention ideas derived from the learning theory were put together to articulate a conceptual model of practice that was outlined by Mosey as what she called the *Acquisitional Frame of Reference*.[33] She visualized this frame of reference as based mainly on principles of operant conditioning and saw the goal of therapy based on the model as to facilitate role acquisition. By role acquisition, Mosey[33-35] means the development of interpersonal skills such as how to relate to people, dating, or applying for a job. She conceptualized those skills as leading to role acquisition and proposed that they were acquired by the client through the teaching-learning process in therapy.

Later, occupational therapy theorists developed a cognitive model for client rehabilitation based on principles derived from a newly emerged science of cognitive psychology whose development was inspired by advances in computer science and neuroscience.[1,21,56] This model addressed "intervening variables" in the "black box" to which Diasio[8] referred. Currently, some occupational therapy authors see the cognitive-perceptual perspective as a separate conceptual model of practice.[24] Others combine behavioral and cognitive principles to form what may be referred to as "learning perspectives,"[19] behavioral cognitive model,[6] or the *Acquisitional Frame of Reference*.[36] This book adopts the idea of discussing the learning perspective in general rather than separating behavioral, cognitive, and information-processing principles. Therefore we will discuss the three principles under what is referred to in the book as the *Behavioral/Cognitive-Behavioral conceptual model of practice.*

Scientific Base

Constructs that are used as building blocks for the Behavioral/Cognitive-Behavioral conceptual model of practice are derived from behavioral psychology, particularly B.F. Skinner's operant conditioning theory, cognitive and cognitive-behavioral principles, including Ellis's Rational Emotive Behavior Therapy, Beck's Cognitive Therapy, Bandura's Cognitive Social Learning Theory, and the information-processing theory.[*] These psychological theories are discussed in detail in Chapter 3. In this chapter, we will present a summary of the theoretical core of the conceptual practice model, as gleaned from occupational therapy literature.

The Theoretical Core of the Conceptual Model of Practice

The Behavioral/Cognitive-Behavioral conceptual model of practice may be conceptualized as

*References 1,6,10,19,36,56.

illustrated in Figure 10-1. It is suggested here that the human adaptive process begins with action or behavior, which includes occupational behavior. Consistent with operant conditioning principles, this behavior is learned.[3,45] Learning occurs through the process of operant conditioning where adaptive behavior is reinforced by one's environment. Reinforcement (reward) of behavior increases the likelihood of it being repeated. As the behavior is repeated over and over, it becomes habitual and therefore learning occurs. When adaptive behavior is learned, it leads to ability to participate in occupations that a person wants, is expected to do, or needs to do, including self-care, pursuit of meaningful leisure activities, and work/productive activities.

In this perspective, learning depends on the environmental response to behavior. However, a person's interpretation of environmental feedback to behavior ultimately determines whether or how behavior is repeated. Therefore, environmental explanation of learning alone is not enough. Some of the factors that determine how a person interprets and responds to environmental feedback include inherent capacities such as how well a person is able to attend to, perceive, and process information and generalize learning; his or her motivation to learn or engage in behavior; and whether beliefs about self and the world are irrational and distorted or rational

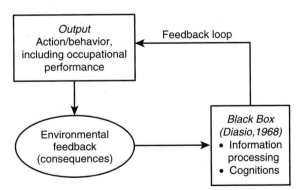

Figure 10-1. The theoretical core of the Behavioral/Cognitive-Behavioral conceptual model of practice.

and realistic.* These individual characteristics fall within what Diasio termed "intervening variables" in the "black box" lying "*between* stimulus and response in the form of cognitive processes" (p. 402)[8] (see Figure 10-1). We will discuss these variables briefly.

Processing Environmental Information as Part of the Learning Process

Learning from environmental feedback depends on one's capacity for "effective sensory reception, brain processing, and motor behavior for either movement or communication. Errors in this information processing system can lead to errors" in behavioral output in response to environmental feedback and therefore to "errors in occupational performance" (p. 254).[19] This proposition can be illustrated as follows. In the United States and in many other countries today, the ability to read and interpret instructions accurately is an essential skill for independent occupational performance. For example, many consumer products (e.g., snow blowers, lawnmowers, stereo systems) come packaged as components with instructions that the purchaser has to follow in order to assemble them. The skill needed to read and follow the instructions so as to assemble and operate such products is therefore culturally meaningful and rewarded by the environment (e.g., by teachers in schools, peers, parents, employers).

However, whether or not one is able to learn skills such as reading, interpreting, and following instructions accurately depends to a large extent on the ability to read, comprehend, think abstractly, use information-organization strategies so that it makes sense, and so on. If an occupational therapy client does not have the above-mentioned cognitive capabilities (either due to brain damage, developmental anomalies, or a learning disorder), he or she may not be able to learn the skill in question irrespective of environmental reinforcement. His or her ability to function independently in the community may therefore be negatively affected. Development

*References 1,19,36,40,56,58.

of the cognitive capabilities to read, interpret, and use information should be addressed in therapy. Similarly, if a client has self-defeating beliefs/thought processes, such as "I am stupid and cannot do such complicated tasks," chances are that he or she may shy away from even trying the tasks. Those cognitions should be addressed before any progress can be made in learning the requisite skills.

The above illustration denotes the need to use cognitive and information-processing strategies to correct any anomalies in the "black box" in Figure 10-1, so that operant conditioning can be effective in facilitating learning of the desired/adaptive behaviors or skills. A person who is deficient in information-processing skills can be taught cognitive strategies that enable him or her to organize information before learning how to interpret and apply it accurately to assemble and operate implements necessary for independent occupational performance. For the client with self-defeating beliefs/thought processes, these beliefs can be brought into his or her awareness and challenged/disputed, so that more adaptive ones can be developed.

Refer to Lab Manual Exercises 6-2 and 6-3 to learn how to begin developing skills in behavioral and cognitive-behavioral therapeutic intervention techniques.

Levels of Information Processing and their Effect on Learning

For learning to result in adaptive behaviors, a person has to be able to commit information to long-term memory and retrieve it for application in solving problems and, subsequently, occupational functioning. In this regard, long-term memory may be viewed as either *declarative* or *nondeclarative*.[19,23,47] *Declarative* memory consists of the "what" type of information, such as the facts, events, and people involved. It is information that results in formulation and declaration of a proposition, such as "This is a reacher. It can be used to help put on a pair of pants without having to bend too far. It is different from a sock aide." *Nondeclarative* memory consists of information about procedures, skills, habits, and so on, such as "In order to make a cup of instant coffee, I need to boil water, pour it into a cup, measure the coffee and put it in the hot water, add sugar or cream to taste, and stir until mixed."

The ability to learn depends on the above two types of memory. Use of learned skills in real-life situations depends on three levels of transferability that are primarily based on the extent to which one is able to generalize skills learned in one context/situation to other contexts/situations: (1) associationism, (2) representation, and (3) abstraction.[1,19,23,47,56]

Associationism

A person associates two events. For example, a child who is repeatedly bullied when he goes to school learns to associate school with unpleasant experiences. Every Sunday evening during the school semester, the child may become anxious in anticipation of going to school the following day. This is the type of learning that was emphasized by behavioral psychologists.[19] People at this level of learning are able to do only what Abreu and Toglia called *"near transfer"* (p. 508).[1] This means that they can transfer skills only to tasks in which one or two surface characteristics present in the original learning task are changed. For example, a client who has had a stroke learns a one-handed technique to chop carrots. He or she can easily transfer this skill to potatoes, cucumbers, and so on. Only the type of vegetable is changed. The skill of chopping is essentially the same.

Representation

In this type of learning, a mental image representing events is formulated and a framework to guide organization and retrieval of events from memory is created.[19] This allows generalization of learning to tasks that share similar characteristics with the original task, but are not readily identifiable. This is what Abreu and Toglia referred to as *"intermediate transfer"* (p. 508),[1] where three to six surface characteristics in the original task have

been changed. For example, a person who learned the one-handed technique of chopping vegetables may use the same skill to cut cooked meat on a plate and eat a steak meal independently. In this case, the type of food is different (meat instead of vegetables), the texture is different (it is cooked meat instead of raw vegetables), and it is on a plate instead of on a cutting board.

Abstraction

In this type of learning, "rules, knowledge, and facts abstracted from events" are stored "independently of spatio-temporal context" (p. 14).[20] This level of abstraction allows articulation of principles underlying a skill, making it possible to transfer it to contexts that are completely different from the original context in which it was learned. Abreu and Toglia called this *"far transfer"* (p. 508).[1] For example, the client with a stroke who learns the one-handed technique of chopping vegetables may eventually abstract this skill into the principle of reduction of food particles into little units before cooking it.

With this principle in mind, the client would be able to transfer the one-handed skill into grating cheese or dicing onions, tomatoes, garlic, and so on. He or she can even improvise in cases in which the utensils needed are different from what is available. This level of learning results in the most adaptive behavior. Furthermore, this ability to generalize skills so that they are the most adaptive can be reinforced using operant conditioning principles. For instance, every time a client applies skills learned in the clinic to his or her life in general, he or she can be rewarded. Eventually this may result in a habitual way of thinking that allows ability to generalize learning.

Postulations About Function, Dysfunction, and Change

Function

According to the above statement of the theoretical core, *function* is the ability to learn adaptive skills that enable one to act and interact with his or her environment in such a way that needs are met, one is living according to values, is independent, and is able to live a pleasurable and harmonious life.[4,10,36,51] It is also the capacity to acquire and process information appropriately so as to learn and generalize knowledge leading to participation in occupations that a person wants, is expected to do, or needs to do.[57] Furthermore, learning and generalization of skills is dependent on having positive beliefs/thought processes that are consistent with function necessary for adaptive occupational functioning.

Dysfunction

In this conceptual model, *dysfunction* is conceived to result from faulty behavior due to maladaptive learning.[4,51] It can also result from limitation in one's ability to process information effectively.[1,14,15,19,56] Self-defeating beliefs/thought processes also contribute to maladaptive behavior that leads to dysfunction. Faulty learning, deficiencies in information-processing ability, and faulty beliefs/thought processes all lead to maladaptive behavior and consequent inadequate occupational functioning. This limits one's ability to meet needs, live according to values, be independent, and thus live a pleasurable and harmonious life.

Change

Therapy based on guidelines derived from the Behavioral/Cognitive-Behavioral conceptual model of practice is expected to cause change in three ways:

1. *Facilitating behavioral change so that the client adopts adaptive behaviors and abandons maladaptive ones (behavior management).*[4] For example, a client with substance abuse problems may among other things experience difficulty keeping a job once discharged from the hospital. This may be due to poor work habits such as arriving to work late due to his or her tendency to prioritize substance-seeking behaviors to the detriment of performance at work. To a certain extent, substance-seeking behaviors may be seen as learned. (Substance

abuse is addictive, which decreases the extent to which a person may be held accountable to control of the behavior. However, it is also a learned behavior that often begins as a social activity.) The goal of therapy in this case would be in part to help the client learn how to structure time by establishing new routines that do not support substance use but instead facilitate meaningful occupational performance.

2. *Helping the client develop adaptive skills.* Elimination of the client's substance-seeking routines described above may be facilitated by teaching him or her leisure skills to enable him or her use time in occupations that can be substituted for substance use. For example, the client may be taught to explore and learn a variety of enjoyable leisure occupations that support adaptive functioning at work and in self-care, and in which he or she can engage preferably with other people, instead of ingesting substances. Learning time management skills such as prioritizing, scheduling tasks, using "to do" lists, and so on may also contribute to the establishment of healthy habits and routines. Consistent engagement in such occupations may lead to development of adaptive habits and routines that support the ability to function independently in all occupational areas (work, leisure, and self-care) constituting what Stoffel and Moyers refer to as *complete lifestyle adjustment.*[53]

3. *Helping the client change irrational and distorted cognitions that impend effective functioning.* For instance, the client described above may be ingesting drugs to self-medicate in an attempt to escape from stress resulting from negative environmental circumstances against which he or she feels helpless. Cognitive distortions may include automatic irrational thoughts such as: "I am not capable of determining the direction of my life," "I am dependent on environmental circumstances," or "Other people's actions cause all my problems." Due to this thought process, the client is likely to view his or her

life as being out of control, leading to a sense of helplessness that necessitates (in his or her view) an escape through ingestion of drugs.

Such thinking would make it difficult for the client to commit to learning new ways of functioning that are consistent with adaptive functioning. In this case, therapy would be geared toward helping the client gain insight regarding how this type of thinking is limiting his or her ability to realize his or her potential and to live a meaningful, healthy, functional life. Helping the client develop this insight may lead to development of awareness so that when such self-defeating thought processes occur, he or she can consciously dispute them, and replace them with more adaptive thought processes, such as, "I have the ability to act, if I choose to, and change my life circumstances."

Therapy based on this model, therefore, aims at helping clients develop skills and performance capabilities and counteract stressful circumstances in their lives so that they can remain functional. This may be achieved by learning skills such as acceptable social behavior, time management, self-control/discipline, relaxation, stress management, and management of reaction to environmental events through cognitive control and biofeedback. Strategies such as modeling, coaching, shaping, and testing cognitions through alternative behaviors are also used to facilitate learning and produce change.[4]

Guidelines for Client Evaluation

Occupational therapy within the framework of the Behavioral/Cognitive-Behavioral conceptual model of practice may be viewed as a teaching/learning process. According to Giuffrida and Neistadt, "Occupational therapy clients spend most of their intervention time *learning* different strategies to become more independent. Consequently, occupational therapy practitioners need to know something about learning and learning theory" (p. 253).[19] Evaluation and intervention based on this model focuses on the

client learning adaptive behaviors and skills. In this perspective, "The teaching/learning process is an interaction between the client and the therapist designed to help the client *acquire new and more adaptive knowledge, strategies, skills, and attitudes*" (p. 443, emphasis mine)[1]; one may also add behaviors. Evaluation of clients and therapeutic intervention focuses on three areas: (1) maladaptive behaviors, (2) information processing and ability to transfer (generalize) learning, and (3) irrational and distorted cognitions that are automatic and self-defeating.

Assessment Guidelines
Identifying Maladaptive Behaviors

Behavior may be either overt or covert.[51] Overt behavior consists of observable actions, while covert behavior involves unobservable processes of the mind. Whether covert or overt, in order to be measurable, behavior needs to be verifiable. Its measurement may be based on intensity, frequency, or duration. Once the faulty behavior/skill that interferes with appropriate occupational performance is identified (e.g., inability to communicate clearly with people, disorganization, inability to complete tasks within an allotted time), it is measured objectively by observing its intensity, frequency, and/or duration of occurrence within a certain period of time (until a stable pattern is established).[4,10,51]

Both behaviors that interfere with and those that are necessary for occupational functioning that leads to healthy adaptation need to be observed and recorded. Moreover,

A detailed description of a problematic [and adaptive] behavior includes an analysis of antecedents (what comes before the event), the behavior itself, and the consequences of the behavior for the individual. Documentation records of this analysis are called '*antecedent-behavior-consequence (ABC) records*' (p. 259, emphasis mine).[14]

A record of incidences of antecedents and responses to them constitute a baseline of behaviors that hinder or facilitate occupational performance in all the areas of a client's life (i.e., work, activities of daily living [ADLs], leisure, and interpersonal relationships). To establish this baseline, both informal observations as well as formal instruments that best meet verifiability criteria are used to gather information.[4,10,51] Examples of observation instruments include behavioral scales, tallies, and checklists. Behaviors can then be recorded in charts and graphed.

Examples of standardized instruments that are used to assess behaviors and skills objectively include the Kohlman Evaluation of Living Skills (KELS)[54,55] and the Scorable Self Care Evaluation (SSCE).[5] These instruments elicit information through a combination of interview (e.g., the client is asked how often he or she takes a bath, combs hair), and observation of the client engaging in samples of daily living tasks (e.g., planning a day's meal, identification of safety hazards from pictures). Other instruments that may be used include the Task Check List (TCL),[27] which is used to assess adult psychiatric clients' learning needs; the Stress Management Questionnaire (SMQ),[49,50] which assesses how clients articulate their stress (by describing symptoms, stressors, and coping activities), and how they manage it; and Rotter's Internal-External Scale,[4] which is used to assess whether an individual has an internal locus of control (attributes consequences to personal actions and efforts), among others. Once a baseline of performance has been established, target behaviors to be encouraged or discouraged and skills to be developed are identified, and treatment goals are established accordingly.

Identifying Information-Processing Difficulties

Some of the skills evaluated include information-processing abilities such as visual/perceptual abilities (e.g., left-right, up-down visual scanning), organizing information (e.g., chunking), relating it to prior experiences (assimilating), prioritizing, planning ahead, and time management.[1,19,56] Of particular importance is assessment of the client's ability to transfer learning. Through careful observation, the therapist determines whether the client is capable of only associative learning, in which skills learned in one context can be transferred only to another task with only one or two characteristics changed; representational learning, in which three to six surface characteristics of a task can be changed; or abstract learning, in which the client grasps the principles underlying learned skills and therefore is capable of improvising to complete tasks whose surface characteristics are completely different from those of the task used to learn the skills.

An example of an instrument used to evaluate information-processing ability is the Cognitive Adaptive Skills Evaluation.[30] A therapist using this instrument assesses cognitive processes such as the following:

- The ability to engage in imitation and circular reactions
- The ability to develop and use object permanence, time concepts, language, images, classifications, and relational and number skills
- The ability to use judgment and engage in moral behavior (p. 280)

Another important area of assessment is metacognition, which includes awareness of strengths and limitations and self-monitoring of performance.[7,26] Included in this category of information processing is the ability to predict self-performance accurately. To evaluate these skills, the therapist helps the client rate himself or herself using checklists that assess awareness of deficits and self-monitoring of performance. Such checklists measure both emergent awareness, which refers to ability to recognize and correct errors and solve problems as they occur, and anticipatory awareness, which refers to the capacity to "foresee problems and prepare to respond accordingly" (p. 53).

Assessment of Cognitions

Finally, the therapist assesses the client's typical appraisal of self, others, and the world, and identifies errors in his or her thinking as indicated by irrational beliefs (e.g., "I must complete every task I try perfectly or I am a failure") as well as cognitive distortions (e.g., "I have always been a failure and will always be a failure").[32,41] The effect of these mistaken beliefs and thoughts on maintenance of occupational performance dysfunction is evaluated.

Guidelines for Therapeutic Intervention

During evaluation as described above, the desired behavior or skill (terminal behavior/skill) is identified. Expected level of learning (associative, representation, or abstract) is established. This is the first step toward intervention. The terminal behavior/skill is the treatment goal. It should be relevant, observable, understandable, measurable, behavioral, and attainable within a reasonable length of time.[6,10,43a,44,51] It should be described operationally so that it can be observed and measured precisely and can be replicated. While setting therapy goals, the therapist should remember that "most current theories include cognition in the definition of observable behavior and acknowledge internal control of the individual" (p. 137).[6] Therefore, cognitive skills such as *metacognition* (awareness of strengths and limitations, prediction, and self-monitoring of performance) are incorporated into therapy goals.[1,15,26,56] The goals are stated in words/actions that are easily observable, heard, or read, and that can be counted, their length of occurrence measured, or their intensity objectively established.

Once the terminal behavior/skill is identified, defined, and stated as a therapeutic goal using observable and measurable actions/words, activities/procedures to facilitate attainment of the behavior/skill are selected (e.g., rehearsal and practice; shaping; chaining; role playing, modeling, and imitation; systematic desensitization).[4,6,10,51] Each of the procedures will be described next.

Rehearsal and Practice

The client is taught to "talk through" new behaviors/skills. Such behaviors/skills are then practiced until they become habitual.[6,10] Skills that are rehearsed and practiced include "self-care, cooking different meals, home maintenance chores, banking, shopping, planning vacations, setting up interviews and doctor's appointments, planning weekly schedules, leisure games and community outings," (p. 55)[26] among others. Sometimes these skills are rehearsed and practiced under supervision of a life skills coach.

Shaping

Behaviors that more and more approximate the target behavior/skill are reinforced successively and mastered until target behavior/skill is attained.[4,6] For example, imagine a student who is having difficulty disciplining himself to be able to focus and study, and complete school assignments. As a result, he is failing in school. The occupational therapy goal for this student might be to help him to develop the self-discipline/control necessary to focus on his studies and school assignments 2 hours every night, and to effectively read and complete all his assignments. To help him achieve this objective, the therapist rewards him initially for sitting and reading for 10 minutes, then rewards him only when able to read continuously for 20 minutes, then for one-half hour while taking notes, and then for 1 hour while taking notes, and finally for 2 hours while taking notes, with a 10-minute break after 1 hour. Each behavior more closely approximates the target behavior of being able to concentrate on his studies and assignments for 2 hours. Also, increasing effort in the direction of the target behavior is required in order to receive the same reinforcement.

Chaining

Chaining is similar to shaping in many respects. In this behavioral therapeutic approach, a task is taught in progressive components, where each component becomes a stimulus that sets in motion the next step.[4,6,61] This technique is especially effective for children and adults with limited cognitive abilities, but it is also used in education in general. For example, think about how you learned to read and write. First, you were taught how to read and write letters of the alphabet. Once that skill was mastered, you were taught how to differentiate vowels, then how to combine them with other letters of the alphabet to make basic sounds. Then you learned how to combine those sounds to make words, then sentences, and finally, you were able to write paragraphs and eventually whole pages. This approach is referred to as *forward chaining*. Learning begins with simple skills, which are then combined to form more complex skills leading to complex operations.

Backward chaining can also be used and is very effective with clients who have limited cognitive skills such that they cannot imagine a complete product. For such clients, beginning with the last step (which gives them a visual image of the final product) acts as reinforcement, making the client want to learn how to complete the entire task.[4,61] For example, a therapist may prepare all the ingredients for a client who is learning how to make an omelet breakfast. The therapist places the eggs in the skillet and at the appropriate time, asks the client to put the rest of the ingredients on top of the eggs and finish making the omelet. The client therefore sees the finished product (the omelet), and this encourages him or her to learn the other steps of the task. Next, the client is asked to scramble the eggs, put them in the skillet, and add the other ingredients. Then, he or she is asked to dice the vegetables, scramble the eggs, place them in the skillet, and add the diced ingredients. Finally, the client is asked to choose the vegetables, prepare and wash them, dice them, break the eggs and scramble them, place them in the skillet, add the diced vegetables, and complete the preparation of the omelet independently.

Role Playing, Modeling, and Imitation

These three techniques are derived from Bandura's Cognitive Social Learning Theory (CSLT) (see Chapter 3 for a detailed discussion of the CSLT).[2] These techniques are based on the idea of *vicarious learning*.[14] This is the type of learning that occurs through observation of others engaged in the desired behavior and the consequences resulting from their behavior. For example, the therapist may demonstrate how to behave in an interview for a job in a role play. The client then imitates the therapist's behavior through similar role play, and feedback is provided regarding the effectiveness of the behavior. In this case, the therapist is using *role play* to *model* desired behavior that the client *imitates*. Another way of teaching the behavior may be by having the client watch a video showing individuals engaging in an interview successfully and getting a desired job. Through the video, the client learns vicariously job interview behaviors that are effective.

Other Cognitive-Behavioral Therapeutic Procedures

Other cognitive-behavioral techniques used by occupational therapists include systematic desensitization/relaxation therapy, biofeedback, and psychoeducation.[4,10,51] Systematic desensitization/relaxation therapy is based on the principle of reciprocal inhibition, which states that one cannot be relaxed and anxious at the same time. Based on that principle, the client is helped to achieve a state of progressive muscle relaxation (e.g., by using a combination of deep breathing and guided visualization while listening to soothing music). While in this state of relaxation, the feared stimulus (e.g., messy occupational therapy media for clients with obsessive compulsive disorders [OCDs]) is gradually introduced. Eventually the client is able to handle the feared stimulus (e.g., working with clay) without experiencing disabling anxiety.

Biofeedback refers to a technique in which technological devices are used to portray physiological processes, such as brain waves. The client uses this visual feedback as a cue to indicate the need to control these physiological processes, such as anxiety.

Finally, in psychoeducation, the client is seen as a student, and the therapist acts as a teacher.

Therapy is organized into educational modules. Clients sit in "class" and receive instruction didactically and through other educational activities. They take notes, are given assignments, and take quizzes and tests. This approach has been found to be effective in teaching a variety of life skills, including social behaviors such as self-expression, "other-enhancement," assertiveness, and communication skills.

Cognitive Approaches

The therapist uses principles of cognitive therapy to teach the client to monitor automatic thoughts that interfere with effective occupational performance, such as "I am helpless," "I cannot do this," "I have never been good at this and will never be able to perform this activity," "I am hopeless," and so on.[9,13,15,32] The therapist may use the *G, ABC, D* model suggested by Albert Ellis (see Chapter 3) as a guide for intervention. *G* refers to the client's goals, *A* to anteceding event(s) that affect attainment of goals, *B* stands for the belief system associated with the event(s), *C* for emotional and behavioral consequences of the event, and *D* for therapeutic intervention that consists of finding and disputing irrational beliefs and replacing them with more realistic ones. By learning the "disputing" skill, the client is able to heighten awareness of mistaken thought processes and replace them with more adaptive ones.[41] By replacing mistaken thought processes, self-imposed limitations to occupational performance are eliminated and the client is more successful in engaging in occupations that he or she wants, is expected to do, or needs to do.

Generally, cognitive interventions consist of facilitating the client's (1) recognition of the relationship between cognition, affect, and behavior (including occupational performance behavior), (2) awareness of thoughts (distortions and automatic thoughts), (3) examination of distortions through reality testing (e.g., using carefully planned exposure to situations eliciting anxiety and gathering evidence both for and against the automatic thoughts [known as experiments]), (4) response to distortions with logic, reasoning, and empirical evidence, (5) substitution of distortions with more balanced thoughts, and (6) making plans to develop new thought processes.[41,48]

Nonsituational Information-Processing Strategies

To facilitate transfer of learning, a multicontextual approach of intervention is used in which the client is taught nonsituational techniques to facilitate increased awareness and performance.[1,26,56] Such techniques include using rating scales to predict performance and then comparing with actual performance after the task, using checklists to enhance self-questioning (e.g. "What did I forget?"), writing down supplies and sequential steps needed to complete tasks on notepads, and so on.

After a suitable intervention strategy is selected, reinforcement and a reinforcement schedule are chosen.[4,6,10,44] The chosen reinforcement should be an activity or object that is important to the client but not contraindicated to therapy goals. Reinforcement may be positive or negative. Positive reinforcement refers to reward for engagement in the desired behavior, such as watching a movie after reading for 2 hours. Negative reinforcement is removal of negative consequences once the desired behavior occurs. For instance, imagine a situation in which a wife constantly nags her husband until he takes out the trash. Nagging is a noxious stimulus for the man. As soon as he takes out the trash (desired behavior), the nagging (noxious stimulus) stops. Therefore, in the future, he takes out the trash spontaneously to avoid nagging. In this case, elimination of nagging is negative reinforcement for the husband.

Punishment may also be used to change behavior. Positive punishment occurs when noxious stimulus, such as pain, is presented following unwanted behavior. Negative punishment is simply ignoring behavior and taking away positive consequences. For instance, an attention-seeking teenager who disrupts the group during therapy in order to get attention may be ignored every time she disrupts the group. Ignoring her takes away the attention that she is seeking. Every time she attends to the group activities appropriately for a defined period of time, the therapist praises her (positive reinforcement).

Reinforcement schedule refers to how often rewards are given for engagement in the desired behavior. In the beginning of learning a new behavior/skill, reinforcement should be continuous, so that every time the behavior occurs it is rewarded.[4] Once behavior is learned, intermittent reinforcement is the most effective way to ensure its maintenance. Intermittent reinforcement is random, so that engagement in the desired behavior may or may not result in a reward. Thus, the client performs the desired behavior in hope that the reward will come at any time.

CASE STUDY: DRAKE

For illustration of the clinical use of this conceptual model, refer to Drake's case introduced in Chapter 6. This analysis occurs after Drake has been released from the hospital, based on the occupational therapist's recommendation, to live in an apartment with minimal daily supervision by a mental health aid, until he is able to reunite with his wife and family. This constitutes a trial period to determine his ability to live independently at home with his family. Illustration of how one of Drake's short-term goals was addressed using the Behavioral/Cognitive-Behavioral conceptual model of practice is shown in Table 10-1. The goal was broken down into discreet subgoals to increase preciseness as required when using this model.

The following progress note (SOAP format) written 1 week after Drake was discharged to an apartment illustrates how reassessment clinical data is compared to the baseline evaluation findings.

S: This morning, Drake stated, "I feel better today than I have felt in a long time."

O: Under the therapist's supervision, the mental health aide worked with Drake this week focusing on meal planning and preparation, making grocery lists, going grocery shopping, and social dining. Drake also attended an outpatient occupational therapy group in which the role of meals in socialization, family relationships, health and well-being, and leisure was discussed. Drake made significant progress toward his goal as follows:

STG	Previous Status	Current Status
By the end of 4 weeks, Drake will demonstrate improved ability to: • Plan 3 balanced meals for a typical day using the criteria provided in the SSCE • Shop for groceries • Independently prepare the meals	During the SSCE evaluation, Drake was not able to: • Plan 3 balanced meals for 2 consecutive days. He indicated that he would eat hamburgers for breakfast, lunch, and dinner. His meal intake chart indicated that before hospitalization, he went for up to 3 days without eating, and when he ate, he consumed mostly junk foods such as popcorn and candy. • Make a grocery shopping list for a day's meal. • Prepare a complete meal: breakfast, lunch, or dinner, even with verbal instructions.	Today, Drake: • Independently planned 3 balanced meals on paper according to the criteria provided in the SSCE. • Made a list of groceries needed for the meals, and the mental health aide shopped for the groceries. • Independently made and ate 3 balanced meals (as specified in the criteria provided in the SSCE) on Monday and Thursday.

Continued

CASE STUDY: DRAKE—CONT'D

A: This week, Drake made significant progress toward the STG as indicated by planning, making, and eating 3 balanced meals (according to the criteria provided in the SSCE, the instrument used in the initial assessment), and eating the meals 2 days of the week.

P: Continue working with Drake as per the treatment plan to help him achieve his long-term goal to take care of himself by making and eating balanced meals independently.

Revisit Lab Manual Exercises 6-2 and 6-3 and complete Exercises 6-4 and 12-1 for further reflec-tion in developing Behavioral/Cognitive-Behavioral skills for use in your clinical practice.

Table 10-1. CLINICAL APPLICATION OF THE BEHAVIORAL/COGNITIVE-BEHAVIORAL CONCEPTUAL MODEL TO GUIDE INTERVENTION TO ADDRESS ONE OF DRAKE'S SHORT-TERM GOALS

Intervention Step	Example of Intervention with Drake
1. Identify target behavior (treatment goal)	By the end of 4 weeks, Drake will demonstrate improved ability to take care of himself as indicated by his ability to do the following: • Plan 3 meals for a typical day based on the criteria provided in the SSCE • Shop for groceries • Make the meals independently
2. Determine behavioral baseline by counting frequency of behavior	The SSCE was used to evaluate Drake's ability to plan 3 balanced meals for 2 consecutive days. He was also asked to list the ingredients for each meal so that he could shop for them in the grocery store. In addition, he was asked to record what he ate for breakfast, lunch, and dinner every day for 7 days before his hospital admission.
3. Select a method of counting and recording behavior	For objective observation and recording of behavior, the therapist opted to use SSCE (a standardized evaluation instrument), listing of meal preparation ingredients, and a chart in which the frequency with which meals with certain nutritional value were consumed. These frequencies were recorded again while the client was living on a trial basis at the apartment and graphed so that a visual track of eating habits before and after hospitalization could be demonstrated.
4. Select an intervention procedure and appropriate reinforcement that is personally meaningful to Drake	The procedures chosen to teach Drake appropriate self-care habits/skills included psychoeducation (to teach him the value of balanced meals and the nutritional value of various foods, cooking, grocery shopping, and so on) and rehearsal and practice of the learned skills. Drake was also taught to monitor his urge to eat unhealthy foods using a checklist where he checked off the nutritional contents of every foodstuff that he ingested. Since Drake enjoys riding his motorcycle, this leisure activity was used as a reward. His daughter was asked to be in charge of the motorcycle so that she could allow Drake to ride for a specified length of time once he made progress and sustained learned skills for a certain period of time.
5. Select a schedule of reinforcement	It is usually recommended that intermittent reinforcement be used to maintain behavior once it has been learned. However, since Drake is already motivated to take care of himself so that he can go home to his family, reinforcement is only used as a means of encouraging him to stick to the process of change especially during challenging times. Therefore, continuous reinforcement was used. Every time he consistently ate 3 balanced meals a day (according to criteria specified in the SSCE) for 1 week, he was rewarded by being allowed by his daughter to ride his bike over the weekend. This method of reinforcement was used until healthy eating became habitual for Drake.

Adapted from Sieg KW: Applying the behavioral model to the occupational therapy model, *Am J Occup Ther* 28:421-428, 1974.

Consistency of the Behavioral/ Cognitive-Behavioral Model with the Occupational Therapy Paradigm

In Chapter 4, it was pointed out that a conceptual practice model is consistent with the occupational therapy paradigm to the extent that it emphasizes an occupation and client-centered perspective and is grounded on a complexity/ chaos theoretical framework. The role of the therapist in this paradigm is conceptualized as that of providing opportunities for occupational performance, environmental modification, assistive devices, and education/counseling in order to facilitate occupational performance necessary for participation in life.

Based on the above criteria, it can be concluded that the Behavioral/Cognitive-Behavioral conceptual model of practice is consistent with the professional paradigm in certain respects but inconsistent in others. One of the major criticisms of behaviorism from the occupational therapy perspective is that it is mechanistic, does not account for wholeness of human experiences and human creativity, and is manipulative and coercive.[51] This criticism indicates that therapy based on behavioral constructs is not collaborative and therefore not client-centered. To that extent, it would not be consistent with the current professional paradigm. This shortcoming has been meliorated by making therapy based on the model more collaborative and based on the client's concerns, rather than what the therapist perceives to be the problems.

Current descriptions of the Behavioral/ Cognitive-Behavioral model (which consists of a combination of techniques and constructs from behaviorism, information processing, and cognitive psychology) indicate that it focuses on issues identified by the client and his or her family as areas of concern.[26] Where the client's level of insight does not allow realistic identification of performance problems, development of awareness becomes a central goal of therapy, based on the recognition that change cannot occur unless the client perceives a need

for it.[7,26,56] Therefore, it is evident that the model, as gleaned from the current description of application in literature, is evolving toward a client-centered perspective.

Furthermore, in interventions based on the model, occupations are used to help clients learn the behaviors/skills needed to function in their everyday life, and the overarching goal is safe occupational functioning. This is clear from the emphasis placed on transfer of learning.[1,19,26,56,57] It can be said, therefore, that in its current form, the model is occupation- and client-centered, and consistent with the occupational therapy paradigm.

The question, however, is whether it is grounded on the complexity/chaos theoretical framework. In order for the model to be consistent with the complexity/chaos theoretical framework, its perspective of the human needs to be that of a complex, dynamic, adaptive system engaged in interaction with its environment, in the process of which increased self-organization and adaptive behaviors emerge (see Chapter 4 for a detailed discussion of the complexity/chaos theoretical perspective). Therefore the role of therapy would be to present challenges to which the client can respond and in the process develop adaptive capabilities.

The Behavioral/Cognitive-Behavioral model, so far, emphasizes clear identification of terminal behavior/skills, and then uses clearly defined strategies to achieve them. This emphasis is not consistent with presentation of challenges to facilitate emergence of adaptive capabilities. However, within the model, a motor-learning perspective is emerging, which is based on the postulation that, "practice produces cumulative changes in behavior and with practice a more appropriate representation of action is developed" (p. 271).[18] In this evolving model, "active involvement of the learner" in the learning process is encouraged, in which the client "receives reduced knowledge of results and performance and encounters difficulty in the practice context" (p. 272).[18]

In the information-processing aspect of the model, the latest developments are deemphasizing specific cognitive abilities in favor of activities in therapy that "elicit and challenge" information-processing capacities (p. 135).[24] This new approach is dynamic and "emphasizes understanding how cognitive-perceptual behavior emerges under different task and contextual conditions" (pp. 135-136).[24] Therefore it is clear that the Behavioral/Cognitive-Behavioral model is evolving to embrace the complexity/chaos theoretical perspective, consistent with the current occupational therapy paradigm.

The role of the therapist using this model is to provide opportunities for the client to engage in occupations that lead to development of behaviors/skills needed to function safely and independently, environmental modification using a variety of cognitive strategies to enhance occupational performance, and education/counseling to encourage the client to identify distorted automatic cognitions that interfere with occupational functioning and replace them with more realistic and functional cognitions, as well as to develop cognitive strategies to facilitate more effective occupational functioning. This model is therefore highly consistent with the occupational therapy paradigm and is evolving to be even more consistent by embracing the motor-control view of therapy.

Consistency with the Philosophy of Pragmatism

Therapists using the Behavioral/Cognitive-Behavioral model recognize the central role of the mind in occupational functioning. That is why clarification and change of the client's cognitions is crucial. Importance of the role of environmental feedback on learning is also recognized, and so is the centrality of habit in maintenance of desired behaviors/skills as indicated by the model's emphasis on rehearsal and practice as techniques of therapeutic intervention. Therapy using this model also depends largely on exposure of the client to situa-

tions that test hypotheses derived from beliefs. Furthermore, it is clear that the theoretical basis of this model has a common origin with functionalism, which was espoused by pragmatists, especially James and Dewey.[51] Thus the model is highly consistent with the philosophy of pragmatism as illustrated by constructs that are common to both.

Consistency with the Complexity/ Chaos Theoretical Scientific Framework

As discussed earlier, this model was originally not consistent with the complexity/chaos theoretical framework. However, it is evolving toward incorporation of constructs from this framework in its theoretical core.

Recommendations for Reinterpretation of the Model

This conceptual model is evolving in the right direction. It would be beneficial to continue developing the model's practice guidelines drawing more from the complexity/chaos theoretical framework and making this link more explicit. Furthermore, common factors between the various components of the model (behavioral, cognitive, and information-processing) need to be made clearer. It is easier to develop it as one model rather than trying to continue to develop each component as a stand-alone conceptual model, as has been the case in the past. After all, behavioral, cognitive, and information-processing constructs and techniques are used in combination in practice, and trying to separate them as independent conceptual models leads to artificial divisions.

Evidence-Based Practice Using the Behavioral/Cognitive-Behavioral Model

The Behavioral/Cognitive-Behavioral conceptual model of practice is one of the most researched models in occupational therapy.* Many of the studies indicate that interventions based on the model result in significant changes in occupational functioning, which are often generalized into all areas of clients' lives, and are often enduring long after termination of therapy. Furthermore, contrary to postulations in literature that suggest that rapid recovery from certain cognitive conditions such as those acquired through traumatic brain injury (TBI) happens in the early stages of rehabilitation and no significant changes are expected after 1 year following injury,[22,37] studies indicate that this model can be used to guide therapy resulting in notable functional changes even 8 years after injury.[26,38]

More recent clinical practice and research studies based on this model are investigating application of electronic technology, for instance, personal digital assistants (PDAs) to enhance clients' use of cognitive strategies to improve occupational functioning and participation in life.† Such technology has proven beneficial in facilitating use of items like checklists and alarms to enhance completion of daily routines, leading to increased independence, compliance with medication, reduced rate of relapse, and improved quality of life. It is evident that this model has much potential to enhance the practice of occupational therapy in a way that is consistent with the current professional paradigm, especially considering that it can be used to guide intervention in all areas of occupational therapy practice (e.g., physical rehabilitation, mental health, long-term care, school system, home health).[6]

SUMMARY

In this chapter, we presented the Behavioral/ Cognitive-Behavioral conceptual model of practice. It was one of the earliest conceptual models to be articulated in occupational therapy, along with the psychodynamic conceptual model. Rather than considering the behavioral, cognitive, and information-processing components

---

*References 16,26,31,38,39,42,52.
†References 12,17,25,28,29,60,62.

to be individual conceptual models of practice, it is more judicious to combine them into one model referred to as the Behavioral/Cognitive-Behavioral model. Indeed, this move to combine them into one comprehensive model is evident from early occupational therapy where attempts at integrating behavioral and cognitive constructs into one perspective are evident. In the comprehensive model, it was emphasized that the behavioral component would focus on the action/behavior-consequence (behavioral change) coupling, while cognitive and information-processing components would explain and provide a rationale for what happens between action and consequence. Sources of constructs forming the model's theoretical core were identified as behavioral psychology, cognitive psychology, and information-processing theory.

We also discussed postulations of the model regarding function, dysfunction, and change. Guidelines for evaluation and intervention based on the model were presented. A case example was provided to illustrate how the model's guidelines may be applied in clinical practice. We found that the model is largely consistent with the occupational therapy professional paradigm and the philosophy of pragmatism. It is also evolving toward increased consistency with the complexity/chaos theoretical framework, with the inclusion of the motor-control perspective and further development of the information-processing view toward increased emphasis on emergent characteristics of cognitive processes. Finally, we observed that there is a remarkable body of research supporting efficacy of this model as a guide to clinical practice. It is therefore a promising model whose further development may be crucial in enhancing the place of occupational therapy in the provision of rehabilitation services.

REFERENCES

1. Abreu BC, Toglia J: Cognitive rehabilitation: a model for occupational therapy, *Am J Occup Ther* 41: 439-448, 1987.
2. Bandura A: *Social learning theory,* New York, 1977, General Learning Press.

3. Boeree CG: B.F. Skinner: 1904-1990. *Personality Theories,* 1998. Retrieved August 2005, from http://www.ship.edu/cgboeree/skinner.html.

4. Bruce M, Borg B: *Psychosocial frames of reference: core for occupation-based practice,* ed 3, Thorofare, NJ, 2002, Slack.

5. Clark EN, Peters M: *Scorable self care evaluation,* Thorofare, NJ, 1984, Slack.

6. Cole MB: *Group dynamics in occupational therapy: the theoretical basis and practice application of group intervention,* ed 3, Thorofare, NJ, 2005, Slack.

7. Crosson B, Barco PP, Velozo CA, et al: Awareness and compensation in post-acute head injury rehabilitation, *J Head Trauma Rehabil* 4:46-54, 1989.

8. Diasio K: Psychiatric occupational therapy: search for a conceptual framework in light of psychoanalytic ego psychology and learning theory, *Am J Occup Ther* 22:400-407, 1968.

9. Duncombe L: The cognitive behavioral model in mental health. In Katz N, ed: *Cognition and occupation in rehabilitation,* Bethesda, MD, 1998, AOTA, pp. 165-191.

10. Early MB: *Mental health concepts and techniques for the occupational therapy assistant,* New York, 2000, Lippincott Williams & Wilkins.

11. Ellsworth CP, Colman AD: Reinforcement systems to support work behavior: the application of operant conditioning principles, *Am J Occup Ther* 24:562-568, 1970.

12. Gentry T: A brain in the palm of your hand: assistive technology for cognition, *OT Practice* 10-12, 2005.

13. Giles GM: Anorexia nervosa and bulimia: An activity oriented approach, *Am J Occup Ther* 39:510-517, 1985.

14. Giles GM: Behaviorism. In Crepeau EB, Cohn ES, Schell BA, eds: *Willard & Spackman's occupational therapy,* ed 10, New York, 2003, Lippincott Williams & Wilkins, pp. 257-259.

15. Giles GM: Cognitive therapy. In Crepeau EB, Cohn ES, Schell BA, eds: *Willard & Spackman's occupational therapy,* ed 10, New York, 2003, Lippincott Williams & Wilkins, pp. 259-261.

16. Giles GM, Ridley JE, Dill A, et al: A consecutive series of adults with brain injury treated with a dressing retraining program, *Am J Occup Ther* 51:256-266, 1997.

17. Giles GM, Robinson K: The effectiveness of an electronic memory aid for a memory impaired adult of normal intelligence, *Am J Occup Ther* 43:409-411, 1988.

18. Giuffrida CG: Motor learning: an emerging frame of reference for occupational performance. In Crepeau EB, Cohn ES, Schell BA, eds: *Willard & Spackman's occupational therapy,* ed 10, New York, 2003, Lippincott Williams & Wilkins, pp. 267-272.

19. Giuffrida CG, Neistadt ME: Overview of learning theory. In Crepeau EB, Cohn ES, Schell BA, eds: *Willard & Spackman's occupational therapy,* ed 10, New York, 2003, Lippincott Williams & Wilkins, pp. 253-257.

20. Goldstein LH, Oakley DA: Expected and actual behavioral capacity after diffuse reduction in cerebral cortex: a review and suggestions for rehabilitative techniques with the mentally handicapped and head injured, *Br J Clin Psychol* 24:13–24, 1985.

21. Hergenhahn BR: *An introduction to the history of psychology,* ed 3, Pacific Grove, CA, 1997, Brooks/Cole.

22. Jennett B: The measurement of outcome. In Brooks N, ed: *Closed head injury: psychological, social and family consequences,* Oxford, 1984, Oxford University Press, pp. 37-43.

23. Kandel ER, Kupfermann I, Iversen S: Learning and memory. In Kandel ER, Schwartz JH, Jessell TM, eds: *Principles of neuroscience,* New York, 2000, McGraw Hill, pp. 1227-1245.

24. Kielhofner G: *Conceptual foundations of occupational therapy,* ed 3, Philadelphia, 2004, FA Davis.

25. Kim HJ, Burke DT, Dowds MM, et al: Electronic memory aids for outpatient brain injury: follow-up findings, *Brain Injury* 14(2):187-196, 2000.

26. Landa-Gonzalez B: Multicontextual occupational therapy intervention: a case study of traumatic brain injury, *Occup Ther Internat* 8:49-62, 2001.

27. Lillie M, Armstrong H: Contributions to the development of psychoeducation approaches to mental health service, *Am J Occup Ther* 36:438-443, 1982.

28. LoPresti EF, Mihailidis A: Assistive technology for cognitive rehabilitation: state of the art, *Neuropsych Rehabil* 14(1/2):5-39, 2004.

29. Lynch W: Historical review of computer-assisted cognitive retraining, *J Head Traumatic Rehabil* 17(5):446-457, 2002.

30. Masagatani GN: The cognitive adaptive skills evaluation. In Hemphill-Pearson BJ, ed: *Assessments in occupational therapy mental health: an integrative approach,* Thorofare, NJ, 1999, Slack, pp. 279-284.

31. Mathiowetz V, Haugen J: Motor behavior research: implications for therapeutic approaches to central nervous system dysfunction, *Am J Occup Ther* 48:733-745, 1994.

32. McMullin RE: *The new handbook of cognitive therapy techniques,* New York, 2000, Norton.

33. Mosey AC: *Three frames of reference for mental health,* Thorofare, NJ, 1970, Slack.

34. Mosey AC: *Activities therapy,* New York, 1973, Raven.

35. Mosey AC: *Psychosocial components of occupational therapy,* New York, 1987, Raven.

36. Mosey AC: *Psychosocial components of occupational therapy,* New York, 1996, Lippincott Williams & Wilkins.

37. Neistadt ME: The neurobiology of learning: Implications for treatment of adults with brain injury, *Am J Occup Ther* 48:421-430, 1994.

38. Nelson DL, Lenhart DA: Resumption of outpatient occupational therapy for a young woman five years after traumatic brain injury, *Am J Occup Ther* 50: 223-228, 1996.

39. O'Neill ME, Gwinn KA, Adler CH: Biofeedback for writer's cramp, *Am J Occup Ther* 51:605-607, 1997.

40. Patterson CH: *Theories of counseling and psychotherapy*, New York, 1980, Harper & Row.

41. Rodebaugh TL, Chambless DL: Cognitive therapy for performance anxiety, *J Clin Psychol* 60:809-820, 2004.

42. Romano JM, Jensen MP, Turner JA, et al: Chronic pain patient-partner interactions: Further support for a behavioral model of chronic pain, *Behavior Ther* 31: 415-440, 2000.

43. Rugel RP, Mattingly J, Eichinger M, et al: The use of operant conditioning with a physically disabled child, *Am J Occup Ther* 25:247-249, 1971.

43a. Sames KM: *Documenting occupational therapy practice*, Upper Saddle River, NJ, 2005, Pearson/Prentice-Hall.

44. Sieg KW: Applying the behavioral model to the occupational therapy model, *Am J Occup Ther* 28:421-428, 1974.

45. Skinner BF: *About behaviorism*, New York, 1974, Knopf.

46. Smith AR, Tempone VJ: Psychiatric occupational therapy within a learning theory context, *Am J Occup Ther* 22:415-420, 1968.

47. Squire LR: Memory and the hippocampus: a synthesis from findings with rats, monkeys, and humans, *Psychol Rev* 99:195-231, 1992.

48. Squires G: Using cognitive behavioral psychology with groups of pupils to improve self-control of behavior, *Educ Psychol Practice* 17:317-335, 2001.

49. Stein F, Bentley DE, Natz M: Computerized assessment: the stress management questionnaire. In Hemphill-Pearson BJ, ed: *Assessments in occupational therapy mental health*, Thorofare, NJ, 1999, Slack.

50. Stein F, Cutler SK: *Psychosocial occupational therapy*, San Diego, CA, 1998, Singular.

51. Stein F, Cutler SK: *Psychosocial occupational therapy: a holistic approach*, ed 2, Albany, NY, 2002, Delmar Thomson Learning.

52. Stein F, Nikolic S: Teaching stress management techniques to a schizophrenic patient, *Am J Occup Ther* 43:162-169, 1989.

53. Stoffel VC, Moyers PA: Occupational therapy and substance use disorders. In Cara E, MacRae A, eds: *Psychosocial occupational therapy: a clinical practice*, Clifton Park, NY, 2005, Thomson Delmar Learning, pp. 446-473.

54. Thomson LK: *The Kohlman evaluation of living skills*, Bethesda, MD, 1992, AOTA.

55. Thomson LK: The Kohlman evaluation of living skills. In Hemphill-Pearson BJ, ed: *Assessments in occupational therapy mental health: an integrative approach*, Thorofare, NJ, 1999, Slack, pp. 231-242.

56. Toglia JP: Generalization of treatment: a multicontextual approach to cognitive perceptual impairment in the brain injured adult, *Am J Occup Ther* 45:505-516, 1991.

57. Toglia JP: Multicontext treatment approach. In Crepeau EB, Cohn ES, Schell BA, eds: *Willard & Spackman's occupational therapy*, ed 10, New York, 2003, Lippincott Williams & Wilkins, pp. 264-267.

58. Weinrach SG: Cognitive therapists: a dialogue with Aaron Beck, *J Couns Dev* 67:159-164, 1988.

59. Weinrach SG: Nine experts describe the essence of rational-emotive therapy while standing on one foot, *J Couns Dev* 74:326-331, 1996.

60. Wilson BA, Emslie HC, Quirk K, et al: Reducing every day memory and planning problems by means of a paging system: a randomized control crossover study, *J Neurol Neurosurg Psychiatr* 70:447-482, 2001.

61. Wilson M: *Occupational therapy in long term psychiatry*, New York, 1983, Churchill Livingstone.

62. Wright P, Rogers N, Hall C, et al: Comparison of pocket-computer memory aids for people with brain injury, *Brain Injury* 15:787-800, 2001.

11

The Cognitive Disabilities Conceptual Model of Practice

Preview Questions

1. Discuss the interdisciplinary basis of the Cognitive Disabilities model of practice. Explain how Piaget's theory of cognitive development relates to the model.
2. Concisely state the theoretical core of the Cognitive Disabilities model of practice.
3. Explain the postulations of the Cognitive Disabilities model about the following, and use the Allen Cognitive Levels to explain the postulations.
   a. Function
   b. Dysfunction
   c. Change
4. Describe the model's guidelines for clinical assessment and intervention.
5. Discuss the consistency of the Cognitive Disabilities model with each of the following:
   a. The occupational therapy paradigm
   b. The philosophy of pragmatism
   c. The complexity/chaos theoretical framework
6. Discuss available empirical evidence supporting clinical effectiveness of the Cognitive Disabilities model as a guide to intervention in occupational therapy practice.
7. Suggest any modifications that may improve the model.

The Cognitive Disabilities conceptual model of practice was developed by Claudia Allen, one of the most influential occupational therapy theorists in the last quarter century. By virtue of its focus on the cognitive processes, it is closely related to the Behavioral/Cognitive-Behavioral model. However, as we will see later, while the latter strives to change human function by facilitating learning of adaptive behaviors and cognitive strategies, the former aims at compensating for cognitive dysfunction. While working as a psychiatric occupational therapist, Allen realized that many of the psychotic patients with diagnoses such as schizophrenia seemed to have similar problems to children with cerebral palsy or mental retardation. In both cases, there was evidence of inability to process information to be able to follow more than one direction at a time. This was the beginning of her formulation of what was later to be published as the Cognitive Disabilities conceptual model of practice.[2,3]

Interdisciplinary Scientific Base

Based on her conclusion that people with psychotic disorders such as schizophrenia had cognitive processing problems that were similar to children with mental retardation, Allen postulated that the source of their maladaptive functioning was cognitive dysfunction originating from defects in the brain organ.[2,3] Therefore these dysfunctions were biological and structural, and any changes could only be attributed to medical intervention or natural progression of the disease process. Based on this view of cognitive disability, Allen did not think that occupational therapy could change cognitive function.[33] The role of occupational therapists, she argued, was to change the environment and activities so that the client was able to function optimally with residual cognitive abilities.[3,4,31-33]

Allen developed the Cognitive Disabilities model in an attempt to achieve this objective (matching the environment/activities to clients' cognitive abilities). She initially borrowed constructs from Piaget's cognitive development theory, later incorporating constructs from the Soviet psychology,[33] which was probably based on Pavlov's physiological approach to the study of behavior (see Chapter 3). The influence of Piaget's theory on Allen's thinking is obvious in her statement in the first paper published on this model:

> Our observations of changes in behavior, seen during the course of improvement of psychiatric patients, suggested some functional units of behavior. Patients vary in the things they pay attention to, that is, some physical elements of the environment capture and sustain their attention, whereas other elements are ignored. *These observations are supported in the Piagetian literature* (p. 732, emphasis mine).[2]

Initially Allen's cognitive levels (discussed below), were based on Piaget's cognitive psychology. However, Allen also thought that the central domain of concern for occupational therapy was human activity, and Piaget's psychology was not adequate in addressing this concern. Therefore she proposed that,

> The only branch of the social sciences that has used the concept of activity as a central focus of study is Soviet psychology. During the last few years, a lot of conceptual material has been translated into English, providing a rich resource of 60 years worth of conceptual experience and critical analysis. These translations allow us to profit from the Soviets' experience (p. 564).[4]

From the Soviet psychology, she borrowed the constructs of limitations (referring to loss of capability due to disease), assets (residual capabilities), capacity (present capacity and ability to develop new capabilities), competence (ability to act and produce results), prognosis (expected change after disease onset), and community support. Allen also incorporated constructs from the neurosciences.[4,11,29,33]

Propositions About Function, Dysfunction, and Change

Function

Allen defined *cognitive disability* as "a restriction in voluntary motor action originating in the physical or chemical structures of the brain and producing observable limitations in routine task behavior" (p. 31).[3] This definition implies that function is "competence, which means the ability to handle one's own affairs" where "competence or incompetence is generally based on the ability to make sound judgments and reasonable decisions about those activities that the individual intends to do" (p. 186).[27] Competence here denotes that *function* is the ability to use motor actions to engage in activities, guided by cognition that enables one to make sound judgments and decisions, leading to performance of tasks effectively and safely.

Function can also be defined as use of mental energy in terms of cognitions necessary to make judgments and decisions and to guide motor and speech functions in a changing environment, leading to adaptation. The extent to which one is able to adapt, in Allen's view, is determined by a person's ability to effectively perceive and process new information.[7,31] In a more recent definition, Allen includes deficits in communication abilities as another manifestation of cognitive disability.[40]

Dysfunction

Dysfunction may be conceptualized as restriction in motor function that originates from a deficiency of cognitive abilities due to structural damage of the brain resulting from physical injury, degeneration of the brain organ, or chemical imbalance in the central nervous system (CNS). This cognitive disability, which can also be defined as "An impairment in task behavior relative to cognitive skill" (p. 262),[33] presents in a function/dysfunction continuum that is outlined in six cognitive levels, originally developed to follow closely Piaget's stages of cognitive development.[3,4,7] The definition and mapping of the six levels on Piaget's cognitive schema are illustrated in Table 11-1.

Mapping Allen cognitive levels on Piaget's stages of cognitive development is only approximate. There is no precise correspondence between the two entities. For one, Allen cognitive levels were designed to evaluate the cognitive functioning of older children and adults whose information-processing capacity was lost due to disease, injury, or developmental malady. Therefore past experience affects their functioning, in addition to their cognitive deficits. Piaget's stages, on the other hand, simply describe cognitive development of children. Furthermore, Allen cognitive levels focus on the effects of cognitive processes on activity performance (by *activity* meaning *occupations*),

Table 11-1.   ALLEN COGNITIVE LEVELS AND THEIR RELATIONSHIP TO PIAGET'S STAGES OF COGNITIVE DEVELOPMENT

Allen Cognitive Level	Piaget's Stages of Cognitive Development
LEVEL 1: AUTOMATIC ACTIONS • Motor actions are reflexive and automatic • Withdraws from noxious stimuli • Responds to hunger, thirst, and discomfort (automatic survival responses)	**SENSORIMOTOR STAGE: 0-2 YEARS** **SUBSTAGE 1: REFLEXIVE—0-1 MONTH** • Reacts to stimuli (e.g., by sucking and kicking [reflexive patterns]) **SUBSTAGE 2: PRIMARY CIRCULAR REACTIONS—1-4 MONTHS** • Able to repeat interesting actions voluntarily
LEVEL 2: POSTURAL ACTIONS • Has postural motor responses (such as moving body to attain sitting, standing, or walking position) • Approximately imitates motor actions • Attends to cues related to body movement, position in space and response to gravity, posture, gesture, and motion	**SUBSTAGE 3: SECONDARY CIRCULAR REACTIONS—4-8 MONTHS** • Acts more on objects in order to make interesting actions last longer
LEVEL 3: MANUAL ACTIONS • Manual but not goal-directed actions • Manipulates, touches, and picks up objects • Follows one-step cues when activities are familiar • Can string beads • Responds to tactile cues and therefore can work with objects that can be touched and moved	**SUBSTAGE 4: COORDINATION OF SECONDARY CIRCULAR REACTIONS—8-12 MONTHS** • Able to use objects instrumentally to accomplish a goal • Demonstrates intentionality • Acquires the concept of object permanence (things continue to exist even when out of sight)
LEVEL 4: GOAL-DIRECTED ACTIONS • Able to copy and reproduce actions • Rote learning is possible (i.e., can relearn to perform highly familiar tasks to accomplish a goal) • Can perform activities such as chopping carrots, sanding wood, and so on. • Responds only to visible cues (things that are out of sight are ignored) • Can respond to sensations related to color, size, and comfort	

Table 11-1. ALLEN COGNITIVE LEVELS AND THEIR RELATIONSHIP TO PIAGET'S STAGES OF COGNITIVE DEVELOPMENT—CONT'D

Allen Cognitive Level	Piaget's Stages of Cognitive Development
LEVEL 5: EXPLORATORY ACTIONS • Uses experimentation/trial and error to solve problems • Able to learn new knowledge by remembering effects of previous actions • Able to grasp the relationship between two cues • Able to respond to cues such as overlapping objects, mixing colors, spatial relationships, and so on	**SUBSTAGE 5: TERTIARY CIRCULAR REACTIONS—12-18 MONTHS** • Can solve problems by trial and error **SUBSTAGE 6: INVENTION OF NEW MEANS THROUGH MENTAL COMBINATIONS—18 MONTHS TO 2 YEARS** • Can plan ways of manipulating the environment without overt experimentation **PREOPERATIONAL STAGE: 2-7 YEARS** • Able to use signs and symbols to represent something else, and therefore begins developing sophisticated use of language • Egocentricity: Unable to see another person's point of view, and therefore tends to think that if he or she cannot see another person in a hide-and-seek game, the person cannot see him or her • Focuses on salient aspects of a stimulant, ignoring all others • Unable to see reversibility of actions **CONCRETE OPERATIONS** • Begins to understand reversibility of actions • Able to grasp mathematical concepts • Able to grasp the concept of identity (i.e., things are the same irrespective of spatial orientation, shape, size, and so on) • Understands concepts of time, speed, distance, and so on
LEVEL 6: PLANNED ACTIONS • Actions are initiated without demonstration • Able to work with abstract or symbolic stimuli/concepts such as energy, time, gravity, and so on. • Thinks of actions and conceptualizes plans before acting • Able to perform tasks such as budgeting, building something following a diagram and directions, and so on	**FORMAL OPERATIONS: 12 YEARS AND OVER** • Able to apply scientific principles and to systematically collect data to validate previous knowledge • Engages in hypothetico-deductive reasoning • Visualizes possibilities and anticipates outcomes • Able to plan and imagine consequences of behavior without having to act first • Has highly evolved symbolic thought and representation

Data from Allen CK: Independence through activity: the practice of occupational therapy in psychiatry, *Am J Occup Ther* 36:731-739, 1982; Allen CK: *Allen Cognitive Level Screen (ACLS) test manual,* Colchester, CT, 2000, S&S Worldwide; Early MB: *Mental health concepts and techniques for the occupational therapy assistant,* ed 3, Philadelphia, 2000, Lippincott Williams & Wilkins; Grant S: Cognitive disability frame of reference. In Crepeau EB, Cohn ES, Schell BA, eds: *Willard and Spackman's occupational therapy,* New York, 2003, Lippincott Williams & Wilkins, pp. 261-264; and Mandich M: Theoretical framework for human performance. In Cronin A, Mandich M, eds: *Human development and performance throughout the lifespan,* Clifton Park, NY, 2005, Thomson Delmar Learning, pp. 22–24.

whereas Piaget's theory describes cognitive development in general, emphasizing language and abstract thinking in particular. The mapping of Allen cognitive levels on Piaget's stages of cognitive development is therefore only approximate and should be viewed with caution.

According to the continuum illustrated in Table 11-1, individuals below level 1 are basically in a coma. Level 6 was conceptualized to represent absence of cognitive disability. Allen stated that "Theoretically, Level 6 is designed to describe capabilities of normal adults (80% of a control sample). Most of the social science information processing literature assumes that human beings are at Level 6" (pp. 566-567).[4] Therefore this tautology states that people at cognitive levels 0 to 5 have cognitive deficits that limit their ability to process information effectively to be able to adapt to their environment, and they demonstrate capability deficits that characterize dysfunction.

Furthermore, people in levels 1 and 2 "do not work with objects" (p. 2)[5]; occupational therapy intervention for such clients is limited in terms of activities that can be used in therapy. It is for people in levels 3 to 5 that "the special knowledge and skill of the occupational therapist is required" (p. 2).[5] Specifically, "Those functioning at levels 1 to 4 have difficulty living unassisted in the community because they cannot perform necessary routine tasks, such as paying bills, obtaining adequate nourishment, and finding their way to an unfamiliar place" (p. 75).[32]

People at level 5 tend to portray characteristics that may be interpreted as depicting carelessness because of their difficulty in foreseeing the consequences of their actions. For example, they may cause an accident by driving too fast in wet weather or in the dark, because they cannot foresee that those conditions may make it difficult to stop quickly in an emergency. "Allen believes that level five is sufficient for a person of lower educational and occupational background to function in the community, although she warns that the level 5 person may not take ordinary and reasonable care regarding the rights of others" (p. 79).[32]

Later, the six levels were expanded to include 26 modes of functioning, using a decimal system, in order to be more sensitive to differences in performance.[7] In this expanded version, 5.8 indicates the level at which most "normal" people function for most of the time, except when faced with novel situations requiring them to heighten their level of information processing (e.g., when learning a new task).

Change

Because occupational therapy, within the Cognitive Disabilities model perspective, is not seen as an intervention that can affect the clients' cognitive levels, change is not conceptualized as a suitable therapeutic goal. Rather, the role of occupational therapy intervention is viewed as to assist the medical doctor/psychiatrist in making a diagnosis, being supportive, monitoring cognitive changes, and when a stable cognitive level is attained, providing compensation so that the client is able to function optimally with residual cognitive abilities.[2-4,33] In 1992, Allen acknowledged that some conditions can go into remission leading to a change in cognitive level.[29] This acknowledgement has led to more emphasis on monitoring cognitive changes in therapy. However, the major thrust of therapy based on this model remains compensation for lost cognitive skills rather than change in cognitive abilities.

Guidelines for Client Evaluation and Therapeutic Intervention

Client Evaluation

Allen believed that occupational therapists must maintain the strength of their practice, which she thought was grounded on activities, including crafts and routine tasks.[2,29] She postulated that one can assess cognitive functioning by observing the client's motor actions during tasks and inferring sensory cues to which he or she is responding. Furthermore, "a person's mental disorganization can impair performance of tasks such as leather lacing and getting dressed" (p. 74).[32] Because crafts and daily living activities are made possible by the same cognitive-processing skills, cognitive deficits observed while a client is engaged in a craft such as leather lacing can give an indication of how one is likely to function in other areas of life.

In addition, according to the model, cognitive functioning is based on the ability to learn and process new information.[2-4,32,33] Allen reasoned that the best task to assess clients' cognitive level was one with which they were not familiar, otherwise, the therapist would be testing ability to engage in familiar routines rather than to process new information. Therefore in this model, "crafts are used" to evaluate clients "precisely because they are unfamiliar to many people" (p. 74).[32] The evaluation tools developed in conjunction with this model are largely based on activity analysis, which Allen sees as the unique strength of an occupational therapist.[4]

The first cognitive screening instrument to be developed by Allen was the Allen Cognitive Level Screening test (ACLS).[3,42] The ACLS is a kit consisting of a 3¼-by-4¾-inch punched oval piece of leather, a blunt sewing needle, leather lace, two Perma-lok lacing needles, waxen linen thread, and an instruction manual (Figure 11-1).[7]

The client is first asked whether he or she has ever done something similar to the leather-lacing task. If he or she has, the therapist uses another tool to test him or her because the ACLS would no longer be testing ability to learn and process new knowledge.

The client is asked to complete three progressively difficult stitches. The first is a running stitch, which is demonstrated and the client asked to replicate. The second stitch (whip stitch) is also demonstrated and the client is asked to do a similar one. Then, the therapist makes a cross in the back of the stitch by holding the lacing below the hole in the back and pushing the needle through from front to back. The client is asked if he or she can recognize the mistake and correct it. If he or she can, the therapist twists two stitches and asks the client if he or she can find and correct the mistake. If the mistake is located and corrected, the client is next asked to figure out and replicate a cordovan stitch (the most complicated stitch in the test) by

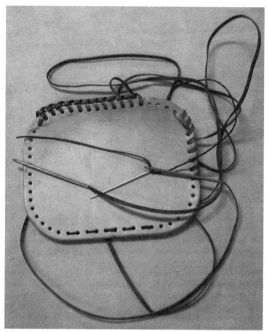

Figure 11-1. The Allen Cognitive Level Screening Test (ACLS) is a standardized screening tool used by occupational therapists. The ACLS kit consists of a punched oval piece of leather, a blunt sewing needle, leather lace, two lacing needles, waxen linen thread, and an instruction manual. A larger version is also available and is useful for therapists working with the elderly and other visually impaired populations.

looking at some stitches previously made by the therapist. The test is scored according to criteria provided in the test manual, based on the most complicated stitch the client was able to complete and the type of mistake(s) made. This test evaluates only cognitive levels 3 to 5.8. If he or she can complete three consecutive cordovan stitches correctly without assistance, a score of 5.8 is given.

The Allen Cognitive Level test (ACL) was developed in the 1970s, and the standardized version was published in 1978.[42] Originally it was the only test available to evaluate the cognitive levels based on the Cognitive Disabilities model. Other tests were developed later, and currently it is proposed that the ACL be used only as a screening tool.[7,33,34] It is now referred to as the Allen Cognitive Level Screening test (ACLS), whose purpose is to provide a quick appraisal of the client's level of cognitive functioning. If a score of 3.0 or above is achieved, the therapist chooses one of the other instruments to assess the client further.

Also, since the purpose of the ACLS is to screen for cognitive dysfunction, accommodations should be made for individuals with visual and fine-motor coordination difficulties, so that they do not interfere with functioning in the test. For this purpose, the large version of the ACLS (LACLS) was developed for clients with visual and coordination deficits.[7,32] Other instruments developed within the Cognitive Disabilities model include the Routine Task Inventory (RTI),

Cognitive Performance Test (CPT), and the Allen Diagnostic Module (ADM).[8,31-33,42]

The RTI was introduced in 1982.[2,42] This is a tool consisting of tasks, which Allen defined as bearing "a striking resemblance to the activities of daily living (ADL)" (p. 734).[2] These include "wearing clothing, preparing food, using transportation, altering the environment for sheltered living, sanitary disposal of body wastes, and earning and spending money. A routine task is one that is done on a daily or weekly basis, year in and year out" (p. 734).[2] The current version of the test is the RTI-2.[32] It consists of tasks that are analyzed so that they are presented as behavioral disabilities in the following categories: self-awareness disability, situational awareness disability, occupational role disability, and social role disability (Box 11-1).

| **Box 11-1** | Routine Tasks Constituting the Routine Task Inventory: Analyzed and Presented as Behavioral Disabilities |

10: Self-Awareness

.0 Grooming
.1 Dressing
.2 Bathing
.3 Walking
.4 Feeding
.5 Toileting
.6 Taking medications
.7 Using adaptive equipment
.8 Other
.9 Unspecified

11: Situational Awareness

.0 Housekeeping
.1 Obtaining, preparing food
.2 Spending money
.3 Shopping
.4 Doing laundry
.5 Traveling
.6 Telephoning
.7 Adjusting to change
.8 Other
.9 Unspecified

12: Occupational Role Disability

.0 Planning, doing major role activities
.1 Planning, doing spare time activities
.2 Pacing and timing actions
.3 Exerting effort
.4 Judging results
.5 Speaking
.6 Following safety precautions
.7 Responding to emergencies
.8 Other
.9 Unspecified

13: Social Role Disability

.0 Communicating meaning
.1 Following instructions
.2 Contributing to family activities
.3 Caring for dependents
.4 Cooperating with others
.5 Supervising independent people
.6 Keeping informed
.7 Engaging in good citizenship
.8 Other
.9 Unspecified

Data from Early MB: *Mental health concepts and techniques for the occupational therapy assistant*, ed 3, Philadelphia, 2000, Lippincott Williams & Wilkins, p. 78.

The therapist completes the RTI-2 by asking either the client or the caregiver how the client performed the listed activities, or by observing the client while engaging in them.[32] This is a structured interview through which the therapist is able to determine activities that the client is able to complete safely and independently.[10] Thirty-two activities are included in the inventory,[40] each described according to the six cognitive levels. The client's observed or reported behavior while performing each task is matched with the description under the task; this enables the therapist to determine the cognitive level of the client on that task.

The Cognitive Performance Test (CPT) "was initially developed as a research instrument to provide a measure of global function in individuals with Alzheimer's Disease (AD) and to track change over time" (p. 1).[17] Six commonly used activities of daily living (ADLs) (dressing, shopping, making toast, using the telephone, washing, and traveling) comprise the test. Recently, the task of managing medication was added. Based on the level of information processing capacity the client uses to complete the tasks, a score is obtained for each task, and the average score for all tasks determines the cognitive level and mode of functioning. Although originally developed for research purposes, the test is currently being used in the clinics.

The Allen Diagnostic Module (ADM) is a craft-based assessment.[12] One problem with the ACLS is that it cannot be used to track cognitive changes for clients functioning at higher cognitive levels (5 and above) because they can learn the stitches, making the test invalid as an evaluation of ability to learn new skills. Other tests such as the RTI-2 and CPT are based on ADLs, which are familiar to most clients, and are therefore not reliable methods of assessing new learning. Thus Allen and Reyner developed the ADM such that it is not possible to learn its activities and therefore it can be used for reassessment to track changes in cognitive levels of clients. It consists of 29 activities (crafts) that have been tested and retested against 52 modes

of functioning. The ADM can be administered as a comprehensive assessment, or selected tasks can be used to verify the quick appraisal of the client's cognitive level obtained using the ACLS.

Thus the ideal assessment of a client when a therapist is using the Cognitive Disabilities model would include a quick appraisal of the client's cognitive level of functioning using the ACLS, followed by verification using selected tasks from the ADM, and then using both the RTI-2 and the CPT to assess actual performance in ADLs. Based on the information obtained from these assessments, intervention can then be planned. For cognitive levels 3.0 to 4.0, the ACLS can be used to re-evaluate the client regularly to determine changes in cognitive functioning, because repetition is not expected to result in learning the tasks. For those at higher cognitive levels, the ADM can be used for regular reassessment.

Refer to Lab Manual Exercises 13-1 and 13-2 to learn how to use some of the evaluation instruments associated with the Cognitive Disabilities model.

Therapeutic Intervention

Three concepts regarding performance based on the Cognitive Disabilities model guide intervention to help clients function optimally and safely in their environment. These are views about what the client can, will, or may do.[33] What a client *can do* is determined by biological factors and, specifically, the cognitive level of functioning as measured on the Allen Cognitive Levels. What he or she *will do* is related to psychological factors such as motivation, belief in personal abilities, meaningfulness of the task, and so on. What the client *may do* depends on the support systems available in the environment to facilitate ability to engage in tasks within one's capability and interest, given residual cognitive abilities. Based on the above concepts and the postulations of the model about cognitive change, three intervention strategies are proposed: *expectant* (in which the therapist tracks remission of a client's symptoms through observation of his or her engagement in various tasks); *supportive* (using diversional activities to support the client during the acute phase of illness); and *compensatory* (changing the task or environment to facilitate the client's optimal performance within the environment.[2,10]

Specifically the role of the therapist is to identify the client's cognitive level, monitor changes of cognitive functioning that are proposed to result from the natural progression of disease or medical intervention, and modify the task or environment to facilitate optimal functioning by the client. Intervention is divided into phases according to progression of the disease[10,32,37]:

1. During the *acute phase,* the client is evaluated to determine the cognitive level. Further intervention may consist of alleviation of discomfort through positioning for clients in lower cognitive levels, and supportive (diversional) activities for those at higher levels (levels 3.0 and 4.0).

2. In the *expectant phase,* intervention is mostly palliative. Caretakers are educated regarding how to cue the client for optimum performance. Monitoring cognitive changes continues hand in hand with recommendations to caretakers for the level of assistance needed during this phase.

3. In the *residual* (rehabilitative) phase, the therapist determines the current level of cognitive functioning that is expected to remain stable and plans discharge accordingly. No more cognitive changes are expected at this stage. Emphasis is on optimizing performance by providing assistive devices, modifying the environment, and training caregivers on how to cue the client for optimal safe functioning.

Furthermore, based on the predictions of the Cognitive Disabilities model, in discharge planning, clients functioning at cognitive levels 1.0 to 4.0 are not expected to be able to live independently in the community because of inability to complete tasks such as paying bills, obtaining adequate nourishment, and commu-

nity mobility safely. Those at cognitive level 5.0 may need supervision to live in the community safely because of their impulsiveness, inability to think ahead and foresee problems, and their trial-and-error mode of information processing. This makes safety a big concern for them. Therefore discharge recommendations based on ACL evaluations are made with those precautions in mind.

Recently, attempts have been made to develop extensive caregiver guidelines based on the ACL.[18-23] According to these guidelines, clients functioning at levels 2.4 to 3.8 require 24-hour on-site supervision; those at levels 4.0 to 4.4 require 24-hour supervision that may or may not be onsite; and those at 4.6 to 4.8 can live in the community on their own with environmental modifications for safety and establishment of a routine and rehearsed safety plans, with daily or weekly supervision. Clients at levels 5.0 to 5.2 can live alone in the community with weekly supervision and modification of the environment for safety, and a well-rehearsed safety plan. Specific guidelines are also provided regarding the level of assistance needed at each level during the client's performance of ADLs including handling medication, eating, bathing, dressing and personal hygiene, toileting, safety, mobility and positioning, money and time management, transportation, and leisure.

Guidelines have also been developed suggesting activities to be used by therapists for sensory stimulation of clients at cognitive levels 3.0 and 4.0.[24-26,28] Such activities include use of rocking chairs, bubble lumps, musical instruments, weighted blankets, and so on. Such activities are based on the tactile and visual cues that clients are attentive to according to the criteria provided by Allen, Earhart, and Blue,[10] and Allen.[6]

Consistency of the Cognitive Disabilities Model with the Occupational Therapy Paradigm

The model's assessment instruments such as the RTI-2 and the CPT are based on occupations

CASE STUDY: SARA

Sara, a 76-year-old Caucasian female, was admitted to the subacute rehabilitation facility following a fall from her wheelchair. Prior to admission, she was living in a long-term care facility. Available history at admission indicated that before commitment to long-term care, Sara was living alone at home. Her husband had died about 10 years earlier. Together, they had four children: three daughters and one son. All the children were married and had their own families. They visited her regularly. Gradually, they started noticing that her memory was worsening and she was unable to prepare meals and take care of herself. They decided as a family to take her to a long-term care facility. Within 2 months after commitment to the facility, Sara's cognitive functioning had deteriorated to the point where she was wheelchair bound, incontinent, and dependent in all self-care activities.

Occupational therapy evaluation revealed that Sara could maintain visual contact and tracking. She was disoriented with regards to time and place, but when her name was called she responded by looking at the therapist. She did not comprehend any directions. When placed on the wheelchair, Sara demonstrated antero-lateral trunk flexion. She had poor sitting endurance, not being able to tolerate sitting on the wheelchair for more than 10 minutes, and clung to the wheelchair arms the whole time, as if she was afraid of falling. She could not stand or communicate verbally.

The therapist's observations using RTI-2 and based on Allen's description of the six cognitive levels (see Box 11-1 and the description of client responses in Chapter 13 of the Laboratory Manual) led her to conclude that Sara was functioning at cognitive level 1.0. She responded to her name, demonstrated eye tracking, and withdrew from noxious stimuli. Thus her reactions were those associated with basic survival, which is consistent with Allen Cognitive Level 1.0. Recommended intervention for this client was largely palliative. Caregivers were trained regarding appropriate positioning both on the wheelchair and in bed, with emphasis on fall prevention and making the client feel safe.

A sensory diet consisting of music, touch, and activities requiring the client to reach out was suggested to encourage active range of motion and prevent contractures. Pictures and other artifacts from the client's home were incorporated in the sensory diet, as were scented lotions and a variety of aromas, and actions such as drinking using straws. Caregivers and family members were trained on how to approach the client and how to use the sensory diet to keep her stimulated and to make it easier to assist her to participate optimally in her ADLs, such as feeding and dressing. Once caregivers and family members were adequately trained, and positioning equipment such as the weighted lap pad were obtained to increase safety while in the wheelchair, the client was discharged back to the long-term care facility.

 Refer to Lab Manual Exercise 13-2 to learn how to use the Cognitive Disabilities model in clinical practice.

such as the ADLs, occupational roles, and social roles. The overarching goal of the model is to facilitate optimal occupational functioning with residual cognitive abilities. One may therefore conclude that the model is occupation-based both in its assessments and desired outcome of therapy. However, although there is some reference to meaningfulness of activities as a central factor in motivating the client,[2,33] collaboration with the client is not explicitly emphasized. Allen states that "A person with disability must be given the right to select his or her own task content" (p. 734).[2] However, she also asserts that "For the cognitively disabled, each cognitive level is accompanied by a task analysis that acts as a guideline for therapists in selecting and designing activities that correspond to the patient's level of ability" (p. 734).[2]

Therefore it seems that the right for the client to choose the task context is secondary to the therapist's exercise of his or her expertise in analyzing and designing tasks for the client. It seems that the model's view of therapy is that of a therapist bearing in mind the meaningfulness of activities while he or she chooses tasks for the client. Collaboration is not explicitly placed at the forefront in the model's theoretical core, although therapists who use it probably in practice collaborate very closely with clients and their families in the design of therapeutic plans and choice of therapeutic activities. To that extent, it can be said that the model is occupation-based, which is consistent with the occupational therapy paradigm. However, unlike the professional paradigm, the collaborative, client-centered approach to therapy is not categorically emphasized in the model's theoretical core.

Also, the model is consistent with the professional paradigm in that the roles of the therapist are viewed as consisting of environmental modification, providing assistive devices, and educating both the client and caregivers to facilitate optimum occupational functioning. However although Allen emphasizes the need to use crafts and activities that are of interest to clients in order to motivate them to engage in therapy, providing opportunities for client participation in meaningful occupations as defined in the *Occupational Therapy Practice Framework*[13] is not emphasized.

Based on the above analysis, it can be concluded that the model is consistent with the occupational therapy paradigm in that it is occupation-based, and specifies the therapist's role as environmental modification, providing assistive devices, and client/caregiver education to facilitate the client's optimum functioning. Its consistence with the paradigm could be enhanced by explicitly and categorically emphasizing within it's theoretical core and practice guidelines collaboration and client-centeredness, and providing opportunities for client engagement in meaningful occupations.

Consistency with the Philosophy of Pragmatism

Like the philosophy of pragmatism, the Cognitive Disabilities model's focus is on the client's active doing, as indicated by the overarching goal of optimum functioning within his or her environment given residual cognitive abilities. The model's interest in cognitive abilities is only in as far as those abilities guide motor action and verbal communication.[*] Also, consistent with the philosophy of pragmatism, within the model, the human being's interaction with his or her environment through occupational functioning is valued. However, unlike pragmatism, the model does not underscore human agency through choice and self-determination. Consistent with the medical model, the therapist guided by this model sometimes chooses activities for the client and makes recommendations based on what he or she sees as appropriate and safe performance, based on activity analysis.

Furthermore, because of the hypothesized inability of the client with cognitive disabilities to have the information processing capability necessary to connect action with consequences, the role of belief as a rule for action (which is one of the central tenets of pragmatism) is deemphasized. Consequently, the whole notion of instrumentalism, which has been suggested in this book as the basic pragmatic construct that can be operationalized for application in clinical practice, is not applicable to the Cognitive Disabilities model. Although cognition is viewed as the primary guide for motor action and therefore for occupational functioning, the idea of instrumental use of the mind as a means of fashioning one's environment and attaining meaningful existence is missing in the goals of therapy guided by the model.

[*]References 2,4,10,29,32,33.

The above-discussed constructs, among others, indicate significant inconsistencies between the model and the philosophy of pragmatism.

Consistency with the Complexity/Chaos Theoretical Framework

The core theoretical argument of the Cognitive Disabilities model is that once damage to the brain has occurred, some cognitive function can be recovered through natural progression of the healing process. Further cognitive recovery may be achieved through medication, which alters the actual brain physiology. Through the combination of medication and natural progression, a stable state of cognitive functioning is reached. It is at this point that occupational therapy becomes useful, by providing environmental modification and education to the client and caregivers that is necessary to enable the client to function optimally with residual cognitive abilities. Thus meaningful occupation is not envisaged in this model as a means of changing the brain structure. Consequently, occupational participation is not expected to improve cognitive abilities. This argument is contrary to the premise of complexity/chaos theory that interaction of the client with his or her environment through meaningful and challenging occupations would lead to increased self-organization resulting in emergence of adaptive cognitive abilities.[43] Thus the Cognitive Disabilities model is not consistent with the complexity/chaos theoretical framework.

Recommendations for Reinterpretation of the Model

The Cognitive Disabilities model has much to offer clinical intervention in occupational therapy. Although it does not explain etiology,[40] it gives a detailed description of the manifestations of cognitive disability in occupational functioning and methods of observing and measuring such manifestations precisely. One concern to occupational therapists might be the model's insistence that occupational therapy has no effect on change in cognitive functioning. Such an assertion has far-reaching implications regarding practice. It is for this reason that the model restricts the role of the occupational therapist to monitoring of cognitive changes, environmental modification, and caregiver education. It is proposed in this book that the Cognitive Disabilities model may be strengthened by desisting from the basic argument that engagement in occupations does not affect change in organic brain structure until more research evidence is available to provide direction one way or the other as will become apparent in the discussion that follows.

Assertion that engagement in occupations does not affect change in cognitive functioning was probably founded on postulations in literature that suggested that improvement in cognitive functioning following brain damage occurs in early stages of rehabilitation, and no changes are expected after 1 year following injury.[38,46] Although this view is still prevalent in literature, some studies have since yielded evidence indicating that rehabilitation can result in significant positive cognitive functioning changes even 5 years or more after injury.[41,47] Furthermore, there is also increasing evidence that physical activity affects the organic and chemical neural structures.

For instance, even in utero, it has been found that intrauterine environmental activity stimulates and modifies development of neurons.[45] Similarly, it has been found that exercising the brain by engaging in challenging activities, especially those that are socially stimulating, helps deter brain deterioration that is usually associated with the aging process.[30] Other studies have indicated that thinking happy thoughts changes the frontal cortex structure of the brain as measured on EEG brainwave biofeedback protocol using Positron Emission Tomography (PET), which would suggest that engaging in occupations that generate happy thoughts has the potential to change brain structure.[14] In another study, it was found that negative experiences such as rape change both the brain structure and function in children and adults.[16] These and many other studies increasingly indicate that physical activity has the potential to change brain structure either positively or negatively, which implies that occupational therapy can impact the biological structure of the brain.

Certainly, the debate regarding the effect of engagement in occupations on physiological functioning will continue until the issue is settled one way or the other as more empirical evidence becomes available. For the moment, given research findings that continue to emerge, it may be better to keep an open mind even while engaging in further research to investigate the issue. This is why

> Some take issue with the assertion that biological change is the exclusive domain of medicine. Certainly, many of the models...assert that participation in occupation can influence biological changes (e.g., muscle fiber size and synaptic connections) that are also manifest as functional changes (e.g., strength, sensory and perceptual abilities) (p. 112).[40]

Closely related to the argument for change in perspective regarding the role that occupational therapy can play in cognitive rehabilitation is the recommendation for the model to adopt the complexity/chaos theoretical framework as a scientific guide. Even though there is not enough research evidence to support the chaos theoretical constructs, given that physical activity seems to be indicated in changes of the brain structure according to some of the recent research findings, it is not difficult to make the leap to the proposition that dynamic interaction with the environment through occupational performance has the potential to lead to higher cognitive self-organization through establishment of new neural connections.[43]

Allowing such a postulation would open new doors to an investigation of how occupational therapy may affect the biological structure of the brain. Indeed, this view is being adopted by other related conceptual models such as the Cognitive-Perceptual Model (CPM),[40,52] which was discussed as part of the Behavioral/Cognitive-Behavioral model in this book. In the

CPM, "Cognitive processing, cognitive strategies, and metacognition" are now being considered to be "emergent phenomena that are influenced by environmental and task parameters" (p. 132).[40]

Accepting the proposition that occupational functioning can change the biological brain structure and adopting the complexity/chaos theoretical framework as a guide to understanding the outcome of the interaction between humans and the environment through occupational performance would allow the Cognitive Disabilities model to develop new practice guidelines. Such guidelines would allow the occupational therapist to design meaningful occupations for intervention aimed at changing cognitive functioning of clients. The model's well-developed assessment capacity would then be enhanced by its ability to guide cognitive change, which would greatly strengthen occupational therapy as a profession.

Evidence-Based Practice Using the Cognitive Disabilities Model

The Cognitive Disabilities model is one of the most used, taught, and researched conceptual models of practice in occupational therapy. Allen's Cognitive Levels have even been recommended as a guide for the entire rehabilitation team in cognitive rehabilitation.[15] Blue Shield of Texas now requires use of the CPT codes for treatment modalities for clients with cognitive disabilities.[9] Further, "A new National Medicare CPT Code: 975X1 is to be established in the USA using the Allen Cognitive Levels" (p. 5).[1] The model is being taught in most occupational therapy programs in the United States. Thus the Cognitive Disabilities model has been very influential in the profession.

Extensive research associated with this model has been devoted to establishment of the parametric properties of assessment instruments. The ACLS, which has been used extensively by occupational therapists as a cognitive functioning screening tool in North America, Australia, and Israel,[39] is one of the occupational therapy assessment tools that have been most investigated in research. It has been found to have very good interrater reliability, ranging from $r = .90$ to $.99$.[10,36,44,48] Concurrent validity of the tool has also been investigated by comparing it with other instruments. In this regard, Keller and Hayes found a moderate correlation between the ACL-90 and the Life Skills Profile (LSP): $r(56) = .54, p < .01$.[39]

The LSP, which is composed of 39 items in five subscales—communication, nonturbulence, responsibility, self-care, and social contact—"is an internationally accepted measure of the adaptive functioning of persons with schizophrenia, who are known to have deficits in this area" (p. 853).[39] In another study by Secrest, Wood, and Tapp, it was found that the ACL is correlated with the Wisconsin Card Sorting Test (WCST), which measures manifestations of cognitive dysfunction such as "problem solving, abstract thinking, and mental shift in set and is specifically sensitive to frontal lobe brain lesions" (p. 130).[51] The WCST was also correlated to the Routine Task Inventory (RTI). These correlations indicate that both the ACL and RTI have the same ability as the WCST to measure clients' cognitive executive functioning. The RTI has also been found to have excellent interrater reliability ($r = .987$) and test-retest reliability ($r = .907$).[35] Published research investigating the CPT and ADM is limited.

Outcome research is not conclusive regarding the ability of the Cognitive Disabilities model to predict community functioning.[50,53] Some studies indicate moderate relationship between cognitive levels as measured on the ACL and RTI and community functioning. A study by Henry and colleagues indicated that ACL scores combined with involvement of clients with schizophrenia in the homemaker role predicted possible discharge to independent living situation.[37] Other studies indicate that cognitive levels are poorer predictors of community functioning than other factors such as sex, age, work history, marital history, and so on.[50,53] This raises the question of the accuracy of using cognitive levels to predict community adjustment of clients. An experimental study by Raweh and Katz indicated that intervention guided by the Cognitive Disabilities model yielded greater increase in functioning of clients in the experimental group as evaluated using the RTI compared to those in the control group.[49]

It is therefore clear from available research evidence that the Cognitive Disabilities model instruments have good validity and reliability. However, more research is indicated to further establish the predictive validity of the model. This is important considering that the essence of the model is to predict discharge placement of clients with cognitive disabilities based on the cognitive level.

SUMMARY

The Cognitive Disabilities model is based on the core proposition that cognitive disability is a result of direct physical or chemical insult to the brain. The disability is manifested in motor and communication limitations because cognitive functions determine physical and verbal/communication processes. Furthermore, the same cognitive processes mediate engagement in crafts and daily life activities. Observation of a client's performance in crafts can indicate his or her functioning in other areas of life. Therefore crafts can be used to assess cognitive abilities necessary for safe and independent performance of activities of daily life.

Cognitive abilities are conceptualized to be in a function-dysfunction continuum, which is presented in an ordinal scale of levels, ranging from coma (level 0.0) to planned activities demonstrated through processing of abstract information (level 6.0). These levels were originally modeled along Piaget's stages of cognitive development. Cognitive functioning is evaluated using a variety of instruments including the Allen Cognitive Level Screening test (ACLS), which is one of the most widely used assessments in occupational therapy, the Cognitive Performance Test (CPT), the Routine Task Inventory (RTI), and the Allen

Diagnostic Module (ADM). Once the cognitive level of the client is established, intervention is designed. Such intervention may be expectant (the therapist tracks changes in the client's cognitive function), supportive (activities are designed to give the client courage and strength during the acute phase of illness), and compensatory (the environment or task is changed to facilitate maximum functioning given residual cognitive abilities, when it is determined that no more cognitive improvement is expected).

The Cognitive Disabilities model is one of the most researched conceptual models of practice in occupational therapy. Extensive research directed toward investigating the parametric properties of the instruments associated with the model has been conducted. It has been found that both the ACLS and the RTI have excellent validity and reliability. Outcome research indicates that the model's ability to predict a client's level of functioning in the community is mixed, with some research evidence indicating good predictive ability of the model and other evidence indicating that other factors such as age, sex, marital status, and so on, are better predictors of community adjustment following discharge than the Allen Cognitive Level status. Finally, we recommended that the model may be strengthened by revising the position that engagement in occupations does not affect change in cognitive functioning, and incorporating constructs from the complexity/chaos theoretical perspective, which would lead to the view that cognitive abilities emerge from the client's interaction with the environment through challenging occupations.

REFERENCES

1. ACL International: *History and development of the Allen cognitive levels,* 2005. Retrieved October 2005, from http://www.allenCogadvisor.com/general/history.htm.
2. Allen CK: Independence through activity: the practice of occupational therapy in psychiatry, *Am J Occup Ther* 36:731-739, 1982.
3. Allen CK, ed: *Occupational therapy for psychiatric diseases: measurement and management of cognitive disabilities,* Boston, 1985, Little Brown & Company.
4. Allen CK: 1987 Eleanor Clarke Slagle lecture—Activity: occupational therapy's treatment method, *Am J Occup Ther* 41:563-575, 1987.
5. Allen CK: *Structures of cognitive performance modes,* Ormond Beach, FL, 1996, Allen Conferences.
6. Allen CK: *Structures of the cognitive performance modes,* Ormond Beach, FL, 1999, Allen Conferences.
7. Allen CK: *Allen Cognitive Level Screen (ACLS) test manual,* Colchester, CT, 2000, S&S Worldwide.
8. Allen C: *Cognitive disabilities frame of reference,* 2005. Retrieved October 2005, from http://www.fiu.edu/~otweb/Courses/allen.htm.
9. Allen Conferences, Inc: The official web site of Allen Cognitive Levels, 2000. Retrieved October 2005, from http://www.allen-cognitive-levels.com/.
10. Allen CK, Earhart CA, Blue T: *Occupational therapy treatment goals for the physically and cognitively disabled,* Rockville, MD, 1992, American Occupational Therapy Association.
11. Allen CK, Earhart CA, Blue T: *Understanding cognitive performance modes,* Ormond Beach, FL, 1995, Allen Conferences.
12. Allen CK, Reyner A: *How to start using the Allen Diagnostic Module: a guide to introducing Allen's theories into your practice,* ed 2, Colchester, CT, 1996, S&S Worldwide.
13. American Occupational Therapy Association: Occupational therapy practice framework: domain and process, *Am J Occup Ther* 56:609-639, 2002.
14. Baehr E, Rosenfeld JP, Baehr R: *Frontal asymmetry changes reflect brief mood shifts in both normal and depressed subjects,* Paper presented at the International Society for Neuronal Regulation, 2002 Conference, Phoenix, AZ, 10th Annual Conference. Abstract Retrieved October 2005, from http://www.snr.jnt.org/newspluss/2002/papers2002.htm.
15. Bertrand C: *Interdisciplinary benefits of the Allen's cognitive levels in geriatric rehabilitation,* Paper presented at the National Geriatric Rehab Conference, Boston, 1997.
16. Black L, Herrington R, Hudspeth B, et al: *Effects of childhood sexual abuse on adult brain plasticity as measured by quantitative electroencephalogram,* Paper presented at the International Society for Neuronal Regulation, 2002 Conference, Phoenix AZ, 10th Annual Conference. Abstract Retrieved October 2005, from http://www.snr.jnt.org/newspluss/2002/papers2002.htm.
17. Burns T: Cognitive performance update, 2003. Retrieved October 2005, from http://CPT/Update.htm.
18. Champagne T: Occupational therapy levels 5.0-5.2: caregiver guide, 2001. Retrieved October 2005, from http://www.ot-innovations.com/pdf_files/LEVELS_5.0-5.2_CAREGIVER_GUIDE.pdf.
19. Champagne T: Occupational therapy levels 2.4-2.8: caregiver guide, 2003. Retrieved October 2005, from

http://www.ot-innovations.com/pdf_files/Caregiver-Guide24-28.pdf.

20. Champagne T: Occupational therapy levels 3.0-3.4: caregiver guide, 2003. Retrieved October 2005, from http://www.ot-innovations.com/pdf_files/Caregiver-Guide30-34.pdf.

21. Champagne T: Occupational therapy levels 3.6-3.8: caregiver guide, 2003. Retrieved October 2005, from http://www.ot-innovations.com/pdf_files/Caregiver-Guide36-38.pdf.

22. Champagne T: Occupational therapy levels 4.0-4.4: caregiver guide, 2003. Retrieved October 2005, from http://www.ot-innovations.com/pdf_files/Caregiver-Guide40-44.pdf.

23. Champagne T: Occupational therapy levels 4.6-4.8: caregiver guide, 2003. Retrieved October 2005, from http://www.ot-innovations.com/pdf_files/Caregiver-Guide46-48.pdf.

24. Champagne T, Schubmehl J: Allen cognitive level 2: sensory diet guide, 2003. Retrieved October 2005, from http://www.ot-innovations.com/pdf_files/SensoryDietGuidesUpdate.pdf.

25. Champagne T, Schubmehl J: Allen cognitive level 3: sensory diet guide, 2003. Retrieved October 2005, from http://www.ot-innovations.com/pdf_files/SensoryDietGuidesUpdate.pdf

26. Champagne T, Schubmehl J: Allen cognitive level 4: sensory diet guide, 2003. Retrieved October 2005, from http://www.ot-innovations.com/pdf_files/SensoryDietGuidesUpdate.pdf

27. Cole MB: *Group dynamics in occupational therapy,* ed 3, Thorofare, NJ, 2005, Slack.

28. Cooley-Dickinson Hospital-West 5 Occupational Therapy Department: *Create your own personalized sensory diet form: check off the things that are helpful to you! Sensory stimulation,* 2003. Retrieved from http://www.ot-innovations.com/pdf_files/SensoryDietGuidesUpdate.pdf.

29. Donohue MV: Claudia Allen. In Miller RJ, Walker KF, eds: *Perspectives on theory for the practice of occupational therapy,* Gaithersburg, MD, 1993, Aspen, pp. 219-245.

30. Dye L: Study finds being social late in life helps keep the mind fresh [Electronic version], ABC News, October 31, 2002. Retrieved October 2005, from http://printerfriendly.abcnews.com/printerfriendly/print?fetchFromGLUE=true&GLUEService=ABCNewsCom.

31. Earhart CA, Allen CK, Blue T: *Allen diagnostic module instruction manual,* Colchester, CT, 1993, S&S Worldwide.

32. Early MB: *Mental health concepts and techniques for the occupational therapy assistant,* ed 3, Philadelphia, 2000, Lippincott Williams & Wilkins.

33. Grant S: Cognitive disability frame of reference. In Crepeau EB, Cohn ES, Schell BA, eds: *Willard and Spack-*

man's occupational therapy, New York, 2003, Lippincott Williams & Wilkins, pp. 261-264.

34. Hayes RL, Keller SM: Why won't Australian occupational therapists adopt Allen's cognitive disability theory? *Austr Occup Ther J* 46:188-192, 1999.

35. Heimann NE, Allen CK, Yerxa EJ: The routine task inventory: a tool for describing the functional behavior of the cognitively disabled, *Occup Ther Pract* 1(1):67-74, 1989.

36. Henry A: Predicting psychosocial functioning and symptomatic recovery of adolescents and young adults with a first psychotic episode: a six-month follow-up study, unpublished doctoral dissertation, 1994, Boston University.

37. Henry AD, Moore K, Quinlivan M, et al: The relationship of the Allen Cognitive Level test to demographics, diagnosis, and disposition among psychiatric inpatients, *Am J Occup Ther* 52:638-643, 1998.

38. Jennett B: The measurement of outcome. In Brooks N, ed: *Closed head injury: psychological, social and family consequences,* Oxford, 1984, Oxford University Press, pp. 37-43.

39. Keller S, Hayes R: The relationship between the Allen Cognitive Level Test and the Life Skills Profile, *Am J Occup Ther* 52:851-856, 1998.

40. Kielhofner G: *Conceptual foundations of occupational therapy,* ed 3, Philadelphia, 2004, FA Davis.

41. Landa-Gonzalez B: Multicontextual occupational therapy intervention: a case study of traumatic brain injury, *Occup Ther Internat* 8:49-62, 2001.

42. Lazzarini I: A historical perspective of the Allen Cognitive Levels (ACL), Cognitive Assessments: A focus on the history, 2003. Retrieved October 2005, from http://www.ot-innovations.com/acl-paper.html.

43. Lazzarini I: Neuro-occupation: the nonlinear dynamics of intention, meaning and perception, *Br J Occup Ther* 67(8):342-352, 2004.

44. Moore D: *An occupational therapy evaluation of sensorimotor cognition: initial reliability, validity, and descriptive data for hospitalized schizophrenic adults,* unpublished master's thesis, Los Angeles, 1978, University of Southern California.

45. Nathanieisz PW: Fetal and neonatal environment has influence on brain development (Electronic version), *Lancet* 347:1-3, 1996. Retrieved October 2005, from http://www.EBSCOhost.htm.

46. Neistadt ME: The neurobiology of learning: implications for treatment of adults with brain injury, *Am J Occup Ther* 48:421-430, 1994.

47. Nelson DL, Lenhart DA: Resumption of outpatient occupational therapy for a young woman five years after traumatic brain injury, *Am J Occup Ther* 50:223-228, 1996.

48. Penny NH, Mueser KT, North CT: The Allen Cognitive Level Test and social competence in adult psychiatric patients, *Am J Occup Ther* 49:420-427, 1995.

49. Raweh DV, Katz N: Treatment effectiveness of Allen's cognitive disabilities model with adult schizophrenic outpatients: a pilot study, *Occup Ther Mental Health* 14(4):65-77, 1999.

50. Roitman DM, Katz N: Predictive validity of the Large Allen Cognitive Level test (LACL) using the Allen Diagnostic Module (ADM) in an aged, non-disabled population, *Phys Occup Ther Geriatrics* 14(4):43-57, 1996.

51. Secrest L, Wood AE, Tapp A: A comparison of the Allen Cognitive Level test and the Wisconsin Card Sorting Test in adults with schizophrenia, *Am J Occup Ther* 54:129-133, 2000.

52. Toglia JP: A dynamic interactional model to cognitive rehabilitation. In Katz N, ed: *Cognition and occupation in rehabilitation: cognitive models for intervention in occupational therapy,* Bethesda, MD, 1998, American Occupational Therapy Association, pp. 5-10.

53. Velligan DI, Bow-Thomas CC, Mahurin RK, et al: Concurrent and predictive validity of the Allen cognitive levels assessment, *Psychiatry Res* 80:287-298, 1998.

12
The Model of Human Occupation

Preview Questions

1. Discuss the interdisciplinary basis of the Model of Human Occupation and particularly the use of systems theory to provide its framework.
2. Concisely state the theoretical core of the Model of Human Occupation. Differentiate between the constructs *hierarchy* and *heterarchy,* and state the implications of each to occupational therapy intervention planning.
3. Explain the postulations of the Model of Human Occupation about the following:
   a. Function
   b. Dysfunction
   c. Change
4. Describe at least four of the model's assessments, at least two of which should be observation based. Explain how each of them is used and how information derived from it is used for treatment planning.
5. Give an example of a short-term treatment goal targeting each of the four components of the human system as conceptualized from the model's perspective.
6. Discuss the consistency of the Model of Human Occupation with each of the following:
   a. The occupational therapy paradigm
   b. The philosophy of pragmatism
   c. The complexity/chaos theoretical framework
7. Discuss available empirical evidence supporting clinical effectiveness of the Model of

Human Occupation as a guide to intervention in occupational therapy practice.

The Model of Human Occupation (MOHO) was originally developed by Gary Kielhofner and two other therapists in the 1970s and was first published in 1980.[26,27,32,33] Kielhofner's interest in occupational therapy started with his experiences early in life when his grandmother's leg was amputated.[51] He watched her spend her remaining years in a wheelchair as a result of poor rehabilitation efforts. While running a recreation program in an occupational therapy department, he became interested in occupational therapy and decided to pursue it as a career.[13]

However, Kielhofner's initial experiences studying occupational therapy were disappointing, and he contemplated pursuing a different career. At this time, he met Mary Reilly at an AOTA presentation and heard her speak.[13,51] He was so impressed with Reilly's way of thinking and processing ideas that he decided to transfer to the University of Southern California where she was teaching. Kielhofner expresses Mary Reilly's initial influence on him as follows: "There was something about the way that Reilly thought and the way that she processed ideas that I really got! And that I liked!" (p. 46).[13]

Kielhofner attributes the basic ideas that he used to formulate MOHO to Reilly. He states that in the course of 2 years that he spent studying with Reilly, she took the position that "occupational therapy needs to define what its business is, and that its business is dealing with people's every day occupational problems and using occupation as a therapeutic media, and all that that means" (p. 181).[51] Furthermore, he states that "Obviously I stand on her shoulders as the foundation of what I believe, and I could not have ever thought or done anything that I did without her training me, although I think I can now say I disagree with her on some points" (p. 182).[51]

Because of Kielhofner's interaction with Reilly, MOHO was highly influenced by the *Occupational Behavior Frame of Reference,* which she developed to help spur the profession back to its roots consistent with her call in her Slagle lecture.[55] She developed the frame of reference based on the premise that "humans have a need to master their environments and occupation is vital to this mastery," and this "Mastery occurs primarily through the continuum of play and work" through which "individuals learn roles needed to become competent in mastery" (p. 15).[1] She saw play, use of tools, the human hand, and the brain as being interrelated factors in human evolution, in which both behavior and morphology underwent contemporaneous change.[56,57] Kielhofner emphasizes that MOHO arose from an attempt to apply constructs from the occupational behavior frame of reference in clinical practice.[51]

Initially, Kielhofner started with what he called the *Temporal Adaptation Conceptual Framework.*[25] In this work, he emphasized Adolph Meyer's proposition[50] that the rhythms of nature organize behavior so that the human is able to live in harmony and balance with his or her environment. This balance was conceptualized to be a result of routine task performance over time. Use of time was seen as a measure of one's adaptation or maladaptation to the environment.

Therefore Kielhofner insisted that "occupational therapy should view patients within the context of time through the unfolding of their lives" (p. 235).[25] This meant that occupational therapy should view the therapist as a caretaker of activities of daily living (ADLs) rather than ADLs constituting merely a checklist of self-care routine. Based on this core proposition, he recommended introduction of the construct of temporal adaptation in occupational therapy as a framework within which the entire spectrum of activities that support health can be described. According to the proposed framework, there would be no separation between consciousness of time and adaptation, because it is through awareness of time that humans are able to perceive change in both themselves and the environment, a phenomenon referred to as *adaptation.* He asserted that:

Armed with temporal consciousness, man is a supreme actor in time. Not only is he aware of changing events, but he is likewise conscious of the fact that he can have some effect on that course of events. The *perception of the self as a cause* comes from *experiencing the results of one's own actions in time.* Man's awareness of time, the awareness of his causative ability, and the potential for consequences are interrelated phenomena. The human condition is transformed by the awareness of the individual that he or she has acted, is acting, and will continue to act. Man's awareness of time makes possible this continuity of experience that transforms the nature of his adaptation. (p. 237, emphasis mine)[25]

In the above statement, the seeds of what came to be the major constructs of MOHO can be seen: the idea of personal causation (perception of self as a cause) and the importance of habits in structuring performance (experiencing the results of one's own actions in time). In Kielhofner's later work, the *Temporal Adaptation Framework* was incorporated into the model of human occupation. This model was initially published in a series of four articles.[26,27,32,33]

Scientific Base

The greatest theoretical influence on MOHO has been the general systems theory.[26,32] Other sources of constructs included occupational therapy literature, particularly Mary Reilly's postulations about occupational behavior,[13,57] anthropology, sociology, and psychology.[30] In this section, we will examine the theoretical base of the model in its current status.[13,26,27,30]

Initial Postulations

Kielhofner and colleagues set out to create a model focusing on occupation and supporting what they saw as a general paradigm of occupational therapy that needed to be articulated. This was evident in their view that the model was "an important step in the development of a more generic paradigm designed to stimulate further practice, theory, and research in occupational therapy" (p. 572).[32] In doing so, they used the general systems theory to organize concepts of occupation.

General Postulations

The original core proposition of the model based on the open systems theory was that the occupational human was an open system in a dynamic interaction with the environment, being affected and affecting the environment, through the process of input, throughput, output, and feedback.[26,32] The output consisted of information and physical, mental, and social action. The output information was understood to be fed into the system as feedback, along with other information from the environment, as input. This information was processed in the throughput, which consisted of three subsystems: *volition, habituation,* and *performance.*

In this view, volition, habituation, and performance were understood to be arranged hierarchically, with the volition subsystem primarily organizing the functioning of both the habituation and the performance subsystems. These ideas have since evolved as concepts in the

general systems have changed. The postulations discussed next are based on the theoretical core of the model as it currently exists.[28,29]

Postulations about Function, Dysfunction, and Change

Function

Interaction of the human with the environment is still viewed as occurring through occupation and mediated by the four components of the human as an occupational system: volition, habituation, performance, and the environment. However, one of the significant changes has been abandoning the view of the interaction between subsystems from a hierarchical perspective (where the volition subsystem controls and organizes other subsystems) to a heterarchical perspective (where all four components of the human system act together, with each contributing to the dynamics of the entire system.[28] In this dynamic systems perspective (also referred to as complexity/chaos in some sections of literature[16]), Kielhofner asserts that we have begun "to address how humans manage complex performance without hierarchical control" (p. 33).[28] In this view, internal factors (volition, habituation, and performance, as well as intrapsychic, neurological, and kinesiological structural functions) are assembled together in response to specific environmental demands.

In addition, the development and process of the volitional component of the system has been further clarified.[29,30] In this enhanced elaboration of the process, "Volitional thoughts and feelings are embedded in a cycle of anticipation, choice, experience while doing, and subsequent interpretation" (p. 149).[30] Anticipation refers to the expectation of success and enjoyment of activities, which determines the likelihood of choosing to engage in those activities.[29] The volition subsystem also determines how we experience whatever we are doing (whether we enjoy it, are bored, are miserable, and so on). Furthermore, experience is an important factor in therapy. It is important that therapy be perceived as a positive experience. Further, volition determines how actions are interpreted. For instance, if an activity is valued, it will be interpreted as something worth pursuing. If it is not valued, the person may just go through the motions in order to get to another more valued activity. Therefore "volition provides us with a framework for making sense of our actions" (p. 58).[29]

Also, the current conceptualization of MOHO emphasizes even more than the earlier version the importance of the environmental context to occupational performance. In addition to this emphasis on the importance of the environment, the construct of emergence has been introduced. In the earlier version of the model, the output was considered to consist of information and action, resulting from processing of input information in the throughput. In the current version, intention to do something, "neurological organization, biomechanics," and the task being done, "become a functional heterarchy, linked together in" (p. 36)[28] the intended action. "The actual movements" required to complete the task "emerge out of their total dynamics" (pp. 36–37).[28]

Thus output is emergence or "spontaneous occurrence of complex actions coming out of the interactions of several components without the benefit of a central control" (p. 35).[28] In this sense, occupation, which is the result of such complex actions, is an emergent phenomenon. Along with occupation is emergence of thoughts and emotions that both maintain behavior and also emerge from it. In other words, "Volition, habituation, performance capacity, and the environment always resonate together, creating conditions out of which our thoughts, feelings, and doing emerge" (p. 39).[28]

Furthermore, in the current status of the MOHO, function is viewed as engagement in occupation, which denotes "a dynamic process through which we maintain the organization of our bodies and minds" (p. 40).[28] In other words, through occupation, we use our minds and bodies and in the process shape them. Engagement in occupation shapes physiological structures, for example, by generation of extra muscle fibers leading to increased strength and endurance, or development of new neural synapses leading to enhanced cognitive functioning. We emerge, so to speak, through engagement in occupation. As a result, occupational adaptation, which is "the construction of a positive identity and achieving competence over time in the context of one's environment," is achieved (p. 152).[30]

Dysfunction

Loss of occupation may lead to deterioration or loss of capacities (e.g., atrophy of muscles due to disuse or loss of cognitive abilities due to lack of challenging intellectual activities). When this happens, one is in a state of *dysfunction*, which "depends not only on the status of inner components, but also a relationship between a person's inner circumstances and the external environment" (p. 38).[28] In other words, dysfunction can result from alteration of internal structures leading to inability to engage effectively in occupation and subsequent emergence of maladaptive behavior, or circumstances in the environment that act as barriers to effective occupational performance (such as an impoverished environment). Therefore dysfunction may be summarized as follows: "When people's identities do not fit with their possibilities for enacting them, or when they become frayed by life circumstances, occupational adaptation is threatened" (p. 153).[30]

Change

For therapists using the MOHO, change constitutes alteration of any component in the heterarchy (volition, habituation, performance capacity, or environmental conditions), in an endeavor to reconfigure their dynamic interaction, leading to emergence of new thoughts, feelings, and actions. In other words, alteration of external circumstances causes a shift in the volition, habituation, performance capacity, or environment (or all four components), leading to emergence of new adaptive thoughts, feelings, and behaviors.

Furthermore, the new thoughts, feelings, and behaviors need to be repeated often enough so that volition, habituation, and performance capacity come together to form their own structure.[28] Thus Kielhofner currently conceptualizes the process of change as follows: (1) when any of the four components of the human system (volition, habituation, performance capacity, or the environment) is altered, new thoughts, feelings, and actions emerge; (2) repetition of the altering conditions enough times leads to a coalescing of the volition, habituation, and performance capacity into a new emergent internal organization; and (3) when the newly emerged internal organization interacts with a stable environment on an ongoing basis, the newly emerged patterns of thoughts, feelings, and actions are stabilized.

Guidelines for Client Evaluation and Therapeutic Intervention

Client Evaluation

Numerous MOHO assessment instruments have been developed. All of them evaluate parts of or the entire human system: performance capacity (particularly motor and process skills that make participation in occupation possible), habituation (habits, routines, and roles), and volition (personal causation, values, and interests). It is not possible to present all of them in this book or to teach them in a basic psychosocial rehabilitation class. Therefore we selected for discussion those instruments of the model that appear regularly in literature and that seem to be popular in other texts. A literature search revealed over 20 research articles based on the MOHO that were published in a variety of scholarly journals.

The articles reported research based on the following evaluation instruments: Assessment of Communication and Interaction Skills (ACIS),[15] Assessment of Motor and Process Skills (AMPS),[10] the Occupational Performance History Interview, Version 2 (OPHI-II),[40] and the Occupational Case Analysis Interview and Rating Scale (OCAIRS)[24] (this instrument has been revised and is now known as the Occupational

Circumstances Assessment-Interview Rating Scale).

Early[6] identifies OPHI-II, the Role Checklist,[54] and the National Psychiatric Institute Interest Checklist (NPI Interest Checklist),[59] which is presented in the MOHO as the modified Interest Checklist.[37] Finally, the following instruments were discussed in Hemphill-Pearson,[21] an edited work presenting evaluation instruments that are commonly used by psychosocial occupational therapists: OPHI-II,[22] the Role Checklist,[2] Watts and colleagues,[62] and the Role Activity Performance Scale (RAPS).[17] These instruments were chosen by occupational therapy faculty as some of the most important assessments in the profession as indicated in a field survey.[21]

We will briefly discuss the above instruments with the exception of the RAPS, which is no longer used in conjunction with the MOHO.[31] For a more detailed discourse, the reader should refer to the references at the end of this chapter.[14,35-37] Also, further information about the instruments can be obtained from the Model of Human Occupation Clearinghouse website, available at www.moho.uic.edu/. Presentation of the assessments will follow the categorization used in the above sources: observational, self-report, interview-based, and multimethod assessments.

Observational Assessments

Assessment of Communication and Interaction Skills

The Assessment of Communication and Interaction Skills (ACIS) is designed to assess performance capacity. Specifically, it is used to evaluate the communication and process skills in varied environmental contexts while the client engages in daily occupations that are meaningful to him or her.[15,44] The ACIS consists of 20 communication and process skills that are grouped into three categories: *physicality, information exchange,* and *relations* (Box 12-1).

There is an accompanying manual providing details of definitions and instructions on how to observe and score the various theoretical

Box 12-1	Sample Domains and Items in the ACIS

Domains and Items for Assessment of Communication and Interaction Skills

Physicality

Contacts—Makes physical contact with others
Gazes—Uses eyes to communicate and interact with others
Gestures—Uses movements of the body to indicate, demonstrate, or add emphasis
Maneuvers—Moves one's body in relation to others
Orients—Directs one's body in relation to others and/or occupational forms
Postures—Assumes physical positions

Information exchange

Articulates—Produces clear, understandable speech
Asserts—Directly expresses desires, refusals, and requests
Asks—Requests factual or personal information
Engages—Initiates interactions
Expresses—Displays affect/attitude
Modulates—Employs volume and inflection in speech
Shares—Gives out factual or personal information
Speaks—Makes oneself understood through the use of words, phrases, or sentences
Sustains—Keeps up social action or speech for appropriate durations

Relations

Collaborates—Coordinates one's action with others toward a common end goal
Conforms—Follows implicit and explicit social norms
Focuses—Directs conversation and behavior to ongoing social action
Relates—Assumes a manner of acting that tries to establish a rapport with others
Respects—Accommodates to other people's reactions and requests

Data from Kjellberg A, Haglund L, Forsyth K, et al: The measurement properties of the Swedish version of the assessment of communication and interaction skills, *Scand J Caring Sci* 17:271–277, 2003.

constructs being assessed. Physicality is indicated by skills such as making contact with other people, using eye contact to communicate, assuming appropriate postures, and using gestures. Information exchange is indicated by articulation and production of clear speech, appropriate self-assertiveness, engagement (ability to initiate interactions), speaking coherently, and other such behaviors. Indicators of the relations category include appropriate collaboration with others to achieve a goal, conformation to established social norms, focus of conversation and behavior on prevailing social action needed to complete a task, and so on.

The client is observed while engaging in an occupation in a social context.[44] A skill that is performed to support ongoing social action, for instance speaking clearly, is rated 4. A rating of 3 indicates that mastery of the skill to the extent that it supports ongoing social action is questionable; 2 means that there is a lack of the skill to the extent that it interferes with social action (for instance the client's speech is disruptive); and a rating of 1 means that the skill is severely deficient to the extent that it causes a breakdown of social interaction. Through observation and scoring of the skills in the three categories, a profile of the client's strengths and challenges in communication and interaction is generated. Administration of the instrument takes 20 to 60 minutes, with observation time ranging between 15 and 45 minutes.[36] A treatment plan is developed targeting the deficient skills.

Assessment of Motor and Process Skills

The Assessment of Motor and Process Skills (AMPS) is designed to assess performance of ADLs with a focus on motor and process skills necessary to complete tasks.[8,9] It consists of a battery of 83 ADL tasks that are standardized, ranging in difficulty from easy to difficult. There are 9 Personal ADL (PADL) tasks and 74 Instrumental ADL (IADL) tasks. PADL refers to activities such as toileting, maintaining personal hygiene, dressing, and so on. IADL includes activities such as cleaning, shopping for groceries, making meals, and so on. The tasks are lineally calibrated such that their level of difficulty can be adjusted. Some of the tasks in the instrument are "putting on shoes and socks, sweeping the floor, changing sheets on a bed, and cleaning a bathroom" (p. 599).[45] Examples of skills that are assessed include stabilization of the body to maintain balance, appropriate positioning of body in relation to the task, coordination, appropriate sequencing of steps and choice of procedures and tools to complete a task, and so on (see example in Table 12-1). They are divided into *motor skills* (referring to execution of motor behavior required to complete a task) and *process skills* (cognitive processes, including accurately following procedures required to complete a task).

Table 12-1. BEHAVIORS OBSERVED IN ADL PERFORMANCE IN RELATION TO AMPS ITEMS

Behavior Observed	AMPS Item
Opens a cupboard	Grips (ADL motor skill)
	Moves (ADL motor skill)
	Calibrates (ADL motor skill)
Searches for glasses	Searches/locates (ADL process skill)
Reaches for glasses	Reaches (ADL motor skill)
	Bends (ADL motor skill)
Grasps the glass	Chooses (ADL process skill)
	Grips (ADL motor skill)
Lifts the glass from the shelf	Lifts (ADL motor skill)
Places the glass on the bench	Calibrates (ADL motor skill)
	Gathers (ADL process skill)
	Organizes (ADL process skill)

From Kottorp A, Bernspang B, Fisher AG: Validity of a performance assessment of activities of daily living for people with developmental disabilities, *J Intellectual Disabil Res* 47:600, 2003.

The AMPS is administered as follows:

1. The client is interviewed to determine activities of daily living (ADLs) that are familiar and important/meaningful to him or her.
2. Four to five standardized occupational forms of appropriate level of difficulty that are close to the identified ADLs are selected from the AMPS list.
3. The client chooses two of the three or four occupational forms.
4. The client is observed while engaging in those occupational forms.
5. Sixteen motor and 20 process skills in the AMPS are scored on a 4-point criterion referenced rating scale in relation to observed performance of the selected occupational forms. The scale is anchored at 4 (competent skill level) and 1 (unacceptable skill level).
6. The raw scores are entered in a computer for analysis using computer software (*FACETS* computer program).[45,47] A report is generated detailing the client's motor and process ability. It indicates whether the client's skill level is adequate (A), there are difficulties (D), or there are marked skill deficits (MD). A treatment plan is established targeting skills in which the client has difficulties or deficiencies.

Self-Report Assessments
Modified Interest Checklist
The Modified Interest Checklist was originally introduced in 1961 at the National Psychiatric Institute (NPI) at the University of California at Los Angeles.[49] It was designed for use with adult psychiatric inpatients. The original NPI Interest Checklist consisted of a list of 80 activities, for each of which the client indicated the level of interest (casual, strong, or no interest). There were two parts to the instrument. Part I consisted of the 80 activities. In Part II, the client was requested to list any other interests. At the time, it was thought that "The raw data can be systematized into a pattern of interests according to the five categories of Manual Skills,

Physical Sports, Social Recreation, ADL and Cultural/Educational, and the three expressions of strength of interest" (p. 327).[49] However, subsequent research indicated no evidence of such clustering of interests.[59]

Since the instrument is used to assess interests, which comprise part of the volitional component of the human system as conceptualized in the MOHO, therapists subscribing to the model adopted it. It was later modified by Scaffa[61] and again by Kielhofner and Neville.[42] The current Modified Interest Checklist (MIC) consists of 68 of the original 80 activities. For each activity, Kielhofner and Neville have added a requirement for the client to indicate the level of interest (strong, some, or no interest) in the past 10 years as well as in the past year. Then the client indicates whether he or she currently participates in the activity, and whether he or she would like to pursue it in the future. The client's ratings of the level of interest, current participation, and intent to pursue activities in future provides information that "is particularly useful for appreciating the impact that disability has had on how the client is experiencing pleasure from an activity or the significance disability has had in altering a client's attraction to particular kinds of activities" (p. 215).[37] This information can be used to facilitate discussion with the client leading to formulation of a treatment plan. Refer to Chapter 14 of your Lab Manual to see a copy of the instrument, or download it from http://www.moho. uic.edu/images/Modified%20Interest% 20Checklist.pdf.

Role Checklist

The Role Checklist is another instrument designed to assess the habituation (patterning of occupations into routines constituting roles that help meet individual and societal needs) and volitional (valuation of occupational roles) components of the human system.[2] It was developed by Oakley,

Kielhofner, and Barris[53] "to obtain information on clients' perceptions of their participation in occupational roles throughout their life and on the value they place on those occupational roles" (p. 231).[37] Consequently, it comprises two parts. Part 1 consists of a list of roles. For each role, the client indicates whether he or she has performed it in the past, is performing it currently, or plans to perform it in the future. The past refers to any time until the last 7 days before administration of the assessment. The present refers to the last 7 days up to the day of administration, and the future refers to the day following administration of the checklist. This part of the assessment provides information about the client's identification with the various roles that are listed on the checklist. In Part 2 of the instrument, the client indicates how much each role is valued (not at all, somewhat, or very valuable).

Instructions for administration of the checklist are as follows[2]:

1. The client is asked to fill out demographic information.
2. The client is then asked to read the instructions, and the therapist inquires about whether they are understood.
3. Time frames are defined for the client as described above.
4. After Part 1 is completed, the client is asked to read the instructions for Part 2, and the therapist inquires about whether they are understood.
5. Variables (definitions of worth assigned to each role) are defined for the client.
6. The therapist instructs the client that he or she is available to provide any required assistance until the client has completed the assessment.

Information obtained from the evaluation assists the therapist to collaborate with the client in identifying "patterns in role selection, preference, and performance" (232–233).[37] These patterns provide insights about the client's life that can be used in treatment planning.

Interview-Based Assessments

Occupational Performance History Interview, Version 2

The Occupational Performance History Interview, Version 2 (OPHI-II) was designed to assess general occupational adaptation, using both quantitative and qualitative data.[39] It originated from research funded jointly by the American Occupational Therapy Association (AOTA) and the American Occupational Therapy Foundation (AOTF) with a mandate to develop "a generic historical interview to be used in occupational therapy evaluation" (p. 260).[41] The result of the investigation was a three-part instrument consisting of 10 items. The three parts were a semistructured interview, a rating scale, and a life history narrative. Thus the instrument was designed to use the life history method of gathering occupational adaptation information.

In its current form, the revised Occupational Performance History Interview-version 2 (OPHI-II) seeks to elicit information about the client's occupational adaptation in the past and present.[40] It consists of three parts that were in the original instrument: Part 1 is a semistructured interview, Part 2 is a rating scale, and Part 3 is a life history narrative. The semistructured interview in Part 1 is guided using recommended questions designed to gather information in each of the following thematic categories: activity/occupational choices, critical life events in the client's life, daily routine, and occupational behavior settings (environmental/social contexts). Part 2 consists of three rating scales consisting of 29 items that provide a quantitative measure of the client's identity (values, interests, and sense of confidence in ability to perform the occupations—volition), sense of competence (ability to sustain a satisfying and productive pattern of occupational participation—habituation), and impact of occupational performance on his or her environmental context from information gathered through the interview. The narrative in Part 3 provides a means of assessing the qualitative aspects of the life history.

Consistent with the design of the instrument, assessment is completed in three parts:

1. The client is interviewed. The interview takes about 45–60 minutes.
2. Each of the 29 items in the three rating scales is scored on a 4-point rating based on criteria describing the client in relation to each item (see Figure 12-1 for an example of one rated item).
3. A life history narrative form is completed. The client's life story is plotted. This gives the therapist a glimpse of the client's life story and particularly the turning points, and indicates his or her identity, competence, and ability to adapt over time.

Occupational Circumstances Assessment-Interview and Rating Scale

Similar to OPHI-II, the Occupational Circumstances Assessment-Interview and Rating Scale (OCAIRS) was designed to assess general occupational adaptation. However, it is shorter than the OPHI-II and focuses on present adaptation rather than the client's entire life. Originally, it was referred to as the Occupational Case Analysis Interview and Rating Scale.[24] Although the original version is no longer used, we will discuss it here because the case example in this chapter is based on it. As of this writing, the author was unable to find an example based on the new version of the instrument. However, it may be advantageous to understand the earlier version because there are several similarities with the current version.

Development of the OCAIRS began with an attempt to generate information from psychiatric clients as part of case analysis, hence the name *case analysis interview*. Gradually the process of conducting the interview was systematized, and a rating scale was developed. It consisted of 14 items (interests, roles, habits, skills, output, physical environment, social environment, feedback, historical, personal causation, values and goals, dynamic, contextual, and system trajectory).

Item	Rating	Criteria
Has personal goals and projects	4	☐ Goals/personal projects challenge/extend/require effort ☐ Feels energized/excited about future goals/personal projects
	3	☐ Goals/personal projects fit strengths/limitations ☐ Enough desire for future to overcome doubt/challenges ☐ Motivation to work on goals/personal projects
	2	☐ Goals/anticipated projects underestimate/overestimate abilities ☐ Not very motivated to work on goals/personal projects ☐ Difficulty thinking about goals/personal projects/future ☐ Limited commitment/excitement/motivation
	1	☐ Cannot identify goals/personal projects ☐ Personal goals/projects are unattainable given abilities ☐ Goals bear little/no relationship to strengths/limitations ☐ Lacks commitment or motivation to the future ☐ Unmotivated due to conflicting/excessive goals/personal projects
Key: **4** = Exceptionally competent occupational functioning; **3** = Appropriate satisfactory occupational functioning; **2** = Some occupational dysfunctions; **1** = Extremely occupationally dysfunctional		

Figure 12-1.   An example of the scoring system for the OPHI-II scale. (Adapted from Kielhofner G, Forsyth K, Clay C, et al: Talking with clients: assessments that collect information through interviews. In Kielhofner G, ed: *Model of human occupation: theory and application,* Philadelphia, 2002, Lippincott Williams & Wilkins, p. 242.)

The instrument was designed to evaluate different subsystems of the MOHO (volition, habituation, and performance capacity) as well as interaction with the environmental context (physical and social). Thus the first three items (interests, roles, and habits) explored the habituation subsystem. The next two items (skills and output) were directed toward performance capacity; the next two items (physical environment and social environment) were directed toward environmental supports available to the client; and the next item (feedback) examined the system's ability to use feedback to adjust itself. One item (historical) examined the client's perception of how he or she was able to adapt in the past. The next two items (personal causation, and values and goals) were directed toward the volitional subsystem.

The final three items (dynamic, contextual, and system trajectory) summarized and synthesized information gathered through the first 11 items. The dynamic item guided the therapist to formulate a profile of the client's ability to generate output that was consistent with adequate interaction between the volitional subsystem (ability to pursue personal interests and goals, guided by personal values, and with a sense of self as an actor in the world) and the habituation subsystem (ability to maintain a lifestyle that supported performance of activities that were consistent with the volitional subsystem). The contextual item assessed adequacy of environmental supports to the client's adaptive functioning and his or her ability to use environmental feedback to adjust performance as necessary. Finally, using the system trajectory item, the therapist generated an assessment of the extent to which the client was in an adaptive or maladaptive cycle, based on a synthesis of information collected through all other items. The therapist also predicted whether the client system was likely to remain in the adaptive/maladaptive cycle and therefore whether occupational therapy was indicated to help the client become or stay adaptively functional.

Each item was rated on a 5-point Likert-type scale that was defined specifically for that item. For example, for item number 1, the client was given a score of 5 if he or she identified four or more satisfying interests and two of the activities mentioned were pursued regularly, in response to the questions: "How do you like to spend your time?" "Do you have any other special interests?" and "How often do you participate?"[24] If the client did not identify any interests, a score of 1 was given for this item. To assist in integration of information and generation of a prediction, data were summarized in a summary form. The scores and prediction were used as a basis for treatment planning.

Haglund and colleagues[20] revised the original OCAIRS and developed the current Occupational Circumstances Assessment-Interview and Rating Scale. The later version still targets the components of the human system as conceptualized in the MOHO and, as mentioned earlier, is similar to the original OCAIRS in many respects. Interview guided by the instrument takes about 40 minutes, and 15 minutes are needed to complete the scale. Furthermore, the instrument was expanded by an additional 6 items, making a total of 20 items. Added items include short-term goals, long-term goals, motor skills, process skills, communication and interaction skills, and previous experiences. Other items were modified to gather more information about the client's functioning and adaptation. For instance, the environmental item was broken into physical environment supports, physical environment opportunities, physical environment demands and constraints, and physical environment fit. The social environment item was similarly divided into several items describing various aspects of social contexts. Occupational participation and occupational adaptation items are now used to assess system functioning and adaptation

instead of the dynamic, contextual, and system trajectory items that were used in the original OCAIRS.

Criteria describing the client are provided for each item. Those that best characterize him or her are checked off, and the scale is used to award a rating on the item (see example in Figure 12-2). The reader will notice that in the later version of the OCAIRS, these criteria are more explicitly defined. For example, while the client was required to identify four or more interests and pursue two of them regularly in order to attain the highest score of 5, the new OCAIRS specifies that he or she must identify and participate in three or more interests *outside of work* in order to obtain the highest score (4) for that item. Also, the new scale provides an indication of the client's state of adaptivity/maladaptivity in relation to each item. Further, it includes a rating of perceived level of interest in a primary occupation/role and satisfaction with performance in that occupation/role as part of the criteria for scoring the item.

In addition to the rating scales for the various items, the summary form was also modified to reflect the increased number of items. Figure 12-3 shows an example of how this form is completed.

All of the above assessments target the three components of the human system as conceptualized in the MOHO: volition, habituation, and performance capacity. Observational assessments (the ACIS and the AMPS) primarily assess skills, which are part of the performance capacity. This is logical since skills can easily be explicitly demonstrated to the therapist through observable behavior. The OPHI-II evaluates occupational adaptation capacity over time. The interest checklist primarily targets volition, and the role checklist targets volition and habituation. The OCAIRS evaluates all three components as well as the client's occupational adaptation capacity. Also, it is important to point out that it is recommended that one receive specialized training in order to be able to administer some of the MOHO instruments (e.g. the ACIS, AMPS).

RATING		DESCRIPTION	COMMENTS
4		Identifies and participates in 3 or more varied interests outside of work	
		Expresses a high level of interest in primary occupation	
		Expresses a high level of satisfaction with both the interest and level of participation	
3		Identifies and participates in 2 interests regularly outside of work	
		Is somewhat interested in primary occupation	
		Expresses satisfaction with either interests and/or level of participation	
2		Identifies 1-2 interests outside of work with inconsistent participation	
		Has little interest in primary occupation	
		Expresses some dissatisfaction with both the interests and/or level of participation	
1		Does not identify or does not participate in any interests	
		Has no interest in primary occupation	
		Expresses strong dissatisfaction with both interests and level of participation	
IM		Unable to obtain information regarding	

Key:

Adaptive | 4 | 3 | 2 | 1 | Maladaptive

IM = Information Missing

Figure 12-2. Sample Item (Interests) from the OCAIRS. (Adapted from Kielhofner G, Forsyth K, Clay C, et al: Talking with clients: assessments that collect information through interviews. In Kielhofner G, ed: *Model of human occupation: theory and application,* Philadelphia, 2002, Lippincott Williams & Wilkins, p. 239.)

	4	3	2	1	IM
Interests		X			
Personal causation				X	
Values			X		
Short-term goals			X		
Long-term goals		X			
Habits				X	
Roles			X		
Motor skills	X				
Process skills			X		
Communication/interaction skills			X		
Previous experiences				X	
Physical environment supports		X			
Physical environment opportunities	X				
Physical environment demands/constraints	X				
Physical environment fit				X	
Social environment supports			X		
Social environment opportunities			X		
Social environment demands/constraints					X
Social environment fit				X	
Occupational participation				X	
Occupational adaptation				X	

Key:
Adaptive | 4 | 3 | 2 | 1 | Maladaptive

IM = Information Missing

Figure 12-3.   An example of a client's ratings on the OCAIRS (revised version). (Adapted from Kielhofner G, Forsyth K, Clay C, et al: Talking with clients: assessments that collect information through interviews. In Kielhofner G, ed: *Model of human occupation: theory and application,* Philadelphia, 2002, Lippincott Williams & Wilkins, p. 239.)

    Refer to Lab Manual Exercise 14-1 to help you learn how to administer choice MOHO assessments.

Therapeutic Intervention

Therapeutic intervention based on the MOHO aims at altering either internal or external components of the heterarchy consisting of the environment, volition, habituation, and performance capacity.[28] It is hypothesized that such alteration would lead to total systemic reorganization, resulting in emergence of new thoughts, feelings, and actions.[28] Consequently, based on evaluation of the client using the instruments described above, therapy goals are established that may be directed toward the environment or any of the other three components. Such goals are consistent with Sames' definition of good therapeutic objectives: relevant, understandable, measurable, behavioral, and attainable within a reasonable length of time.[60] However, some of the goals targeting volition may involve mental processes such as identifying meaningful tasks rather than observable behaviors.

Examples of measurable goals targeting the various components of the human system are as follows:

- Volition—"Within [timeframe], [client] will be *able to identify* [number] of occupational form(s) that are significant to his/her occupational life [or role as a xxx] and which are commensurate with his/her current skills and abilities within [setting] independently [degree]" (p. 341) (emphasis original).[12] Other goals targeting volition may focus on occupational performance, occupational choice, desire to feel a sense of control, and engagement in occupations that are considered valuable.
- Habituation—"Within [timeframe], [client], will be able to *sustain performance* in [name occupational action] involved in reaching their goal, with [degree] support within [setting]" (p. 341) (emphasis original).[12] Other goals targeting this component may aim at facilitating identification of interests to pursue occupations of interest, practicing pertinent skills in order to make them habitual, and development of habits supportive of adaptive functioning.
- Performance—"Within [timeframe], [client] will be able to manage symptoms while engaged in [name the occupational forms] within [setting] independently [degree]" (p. 342).[12]
- Environmental context—"Within [timeframe], [client] will be able to *perform* in the occupational forms they need and/or want to be able to do within [state the physical space] [setting], independently [degree]" (p. 342) (emphasis original).[12] Other goals targeting the environmental context may focus on the client's ability to perform occupations using adaptations needed to overcome physical and social barriers, ability to use caregivers to support one's functioning so as to meet occupa-

tional performance needs, and ability of caregivers to understand the client's occupational performance needs.

Once goals are established, therapeutic intervention is implemented using strategies that are common to occupational therapy and other helping professions such as counseling and psychotherapy. These include "validating, identifying, giving feedback, advising, negotiating, structuring, coaching, encouraging, and providing physical support" (p. 311).[34] These are the same strategies in therapeutic use of relationships discussed in Chapter 7, based on Rogerian client-centered therapeutic principles (see also Chapter 3 in this book and the exercises in Chapters 6 and 8 of the Lab Manual). Interventions target specific components of the human system or the environment as conceptualized in the MOHO. For example, validation may be used to convey respect for the client by demonstrating acceptance of his or her feelings, perspectives, experiences, and so on, as real and important. This addresses the need for the client to feel that he or she is important and has an effect on his or her environment (personal causation, an aspect of volition). Similarly, coaching and encouragement may be used to facilitate

 practice and skill development leading to improved ability to function competently (increasing performance capacity).

Consistency of the Model of Human Occupation with the Occupational Therapy Paradigm

The MOHO is obviously occupation based. Occupational engagement is used as a medium to facilitate system change through emergence of thoughts, feelings, and actions that are adaptive.[34] Intervention using the MOHO is also collaborative since negotiation with the therapist regarding therapeutic goals and interventions is one of the key strategies of therapy using the model. Furthermore, the therapist's role is seen as that of providing an opportunity for engagement in occupation, modifying the environment and educating the client on available environmental resources, providing assistive devices and physical support to facilitate engagement in occupation, and education/counseling by providing feedback, coaching, and so on. Therefore the MOHO is consistent with the current occupational therapy paradigm.

CASE STUDY: JAY

Jay, a 48-year-old Caucasian male, was admitted to the VA hospital with an axis I diagnosis of substance abuse disorder. He and his wife have four children: two sons (ages 28 and 20) and two daughters (ages 26 and 24). Their children are either working or in college. Jay has a very good marriage and lived with his wife in their home of 26 years before admission to the hospital. He spent 8 years in the Navy and is a combat veteran. The medical record indicates that prior to admission at the VA hospital Jay was using cannabis, cocaine, and alcohol almost daily, 20 out of 30 days a month. Eventually, the substance abuse led to impairment in roles. For example, his relationship with his family became strained. However, Jay does not think there is a problem requiring therapeutic intervention for him and his family.

Review of the medical chart revealed that Jay graduated high school and joined the Navy when he was 19 years old. After 8 years in the Navy, he was honorably discharged. Since then, he has worked as a mechanic in a steel plant, a tractor trailer driver, and a construction worker. At the time of the initial interview, Jay was unemployed but was receiving income from the Veterans Disability Administration. In the month before admission, he received $2000 as income from these sources. His wife works as a checkout clerk in a department store and earns about $1000 a month. However, Jay does not think that there is need for intervention to address his worker role. He currently expresses no interest in hobbies/leisure activities, although he played baseball and pool in the past.

Jay has also a history of schizophrenia, depression, and anxiety leading to impairment in cognition as indicated by difficulty remembering, understanding, and concentrating. This is his fifth admission at the hospital. At the initial interview, the therapist found that Jay was able to express himself, although he tended to exaggerate his responses at times. It was also found that Jay had difficulty making decisions on his own and solving complex problems. Even though Jay seems not to have a realistic self-appraisal regarding the extent to which his problem affects his life (e.g., he does not see the strained relationship between him and his family or his lack of employment as a problem), he expresses a strong desire and motivation to change.

Because of Jay's impaired role performance, inability to make decisions, and habits that do not support adaptive occupational engagement, it was determined that the MOHO is the most appropriate conceptual model of practice to help guide his therapy. The OCAIRS[24] was used to evaluate the various components of his person system. A summary of the OCAIRS evaluation is shown in Figure 12-4.

Based on the findings from Jay's evaluation using the OCAIRS, four treatment goals were established for initial intervention (Table 12-2). As Jay progressed in therapy, other goals were established accordingly, until adaptive thoughts, feelings, and actions emerged.

 Refer to Lab Manual Exercise 14-2 to learn about client assessment and treatment planning based on MOHO constructs.

Occupational Case Analysis Interview and Rating Scale

Summary Form

Patient <u>Jay Broom</u>   OT Rater <u>MI</u>   Date <u>9/20/03</u>

Adaptive 5 .... 4 .... 3 .... 2 .... 1 Maladaptive

Personal Causation	2	Jay finds it difficult to make decisions because he has little confidence in his abilities and does not anticipate successful outcome on the basis of his actions.
Values and Goals	1	Jay identified no goals although he is motivated to create change in his life.
Interests	2	States that he used to be interested in baseball and pool and would like to start playing pool again. However, he currently does not actively pursue any leisure activity of interest except ingestion of drugs.
Roles	3	Realistically describes two activities of his role as a husband (working and providing for his family and getting involved in his children's education)
Habits	1	Does not describe a daily schedule of activities
Skills	3	Jay vaguely identifies activities that he may need to do to fulfill his role as a husband and father. He will need skill development, especially in the worker role, which is crucial to his participation in his role as provider for the family.
Output	2	Jay states that he would like to improve his performance but does not seem to be able to integrate skills and routines into competent or satisfying occupational behavior. He does not express dissatisfaction with certain roles such as not being able to have a satisfactory family relationship or being able to work.
Physical Environment	5	Jay has a very supportive wife and children. The Veterans affairs department is also a useful source of support for him.
Social Environment	5	Jay's family is very supportive of his therapy goals.
Feedback	2	Although his family clearly points out problems, Jay does not seem to have insight regarding the gravity of the manifestations of his condition in his life.
Dynamic (Gestalt Functioning)	2	Jay has no clear plan for the future. He is unemployed, his role as a family provider is unfulfilled, and his daily routine consists mostly of substance abuse–related behavior. Thus his performance is very limited.
Historical (Life History Pattern)	3	Jay correctly perceives some of his past functioning (e.g., when he was in the Navy) as adaptive. He is aware that currently he has some problems.
Contextual (Environmental Influence)	2	Jay's environment supports his performance. Therefore he is capable of functioning much better in his environment than he is doing right now.
System Trajectory (Occupational Prognosis)	1	Jay is currently in a continuous maladaptive cycle as indicated by not working, having no healthy leisure pursuits, and having difficulty fulfilling his roles as husband and father.

Figure 12-4. Summary of Jay's assessment using the OCAIRS. Jay's rating is about 2.4 on the adaptive/maladaptive scale as deduced from the average ratings. This indicates that he is clearly in a maladaptive cycle and requires occupational therapy to help him transition to an adaptive cycle.

Table 12-2. Jay's Therapeutic Goals Based on Concepts from the MOHO

Goal	Target System Component
1. Within 2 weeks [timeframe], Jay [client] will be able to identify three possible jobs [occupational forms] commensurate with his experience as a mechanic, tractor trailer driver, and/or construction worker, for which he can apply as a first step toward fulfilling his role as provider for his family.	Volition (identification of relevant activities and making choices)
2. Within 3 weeks [timeframe], Jay [client] will make the choice to engage in a leisure activity such as pool with close friends for at least 1 hour three times a week, having identified this as significant to his establishment of a healthy daily routine of activities that does not involve pernicious use of drug.	Volition and habituation (identification of interests and patterning them into an adaptive routine)
3. Within 2 weeks [timeframe], Jay [client] will be able to spontaneously identify at least three responsibilities for his role as a father and husband during one-on-one therapy sessions with the occupational therapist in the OT department.	Habituation and volition (role-related insight development)
4. Within 3 weeks [timeframe], Jay [client] will develop a detailed resume for each of the three jobs identified in goal #1 that he will use to apply for the job.	Performance capacity (development of job-seeking skills)

Consistency with the Philosophy of Pragmatism

Consistent with the philosophy of pragmatism, the MOHO emphasizes the importance of environmental context in human adaptation. The human system is perceived to function within the environment, which is seen as one of the four factors in a heterarchy of volition, habituation, performance capacity, and the environment. Also, since the initial formulation of the MOHO, volition has been viewed as extremely important. Before revising the model to emphasize heterarchy instead of hierarchy in the human system organization, the volition subsystem was seen as controlling the other subsystems. It consists of personal causation (image of self as an actor or a cause in the environment), ability to make choices, and ability to articulate and pursue interests. Therefore it is clear that this component is consistent with the view in pragmatism of belief as a rule for action since the image of self as an actor, which determines how one chooses and develops interests, constitutes one's beliefs about self, others, and the environment.

Habituation, with its emphasis on habits, roles, and routines, seems to be a direct application of James's view of the central role of habits in human functioning as discussed in Chapter 2. Finally, the emphasis on empowering clients to make choices is consistent with the value of agency in pragmatism. The above few constructs indicate that although not explicitly stated by the originators of the model, the propositions and premises of the MOHO are consistent with those of pragmatism.

Consistency with the Complexity/Chaos Theoretical Framework

From the beginning, systems theory was used as an organizing framework for the MOHO.[32] Systems theory was used to conceptualize the human as a system consisting of three subsystems: volition, habituation, and performance capacity. This focus of the MOHO on the systems perspective has continued to the present. Currently, the organization of the human system is seen as a heterarchical structure consisting of the volitional, habituation, performance capacity, and environmental components.[28,29] Although Kielhofner still refers to this conceptualization as based on the systems theory, it is clear from the current emphasis on the dynamic relationship between the subsystems and emergence of feelings, thoughts, and actions, that the model is now based on the complexity/chaos theoretical framework.

Recommendations for Reinterpretation of the Model

The MOHO is one of the conceptual models of practice in occupational therapy that is consistent with the current occupational therapy paradigm. The only recommendation is that consistency of the model's constructs with pragmatism can be made more explicit. The authors of the model can show how constructs such as volition, habituation, and performance are linked to the philosophy of pragmatism. This direct link can help illustrate the centrality of the model in enhancing the unique identity of the profession. Also, the use of complexity/chaos theory as a theoretical framework for explaining system change can be elaborated. For instance, how could the theoretical framework explain system reorganization that leads to emergence of adaptive thoughts, feelings, and actions? Finally, it may be helpful to develop guidelines of how to choose evaluation instruments. For example, in the cognitive disabilities model, it is clear that the therapist begins with administration of the ACLS. Once it is evident that there are cognitive deficits, other tools (e.g., the ADM, RTI) are used to complete an in-depth evaluation. Such guidance is not so clear in the MOHO.

Evidence-Based Practice Using the Model of Human Occupation

The MOHO is another one of the most researched conceptual models of practice in occupational therapy. Currently, there are over 100 published research papers based on the MOHO, making it the most researched model in the profession, second only to the Sensory Integration model.[31] A significant portion of this research has been directed toward validation of the model's instruments. Some of these instruments have been found to have very good parametric properties. For instance, many studies have indicated that the AMPS is varied and reliable.[3–5,43,48,58]

In a study by Mansson and Lexell,[48] for instance, the concurrent validity of the AMPS was investigated. Scores from 44 clients with multiple sclerosis (MS) on the instrument were compared with those on the Functional Independence Measure (FIM). The FIM is a standardized, commonly used evaluation instrument in rehabilitation, consisting of both motor and cognitive components that measure the level of assistance needed by a client in PADLs. Mansson and Lexell found a significant correlation between the FIM motor and AMPS motor abilities ($r = .38$, $p = .01$), FIM cognitive and AMPS process abilities ($r = .36$, $p = .018$), FIM motor and AMPS process abilities ($r = .46$, $p = .002$), and FIM cognitive and AMPS motor abilities ($r = .14$). In other words, the AMPS scores were significantly positively correlated with FIM scores, indicating that the two instruments measure a similar underlying construct.

In another study involving 20 nondisabled community-living Taiwanese adults, ages 24 to 35 years, Fisher and colleagues found that the AMPS had internal validity for all items except "accommodates," "heeds," and "chooses" as measured and analyzed using the Rasch Mean Square method.[11] There was a good fit of the response patterns for 19 of the 20 participants as predicted, indicating that the AMPS measures process skills as conceptualized. Furthermore, the test-retest reliability of the instrument was found to be excellent ($r = .93$). Finally, they concluded that the process skill scale of the instrument is applicable to the Taiwanese population suggesting that it has cross-cultural relevance.

Outcome studies have also been carried out based on this instrument. For example, in analysis of retrospective data from 348 participants with intellectual disabilities (ID) living in Sweden, the United Kingdom, the United States, Australia, New Zealand, Asia, and Israel, it was found that there were significant differences in performance and motor skills as measured on the AMPS between clients with mild ID compared to those with moderate ID.[45] Individuals with moderate ID had more difficulties in motor and process skills compared to those with mild ID, with an overlap between the two. This indicated that the instrument was able to discriminate between levels of intellectual disability. In another study, Oakley and colleagues compared the ADL functioning of 1213 well older adults living in the community as measured on the AMPS with that of 752 older adults diagnosed with dementia of the Alzheimer's type (DAT).[52] The DAT group was divided into two groups: DAT Min (those with DAT diagnosis and minimum dysfunction) and DAT Max (those with DAT diagnosis and maximum dysfunction). Analysis of Variance (ANOVA) revealed a significant difference in functioning between all the three groups.

Studies have established the validity and reliability of other MOHO assessment instruments. For instance, the older version of the OCAIRS has been found to have good interrater reliability (r = .318 to .812 for all 14 items)[19,23] and good concurrent validity when compared with the Global Assessment Scale (GAS, r = .55).[7] In a later study, Lai and colleagues used Rasch statistics to analyze data collected from 145 psychiatric clients from three psychiatric units.[46] They found that 10 of the 14 OCAIRS items measured the same underlying construct (Occupational Adaptation). Furthermore, they found that Occupational Adaptation seemed to be defined by two constructs: occupational identity and occupational competence. Also, scores on the OCAIRS were able to discriminate between clients with severe psychoses (schizophrenia) and those with less psychotic symptoms (unipolar disorder). The later scored higher than the earlier on the instrument.

The OPHI-II has also been found to have good test-retest reliability (r = .55 to .68) and

interrater reliability (r = .38 to .55) for past occupational behavior.[38] Moderate to poor reliability was established for present behavior. Gray and Fossey found the OPHI-II to be useful for gathering qualitative information regarding occupational performance and changes in performance as a consequence of chronic illness.[18] These examples indicate that the MOHO instruments generally have moderate to good validity and reliability. More information about research investigating the parametric properties of these instruments can be found in Kielhofner,[28-30] Dickerson,[2] Watts and colleagues,[62] and Good-Ellis.[17]

SUMMARY

The Model of Human Occupation was intended to emphasize a focus on occupation in occupational therapy and therefore to support a general professional paradigm whose articulation its authors envisioned as necessary. It was conceived to be based on a general systems theoretical framework in which the human was conceptualized to be an open system. In its initial formulation, it was understood that this system received information from the environment (input). The information was processed in the throughput, and the output was information and action. The throughput was conceived to consist of three hierarchically arranged subsystems: volition, habituation, and performance capacity. The volition subsystem guided choice of occupations, and the habituation subsystem patterned those choices into habits and routines that made efficient role performance possible. The performance capacity subsystem consisted of skills that were necessary for actual performance of occupations. The volition subsystem was seen as being at the top of the hierarchy and controlling other subsystems.

Recently, Kielhofner[28,29] has revised his conceptualization of the model's conceptual framework. The volitional, habituation, performance capacity, and the environmental components of the human system are now seen as constituting a heterarchy in which each part contributes to the overall dynamic of the system, resulting in emergence of thoughts, feelings, and actions that constitute occupational adaptation. In this new view, therapeutic intervention is perceived to be directed toward alteration of any of the four components, leading to reorganization of the entire system.

We also reviewed assessment instruments associated with the model and found that many of the MOHO evaluation instruments have good reliability and validity. We discussed intervention guidelines based on the model, including goal-setting and intervention strategies. Finally, we found that the model is highly consistent with the occupational therapy paradigm, the philosophy of pragmatism, and the complexity/chaos theoretical perspective.

REFERENCES

1. Christiansen C: Occupational therapy intervention for life performance. In Christiansen C, Baum C, eds: *Occupational therapy: overcoming human performance deficits,* Thorofare, NJ, 1991, Slack, pp. 3–43.
2. Dickerson AE: The role checklist. In Hemphill-Pearson BJ, ed: *Assessment in occupational therapy mental health: an integrative approach,* Thorofare, NJ, 1999, Slack, pp. 175–191.
3. Doble SE: Test-retest and inter-rater reliability of a process skills assessment, *Occup Ther J Res* 11:8–23, 1991.
4. Doble SE, Fisk JD, MacPherson KM, et al: Measuring functional competence in older persons with Alzheimer's disease, *Internat Psychogeriatrics* 9:25–38, 1997.
5. Duran LJ, Fisher AG: Male and female performance on the assessment of motor and process skills, *Arch Phys Med Rehabil* 77:1019–1024, 1996.
6. Early MB: *Mental health concepts and techniques for the occupational therapy assistant,* New York, 2000, Lippincott Williams & Wilkins.
7. Endicott J, Spitzer RL, Fleiss JL, et al: The global assessment scale. A procedure for measuring overall severity of psychiatric disturbance, *Arch Gen Psychiatry* 33(6):766–771, 1976.
8. Fisher AG: *Assessment of motor and process skills: development, standardization, and administration manual,* ed 4, vol. 1, Fort Collins, CO, 2001, Three Stars Press.
9. Fisher AG: *Assessment of motor and process skills: user manual,* ed 4, vol. 2, Fort Collins, CO, 2001, Three Stars Press.
10. Fisher AG: *The assessment of motor and process skills (AMPS),* ed 3, Fort Collins, CO, 1999, Three Stars Press.
11. Fisher AG, Liu Y, Velozo CA, et al: Cross-cultural assessment of process skills, *Am J Occup Ther* 46:876–885, 1992.
12. Forsyth K, Kielhofner G: Putting theory into practice. In Kielhofner G, ed: *Model of human occupation: theory and application,* Philadelphia, 2002, Lippincott Williams & Wilkins, pp. 325–345.
13. Forsyth K, Kielhofner G: Model of human occupation. In Kramer P, Hinojosa J, Royeen CB, eds: *Perspectives in human occupation: participation in life,* New York, 2003, Lippincott Williams & Wilkins, pp. 45–86.
14. Forsyth K, Kielhofner G, Blondis M, et al: Assessments combining methods of information gathering. In Kielhofner G, ed: *Model of human occupation: theory and application,* Philadelphia, 2002, Lippincott Williams & Wilkins, pp. 263–279.
15. Forsyth K, Salamy M, Simon S, et al: *The assessment of communication and interaction skills (version 4.0),* Chicago, 1998, Model of Human Occupation Clearinghouse, Department of Occupational Therapy, College of Applied Health Sciences, University of Illinois at Chicago.
16. Goldstein J: The tower of Babel in non-linear dynamics: toward the clarification of terms. In Robertson R, Combs A, eds: *Chaos theory in psychology and the life sciences,* Mahwah, NJ, 1995, Lawrence Erlbaum, pp. 34–45.
17. Good-Ellis MA: The role activity performance scale. In Hemphill-Pearson BJ, ed: *Assessments in occupational therapy mental health: an integrative approach,* Thorofare, NJ, 1999, Slack, pp. 205–226.
18. Gray M, Fossey EM: Illness experience and occupations of people with chronic fatigue syndrome, *Austr Occup Ther J* 50:127–136, 2003.
19. Haglund L, Henriksson C: Testing a Swedish version of OCAIRS on two different patient groups, *Scand J Caring Sci* 8:223–230, 1994.
20. Haglund L, Henriksson C, Crisp M, et al: *The occupational circumstances assessment interview and rating scale (OCAIRS) (version 2.0),* Chicago, 2001, Model of Human Occupation Clearinghouse, Department of Occupational Therapy, College of Applied Health Sciences, University of Illinois at Chicago.
21. Hemphill-Pearson BJ, ed: *Assessments in occupational therapy mental health: an integrative approach,* Thorofare, NJ, 1999, Slack.
22. Henry AD, Mallinson T: The occupational performance history interview. In Hemphill-Pearson BJ, ed: *Assessments in occupational therapy mental health: an integrative approach,* Thorofare, NJ, 1999, Slack, pp. 59–70.

23. Kaplan K: Short-term assessment: the need and a response, *Occup Ther Mental Health* 4:29–45, 1984.
24. Kaplan K, Kielhofner G: *Occupational case analysis interview and rating scale,* Thorofare, NJ, 1989, Slack.
25. Kielhofner G: Temporal adaptation: a conceptual framework for occupational therapy, *Am J Occup Ther* 31:235–242, 1977.
26. Kielhofner G: A model of human occupation, part 2: ontogenesis from the perspective of temporal adaptation, *Am J Occup Ther* 34:657–663, 1980.
27. Kielhofner G: A model of human occupation, part 3: benign and vicious cycles, *Am J Occup Ther* 34:731–737, 1980.
28. Kielhofner G: Dynamics of human occupation. In Kielhofner G, ed: *Model of human occupation: theory and application,* Philadelphia, 2002, Lippincott Williams & Wilkins, pp. 28–43.
29. Kielhofner G: Volition. In Kielhofner G, ed: *Model of human occupation: theory and application,* Philadelphia, 2002, Lippincott Williams & Wilkins, pp. 44–62.
30. Kielhofner G: *Conceptual foundations of occupational therapy,* ed 3, Philadelphia, 2004, FA Davis.
31. Kielhofner G: Personal communication, March 13, 2006.
32. Kielhofner G, Burke JP: A model of human occupation, part I: conceptual framework and content, *Am J Occup Ther* 34:572–581, 1980.
33. Kielhofner G, Burke JP, Igi CH: A model of human occupation, part 4: assessment and intervention, *Am J Occup Ther* 34:777–788, 1980.
34. Kielhofner G, Forsyth K: Therapeutic strategies for enabling change. In Kielhofner G, ed: *Model of human occupation: theory and application,* Philadelphia, 2002, Lippincott Williams & Wilkins, pp. 309–324.
35. Kielhofner G, Forsyth K, Clay C, et al: Talking with clients: assessments that collect information through interviews. In Kielhofner G, ed: *Model of human occupation: theory and application,* Philadelphia, 2002, Lippincott Williams & Wilkins, pp. 237–262.
36. Kielhofner G, Forsyth K, de las Heras CG, et al: Observational assessment. In Kielhofner G, ed: *Model of human occupation: theory and application,* Philadelphia, 2002, Lippincott Williams & Wilkins, pp. 191–212.
37. Kielhofner G, Forsyth K, Federico J, et al: Self-report assessments. In Kielhofner G, ed: *Model of human occupation: theory and application,* Philadelphia, 2002, Lippincott Williams & Wilkins, pp. 213–236.
38. Kielhofner G, Henry AD: Development and investigation of the occupational performance history interview, *Am J Occup Ther* 42:489–498, 1988.
39. Kielhofner G, Henry AD, Walens D: *Occupational performance history interview,* Rockville, MD, 1989, American Occupational Therapy Association.
40. Kielhofner G, Mallinson T, Crawford C, et al: *The occupational performance history interview (version 2.0) OPHI-II,* Chicago, 1998, Model of Human Occupation Clearinghouse, Department of Occupational Therapy, College of Applied Health Sciences, University of Illinois at Chicago.
41. Kielhofner G, Mallinson T, Forsyth K, et al: Psychometric properties of the second version of the occupational performance history interview (OPHI-II), *Am J Occup Ther* 55:260–267, 2001.
42. Kielhofner G, Neville A: *The modified interest checklist,* unpublished manuscript, Chicago, 1983, University of Illinois at Chicago.
43. Kirkley KN, Fisher AG: Alternate forms reliability of the assessment of motor and process skills, *J Outcome Measurement* 1:53–70, 1999.
44. Kjellberg A, Haglund L, Forsyth K, et al: The measurement properties of the Swedish version of the assessment of communication and interaction skills, *Scand J Caring Sci* 17:271–277, 2003.
45. Kottorp A, Bernspang B, Fisher AG: Activities of daily living in persons with intellectual disability: strengths and limitations in specific motor and process skills, *Austr Occup Ther J* 50:195–204, 2003.
46. Lai J, Haglund L, Kielhofner G: Occupational case analysis interview and rating scale: an examination of construct validity, *Scand J Caring Sci* 13:267–273, 1999.
47. Linacre JM: *FACETS* version 3.20 [Computer program], Chicago, 1999, MESA.
48. Mansson E, Lexell J: Performance of activities of daily living in multiple sclerosis, *Disabil Rehabil* 26:576–585, 2004.
49. Matsutsuyu JS: The interest checklist, *Am J Occup Ther* 23:323–328, 1969.
50. Meyer A: The philosophy of occupational therapy, *Am J Occup Ther* 31:639–642, 1977.
51. Miller RJ: Gary Kielhofner. In Miller RJ, Walker KF, eds: *Perspectives on theory for the practice of occupational therapy,* Gaithersburg, MD, 1993, Aspen, pp. 179–218.
52. Oakley F, Duran L, Fisher A, et al: Differences in activities of daily living motor skills of persons with and without Alzheimer's disease, *Austr Occup Ther J* 50:72–78, 2003.
53. Oakley F, Kielhofner G, Barris R: An occupational therapy approach to assessing psychiatric patients' adaptive functioning, *Am J Occup Ther* 39:147–154, 1985.
54. Oakley F, Kielhofner G, Barris R, et al: The role checklist: development and empirical assessment of reliability, *Occup Ther J Res* 6:157–170, 1986.
55. Reilly M: 1962 Eleanor Clarke Slagle lecture—Occupational therapy can be one of the great ideas of 20th century medicine, *Am J Occup Ther* 16:1–9, 1962.

56. Reilly M: Defining a cobweb. In Reilly M, ed: *Play as exploratory learning*, Beverly Hills, CA, 1974, Sage, pp. 57–116.

57. Reilly M: An explanation of play. In Reilly M, ed: *Play as exploratory learning*, Beverly Hills, CA, 1974, Sage, pp. 117–149.

58. Robinson SE, Fisher AG: A study to examine the relationship of the assessment of motor and process skills (AMPS) to other tests of cognition and function, *Br J Occup Ther* 59:260–263, 1996.

59. Rogers J, Weinstein J, Figone J: The interest checklist: an empirical assessment, *Am J Occup Ther* 32:628–630, 1978.

60. Sames KM: *Documenting occupational therapy practice,* Upper Saddle River, NJ, 2005, Pearson/Prentice-Hall.

61. Scaffa ME: *Temporal adaptation and alcoholism,* Unpublished master's project, 1981, Virginia Commonwealth University.

62. Watts JH, Hinson R, Madigan MJ, et al: The assessment of occupational functioning—collaborative version. In Hemphill-Pearson BJ, ed: *Assessments in occupational therapy mental health: an integrative approach,* Thorofare, NJ, 1999, Slack, pp. 193–203.

13
The Sensory Processing/Motor Learning Conceptual Model of Practice

Preview Questions

1. Discuss the origin of the Sensory Processing/ Motor Learning (SP/ML) conceptual model of practice in Ayre's Sensory Integration (SI) frame of reference and Rood's Neurodevelopmental Theory (NDT).
2. Explain the rationale for application of the SP/ML model of practice in psychosocial rehabilitation and specifically when working with clients diagnosed with chronic nonparanoid-type schizophrenia.
3. Apart from SI and NDT, explain other interdisciplinary sources of constructs used in the SP/ML conceptual model of practice.
4. Concisely state the theoretical core of the SP/ML conceptual model of practice.
5. Explain postulations of the SP/ML conceptual model of practice about the following:
   a. Function
   b. Dysfunction
   c. Change
6. Outline and explain the SP/ML model's guidelines for client evaluation and therapeutic intervention.
7. Discuss the consistency of the SP/ML conceptual model of practice with each of the following:
   a. The occupational therapy paradigm
   b. The philosophy of pragmatism
   c. The complexity/chaos theoretical framework
8. Discuss available empirical evidence supporting clinical effectiveness of the SP/ML conceptual model of practice as a guide to intervention in occupational therapy practice.

Bruce and Borg discuss what they call the "sensory motor model," which is a combination of sensory integration (SI) theory and constructs from the motor control (MC) tradition.[14] They see the model as

> directed toward an adolescent or adult population identified as having CNS dysfunction, typically having behavior and performance problems, and often having psychiatric diagnoses. This population is believed to have problems with processing sensation into normal, fluid movement, which in turn relates to impoverished body image, confidence, and task and social behavior. Therapeutic occupation is selected according to its neurophysiological properties and its ability to enhance the opportunity for an integrated, organized response (p. 302).[14]

This model is based on King's[23] proposed sensory-integrative approach to the treatment of clients with schizophrenia. Bruce and Borg see approaches from the motor control model as the domain of physical rehabilitation in occupational therapy where they are "termed 'neuromotor,' 'motor learning,' or 'sensorimotor'" (p. 302).[14] However, a literature review reveals that, from the very beginning of the use of SI techniques to treat clients with psychiatric conditions, constructs were borrowed from the Neurodevelopmental Theory (NDT), which is a part of what has evolved into the motor learning/motor control (ML/MC) theory.[26,35,41,42] Rood's approach was in particular central to King's[23] proposed application of SI to treat clients with chronic nonparanoid schizophrenia. Thus SI and ML principles were used in combination in psychosocial occupational therapy rehabilitation. SI interventions can be integrated with contemporary ML approaches consisting of posing environmental challenges in form of occupations to facilitate development of coordinated adaptive movements in the client. It is proposed that the integrated model be referred to as the Sensory Processing/Motor Learning (SP/ML) conceptual model of practice.

The theoretical core of the SP/ML model will be presented as follows: we will discuss the SI theory developed by A. Jean Ayres. We will also examine the Rood approach, which has been mentioned repeatedly in literature discussing application of SI in psychosocial occupational therapy. We will then discuss the combined SI and Rood's NDT approaches, emphasizing incorporation of the current motor control concepts derived from the complexity/chaos theory. We will propose a concise statement of the model's theoretical core integrating constructs from SI, Rood's NDT, and contemporary MC theory. Later we will examine the model's postulations about function, dysfunction, and change. We will also expound the guidelines for evaluation and intervention using the model and their consistency with the current occupational therapy paradigm, the philosophy of pragmatism, and the complexity/chaos theory. Finally, we will evaluate research evidence supporting the clinical validity and effectiveness of the model.

Theoretical Base

Ayres was an occupational therapist as well as a psychologist and neuroscientist. Therefore the SI theory was based on constructs borrowed from developmental psychology, educational psychology, neuroscience, and the theory of evolution. Rood's NDT approach also drew constructs from physiology, neuroscience, and human development. These are the scientific sources of constructs used in the SP/ML model.

Background
Ayre's Sensory Integration Theory

The SI theory was developed for use with children who have developmental and learning disorders.[4-6] While observing these children, Ayres noticed that they exhibited certain clusters of behaviors including distractibility, irritability with sensory stimulation, and hyporesponsiveness or hyperresponsiveness to sensory stimulation, particularly tactile or vestibular sensations. She disagreed with the then prevailing view that the source of these characteristics was visual-perceptual difficulties and hypothesized that they were the result of underlying difficulty of the brain to integrate sensory information and make use of it to generate adaptive responses.

One of the basic propositions of the SI theory is that the nervous system mediates sensory input and enables an individual to interact with the environment. Ayres[2] asserted that the development of the nervous system to its current status (the intelligent human) was an evolutionary process. This assertion was based on the phylogenetic principle that in order to survive, the human organism had to interact successfully with its environment. This denoted that the nervous system had to change continually in order to adapt to the demands of the environment. This means that environmental input modified the human nervous system successively over thousands of years, resulting in the intelligent human that exists today.

According to Ayres, in the development of the nervous system, higher centers developed phylogenetically later and were built on to earlier structures. For this reason, function of the higher centers is dependent on lower centers. For example, the functioning of the cerebral cortex is dependent on the effectiveness of the brainstem in integrating sensory information from the environment. One of her central postulations in SI theory was therefore that the brainstem is responsible for integrating sensory input from the environment so that the cerebral cortex can make use of it. The entire theory of SI is based on this postulation.

In addition to phylogenetic theory, Ayres proposed that the development of the nervous system of the individual is ontogenetic, recapitulating the development of the entire human species through the evolutionary process.[8] Therefore systems that were crucial to the survival of the species, such as the somatosensory systems (tactile, gustatory, olfactory, proprioceptive, and vestibular), develop earlier than those that were initially not so crucial to species survival such as visual-spatial and perceptual systems. Indeed, the earlier systems mature in utero, much earlier than the later. Ayres concluded that the systems that matured earlier (tactile, gustatory, olfactory, proprioceptive, and vestibular) could be used for intervention to help individuals with sensory processing difficulties develop sensory modulation capacity and consequently adaptive behaviors.

Based on Ayres' conclusion, the SI is based on several assumptions:

1. The central nervous system (CNS) is plastic (it can be modified by sensory experiences from the environment).
2. The maturing of SI recapitulates the evolutionary development of the systems, such that those systems that were historically crucial to the survival of human species mature earlier in the developing human baby than the others.
3. The brain functions as a whole integrated unit, with hierarchically organized subsystems, where the higher CNS centers (the cerebral cortex) control the rest of the nervous system. Because the lower centers (e.g., the brainstem) were essential to the survival of the human species, they were designed to be functionally independent and autonomous. Therefore they constrain higher centers.

4. Adaptation to the environment is based on the organism's ability to integrate sensory information. Adaptive responses to environmental demands in turn facilitate development of SI capacity.

Based on the above four assumptions, it can be asserted that the ability to function within the environment (adaptation) is based on the ability to take in sensory information from diverse sources through movement and interaction with the environment, process and integrate the information within the CNS, and use it to plan, organize, and act.[5,15,36] This enables the human to learn from the environment through interaction with it. In other words, through movement, interaction with the environment, and organization of sensory information for use in adaptive behavior, the human forms a picture of self in the world (body schema that subsequently develops into self-concept), which in turn guides performance within the environment. When the ability to receive sensory information and integrate it effectively is impaired, an individual perceives normal sensory information (e.g., tactile sensation, movement) as threatening.[3,40] Alternatively, the sensory information may not be perceived at all. This is manifested as hyperresponsiveness to sensory stimulation (e.g., getting agitated when touched, inability to tolerate movement) or hyporesponsiveness (inability to react or decreased reaction to sensory input).

Ayres[9] particularly emphasized the importance of the vestibular system as an anchor for all other SI systems because of its role in helping the person resolve his or her relationship with gravity. This ability to relate to gravity is the basis of movement, through which perception of all other forms of sensory information is possible. This system therefore is of particular importance in SI-based therapeutic interventions. Manifestations of its dysfunction include defective postrotary nystagmus (which may be either decreased in duration and frequency, or increased dysrhythmic nystagmus).[5,6] According to Ayres, measures of deficits in sensory processing may be grouped into two categories[5,6,24]: (1) direct measure of vestibular response, which consists of nystagmus (postrotary), postural (standing balance, eyes open, and eyes closed), and ocular responses, and (2) indirect measures of vestibular response such as deficits in proprioceptive processing, as indicated by "finger-to-nose" exercises, diodo-chokinesia, and serial opposition.

Ultimately, the functional effects of SI dysfunction include loss of fluidity of movement, which negatively affects body image, right-left discrimination, position in space, visual-perceptual processing, finger identification, motor planning (praxis), ability to recognize objects by touch, perceptual-motor learning, self-confidence, and task and social behavior.[14,15] Based on the theoretical postulations of SI, Ayres developed several instruments to measure SI dysfunction and its manifestations.[6,8] These are the Southern California Sensory Integration Test (SCSIT), which later became the Sensory Integration and Praxis Test (SIPT),[10,40] and the Southern California Post-Rotary Nystagmus Test (PRT). We will discuss sensory integration evaluation using these tests later.

Motor Learning Principles: The Rood Neurodevelopmental Theory Approach

Four neurodevelopmental facilitative therapeutic approaches have been used in occupational therapy for some time, especially in pediatrics and rehabilitation of neurological conditions such as cerebrovascular accident (CVA). These approaches are the Rood approach, the Bobath approach, movement therapy, and the proprioceptive neuromuscular facilitation (PNF) approach.[22] In this chapter, we will discuss the Rood approach in detail since it has been incorporated in the sensory motor approach to the treatment of psychiatric clients since its inception.[14,23,24]

The ML theory in general is based on the basic proposition that development of motor control (MC) is necessary for coordinated movement and thus for effective interaction with the environment. In order for organized movement to take place, one has to be able to take in sensory input from the environment and, using the CNS, process it and use it to generate motor response. One can already see similarities between this argument and SI principles. This is because Ayres derived the principles of SI in part from the NDT.[40] Initially, the ML theory was based on Adams' closed-loop hypothesis[1] based on the concept that motor behavior is based on constant postural adjustments as a response to feedback from the environment and from inside the muscles. The feedback mechanism was perceived to be based on a simple neurophysiological idea of reflexes.

The basic postulation was that for skeletal muscles to function appropriately, the brain needs to be constantly fed with information about the status of those muscles.[25] There is a direct relationship between the brain and the skeletal muscles. The brain exerts its influence on the muscles so that they can maintain a healthy tone, which is defined as "resistance to active or passive stretch at rest" (p. 448).[25]

The continuous interchange between the brain and the muscles depends on the proprioceptors in the skeletal muscles and their tendons. These proprioceptors transmit information to the cerebral cortex via the cerebellum. There are two types of proprioceptors: the *muscle spindles* and the *Golgi tendon organs*. Muscle spindles are found deep within skeletal muscles. They consist of modified skeletal muscle fibers known as the *intrafusal muscle fibers*. The central regions of these fibers do not have myofilaments and therefore are not contractile. They are wrapped by afferent or receptive nerve endings that receive and transmit sensory information to the CNS and therefore act as the receptor surfaces of the spindles. The nerve endings are known as *type Ia sensory fibers*, which are sensitive to the rate and amount of stretch in the spindle.

The second type of nerve endings, known as secondary or *type II sensory fibers*, innervate the ends of the spindles and therefore are sensitive to stretch only. The ends of muscle spindles are the only regions of the fibers that are contractile. They are innervated by efferent or motor fibers known as *gamma efferent fibers,* which originate from the ventral horn of the spinal cord. These nerve fibers transmit stimulation from the CNS to the muscle spindles to maintain their sensitivity. Superficial to the muscle spindles are large, voluntary fibers of the muscles, which contain myofilaments that make them contractile. These fibers are known as the *extrafusal muscle fibers* and are innervated by the *alpha efferent fibers* or *motor neurons.* Excitation of the motor neurons causes contraction of the extrafusal muscle fibers.

Muscle spindles are stimulated either by external stretch, as occurs when one carries a heavy load, or by internal stretch caused by stimulation of the gamma efferent fibers of the contractile ends of the spindles. Irrespective of whether stimulation is external or internal, the stretch in the muscle spindle causes a stimulation of type Ia afferent fibers innervating their midsections. The fibers carry the signals to the spinal cord where they synapse with the alpha motor neurons innervating the extrafusal muscle fibers. The afferent fibers also synapse with the gamma efferent neurons innervating the contractile ends of the muscle spindles. The extrafusal muscle fibers contract to counteract the stretch. The sensory neurons also synapse with branches of the motor neurons innervating antagonistic muscles whose stimulation causes them to relax to allow the agonists to contract. As agonists contract, tension in the muscle spindle decreases leading to a decrease in stimulation of the sensory fibers and subsequent reduction in the firing of the gamma neurons. Through these changes, the brain is constantly informed of the state of tension in the muscle spindle and therefore the contractile status of muscles. Contraction of the agonist and antagonist muscles is balanced, making it possible to achieve smooth movement.

The *Golgi tendon organs* are receptors found in muscle tendons, and their role is to ensure onset and smooth termination of muscle contraction.[25] When a muscle contracts, the Golgi tendon organ senses tension in the tendon and transmits the information to the spinal cord. The information is relayed to the cerebellum and

cerebral cortex. The cortex sends motor signals to the spinal cord that are transmitted to the muscles through the gamma and alpha motor neurons, causing relaxation of the muscles and contraction of the antagonists.

Neuroscientists also suggest that the state of excitation of the reticular formation affects the firing of the gamma and alpha motor neurons and therefore the status of muscle tension and contraction. The word *reticular* is derived from the Latin word *reticulum,* which means "network."[27] Therefore the term *reticular formation* refers to a network of nerve fibers. In the spinal cord, spinal nerves are organized into tracts. Sensory nerves become ascending tracts, and motor nerves originating from the cerebral cortex are descending tracts. The reticular formation (nerve network) begins at the upper part of the spinal cord and then ascends through the medulla, pons, brainstem, and finally part of the limbic system. The formation then fans out so that the network involves most of the brain. The ascending reticular formation, which is made up of sensory nerve fibers, is referred to as the *ascending reticular activating system* (ARAS) and the descending network, consisting of motor neurons, is known as the *descending reticular activating system* (DRAS).

The ARAS regulates and facilitates sensory impulses reaching the cerebral cortex and therefore acts as a sieve that filters sensory information. In this way, it regulates the state of consciousness, wakefulness, and alertness. When there is sensory input, the system is activated and one becomes alert and awake. On the other hand, the DRAS seems to have an inhibitory influence to the nervous system. Therefore when activated, it causes sleep or a slow drift into unconsciousness. Since the network passes through the limbic system, which is closely associated with emotions, it may be safe to deduce that the state of reticular system activation is also dependent on emotions, which would suggest that emotions can either arouse or sedate us.

Based on the neurophysiological activity of the RAS and the proprioceptive receptors as described, occupational therapists using SI and NDT aim at reeducating higher centers of the CNS, in the hope of facilitating their control of motor behavior by modulating lower-level reflexes. A variety of sensory stimulation methods are used to achieve this objective. In sensory integration, tactile, vestibular, and proprioceptive forms of stimulation are provided as an effort to elicit an adaptive response.[36,38] Such sensory input consists of joint compression, brushing, physical positioning, rotating, and so on.[14] The vestibular system is particularly targeted in this approach to therapy because of its perceived central role in modulating sensory information through the RAS, resulting in free, confident, movement.[5,7,9]

Margaret Rood, whose work was cited by proponents of SI techniques in psychiatry,[14,23] developed a neuromuscular facilitation approach to therapy based on the rationale that

> Motor patterns are developed from fundamental reflex patterns present at birth which are utilized and gradually modified through sensory stimuli until the highest control is gained on the conscious cortical level. It seemed to me then, that if it were possible to apply proper sensory stimuli to the appropriate sensory receptor as it is utilized in normal sequential development, it might be possible to elicit motor responses reflexly and by following neurophysiological principles, establish proper motor engrams (p. 74).[39]

In Rood's therapeutic approach, sensory stimulation is used to elicit reflexive motor response by the following:

1. Normalizing muscle tone through brushing, stroking, or icing in order to provide sensory input to muscle spindles and the Golgi tendon organs. The type and rate of sensory input determines whether these proprioceptive receptors are stimulated or inhibited. For instance, light and fast brushing, fast stroking, and icing the muscle belly stimulates the receptors. This type of input is used for clients who are hypotonic. Stimulation of the proprioceptive receptors leads to increased firing of motor fibers synapsing with those receptors, which leads to increased muscle tone in the muscles controlled by those fibers. On the other hand, deep, slow stroking, covering the client with a blanket to increase neutral warmth, and so on, causes relaxation of muscle spindles and Golgi tendon organs and subsequent decrease in tension in related motor fibers with a corresponding decrease in muscle tone in related muscles. This is useful for a client who is hypertonic.

2. Assessing motor control follows normalization of muscle tone. Motor patterns are observed in the same sequence as they occur in normal motor development. For example, in normal development of motor control in a baby, the sequence is usually supine withdrawal, rolling over, pivoting in prone position, neck cocontraction, supporting self on elbows, on all fours, standing, and then walking. In each of those developmental positions, reflex integration hypothetically occurs in order to allow normal movement and postural control appropriate for that developmental level. As an illustration, in order to sustain the supine withdrawal position, the baby needs to integrate the tonic labyrinthine reflex (TLR) to allow contraction of the flexors while antagonists are facilitated to contract reflexly. Without integration of the TLR, the baby would not be able to sustain flexion while in supine position. Evaluation in the Rood approach includes assessment of muscle tone, the degree to which there is voluntary movement, and the extent to which that movement is what would be expected of the prevailing developmental stage. Age-appropriate movement indicates integration of reflexes to allow motor control by higher centers of the central nervous system consistent with that age of development.[39,41]

3. After reflex integration and status of voluntary motor movement have been established, facilitation of motor control (where there are deficits) begins. The client is placed in various developmental positions (e.g., supine, prone, on all fours, standing) as appropriate.

Proprioceptive input such as brushing, icing, and stroking are used as described earlier to normalize the muscle tone so that the client is able to hold the postural position. Once the client is able to hold the developmental position, purposeful activities that require contraction of muscles required for maintenance of that posture while at the same time moving in and out of the posture are provided. For example, a client with CVA may be engaged in a kitchen activity requiring picking up dishes and putting them in the cabinets above her shoulders. This activity requires her to maintain the standing position while moving in and out of the position of balance. Rood believed that this type of intervention facilitates regaining of motor control by higher CNS centers and inhibition of reflexes as indicated.[39,41]

Combined Sensory Integration and Rood's Neurodevelopmental Theory

Rood's techniques constitute one of a group of therapeutic approaches referred to collectively as neurodevelopmental theories (NDT) because they focus on the normal human developmental sequence in their assessments and therapeutic interventions.[43] In recent years, these techniques have undergone at least two substantial changes.

First, the original NDT approaches were based on a closed-loop motor learning theory as proposed by Adams.[1] Motor function was viewed as based on a hierarchical model where higher CNS centers controlled the lower centers. The emphasis in these theories was motor development through integration of reflexes.[26] The environment was perceived to provide feedback (sensory cues from both within the body, i.e., from the muscle spindles and Golgi tendon organs, and from the environment, i.e., environmental conditions). Based on these cues, the CNS guided the musculoskeletal system to make adjustments for well-controlled, smooth movements. Therefore "human movement was the summation or combination of reflexes" (p. 733).[26]

Later, when Schmidt[37] developed an alternative open-loop schema theory of motor learning,

the NDT principles changed accordingly.[26,35,41] The open-loop schema of motor control is derived from the argument that motor control is based on generalized motor programs (GMP) in the cerebral cortex. The schema results from an individual's experiences in the environment. It enables one to anticipate changes in environmental conditions and adjust movement accordingly, even before those conditions are experienced. According to Schmidt, the shortcoming of the theory of feedback is that if movement was based purely on feedback, one would not be able to adapt effectively because many times one needs to adjust behavior before observing its effects in order to avoid possible catastrophic consequences. In other words, in Schmidt's theory, motor control is based on feed-forward rather than feedback as assumed by Adams.[1]

In later NDT approaches, the schema theory has been abandoned altogether in favor of a systems perspective as proposed by Bernstein,[13] where movement is seen as an attempt by the central nervous system to solve the varied degrees of freedom (which refers to movement components that are free to vary) so as to effect smooth functional movement.[35] This is the basis of task-oriented approaches to motor control (MC) therapy that are currently commonly used.[18,26] In this more current view, MC is perceived to be attained through soft assembly of coordinative structures in the process of accomplishing a motor task. Coordinative structures are groups of muscles and neural units that act together in order to achieve the movement needed to accomplish a task. Soft assembly means that the necessary components for the desired movement are assembled in the process of doing something.

The second substantial change is that currently there are two views of NDT[42]:

1. Therapists who view NDT as it was initially conceived see it as "a unique intervention approach" (p. 246).[42] This view is commonly held by pediatric occupational therapists specializing in

cerebral palsy, whose focus is primarily motor control.

2. Other therapists no longer see NDT as a unique conceptual model of practice, but rather as a blended approach consisting of such elements as handling, movement, sensory input, and use of verbal feedback. For these therapists, "A blended approach includes aspects of *sensory integration intervention (somatosensory and vestibular influences on movement),* the use of sensory cues and feedback in adapting movement, the practice of motor skills in functional contexts (motor learning), functional occupation-focused intervention, and consideration of cognitive-emotional-social aspects of motivation and meaning making" (p. 246, emphasis mine).[42] This view seems to be based on a combination of SI and NDT, in a similar manner to what was proposed by King[23] and as being applied currently in psychosocial occupational therapy.[14]

Application of Sensory Processing/Motor Learning Model in Psychiatry

King observed that patients diagnosed with nonparanoid type schizophrenia tended to have some common characteristics: (1) an *S*-curve posture, (2) shuffling gait, (3) inability to raise their arms straight over their head, (4) head and shoulder girdle immobility, (5) flexion, adduction, and internal rotation of arms and legs when in a sitting or standing position, and (6) normal hand dysfunction with weakness of grip.[23]

Based on the above observations, King suggested that the etiology of schizophrenia could be

defective proprioceptive feedback mechanisms, the vestibular component in particular being first underreactive, and second, underactive in its role in the sensorimotor integration process. This defect, whether genetic, developmental, or the result of trauma, constitutes an important etiological or prodromal factor in process and reactive schizophrenia (p. 530).[23]

Drawing from the work of A. Jean Ayres, King concluded that the SI theory can be used to explain the characteristics observed in the nonparanoid type of schizophrenia. For instance, she hypothesized that "The lack of perceptual constancy caused by faulty sensory integration may be the mechanism that produces hallucinations" (p. 532).[23] To support her hypothesis, she cited numerous research studies that seemed to suggest that there was vestibular system involvement in schizophrenia. For example, it was found that patients diagnosed with schizophrenia had underreactive vestibular systems as indicated by abnormalities in postrotary nystagmus, and inability to process both visual and vestibular stimuli at the same time.

Furthermore, King suggested that vestibular involvement could be used to explain the *S*-curve schizophrenic posture, which was probably a regression to primitive labyrinthine reflex, characterized by flexion, internal rotation, and adduction. She concurred with Feldenkrais'[17] suggestion that the *S*-posture had primitive survival value since it placed the organism in the best position to survive in case of a fall. Fear of falling is a typical response manifested as vestibular system dysfunction. Feldenkrais had suggested that fear was the primal source of all anxiety. King continued to cite other research that indicated that movement through space (vestibular stimulation) was associated with pleasure. Another sign of vestibular involvement in schizophrenia was corticalization of movement.

Because of impaired balance, clients with schizophrenia had to think about every movement. In other words, automaticity of movement was impaired. King hypothesized that this impairment was the source of psychomotor retardation, impaired speech, and perseveration of thought, speech, and motor behavior (typical clinical features of schizophrenia). In an attempt to explain the significance of corticalization of movement in motor dysfunction for schizophrenic clients, the influence of Rood's NDT theory on King's thought was evident in her statement: "Rood points out that the phasic muscles, which are largely responsible for willed or cortically directed movement, require nine times as much energy as the tonic or sub cortically directed muscles" (p. 533).[23]

Because of the vestibular involvement and subsequent motor retardation, clients with schizophrenia were unable to engage in activities requiring movement, such as running, jumping, and so on. Poor proprioceptive feedback was also blamed for concrete associations and flat affect because proprioception was responsible for toning the reticular activating system (RAS), which enhanced the level of arousal necessary for abstract thinking and facial expression. Therefore King suggested that activities chosen for treatment of clients with schizophrenia should be those geared toward altering posture and increasing movement. She integrated Rood's NDT principles by recommending that activities requiring heavy work patterns of tonic muscle groups be used (in an attempt to facilitate proprioceptive feedback from joints and tendons). Such activities, she argued, should be subcortical, pleasurable, lead to a feeling of mastery and achievement, provide vestibular stimulation, require bilateral use of tonic muscles against resistance, counter primitive labyrinthine and tonic neck reflexes, provide tactile stimulation, and provide proprioceptive feedback from joints and tendons. The activities used could be recreational, involving objects such as a parachute, balloons, beach balls, and beanbag chairs, or purposeful (task-oriented). She insisted that because clients with schizophrenia lacked motivation and self-confidence, activities requiring competition should be avoided.

Ross[30-32] adopted King's ideas but disagreed with her assertion that cognitive level activities be avoided when designing therapeutic intervention for clients with schizophrenia. Instead, she proposed that activities that were more cognitive, such as verbalization, reflection, and reasoning be used, in addition to those that provided sensory input and evoked

motor response. Some research has been conducted to test some of the ideas of the SP/ML model.[16,24,29] We will discuss these studies later in the chapter.

The Theoretical Core of the Sensory Processing/Motor Learning Model

Based on the background presented above, the theoretical core of the SP/ML model may be stated as follows. Human adaptation is the ability to take in sensory information from both within the body (the muscle spindles and Golgi tendon organs) and from the environment, organize it by inhibiting or facilitating its flow through the nerve junctions as necessary, understand the environment, and use this understanding to build neural pathways that allow free, confident movement. Movement as a result of sensory cues from within and without the body depends on motor skills attained within a person's contexts (motor learning), and the personal, cognitive-emotional as well as social meaning of the task that one aims to accomplish through the movement. Modulation of sensory information and organization of movement (motor response) occurs through soft assembly of coordinative structures. Groups of muscles whose contraction is necessary for the desired movement to be achieved, along with neural pathways necessary for control of contraction of those muscle groups, come together in the process of performing a motor task to effect the movement necessary to accomplish the task.

The etiology of some psychiatric conditions, particularly schizophrenia, may be the CNS dysfunction, specifically, deficits in the vestibular and proprioceptive systems, and sensory integration dysfunction. These deficits make it difficult for them to take in sensory information, organize it, and use it to effect smooth, controlled, and effective movement. Deficits in motor control in turn lead to motor retardation, lack of motivation, poor body-image and self-concept, impaired right-left discrimination and position in space, visual perceptual deficits, finger agnosia, apraxia, astereognosis, and generalized feelings of inadequacy and loss of pleasure.[15,23,24,30–32] Clients with these deficits are maladaptive.

Postulations About Function, Dysfunction, and Change

Function

Function is the ability to take in sensory information from multiple sources, modulate it, and use it to generate movement necessary to perform required tasks and engage in occupations and roles adequately and effectively in order to adapt to the environment. This means that a functional individual is one who is able to use sensory information to organize coordinative structures and produce controlled motor activity in order to meet challenges from both physical and social environments.

Dysfunction

Dysfunction, as viewed in this model, is inability to modulate sensory information from multiple sources, organize it, and build neural pathways that facilitate free, confident movement. Deficiency in sensory modulation ability leads to decreased capacity to organize coordinative structures as necessary for effective motor control required for planning and producing adaptive motor behavior. This lack of motor control results in retarded functional movement and inability to respond to environmental challenges through engagement in occupations and roles as appropriate.

Change

The view of change in this model is based on several assumptions[14]: (1) psychiatric problems are neurologically based, (2) psychiatry clients are capable of learning, and (3) learning denotes ability to modulate sensory input, make sense of it, and generate functional movement. Therefore therapeutic intervention aims at mediating sensory integrative problems by providing controlled sensory input that does not overwhelm the client and can be processed adequately in order to produce an adaptive motor response.

Guidelines for Client Evaluation and Therapeutic Intervention

Client Evaluation

Ayres hypothesized that body schema is the basis for movement and it depends on accurate visual-spatial perception and perception of proprioceptive and cutaneous sensations.[5] Based on this hypothesis, she developed the Southern California Sensory Integration Test (SCSIT). This instrument consisted of several subtests that assessed perception of form in space, motor accuracy, tactile sensation, figure-ground perception, imitation of body postures, bilateral motor coordination, crossing body midline, standing balance, and right-left discrimination. She also developed the Southern California Post Rotary Nystagmus Test (SCPRNT),[8] which was specifically designed to evaluate the functioning of the vestibular system. The Southern California Sensory Integration Test has since been renormed and refined several times, evolving into what is currently known as the Sensory Integration and Praxis Test (SIPT).[11] A detailed description of the contents of these tests can be found in the original tests and in many occupational therapy pediatrics textbooks.

The above discussed tests were developed for evaluation of sensory integration capacity for children with learning disabilities.[5,7–9,11] Not many SI assessments are available for adults. This is one of the reasons that application of SI in the treatment of adult clients has been criticized.[14] Parts of the SCSIT have been used to evaluate the postural and bilateral integration of clients with schizophrenia.[16] Other assessments that have been used include a "draw-a-person" test to evaluate body schema and a "step" test to evaluate balance and motor coordination.[29] The Draw-A-Person test consists of asking the client simply to draw a person. The step test consists of the client being asked to step on and off an 18-inch-high stool as fast as possible for 30 seconds. Later, Ross and Burdick[34] developed a training manual for use by therapists and teachers working with regressed psychiatric and geriatric clients. Evaluation of motor control is accomplished by observing the client to determine if there is persistence of primitive reflexes such as the tonic labyrinthine reflex[16] and noting the client's posture and gait.[29]

According to Lindquist,[24] psychiatric client evaluation using this model consists mainly of both direct and indirect measures of the vestibular system. The Vestibular Function Inventory (VFI) is used to provide a direct measure. It includes observation of duration, frequency, and rhythm of postrotary nystagmus, and postural response to vestibular stimulation as measured by duration of standing balance, both with eyes open and closed. The indirect measure of vestibular response is proprioception, which is assessed by observation of motor coordination in the finger-to-nose test, test of diodochokinesis (ability to perceive distances correctly and reach for objects with accuracy), and serial finger opposition. It is however clear that the assessment instruments based on this conceptual model for use with adult psychiatric clients are not well developed.

Therapeutic Intervention

The overarching goal of therapy guided by this model is "to bring about an organized, adaptive whole-person response" (p. 314)[14] of the client to environmental challenges. To achieve this goal, intervention activities are chosen for their ability to elicit movement, provide pleasurable experiences, present an opportunity for social interaction, and develop skills. Examples of such activities include games, gardening, sharing experiences in a group, and so on. Other activities are used to help modulate sensory information.[32] Such activities may provide tactile, visual, auditory, gustatory, or taste sensations, or vestibular and proprioceptive sensory input. Depending on how such activities are presented in therapy, they may help increase the client's state of arousal versus calmness, or they may be soothing. Activities involving rotation, turning the head, jumping, and so on, are used to provide vestibular and proprioceptive stimulation.

In a pilot study by Rider,[29] therapeutic intervention for chronic nonparanoid schizophrenic clients was conducted. Clients participated in 1-hour sessions, 5 days a week for 6 weeks. Each session consisted of a warm-up exercise designed to facilitate body awareness,[20] such as tapping fingers on the head and examining one's palms of the hands. Then activities such as throwing a ball, jumping rope, walking on a table while touching the ceiling, walking a balance beam, and spinning on a chair followed. The activities "were selected to elicit specific, desired responses, such as raising the arms above head, protective extension responses, standing on one foot, jumping, and improved standing balance" (p. 453).[29] It is evident that the above activities provided vestibular stimulation through movement (e.g., walking on a table while touching the ceiling, jumping rope, spinning in a chair) and proprioceptive input through jumping, standing balance activities, and so on, which stimulated muscle spindles and Golgi tendon organs.

One of the most developed therapeutic approaches for psychiatric clients based on this model is the five-stage group intervention developed by Ross.[30,31,33] The five stages in this group protocol are orientation, movement, visual-perceptual activities, cognition, and closure. These stages are summarized in Table 13-1.

The following case study is used to illustrate clinical application of this model because it meets some of the major criteria specified by King[23] for clients with schizophrenia who may benefit from intervention based on SP/ML approaches: nonparanoid type of schizophrenia, postural features (he has a slightly kyphotic posture), a shuffling gait, and chronicity (has had this condition for at least 7 years).

Consistency of Sensory Processing/ Motor Learning Model With the Occupational Therapy Paradigm

As far as the current professional paradigm's emphasis on meaningful occupation is concerned, the SP/ML model is not fully consistent with

Table 13-1. ROSS'S FIVE-STAGE OCCUPATIONAL THERAPY GROUP INTERVENTION BASED ON THE SP/ML CONCEPTUAL MODEL OF PRACTICE

Group Stage	Activities
Stage I: Orientation	Introductions are done, and group members acknowledge each other's presence. Activities involving touching and handling a variety of media are used to provide sensory input for the purpose of increasing the level of alertness. Examples of objects used may be musical instruments with which clients can experiment, scented soaps and candles, and so on.
Stage II: Movement	Activities incorporating gross-motor movement are introduced. The activities should be designed to encourage maximum physical exertion through movement in horizontal, vertical, and sagittal planes. Such activities may include various types of games, dancing, exercising, and so on. They should preferably encourage communication among clients (social interaction) and should be pleasurable.
Stage III: Visual-Motor Perceptual Stage	Activities that are less physically exerting but that require more focused attention and judgment are introduced. At this stage, activities requiring accomplishment of a task, which may be competitive, are preferred. Examples of such activities include safe darts, hokey-pokey, Simon Says, and identifying and naming objects.
Stage IV: Cognitive Stage	Cognitively stimulating activities, such as memory games, poetry, storytelling, and verbal sharing are introduced.
Stage V: Closure	The therapist uses his or her judgment to prepare a closure that instills in group members a sense of accomplishment and inner calm. The proceedings of the group session are summarized, statements of satisfaction with the group proceedings are verbalized, the date for the next session is stated, refreshments are served, and group members say goodbye to each other.

CASE STUDY: LEO

Leo is a 31-year-old African-American male with a diagnosis of schizoaffective disorder, depressive type. Leo also has a secondary diagnosis of cannabis abuse. Leo is scheduled for the day program to assist in his transition from the acute care hospital back to the community and his job. Leo was hospitalized for a little more than 3 weeks with symptoms of auditory hallucinations, withdrawal and isolation, hypersomnia, and psychomotor retardation. Leo's hallucinations cleared, but he still exhibits the other symptoms, only to a lesser degree.

Leo has had multiple hospitalizations because of his schizoaffective disorder. Sometimes stressors in his life precipitate his hospitalizations, and other times he simply stops taking his medications. Occasionally, the onset of the acute symptoms of his illness do not appear linked to any factor at all. This is one of those times.

Leo was admitted to the hospital at the request of his case manager after several weeks of auditory hallucinations, which included voices talking about him negatively, sirens, and loud music. Leo became depressed when the voices spoke badly of him and

CASE STUDY: LEO—CONT'D

began to sleep more, eat less, and grow increasingly isolative. The staff from the group home noticed his behavior changes and notified Leo's case manager, who, in turn, called his psychiatrist. Leo's doctor recommended admission.

Leo's case manager, Amelda, has been working with him for 7 years. Leo trusts both her and his psychiatrist, Dr. Ramkasoon, and rarely disagrees with their recommendations. Leo does not like to go to the hospital, but he dislikes the auditory hallucinations even more.

Leo lives in a group home with three other men with similar diagnoses. Leo has been living there for several years. Amelda arranged it for him because his situation at home seemed to be too stressful and unhealthy for him. Leo's parents are divorced. Leo's father is schizophrenic and is occasionally found wandering and sleeping on the streets. Though not homeless, Leo's father often leaves his rooming house to later be picked up by the police for sleeping on other people's property. Leo's mother drinks heavily and regularly. She lets Leo stay at her house when she is sober. Otherwise, she makes Leo stay out in the garage. Leo has only one sibling, a sister, who is not involved with the family at all.

Leo does well at the group home. He does his own care with occasional reminders and participates in the chores around the house. Leo is responsible for setting and clearing the table and taking out the trash weekly.

Leo works approximately 8 to 10 hours a week with a cleaning company that contracts to clean offices at night. The supervisor picks Leo up on Tuesday nights at 9 P.M. and drives with him and another employee to the one or two locations that need service that night. The men work until the jobs are finished and the supervisor drives Leo home. That is the only night Leo works. Many Tuesdays, the supervisor has to wake Leo up to get him to work, but Leo has never refused. He has had this job for the past 8 months and appears

committed to keeping it. His supervisor, Scott, feels that even though Leo works slowly, he is a good employee and more reliable than most.

Leo is to attend the day program 5 full days a week. The plan is for him to use the program supports to transition back to work. His doctor anticipates that Leo will only need the program for 2 weeks, maybe less. Leo is scheduled for an occupational therapy evaluation on his first day at the program.

Occupational Therapy Evaluation

Upon evaluation, Leo presents as withdrawn and minimally interactive. He is appropriately groomed and dressed. He speaks when spoken to, but answers in one- or two-word sentences. There is a delayed response when he answers, and his speech is slow and labored. He rarely makes eye contact and stares down at his shoes throughout most of the evaluation.

Leo does not appear to have visual or hearing deficits. He exhibits decreased problem solving, short-term memory, attention span, and immediate recall. He also shows decreased organizational skills. He does not have any apparent sensory perceptual deficits.

Leo's posture is slightly kyphotic, his hips are in a posterior tilt, and he shuffles a bit when he ambulates. His ambulation is slow, but he has no balance problems. His Active Range of Motion (AROM) and strength are Within Functional Limits (WFL), but his coordination is slow and his dexterity is impaired bilaterally. Leo says, "I feel stiff. I can't move right," when asked to perform simple manual tasks. He reports doing his own self-care and nods yes when asked if it takes longer than it used to. He shakes his head no when asked if he has resumed his chores at the group home. Leo states he has no pain. He also has no edema or skin changes.

Leo says he likes his work and wants to get back to it. He likes his group home and the people he lives with. He says he spends most of his free

Continued

CASE STUDY: LEO—CONT'D

time watching TV, sleeping, or walking around the neighborhood because he likes "being alone."

Leo agrees to participate fully in the schedule at the day program. He is concerned about it interfering with his appointments with Dr. Ramkasoon, and is reassured that those appointments take precedence over the groups at the day program. Leo has participated in occupational therapy in the past and is vaguely familiar with its purpose. He says his goals for occupational therapy are to get back to work and feel better.*

Suggested SP/ML Assessment for Leo

Apart from the evaluation completed by the therapist as described above, the following additional assessments may be administered:

1. Evaluate direct vestibular function as follows: standing balance—one leg, eyes open and eyes closed (ask Leo to stand straight on one leg, arms stretched out to the side and parallel to the ground, with forearms in pronation, eyes open, then eyes closed; note the duration—In seconds or minutes, that Leo is able to maintain balance), repeat the test with Leo standing on the other leg, then on both legs. Therapists trained in the use of SI methods may also test Leo's vestibular functioning by rotating him on a desk chair and then recording the duration, frequency, and rhythm of postrotary nystagmus.

2. Leo's vestibular functioning can be measured indirectly by assessing his proprioception as indicated by motor coordination. (a) Ask Leo to touch his left index finger with his right index finger and then touch his nose as fast as possible (finger-to-nose test). Repeat the test with Leo touching his right finger with his left finger and then touching his nose. (b) Ask Leo to hold the thumb against the index finger as if picking a pea (finger-thumb opposition). Ask him to repeat the grip with the thumb against each of the other fingers sequentially (serial opposition). Do the test for each of the upper extremities. (c) Ask Leo to reach for an object on the table with each

of the upper extremities (diodochokinesis). Note any overshooting or undershooting of reach (dys-diodochokinesis). (d) Leo's gait and posture are already known (see evaluation by the occupational therapist). He has a kyphotic posture and a shuffling gait. Based on the findings from the above-suggested evaluations, treatment goals for Leo, reflecting both his SP/ML and functional needs, may be stated as follows:

Short-Term Goals

1. By the end of 4 weeks, Leo's speech will have improved significantly as indicated by initiating and holding conversation with other clients, making eye contact as appropriate, while engaging in a group activity at least three out of five times a week.

2. By the end of 3 weeks, Leo's problem-solving ability, short-term memory, and attention span will improve significantly as indicated by his ability to complete a simple unfamiliar craft activity (such as making a paper weight) in the occupational therapy department with minimal verbal cuing after one demonstration by the therapist.

3. By the end of 4 weeks, Leo's standing posture will improve as indicated by decreased kyphosis to enable him to reach for objects above shoulder level with smooth and coordinated movements as noted while Leo participates in standing activities in the occupational therapy department three out of five times a week.

4. By the end of 4 weeks, Leo's gait will have improved significantly as indicated by decreased shuffling while walking.

Long-Term Goals

1. By the end of 6 weeks, Leo will resume his chores as appropriate at the group home.

2. By the end of 6 weeks, Leo's level of activity will increase as indicated by maintaining a balanced repertoire of meaningful activities including work, leisure, and rest, rather than just watching TV and walking around without objective.

CASE STUDY: LEO—CONT'D

The choice of 6 weeks as the length of time needed to attain the intervention goals was based on Rider's[29] pilot study in which notable changes were documented in clients with chronic schizophrenia after 6 weeks of intervention using SP/ML methods. Interventions may include gross-motor activities such as throwing and kicking a ball, playing balloon volleyball, dancing, a variety of exercises (which are hypothesized to impact proprioceptive as well as vestibular responses through resistive movements), and so on. These activities should preferably be done in a group setting to afford interaction with other clients. Craft activities that require problem solving, short-term memory, organizing, and focus should be incorporated as a way of posing environmental challenges out of which sensory integration and motor control may emerge. The protocol for group sessions in which Leo would participate may be prepared using Ross's[31] five-stage group process outline (see Table 13-1).

 Refer to Lab Manual Exercise 15-1 to practice client assessment and treatment planning using SP/ML guidelines.

---

* This case study is reprinted with permission from Halloran P, Lowenstein N: *Case studies through the healthcare continuum: a workbook for the occupational therapy student*, Thorofare, NJ, 2000, Slack, pp. 297–298.

---

it. The model's focus is on the use of activities directed toward stimulation of the vestibular and proprioceptive systems, rather than direct emphasis on participation in meaningful occupations. It can be argued that the model is to a certain extent consistent with the occupational therapy paradigm with regard to being client-centered in that it advocates being cognizant of what is interesting and within the client's capability. However, collaboration with the client in designing therapeutic intervention and selecting therapeutic media does not seem to be a strong focus of the model.

Later formulations of the model incorporate the ML principle of posing environmental challenges as a way of encouraging self-organization that is expected to result in more controlled, adaptive movement. This is illustrated in statements to the effect that the SI model is based on the neurobehavioral assumption that "When people experience a challenge but not overwhelming level of sensory stimulation to their CNS (i.e., just the right amount of challenge) and successfully respond to it, an adaptive response takes place, which contributes to the development of sensory integration" (p. 248).[12] This assumption seems to suggest that both the adaptive response and sensory integration emerge from the interaction between the person and the environment in an effort to respond to environmental challenges.

Similarly, Giuffrida states that "Learning occurs when performers are encouraged to develop their own movement solutions" (p. 271).[19] She continues to state that motor learning also "means providing or altering the practice context so that the client receives reduced knowledge of results and performance and encounters difficulty in the practice context" (p. 272).[19] This emphasis on posing environmental challenges and emergence of capacities resulting from the interaction between a person and the environment in an attempt to meet the challenges are important constructs in the complexity/chaos theory. Therefore it can be argued that the current formulation of SP/ML model prescribes to the complexity/chaos theoretical view and therefore is consistent with the occupational therapy paradigm in this regard. However, this complexity/chaos theoretical view of the model does not seem to be emphasized in the model's current application in psychosocial intervention as outlined by Ross[31,32] and Ross and Bachner.[33]

The role of the therapist in the SP/ML model is to modify the environment so as to control environmental stimulation so that the client gets just the right amount of sensory input necessary to modulate his or her sensory integration capacity.[14] Another role of the therapist is to provide activities designed to elicit movement, provide opportunity for social interaction, develop skills, organize behavior, and facilitate an adaptive response. Therefore consistent with the current occupational therapy paradigm, the role of the therapist in the SP/ML model is to provide environmental modification to facilitate participation in occupation. However, the model does not emphasize affording opportunities for engagement in meaningful occupations, providing assistive devices, or education/counseling to facilitate participation in meaningful occupations.

It can therefore be argued that the SP/ML model is consistent with the current occupational therapy paradigm in certain aspects (it is client-centered to a certain extent, and one of the therapist's roles according to this model is environmental modification). However, in many ways, the model is not consistent with the professional paradigm. For example, it does not emphasize collaboration with the client, the complexity/chaos theoretical perspective, or the role of the therapist to provide opportunities for participation in occupation, assistive devices, or education/counseling to facilitate engagement in meaningful occupation for participation in life.

Consistency With the Philosophy of Pragmatism

Consistent with the philosophy of pragmatism, the SP/ML model values *active doing* as a means of interacting with the environment in order to access environmental stimulation and develop effective motor control. However, it seems that *doing* is designed by the therapist and the client mostly follows the therapist's directions. This minimizes the client's agency (active engagement by making choices about what to do), which is contrary to the principles of pragmatism. Similar to pragmatism, in the SP/ML model, the environmental context is valued since it is seen as the source of sensory information. Also valued is

individualization since the circumstances of each client are considered individually in the design of therapy, and historicity since the model has a developmental perspective. The role of beliefs in determining action is also indirectly acknowledged in the model's emphasis on body image, self-concept, and self-image. Thus it can be said that the model is consistent with the principles of the philosophy of pragmatism in certain ways and inconsistent in other respects. The greatest inconsistency is in the model's seeming understatement of the importance of the client's agency as an important factor in adaptation.

Consistency with the Complexity/Chaos Theoretical Framework

As mentioned earlier, the complexity/chaos theoretical framework is being increasingly incorporated in the current SI and ML conceptual models. However, this theoretical framework does not seem to have been adopted in the current SP/ML model's application in psychosocial occupational therapy practice.

Recommendations for Reinterpretation of the Model

To make the model more consistent with the current occupational therapy paradigm and the philosophy of pragmatism, it might be useful to reformulate its guidelines for practice to emphasize more client participation in meaningful occupations. For instance, the activities chosen to provide vestibular and proprioceptive input could be those that constitute current and anticipated meaningful occupations for the client. For a client whose background is a construction worker for example, tasks involving repairing things, woodworking crafts, and so on could be used. Such tasks could provide the resistance necessary for proprioceptive stimulation and movement (e.g., bending over, standing up, climbing a ladder) to provide vestibular input, while at the same time reconnecting the client to a meaningful occupation. Furthermore, to make the model more collaborative and client-centered, goal setting, and choice of those intervention activities could be done in collaboration with the client.

The occupations in question could also be presented as environmental challenges that the client has to solve. Because they are meaningful to the client, he or she would be actively invested in the *doing* process, and sensory integration and coordinated movement would emerge from this interaction with the environment through doing. This approach would make the model more consistent with the complexity/chaos theoretical framework. Moreover, giving the client a chance to actively make choices would bring to the forefront agency, making the model more consistent with pragmatic principles, and giving the client an opportunity to choose occupations to be used in therapy would constitute providing opportunities for engagement in meaningful occupation, making the model even more consistent with the current professional paradigm.

Finally, education/counseling of the client to help him or her understand the relationship between engagement in meaningful occupations and ability to process sensory information and produce coordinated movement (leading to more effective role performance) could be made more central to the model's principles. Granted that many of the clients for whom this model was formulated are considered to have cognitive deficits that make meaningful choice of occupations and understanding of the connection between performance and outcome difficult. Nevertheless, it is important to make all attempts to involve the client as actively and meaningfully as possible, because this is a central premise of the current occupational therapy paradigm. Also, this effort would validate the model's belief in plasticity of the CNS since it would be based on the assumption that irrespective of the client's cognitive deficits, input of the right kind of sensory stimulation combined with the client's active involvement is likely to result in self-organization of the CNS and subsequent emergence of improved cognitive, sensory integrative, and motor-functioning capacities.

Evidence-Based Practice Using the Sensory Processing/Motor Learning Conceptual Model of Practice

There is a paucity of research investigating application of the SP/ML model in psychosocial occupational therapy practice. In a literature search conducted using the "OT Search," over 20 studies were found that investigated various aspects of SP/ML theory. However, out of these studies, only four focused directly on the use of the model for intervention with adult psychiatric clients.[16,24,28,29] Three studies explored the use of the model for intervention with clients with a diagnosis of schizophrenia, and one was a case study describing the use of the model with an adult client with intellectual disability. The most recent study found in the search on this topic was conducted in 1993. The four studies can be grouped into those that tested the theoretical propositions of the model,[16,24] and outcome studies.[28,29] We will now discuss these studies in detail.

Endler and Eimon[16] conducted a correlational study to test the hypothesis that reflex and postural integration of clients with chronic schizophrenia was different from that of normal controls. They also wanted to find out whether there was a difference in reflex and postural integration between paranoid and nonparanoid clients with schizophrenia as hypothesized by King.[23] To test the two hypotheses, they examined the relationship between reflex integration and performance on parts of the Southern California Sensory Integration Test (SCSIT) measuring postural and bilateral integration.

Twenty-nine individuals participated in the study. They were divided into three groups: Ten participants with chronic nonparanoid schizophrenia, nine with chronic paranoid schizophrenia, and a control group consisting of 10 normal hospital employees. Reflex integration was evaluated for all participants using the Reflex Testing Score Sheet, which was used to examine the asymmetrical tonic neck and labyrinthine tonic neck reflexes. The SCSIT was used to measure postural and bilateral integration. Premorbid status was established using the Ullman-Giovannon Scale, which is a self-administered paper-and-pencil questionnaire.

The findings of the study indicated that there was significant difference between schizophrenic participants and normal controls on the tonic labyrinthine reflex and five out of the six measures of postural and bilateral integration as measured on the SCSIT. No significant differences were found between the paranoid and nonparanoid schizophrenic participants. The researchers concluded that postural and bilateral integration dysfunctions are likely associated with schizophrenia as indicated by the findings of the study. However, if the measured variables were indicators of vestibular and proprioceptive functioning, then the study findings would suggest that there was no difference between paranoid and nonparanoid clients with schizophrenia on vestibular and proprioceptive functioning as postulated by King.[23] Both types of schizophrenia were associated with dysfunctions in reflexive, postural, and bilateral integration.

In another study,[24] Lindquist tested the hypothesis that clients with chronic schizophrenia present with vestibular dysfunctions. She used an experimental design with 40 participants divided into four groups with 10 participants each. Group one comprised participants diagnosed with nonparanoid-type schizophrenia, group two comprised clients diagnosed with mania, group three comprised clients diagnosed with chronic spinal pain, and group four comprised 10 normal participants consisting of therapists and staff members drawn from the community. Data gathered included demographics such as age, gender, medication, length of illness, and hand dominance. The level of physical activity was assessed using the Physical Activity Scale (PAS), which is an interview instrument. The Vestibular Function Inventory (VFI) was used to measure vestibular response using indicators such as "duration of PRN [Postrotary Nystagmus], duration of standing balance with eyes open and eyes closed, finger to nose motor coordination, diodochokinesia, and serial opposition" (p. 61).[24]

Findings indicated that all the suggested indicators of the vestibular and proprioceptive functioning except for the PRN were affected by neuroleptic medication. This was indicated by similar performance on those indicators between schizophrenic and manic clients, who were all on such medications, but not with the chronic pain or the normal control participants who were not on the medications. This finding implied that without being able to control for the effects of medication, the only viable measure of vestibular response in the study was the PRN. On subsequent analysis, it was found that the scores of participants with schizophrenia on the PRN were not significantly different from those in other groups. However, the differences, though not significant, were in the expected direction. Furthermore, the scores of schizophrenic and spinal pain groups were significantly similar. The PRN was also found to be significantly correlated with the level of activity as measured on the PAS. These findings led to the question as to whether the level of activity associated with SI treatment may account for observed effects of the treatment rather than the hypothesized modulation of sensory integration capacity as a consequence of SI interventions.

In another study, Rider[29] investigated the hypothesized improvement in posture and movement patterns and the decrease in psychotic behavior among chronic nonparanoid schizophrenic clients as a result of SI treatment. The researcher utilized a multiple case study design with each participant acting as his or her own control. Five clients with a diagnosis of chronic nonparanoid type schizophrenia participated in the study. The "Draw-A-Person" test was used to evaluate body image and self-concept. The step test was used to test balance and physical endurance. Psychotic behavior was assessed using the Nurses Observation Scale for Inpatient Evaluation (NOSIE), an observation-based instrument that evaluates positive client factors (social competence, social interest, and neatness) and negative factors (irritability, manifest psychosis, and motor retardation). Postural assessment was completed using the Bancroft Plumb-line test which consists of using a plumb-line to measure body alignment in standing position.

The SI treatment consisted of warm-up exercises followed by gross-motor activities. Treatment was conducted in six 1-hour sessions, one session per week. All evaluations were repeated upon conclusion of SI treatment. Evaluation following SI intervention demonstrated inconsistent positive changes in positive participant factors. For some participants, there was improvement, while for others there was a decline in these factors. This was the case for all factors except "neatness," which did not change for any of the clients. Psychosis and irritability decreased for all participants, and activity levels increased. There was improved body image as indicated by person-drawings that were more representative and recognizable as human figures than they were before intervention. Also, gait improved for all participants, but the improvement was not sustained over time. No significant changes were observed in posture.

Finally, Reisman[28] presented a case study demonstrating the effect of SI/proprioceptive intervention on self-injurious behavior (SIB) of a 41-year-old woman with profound intellectual disability, impaired vision, and cerebral palsy. Her SIB included hitting her face with her hand and digging her nails into her skin causing skin lacerations. Because of this SIB, she was placed in restraints. To establish a baseline, the number of minutes that she spent in restraint per day and the number of SIBs per minute were recorded over several days. This data-gathering phase was followed by assessment to determine the type of sensory stimulation that she responded to positively. SI interventions consisted of holding her hand, gently rocking her wheelchair with her arms co-contracted, and slow downward stroking on the arms, legs, and back with surgical gloves 5 minutes per day, followed by attempts to engage her in social interaction and object manipulation.

A steady decrease in time spent in restraints and the number of SIBs per minute was noted soon after initiation of therapy. Other characteristics observed that were not noted in the baseline data were smiling, laughing, maintaining eye contact with staff members, vocalizing, and imitating motions and sounds. All the above studies indicated that the postulated characteristics suggestive of sensory modulation dysfunction for clients with schizophrenia may actually be present. However, the findings were mostly inconclusive.

One of the shortcomings of the studies is that either they were case studies without adequate controls for extraneous variables or the samples in the experimental studies were small, decreasing the power of the studies. Due to these limitations, as Lindquist[24] noted, the changes observed in mental health clients as a result of SP/ML-guided interventions cannot be conclusively attributed to these interventions. The changes could be a result of increased activity levels that are naturally associated with such interventions rather than due to modulation of sensory integration as hypothesized. This possibility is given credence by Lindquist's finding that there was a strong correlation between PRN and activity levels in participants with chronic schizophrenia as well as those with spinal pain. It is clear that if this conceptual model of practice is to be used in psychosocial occupational therapy, more research is needed to determine its validity and effectiveness in this area of practice. It is also clear that SP/ML assessment instruments for use with adult clients with psychosocial problems need to be developed and validated.

SUMMARY

In this chapter, we presented the SP/ML conceptual model of practice. We noted that the model is a combination Jean Ayres' SI and ML principles, particularly those of Margaret Rood. This combination was apparent from the very beginning of this model as developed by King.[23] We discussed the SI and ML principles contributing to the model, the theoretical core of the model, and the model's postulations about function, dysfunction, and change. Function is the ability to take in sensory information both from within the individual and from the environment, process the information so as to make sense of the environment, and generate a coordinated adaptive motor response. Dysfunction is the inability to process sensory information and generate smooth, coordinated, adaptive motor response. The role of therapy is to help facilitate ability to modulate and integrate sensory information and attain motor control necessary to generate adaptive movement. This role of therapy is based on the assumption that the CNS is plastic (it can reorganize itself and change as a result of an individual's interaction with the environment).

We discussed client assessment and therapeutic intervention guided by the model. We illustrated the model's assessment and intervention guidelines using a case study. We also noted that the model is consistent with the current occupational therapy paradigm, the philosophy of pragmatism, and the complexity/chaos theoretical perspective in some respects, but it is inconsistent in others. We then suggested revisions that would make the model more consistent with the professional paradigm, the philosophy of pragmatism, and the complexity/chaos theoretical framework. Finally, we discussed research evidence demonstrating the clinical validity of the model. Since there is not enough research to strongly support the model's application in psychosocial practice, we suggested that more research is needed. Also, since most of the available evaluation instruments associated with this model were developed for use with children with developmental problems, we proposed the need to develop and validate model assessment instruments for use with adult clients with psychiatric conditions.

REFERENCES

1. Adams JA: A closed-loop theory of motor learning, *J Motor Behavior* 3:111–150, 1971.
2. Ayres AJ: The development of perceptual-motor abilities: a theoretical basis for treatment of dysfunction, *Am J Occup Ther* 17:221–225, 1963.
3. Ayres AJ: *Southern California Motor Accuracy Test,* Los Angeles, 1964, Western Psychological Services.
4. Ayres AJ: *Southern California Perceptual-Motor Tests,* Los Angeles, 1968, Western Psychological Services.
5. Ayres AJ: Improving academic scores through sensory integration, *J Learning Disabil* 5:24–28, 1972.
6. Ayres AJ: *Sensory integration and learning disorders,* Los Angeles, 1972, Western Psychological Services.
7. Ayres AJ: An interpretation of the role of the brain-stem in intersensory integration. In Cottrell H, ed: *The body senses and perceptual deficit,* Boston, 1973, Boston University Press.
8. Ayres AJ: *Southern California Postrotary Nystagmus Test,* Los Angeles, 1975, Western Psychological Services.
9. Ayres AJ: *Sensory integration and the child,* Los Angeles, 1979, Western Psychological Services.
10. Ayres AJ: *Southern California Sensory Integration Tests—Revised,* Los Angeles, 1980, Western Psychological Services.
11. Ayres AJ: *Sensory Integration and Praxis Tests,* Los Angeles, 1989, Western Psychological Services.
12. Baloueff O: Sensory integration. In Crepeau EB, Cohn ES, Schell BA, eds: *Willard and Spackman's occupational therapy,* ed 10, New York, 2003, Lippincott Williams & Wilkins, pp. 247–252.
13. Bernstein N: *The coordination and regulation of movements,* Elmsford, NY, 1967, Pergamon.
14. Bruce MA, Borg B: *Psychosocial frames of reference: core for occupation-based practice,* ed 3, Thorofare, NJ, 2002, Slack.
15. Bumin G, Kayihan H: Rehabilitation in practice: effectiveness of two different sensory-integration programs for children with spastic diplegic cerebral palsy, *Disabil Rehabil* 23:394–399, 2001.
16. Endler PB, Eimon MC: Postural and reflex integration in schizophrenic patients, *Am J Occup Ther* 32:456–466, 1978.
17. Feldenkrais M: *Body and mature behavior—anxiety, sex, gravitation, and learning,* New York, 1966, International Universities Press.
18. Flinn N: A task-oriented approach to the treatment of a client with hemiplegia, *Am J Occup Ther* 49:560–569, 1995.
19. Giuffrida CG: Motor learning: an emerging frame of reference for occupational performance. In Crepeau EB, Cohn ES, Schell BA, eds: *Willard and Spackman's occupational therapy,* ed 10, New York, 2003, Lippincott Williams & Wilkins, pp. 267–275.
20. Gunther B: *Sense relaxation below your mind,* New York, 1968, Collier Books.
21. Halloran P, Lowenstein N: *Case studies through the healthcare continuum: a workbook for the occupational therapy student,* Thorofare, NJ, 2000, Slack.
22. Kielhofner G: *Conceptual foundations of occupational therapy,* ed 3, Philadelphia, 2004, FA Davis.

23. King LJ: A sensory-integrative approach to schizophrenia, *Am J Occup Ther* 28:529–536, 1974.

24. Lindquist JE: Activity and vestibular function in chronic schizophrenia, *Occup Ther J Res* 1(1):56–78, 1981.

25. Marieb EN: *Human anatomy and physiology,* Menlo Park, CA, 1992, Benjamin/Cummings.

26. Mathiowetz V, Haugen JB: Motor behavior research: implications for therapeutic approaches to central nervous system dysfunction, *Am J Occup Ther* 48: 733–745, 1994.

27. McKeachie WJ, Doyle CL: *Psychology: the biological background of behavior,* New York, 1966, Addison-Wesley.

28. Reisman J: Using a sensory integrative approach to treat self-injurious behavior in an adult with profound mental retardation, *Am J Occup Ther* 47:403–411, 1993.

29. Rider B: Sensorimotor treatment of chronic schizophrenics, *Am J Occup Ther* 32:451–455, 1978.

30. Ross M: *Integrative group therapy: the structured five-stage approach,* ed 2, Thorofare, NJ, 1991, Slack.

31. Ross M: *Integrative group therapy: mobilizing coping abilities with the five-stage group,* Bethesda, MD, 1997, American Occupational Therapy Association.

32. Ross M: A five-stage model for adults with developmental disabilities. In Ross M, Bachner S, eds: *Adults with developmental disabilities: current approaches in occupational therapy,* Rockville, MD, 1998, American Occupational Therapy Association.

33. Ross M, Bachner S, eds: *Adults with developmental disabilities: current approaches in occupational therapy,* ed 2, Rockville, MD, 2004, American Occupational Therapy Association.

34. Ross M, Burdick D: *Sensory integration: a training manual for therapists and teachers for regressed, psychiatric, and geriatric patient groups,* Thorofare, NJ, 1981, Slack.

35. Sabari JS: Motor learning concepts applied to activity-based intervention with adults with hemiplegia, *Am J Occup Ther* 45:523–530, 1991.

36. Schaaf RC, Miller LJ: Occupational therapy using a sensory integrative approach for children with developmental disabilities, *Mental Retardation Developmental Disabil Res Reviews* 11:143–148, 2005.

37. Schmidt RA: A schema theory of discrete motor skill learning, *Psychological Review* 82:225–260, 1975.

38. Tickle-Degnen L: Perspectives on the status of sensory integration theory, *Am J Occup Ther* 42:427–433, 1988.

39. Trombly CA: *Occupational therapy for physical dysfunctions,* Baltimore, MD, 1983, Williams & Wilkins.

40. Walker KF: A. Jean Ayres. In Miller RJ, Walker KF, eds: *Perspectives on theory for the practice of occupational therapy,* Gaithersburg, MD, 1993, Aspen, pp. 103–154.

41. Warren M: Strategies for sensory and neuromotor remediation. In Christiansen C, Baum C, eds: *Occupational therapy: overcoming human performance deficits,* Thorofare, NJ, 1991, Slack, pp. 633–662.

42. White BP: Neurodevelopmental theory. In Crepeau EB, Cohn ES, Schell BA, eds: *Willard and Spackman's occupational therapy,* ed 10, New York, 2003, Lippincott Williams & Wilkins, pp. 245–247.

14
The Developmental Conceptual Model of Practice

Preview Questions

1. List and discuss the theoretical sources of constructs used in the Developmental conceptual model of practice as applied in adult psychosocial occupational therapy.
2. Discuss the models of human development that are relevant to occupational therapy.
3. Concisely state the theoretical core of the Developmental conceptual model of practice.
4. Explain postulations of the Developmental conceptual model of practice about the following:
   a. Function
   b. Dysfunction
   c. Change
5. Outline and explain the Developmental model's guidelines for client evaluation and therapeutic intervention.
6. Discuss the consistency of the Developmental model of practice with each of the following:
   a. The occupational therapy paradigm
   b. The philosophy of pragmatism
   c. The complexity/chaos theoretical framework
7. Discuss available empirical evidence supporting clinical effectiveness of the Developmental conceptual model as a guide to intervention in occupational therapy practice.

The developmental approach was one of the earliest conceptual models of practice in occupational therapy. It was one of the three frames of reference articulated by Mosey in her book, *Three Frames of Reference for Mental Health*.[65] In this conceptual framework, she postulated that humans have an inherent drive to develop basic skills, which she argued were learned successively, each skill building on to the previous one. She advanced the argument that therapy recapitulated "ontogenesis, the normal sequence of individual development," and enabled "the patient to complete that sequence" (p. 45).[55] Gilfoyle, Grady, and Moore,[37] and Llorens,[51] among others, were other occupational therapists that contributed significantly to the development of this model.

The sensory integration and neurodevelopmental therapies discussed in Chapter 13 were among a group of occupational therapy theories related to this frame of reference. They belonged to a linear, hierarchical, and biological view of human development based on the principles of the central nervous system (CNS) maturation.[9] Although Bigsby considers this model of development to be linear, it is proposed in this book that it can also be conceptualized as a spiral because of the typically observed regression (loss of previously acquired skills) followed by reintegration of skills at a higher level of performance. The predominant conceptualization in this view was that development occurs in a cyclical progression with maturation and growth followed by temporary decline and regression and then resumption of maturation and growth.[75]

However, this conceptual framework was found to be inadequate in explaining motor and cognitive development variability that was found among typically and atypically developing children. Therefore another view based on the concept of adaptation was adopted in occupational therapy. In this theoretical framework, based on the work of Erikson,[30,31] Erikson and Erikson,[32] and Piaget,[69] among others, it was postulated that new skills, behaviors, and experiences were assimilated to previously learned skills, behaviors, and experiences, leading to development of higher levels of functioning, or what was perceived to be adaptation (see Chapter 3 for a detailed discussion of these developmental psychological theories). Llorens,[51] Gilfoyle, Grady, and Moore,[37] Ayres,[3-5] Fidler and Fidler,[34] and Mosey[65] among other occupational therapists, subscribed to this view. This was the stage theory of development.

The problem with the stage theory, however, is that it did not explain the variability of child development as well as the temporary loss of previously acquired skills as described above. In response to this shortcoming of the stage theory, a new conceptual framework based on a dynamic systems perspective is emerging, based mainly on the work of Bernstein.[8] In this framework, development is conceptualized to emerge from a dynamic interaction between age; maturation and growth; human agency; and social, cultural, and environmental context.[74]

Evolution of the Conceptual Model

Linear, Biological, and Hierarchical Perspective

This perspective was based on the biological view of development, beginning with conception through old age and death.* Research in biological sciences has led to increased understanding of how organs form and develop in utero (organogenesis);[83] development of the infant and young child after birth including integration of reflexes, attaining motor control (fine- and gross-motor skills), posture, and other physical characteristics; and the corresponding cognitive development as a result of CNS maturation.[22,23,57,58] Research in late adult life has led to inclusion within the framework of the physical and cognitive changes that occur

in later stages of life. These changes include decreased functioning of the cardiovascular, pulmonary, and other systems of the body, sensory deficits (visual, auditory, vestibular, and gustatory), deteriorating memory and attention, movement difficulties, and so on.[71]

The biological perspective of human development was further developed by Arnold Gessell (1880–1961), a pediatrician associated with the Yale Clinic for Child Development.[56] Gessell perceived development to proceed as follows[56]:
1. In cephalocaudal direction, gaining control of the head, shoulders, down the spine, and the lower legs progressively.
2. Proximal to distal, gaining control of shoulder and hip before the hand and foot.
3. Medial to lateral, which is similar to proximal to distal (e.g., in the hand, development of grasp moves from ulnar [medial] to radial [lateral]).
4. Up against gravity, progressing from completely prone to prone on elbows, then supported by the hands, then by all four limbs, and finally standing and walking (pp. 28-29).

Gessell's principles have been the conceptual basis of assessment of reflexes and motor functioning in occupational therapy for many years.[21] These principles also form the early conceptual foundations of Rood's Neurodevelopmental Theory (NDT) and Ayre's Sensory Integration (SI) theory, which are discussed in Chapter 13 (see also Warren[85]). In addition, knowledge developed from recent studies focusing on changes occurring during old age has been used by occupational therapists to develop assessment and intervention programs in geriatrics.[20,27,28,81]

The Stage Theory of Development

The stage theory of development in occupational therapy is derived mostly from the works of Freud, Erikson, Havighurst, and Piaget. Moral theories of Kohlberg and Gilligan are also often mentioned in occupational therapy but are not commonly used in clinical practice. In Chapter 3, we discussed these theories and pointed out

*References 22,23,57,58,71,76,79,83,87.

that they all view development as acquisition of increasingly complex behaviors and skills with growth and maturation.

In these theories, behaviors and skills are understood to occur in different domains of human functioning. For instance, for Jung, they constituted individuation (development of identity and self-expression in the world as an integrated individual). Havighurst saw development as the acquisition of specific tasks at each stage of life from infancy through adolescence and beyond. Erikson conceptualized development to constitute psychosocial growth consisting of eight stages from infancy through old age. At each stage, the individual resolved conflicting instincts, successful resolution of which was an important step for negotiation of the next stage. Finally, Freud saw development as consisting of psychosexual stages ranging from primarily seeking oral gratification in infancy to mature sexual functioning in adolescence and adulthood.

For all the above-mentioned theorists, the primary proposition was that development was cumulative and adaptive, and skills or behaviors were its building blocks. Each skill or behavior was added to the previously existing skills or behaviors in the process of development; this is what they termed *adaptation*. If skills/behaviors acquired at an earlier stage were faulty (maladaptive), subsequent developmental stages were negatively affected and also likely to be maladaptive. See Chapter 3 for details of these theoretical propositions.

Many occupational therapists seemed to integrate the stage theory, principles of evolution (probably due to the historical influence of pragmatism),[12] and the biological view of development discussed earlier[6,48,51,65] in their formulation of the Developmental conceptual model of practice. They all seemed to subscribe to the construct of adaptation through interaction with the environment. Moreover, they distinguished between evolution of the human species (which takes thousands or even millions of years for significant change to be noticed)[12] and individual

adaptive changes as a function of active response to environmental challenges.

However, they all subscribed to the principle that ontogenesis recapitulates phylogenesis. This meant that individual development followed the same stages and occurred in the same sequence as human evolution occurred over millions of years. For example, Ayres[6] postulated that during human evolution, the somatosensory system of the CNS developed earliest because it was crucial to successful interaction with the environment and to species survival. Development of the brainstem and associated structures followed, and the neo-cortex was the last to evolve. The individual human's development follows the same sequence with tactile sensations developing in utero and cortical functions maturing many years later. Ayres further argued that development of movement followed the same sequence through which the human species evolved, with movements of extremities similar to those used in swimming developing first and bipedal ambulation last.[2]

The best illustration of how developmental occupational therapists subscribed to the stage theory in addition to the biological view of development is the work of Lela Llorens.[51,52,77] She argued that development occurred both horizontally across many domains (physical, psychological, social, and language) and longitudinally as one progressed in time from birth to mature age. As an individual traversed each developmental stage over time, horizontal development of a variety of skills occurred at the same time, so that one demonstrated complexity of performance with chronological maturity. In the early stages, one had only few skills performed with poor coordination. Later in life, the number of skills was large and the coordination with which they were performed was high. In this sense, Lloren's view of development resembled an upside-down pyramid with the base representing the number of skills and the axis temporal maturity.

Other occupational therapy developmental theorists such as King[48] subscribed to similar principles. Their therapeutic interventions were also planned accordingly, where it was suggested that therapy recapitulate ontogenesis.[55] This meant following the sequence of human development in therapy, with mastery of skills at the earliest stages of development being the focus of therapy and those at later stages being added as the client progressed in therapy. As mentioned earlier, however, the stage theory of development did not adequately account for the variability and flexibility of motor and cognitive behavior seen in both typically and atypically developing individuals.[9] Consequently, a dynamic systems view of development is emerging and is being integrated in occupational therapy literature.

The Dynamic Systems Perspective of Human Development

The dynamic systems view of human development is not yet fully articulated. However, emerging ideas, originating from the work of Bernstein,[8] indicate that development is increasingly being conceptualized as a phenomenon emerging from a dynamic interaction between age, maturation, human agency or active participation, and physical/social environmental context.[9,74] Therefore it is a transactional view, which "acknowledges potential effects of socioeconomic status, social support...and individual behavior characteristics" (p. 244).[9] Because of this transactional perspective, the dynamic systems view integrates the biological approach and stage theory.

For example, the CNS ontogenetic theory of Gessel,[56] the developmental-task construct advanced by Havighurst, and the stage theory of Piaget and others (see Chapter 3) can be integrated as follows: The construct *development* refers to adaptation of individual humans by coping with developmental tasks.[82] A "developmental-task is a task which an individual has to and wants to solve in a particular life-period" which "assumes an active learner interacting with an active...environment." Furthermore, "The idea of the concept is that...people want to solve problems themselves (the active learner)" (p. 55).[82]

Developmental task as defined above may be motor (e.g., walking, playing basketball), cognitive (e.g., language development, reading skills) or social (e.g., observing social norms like keeping time, delaying gratification). This broad definition of a developmental task includes the biological perspective of development. Reference to a particular life period denotes consistency with the stage theory of development since a life period may be understood as a developmental stage, marked by milestones such as walking, going to school, going on a first date, getting married, and so on. Skills can only be integrated when the individual is developmentally ready to integrate them. Finally, the transactional idea of an active learner in dynamic interaction with the environment is consistent with the dynamic systems perspective of a complex, dynamic, adaptive system.[42,43] In this conceptualization, development may be understood to emerge from dynamic interaction of an active learner with the physical and social environment resulting in integration of motor, cognitive, and social skills consistent with the individual's developmental stage, and consequent attainment of mastery of the environment consistent with that developmental level.

One of the best illustrations of how occupational therapists are trying to integrate the dynamic systems perspective can be found in the spatiotemporal adaptation theory developed by Gilfoyle, Grady, and Moore in which they wrote that

Spatiotemporal adaptation theory proposes that children acquire sensorimotor skills through a *transactional process* as they develop movement patterns to adapt to their environments of space and time. *Adaptation occurs through developmental and purposeful sequences of activity with developmental sequences emanating essentially from innate, genetically determined behavior, and purposeful sequences evolving from a child's intention to accomplish a goal.* Both developmental and purposeful sequences make use of neuromuscular functions to produce movement. Developmental sequences *direct maturation of automatic responses,* which culminate in patterns of controlled movement, used primarily for moving about in space and for developing reaching and grasping. Purposeful sequences make use of developmental patterns of movement by adapting them to new experiences motivated by intention. As basic functions are adapted to increasingly complex developmental or purposeful activities, *higher level functions emerge* (p. 15, emphasis mine).[37]

Although the spatiotemporal adaptation theory was developed for use in pediatrics, the above statement pertains to all ages and all forms of development in addition to movement. At any stage in any age, skills (whether sensorimotor, cognitive, or social) may be seen as being acquired through a transactional process as individuals strive to interact and adapt to their environment. This interaction with the environment emanates from the innately programmed desire to attain goals and mastery. This process leads to integration of new skills into increasingly complex developmental behaviors and skills leading to emergence of higher levels of function.

The above transactional, dynamic systems perspective, however, does not seem to have been widely adopted in psychosocial occupational therapy. In this area of practice, the stage theory seems to be prevalent, both in the literature and in clinical practice.[13,19,66] The developmental theories of Jung, Erikson, and Levinson seem to be used most frequently by occupational therapists in psychosocial practice.[13,19] Of course, in the Sensory Processing/Motor Learning (SP/ML) theory discussed in Chapter 13, Piaget's theory of cognitive development is well-integrated. See Chapter 3 for a discussion about Jung's analytical psychology and Erikson's psychosocial stages of human development.

As mentioned, Jung[45-47] considered human development to constitute the process of individuation. According to him, the human went through four stages in the process of individuation: childhood, youth, midlife, and old age. In childhood, one had no identity apart from that of the parents and significant other people in his

or her environment. The child's world was nothing apart from the world of his or her parents. A sense of "I" was shaped by parents' beliefs, values, and so on. As the child reached adolescence, a stage in which initiation took place in some cultures, this marked an important transition to adulthood. This was the stage in which consciousness of self as a member of a "we-group" as well as self-identity as an individual who was separate from parents developed.

After transition through adolescence, young adulthood emerged. At this stage, one adapted to social demands to select a career, get married and establish a family, and develop status and recognition by peers. This stage ended with the midlife crisis in which the individual began questioning his or her accomplishments and the hitherto held values. This transition could either be a time of constructive reflection if one felt a sense of accomplishment in young adulthood, or a time of crisis if one felt as if adulthood had been a time of futility. Middle age began around 35 to 40 years of age (what Jung referred to as the afternoon of life). At this stage, if the transition was negotiated successfully, one developed a deeper knowledge of self, and had a tendency to respond to inner drives rather than societal expectations.

It was at this time that unexpressed polar parts of oneself (see discussion about Jung in Chapter 3) began to emerge and develop, leading to further integration and individuation. Individuals at this stage had a tendency to respond to spiritual rather than material values, and therefore philosophy and understanding of belief systems tended to be more appealing than materialism. One began to move toward an ultimate development of selfhood, which Jung referred to as *transcendence*. Finally, at extreme old age, the individual became infirm and increasingly required care from others. He or she now contemplated death, and the prospects of life after death (which Jung believed to be archetypal) became the preoccupying theme. This was thus a stage in which one gradually detached from life in preparation for transition to the afterlife.

As discussed in Chapter 3, Erikson conceptualized eight stages of psychosocial development (see Table 3-2).[30-32] Each stage was understood to constitute a conflict of opposing instincts, such as trust versus mistrust, industry versus inferiority, and so on. Depending on how each stage was negotiated, subsequent stages were either adaptive or maladaptive. The ultimate drive in all eight stages, according to Erikson, was to develop a sense of identity.

Levinson[50] subscribed to Jung's view of development. However, he expanded Jung's theory by emphasizing further the stages of late teens, early and middle adulthood, and the early forties. His theory was based on a longevity research study that he conducted involving 40 men, all 35 years of age, from four different occupational groups. He followed these men until they were 45 years of age. Therefore the focus of his study was on what Jung had referred to as the midlife transition. Based on the findings of his research, Levinson discussed male choice making, expounding on how those choices were related to their roles. He also delineated a sequence of adult development consisting of alternating stable and transitional stages. According to Levinson, each of the stable stages of adulthood (early adulthood [ages 22 to 40], middle adulthood [ages 45 to 60], and late adulthood [ages 65 and over]) lasted between 5 and 7 years. During each of these periods, the individual committed to the developmental tasks typical of the developmental stage, by assuming social and occupational roles specific to the stage (e.g., career and family during early adulthood, mentoring the younger generations during middle adulthood).

According to Levinson, the transitional stages lasted 3 to 5 years and were the periods during which the individual reviewed his or her life, made decisions to abandon elements of the previous stage that were not meaningful in the forthcoming stage, and retain those that were meaningful to the emerging stage. Thus they were stages of conflict whose resolution enabled one to progress toward assumption of the tasks and roles of the next stage of life. These transitional stages were early adult transition (ages 17 to 22), midlife transition (ages 40 to 45), and late adult transition (ages 60 to 65). The early adult transition constituted separation from parents so as to establish a separate identity and assume adult responsibilities of working and establishing a family.

This transition stage involved formulation of a dream about settlement in the adult world (e.g., imagination of the type of career that one would be involved in, the type of family one would like to have). Establishment of the dream was important for successful transition to the adult role. During the midlife transition, the person worked out the various internal polarities such as destruction versus creation, femininity versus masculinity, and attachment versus separation. During the late-life transition, one began to confront his own morality (remember that all participants in Levinson's study were men). He grieved what he must give up and was anxious about the future given the significance of the predominant theme of symbols about death and rebirth typical of this stage.

Levinson[50] introduced three concepts that have been used by occupational therapists in psychosocial practice: *mentorship, transitional stress,* and *developmental tasks.* Mentoring was conceived by Levinson as a complex relationship that occurred especially during early adulthood. The *mentor* was seen as a transitional figure, usually several years older than the protégé, but not old enough to be the protégé's parent. The mentor acted as a teacher, sponsor, inspirer, advisor, role model, and guide. *Transitional stress* referred to the stress associated with these stages of uncertainty, making it necessary for the individual to require assistance from others.

Levinson asserted that if one was unable to deal successfully with developmental tasks at a certain stage, issues surrounding those tasks tended to resurface frequently during subsequent transition stages. We discussed Freud's psychosexual stages of development in Chapter 3. As mentioned earlier, Kohlberg's and Gilligan's stages of moral development do not seem to be prevalently used in occupational therapy.

Other social scientists developed their own theories of human development based on the work of those early leaders in conceptualization of the human developmental framework. Loevinger[53] is an example of such a theorist whose work has inspired much research that has led to the evolvement of the lifespan developmental perspective.[16,36,39,59,61] According to Loevinger, stability of ego development attained by the end of adolescence was maintained throughout adulthood. She described ego development as "that aspect of the mind or personality that organizes and integrates the individual experiences and tendencies" (p. 220).[64] It constituted development of self-awareness and attainment of what she referred to as the *modal self-aware level*.[53] She asserted that development of the ego (or the self) was a holistic process that was imperfectly coherent and unitary consisting of striving, perception, beliefs, and attitudes. It was also more or less synonymous with intellectual development in that part of ego development was cognitive integration. She conceived it to be "promoted by growth in cognitive complexity, tolerance of ambiguity, individuation, and autonomy" (220).[64]

According to Loevinger, each stage of ego development represented a typology corresponding to a specific age in the lifespan developmental framework. This typology stabilized and predicted growth throughout the lifespan. It consisted of nine levels, which could roughly be divided into three phases:

- Phase 1: Symbiotic, impulsive, self-protective (childhood to beginning of adolescence, just before college). In this phase, the individual learned to control impulses. Cognitive processes that were used were rather simplistic. The interpersonal style was manipulative and controlling in attempt to protect self. Blame was often externalized.
- Phase 2: Conformist, self-aware, and conscientious (adolescence through early adulthood).

This phase was characterized by a desire to belong and preoccupation with appearance and being acceptable (hence, the dangers of negative peer pressure). The individual also began to develop awareness of alternatives to behavior and a sense of choice. The interpersonal style was characterized by a desire for enhanced communication.

- Phase 3: Individualistic, autonomous, and integrated (young adulthood). In this phase, there was a heightened sense of individuality, tolerance for ambiguity, and individual identity.

Loevinger considered ego development to stabilize at this stage and to remain more or less the same throughout the rest of a person's life. Research evidence has been elicited that challenges this hypothesis and supports the argument for continued development even into late adult life. This research will be discussed later in this chapter. Such evidence of continued human development throughout the lifespan has been an important source of justification for involvement of occupational therapy in later adulthood, including geriatrics.[29]

The Theoretical Core of the Developmental Conceptual Model

The Developmental conceptual model of practice, as it is currently used in psychosocial occupational therapy, may be stated as follows[13,14,19]: An individual is a physical and psychosocial being with organically determined drive for growth that leads to progressively increasing complexity through physical maturation combined with a need to experience all aspects of oneself and expand one's intellectual prowess. Development denotes change. Since change includes going through transition, and transitions constitute crises, therefore development consists of regular periods of crisis or tension throughout the lifespan. Response to this tension associated with change is what leads to adaptation or maladaptation. Adaptation may be understood as acquisition of adaptive skills necessary to accomplish stage-specific tasks of life. This acquisition of skills is sequential and invariable. This means that skills build on to each other.

Postulations About Function, Dysfunction, and Change

Function

Based on the above core theoretical statement, it follows that, according to the Developmental conceptual model of practice in psychosocial occupational therapy, function is the ability to adapt. This means being able to acquire essential adaptive skills necessary to perform stage-appropriate developmental tasks and interact appropriately with the environment. For example, the adolescent is able to separate from parents as appropriate and emerge as a young adult who is able to establish an individual identity; have a career or means of earning a livelihood; be productive; contribute meaningfully to the economic, social, spiritual, and cultural well-being of the community; have a family; establish status among peers, and so on.

A middle-aged person is able to feel centered by an internal sense of integrity through reflection, which means being comfortable with who he or she is, having a healthy drive to provide mentorship and nurturing to younger generations, and so on. The older adult is able to look back at his or her life and experience satisfaction with what he or she has accomplished, detach from the need to be in authority and to be materially productive as part of self-definition, and look forward to the inevitable transition to the afterlife.

Dysfunction

Disability, according to this model, is the inability to acquire the adaptive skills necessary to accomplish developmental stage-appropriate tasks and to interact effectively with the environment. Requisite skills may not be acquired due to developmental delays for any number of reasons, including brain damage at birth, physical disabilities, or environmental barriers that make it difficult to acquire the skills. Previously

acquired skills may also be lost, for instance as happens in the case of traumatic brain injury of an adult. Sometimes, "just the normal tasks at each transitional stage may be enough to cause a crisis situation" (p. 212),[19] leading to disruption in development and inability to acquire the necessary adaptive skills.

Barriers to development may be situational (lack of time, funds, or information necessary to develop required skills), dispositional (biological or physical limitations to performance, negative attitudes or perceptions associated with a task or past negative experiences with task performance), or institutional (institutional policies that limit certain people). Whether skills were never developed or they were lost, however, the end result is the same; the person is unable to accomplish developmental tasks appropriate for his or her developmental stage.

Change

According to adherents of the Developmental conceptual model of practice, change means helping the client to acquire adaptive skills that were either never attained due to developmental delays, or were lost as a result of illness, injury, and so on, so that he or she is able to accomplish developmental stage-appropriate tasks. This is done by evaluating the client to determine his or her current developmental skill level, and then either constructing a development-facilitating environment, teaching the client the required skills, or both. Skills are usually taught in the same sequence as they naturally occur, beginning with those that the client currently possesses and progressing to those that he or she is supposed to have at his or her age (what Mosey referred to as recapitulation of ontogenesis[65]).

Guidelines for Client Evaluation and Therapeutic Intervention

Client Evaluation

Developmentally-based instruments are used to evaluate the client to determine how he or she is functioning according to stage-specific expectations. However, as Bruce and Borg state,

To date, no standardized occupational therapy tests accurately reflect adult skill performance based on a continuum of normal life span development. Standardized tests are available to assess enabling skills primarily in the area of sensorimotor-integration function, but most have been standardized only for the child population and in the area of cognitive dysfunction (p. 134).[13]

In the absence of many standardized instruments, occupational therapists rely mostly on observation of clients while they are engaged in activities and then interviewing them to determine the developmental skill level. In these observations and interviews, therapists seek to understand clients' life history as well as current performance. Understanding of the developmental theories discussed in Chapter 3 is essential in order for the therapist to be able to structure and interpret the observations. For example, a 28-year-old client who has difficulty socializing with peers and is unable to maintain a long-term romantic relationship may be understood to have a problem negotiating the conflict between intimacy and isolation according to Erikson's psychosocial theory. The therapist would observe the client and note deficient social skills, signs of isolation, and so on. A 42-year-old client who is cheating on his wife by having an affair with a 20-year-old woman may be understood to be experiencing midlife crisis as described in Jungian analytic psychology. This would suggest to the therapist that this client may be having difficulty with appraisal of his life, and integration of his feelings and his reflective nature, which is a task of the second half of life for a man. The therapist therefore uses the cognitive schema informed by theoretical knowledge of clinical reasoning to notice clinical cues, appropriately interpret them, and define the problem accurately. The outline of life developmental tasks[67] may be helpful in guiding the therapist through this process (refer to Chapter 16 of your Lab Manual for more information).

In addition to unstructured observations, two standardized instruments have been identified that may be used to assess developmental skills.[40] In Chapter 9, we discussed the Build a City projective task[18] associated with the psychodynamic model. Observation of how clients handle the media used to construct a city and their interactions during the task may indicate their developmental skill levels. For example, if a client gives opinions and orientation to the group (characterized by analysis, clarification of information, and so on) during the task, the therapist may infer that he or she is in Piaget's formal operations cognitive level since this would be a sign of abstract thinking. On the other hand, if the client consistently shows antagonism, this may be a sign of inability to work cooperatively with others, which is a characteristic of the preoperational cognitive level stage where egocentricity predominates (see Piaget's stages of cognitive development in Table 3-3).

The Cognitive Adaptive Skills Evaluation (CASE)[60] is another instrument that was specifically designed to evaluate the cognitive developmental level of psychiatric clients. It was meant to assess performance-based cognitive skills with the objective of identifying thought processes used by clients and their responses to questions inquiring about their performance. The instrument is a cognitive skill inventory that is based on information obtained through a combination of observation and interview. It was designed to evaluate the following:

- The ability to engage in imitation and circular reactions
- The ability to develop and use object permanence, time concepts, language, images, classifications, and relational and number skills
- The ability to use judgment and engage in moral behavior (p. 280)[60]

In the evaluation, the client is asked to make a 1-week (7-day) calendar and is observed while engaging in the task to determine how he or she follows directions, plans the activity, understands what a calendar is, follows rules, and so on. After the task, the client is asked a set of questions regarding his or her understanding of what a calendar is, how he or she decided what materials to use, whether or not there was a plan for making the calendar, and so on. Then the client is asked to make another 1-week calendar and is observed again, then asked questions about the meaning of the word *another,* how his or her calendar was similar to or different from other calendars, how calendars are used, and so on (refer to Lab Manual Chapter 16 to see the instrument along with the administration instructions).

Accompanying the instrument is a summary sheet. Categories of cognitive behaviors observed are listed in the top row, and cognitive levels (which are based on Mosey's[65] subskills of cognitive development) are listed in the left column. In the administration protocol, rating criteria are provided for each observed behavior, identifying the cognitive level under which the behavior would fall. For example, "willingly responds to directions" is assigned to cognitive level 9, "Concrete Operational Thinking" (p. 280).[60] Based on observations during task performance and the client's answers to questions following the task, behaviors are checked off on the protocol regarding whether they are observed (checked "yes") or not (checked "no"). After the evaluation, the checkmarks are transferred to the summary sheet where each is recorded in the box corresponding to behavioral category and cognitive level.

The data on the summary sheet are analyzed according to the following criteria[60]:

- Repetition of skills or behaviors demonstrated
- Clustering of behaviors demonstrated
- Scattering of behaviors demonstrated
- Categories of behaviors demonstrated (p. 283)

Repetition of skills and behaviors suggests that those skills and behaviors are integrated or are being currently used. Clustering of behaviors

around a particular cognitive level indicates that the individual is functioning at that cognitive development subskill level, and scattering of behaviors throughout cognitive levels may be viewed as chance occurrences rather than indicative of integrated cognitive development. Through analysis of the categories of behaviors demonstrated, the therapist is able to advance a hypothesis regarding the client's quality of cognitive skills "such as decision making, use of language, and having and using images" (p. 283).[60] Through this analysis, the therapist is able to delineate the client's cognitive strengths and weaknesses; this delineation provides direction regarding a possible plan of intervention.

Irrespective of whether standardized instruments or unstructured observations are used, the goal of evaluation is to identify deficient or weak adaptive developmental skills. It is also important that the therapist identify barriers to skill development and task accomplishment that may be the cause of lack of acquisition of stage-appropriate skills. While evaluating the client, it is also important that the therapist be cognizant of his or her age, interests, and culture,[19] since these are the variables that determine the meaningfulness and developmental appropriateness of tasks.

Therapeutic Intervention

For therapeutic intervention using the Developmental conceptual model of practice, the therapist makes behavioral goals related to learning developmental stage-specific behaviors/skills. Intervention may be the objective where development of skills is delayed or the skills are lost, while prevention may be the focus for clients who are at risk of losing skills (e.g., an 18-year-old who is at risk of becoming deficient in early adult skills due to the impoverished environment of a psychiatric hospital after first admission).[13] The goals should be written in the RUMBA (Relevant, Understandable, Measurable, Behavioral, and Attainable) format.[73] This means that target behavioral/performance skills/subskills should be specified and then used as the basis for goal development (see the case study following this section).

Once goals are established, occupational tasks are selected for use as therapeutic media, based on their potential to help the client catch up with developmental skills. The tasks should be meaningful in that they should be "an optimum match with what the client…sees as right for him- or herself at the current time in his or her life" (p. 39).[14] The client should be able to manage them with his or her current repertoire of skills while also learning new skills. Therefore the tasks should be viewed as learning experiences affording experimentation, repetition, practice, and refinement, while the client experiences a sense of meaningfulness from engaging in them. Examples of such tasks include learning to make a budget, meal preparation, interaction in social situations, and job-skill training.

Sometimes the therapist needs to modify the environment so that it affords the client opportunities and experiences to promote learning of the required behaviors/skills. In other words, the therapist uses the client's context as a therapeutic modality by "setting up a growth-facilitating environment" (p. 213).[19] Group processes may be used for this purpose, especially Mosey's[65] developmental groups (see Chapter 7 for a discussion of Mosey's therapeutic groups). In this regard, Cole[19] observes that occupational therapy groups are primarily homogenous, and organized at various developmental levels. For clients in lower levels, activities that stimulate sensorimotor or cognitive skill development are used, while at higher levels, those that facilitate successful transition through various developmental stages are used. Such activities may be used as a means for exploration of work/career choices for adolescents preparing to transition to adulthood, evaluation of personal values for those in midlife transition, or preparation for retirement for those anticipating becoming older adults.

CASE STUDY: KEN

Ken is an 18-year-old young man who was discharged from Mathari Mental Hospital (the national mental hospital in Nairobi, Kenya). He came to the outpatient occupational therapy clinic as part of his continued care by a community-based interdisciplinary mental health team after discharge. During the initial meeting with the therapist, he presented as a well-kempt young man. He was quiet and responded to the therapist's questions with "yes" or "no" answers or short phrases. He did not maintain eye contact with the therapist.

Ken was the oldest of three children in his family—two boys and a girl. His brother and sister were doing well in school. Both his parents were small-scale farmers whose main source of livelihood was coffee and dairy farming. He had a typical childhood, and there was no history of health or developmental problems until he was 16 years old, at which time his friends reported that he was behaving "oddly." According to them, he kept very

much to himself and did not seem to be interested in activities in which they participated. His parents did not think there was a problem, attributing his behavior to typical teenage characteristics. This behavior went on for about 2 years. He was in a day secondary school in form 2 (the equivalent of grade 10) at the time. His grades deteriorated and he became quite isolated.

About 2 weeks after Ken turned 18, he became completely withdrawn and would not come out of the house. Friends who visited him reported that he was talking to himself and laughing for no apparent reason. He did not seem to be aware of their presence. Two days later, he started shouting and throwing stones at the house, breaking windows and threatening to kill his father, accusing him of planning to take him to prison and get him killed. His father called the police who arrested Ken and took him to the hospital. He was diagnosed with schizophrenia and admitted. He was at the hospital for 6 weeks after which he was discharged to continue with therapy and medication as an outpatient. During the first interview, Ken told the therapist that he felt as if he did not fit anywhere in society, and this feeling was overwhelming. He was anxious about what would become of his life.

Evaluation

Based on the history, which suggested that Ken had problems with peer relationships and school tasks since he was 16, and his statement that he did not feel that he belonged anywhere, the therapist hypothesized that his transition through adolescence had been disrupted, which suggested that he had not acquired stage-appropriate developmental skills. This disruption was likely to lead to further inability to accomplish developmental tasks of early adulthood such as establishing a career or means of earning a livelihood. The therapist decided to evaluate and plan therapeutic intervention for Ken based on the Developmental conceptual model of practice.

At the time Ken was treated, the therapist did not use standardized instruments to evaluate him. He used Newman and Newman's *Life Development Tasks* outline[67] (see Lab Manual Chapter 16) to structure his observations, the report from the occupational therapist who treated him at the hospital, and data obtained from interviewing both Ken and his family. Through these data-gathering methods, he noticed that Ken's skills were mostly at middle-school–age level (8 to 12 years). He did not seem to have mastered early adolescence skills. For example, during the interview, he had expressed interest in learning tailoring, which he could use to earn a living. Therefore the therapist tested his aptitude for this occupation by asking him to make a paper pattern of a little boy's shirt using a sample given by the therapist of a similar shirt for an adult person who was twice the boy's size. Ken was unable to figure out how to accurately reduce the pattern to scale. This in-

ability suggested that he had not mastered Piaget's formal operations skills, which are required for the abstract thinking necessary to complete the task successfully. Similarly, history obtained by interviewing Ken and his family indicated that he did not currently have any close friends, and had never been able to have a girlfriend or to relate to girls his age. This suggested that he had difficulty with the peer group and romantic relationship skills typical of the early adolescent transitional stage (13 to 17 years).

Apparently, before the onset of his withdrawal symptoms, Ken was said to have had a very good sense of humor and to be fun, and he had many friends. This suggested that he had been able to establish the social cooperation and team play skills typical of the middle school age. The therapist therefore inferred that Ken had acquired some skills that were specific to the middle-school age (development of a sense of industry according to Erikson's psychosocial stages and concrete operations according to Piaget). However, he was deficient in early adolescence skills (group identity according to Erikson, formal operations according to Piaget, separation from parents and establishment of a separate identity according to Levinson).

Treatment Plan

Based on Ken's evaluation, the therapist, in collaboration with Ken, identified the following as the skills that Ken probably needed to acquire: formal operations (solving problems through abstract reasoning, which was necessary for competent accomplishment of tasks necessary for the adult worker role), social interaction, and romantic interaction. Crucial to therapeutic intervention was facilitating Ken's participation in occupations that enabled him to experience a sense of belonging among his peers, in his family, and in the larger social context. Information gathering during evaluation also revealed that given the fact that Ken had been out of school for almost 1 year and his family's poor economic

Continued

CASE STUDY: KEN—CONT'D

status and limited ability to pay for his education, it was not realistic that he would be able to resume formal education. He therefore needed to learn a trade that would enable him to earn a living as a young adult. His interest in tailoring was a beginning point for this endeavor. Through collaboration between Ken and the therapist, the following intervention goals were established:

Short-Term Goals

1. By the end of 4 weeks, Ken will demonstrate improved abstract problem-solving skills to be able to successfully complete a scaled paper pattern of a shirt with no more that three verbal cues and one demonstration by the therapist.
2. By the end of 3 weeks, Ken's social skills will have improved significantly as indicated by spontaneously participating in a leisure activity of his interest with at least two friends three times a week.
4. By the end of 5 weeks, Ken will demonstrate improved romantic interaction skills as indicated by asking a woman his age and going out for at least two successful dates.

Long-Term Goals

1. By the end of 8 weeks, Ken will demonstrate a beginning occupational repertoire typical of early adulthood comprising mastery of a skill he can use to earn a living and a balanced daily routine consisting of productive and leisure activities, and rest.
2. By the end of 6 weeks, Ken will demonstrate romantic interaction skills necessary for eventual establishment of a family as indicated by having a regular dating relationship with a woman his age.

Based on the above-listed goals, both individual and group interventions were used for treatment. Group activities included social skills training. Group members participated in leisure activities and subsequently discussed interaction skills that were necessary for satisfactory completion of the

activities. Role-plays were used to help develop both peer and romantic interaction skills. Individual intervention for Ken included training in dressmaking consistent with his interest to make a living as a tailor. Other job options were explored. By the end of 8 weeks of intervention, Ken had opened a dressmaking shop and was a church youth leader. I was Ken's occupational therapist until this time. When I changed jobs, the new occupational therapist continued to see Ken. I did not follow up to find out how his therapy ended.

It is important to point out that although in this case the Developmental conceptual model was used as an overall organizing framework for therapeutic intervention, therapeutic strategies were based on a variety of conceptual models of practice as well. For example, behavioral techniques such as modeling, shaping, and chaining were used to help Ken learn social skills and to teach him complex procedures such as planning and sequentially following the plan to complete a task such as making a shirt. This is true for other conceptual models of practice as well. Because of clients' diversity of needs, rarely are intervention techniques drawn exclusively from one model. We will discuss in more detail the eclectic integration of conceptual models of practice in Chapter 17.

Other Evaluations

Use of the Cognitive Adaptive Skills Evaluation (CASE)[60] could have yielded more information about Ken's specific strengths and limitations in planning, judging, and decision making, and problem-solving skills. This information would have helped the therapist in planning, in collaboration with Ken, more targeted interventions to help him learn cognitive skills needed to accomplish his goal of developing competency in performance of job-related activities.

 Refer to Lab Manual Exercise 16-1 to enhance your client assessment and therapeutic intervention skills based on the Developmental conceptual model's guidelines.

Consistency of the Developmental Conceptual Model of Practice with the Occupational Therapy Paradigm

Therapists using the Developmental conceptual model of practice may be at risk of focusing on activities directed at developing specific developmental skills rather than using occupation-based interventions. This risk is illustrated in statements such as:

> The chosen activities should address issues to be resolved or specific skills appropriate to the developmental level of the client group. The theorist, the specific stage to be addressed, and the specific task or skill within that stage should be identified. Since most of the theorists have an identified hierarchy of issues, tasks, or skills to be learned at each level, these can easily serve as guidelines for activity choice (p. 214, emphasis mine).[19]

This focus on use of activities and developmental theorists' guidelines regarding tasks and skills to be learned could derail the therapist's cognizance of the need to emphasize intervention using occupations that are meaningful to the client and that facilitate participation in life. To that extent, the model would be inconsistent with the current occupational therapy paradigm, which emphasizes occupation-based, client-centered practice.

Also, although the role of the therapist is specified as facilitating development of stage-specific developmental skills, the role of availing opportunities for participation in meaningful occupations is not explicitly stated in the model. Other roles of the therapist according to the guidelines of the model include creating an environment that provides opportunities for learning stage-specific tasks and skills, helping the client make necessary adaptations to overcome developmental limitations, and teaching requisite skills. All these roles are consistent with those specified in the current occupational therapy paradigm. Therefore it can be concluded that this model is consistent with the current occupational therapy paradigm in as far as the roles of the occupational therapist include environmental modification, facilitating adaptive capacities, and teaching skills. The model's guidelines regarding use of occupation-based, client-centered interventions are not explicit. To that extent, consistency of the model with the current professional paradigm is not clear.

Consistency with the Philosophy of Pragmatism

The Developmental conceptual model is clearly consistent with the process perspective of the philosophy of pragmatism, which conceptualizes one's emergence as consisting of continuity between the past, present, and future (see Chapter 4). Indeed, as Breines[12] informs us, the whole evolutionary principle that "ontogeny recapitulates phylogeny" that is prevalent in occupational therapy's developmental perspective was first articulated by G. Stanley Hall, one of the greatest influences in John Dewey's thought. According to this principle, "Time is the thread that passes from the past to the future. From ancient to modern times, this continuous thread can be understood through the changes that take place *within each lifetime as individuals develop and learn*" (p. 17, emphasis mine).[12] This principle is one of the central tenets of the Developmental conceptual model of practice. Furthermore, to the extent that the client is encouraged to actively learn stage-specific skills, he or she is conceptualized as an agent in his or her own change. This agentic perspective, along with the view of the environment as a source of experiences necessary for learning stage-specific skills, are also consistent with the principles of the philosophy of pragmatism.

Consistency with the Complexity/Chaos Theoretical Framework

As mentioned earlier, there is an emerging transactional approach to therapy in the Developmental conceptual model of practice derived from the dynamic theory, where developmental skills are conceptualized to emerge from a dynamic inter-action between environmental challenges, social economic status, social circumstances, and neu-romuscular maturation.[9,37] However, this con-ceptual approach does not seem to be prevalent in the model's application to adult psychosocial treatment.

Recommendations for Reinterpretation of the Model

A more explicit statement in its guidelines of the need to make occupational therapy interventions occupation-based and client-centered would make the model more consistent with the current occupational therapy paradigm. It is also sug-gested that explicit directions be provided in the model's guidelines regarding use of occupations during intervention as "perturbations" (environ-mental challenges) designed to push the human system away from the current developmental level of performance (equilibrium). This would move the system away from a state of equilib-rium thereby facilitating emergence of skills at the next developmental stage of functioning.[59] It is highly probable that therapists are already intuitively doing this in practice. However, mak-ing this intention of intervention clear would make treatment planning more efficient and its rationale more apparent.

In this regard, incorporation into the model's guidelines of the interactionist framework for occupational development suggested by Davis and Polatajko[26] may be useful. In this frame-work, occupational performance is conceptu-alized to emerge from a dynamic interaction between the person, environment, and occupa-tion. It is suggested here, consistent with the proposition by Davis and Polatajko, that occu-pational development is "the gradual change in occupational behaviors over time, resulting from the growth and maturation of the individual in interaction with the environment" (p. 40).[17] Furthermore, "The interactionist perspective on development provides a way of framing occupa-tional development and identifying the principles that govern the interaction. These principles are continuity, multiple determinicity, and multiple patternicity, and they provide a model of occu-pational development" (pp. 96–97).[26]

Evidence-Based Practice Using the Developmental Conceptual Model

Much research has been conducted particularly in psychology and sociology validating some of the propositions of the Developmental concep-tual framework. We will discuss a few of these studies. Some of them investigated developmen-tal issues within the framework of Erikson's stages of psychosocial development,[11,63,78] some tested Loevinger's propositions about adult ego development,[59,64] and others were nonspecific with regard to the conceptual framework for human development.

Brennan[11] investigated the relationship between stress due to loss of vision, significant stressful events in life, spirituality, and psychoso-cial development based on Erikson's psychosocial stages among middle-aged and older adults. The hypothesis tested in the study was that higher levels of psychosocial development would be predicted by levels of stress, and spirituality and religiosity would mediate the stressful life events and therefore facilitate development. The study sample consisted of 195 participants, 45 years or older. They were divided into two groups. Group 1 (middle age) consisted of 99 participants 45 to 64 years of age. Group 2 (older adults) consisted of 96 participants 65 years or older.

Vision status for all participants was assessed using a functional screening questionnaire, which inquired about the effect of visual loss on func-tion as indicated by inability to read labels on medication bottles, read street signs, recognize faces of people from a distance, and so on. Subjective perception of life stress was mea-sured on a Ranked Life Experience Inventory (RLEI), spirituality and religiosity on a Spiritual Assessment Scale (SAS), and psychosocial devel-opment on an Inventory of Psychosocial Balance (IPB) questionnaire. All data were gathered by telephone. Correlational analysis and analysis of variance led to the conclusion that as hypothesized, spirituality could be seen as a buffer for negative life events and therefore affected development. In other words, spirituality was found to be a strong predictor of psychosocial development. Also, stress was significantly correlated with psychosocial development, suggesting that stressful life events may be facilitators of adult development along Erikson's eight-stage continuum. These findings suggest that occupational therapists using the Developmental conceptual model may do well to bear in mind the spiritual aspects of occupations used in interventions, and also how they can help clients change stressful events into growth-facilitating opportunities.

In a related study,[63] gender differences were found with regard to how generativity was expressed by study participants. It was found that women expressed generativity through communal acts like employment in helping professions such as teaching and nursing, while men expressed their generativity mostly through goal-oriented (agentic) nonhelping occupations such as engineering. Occupational therapists therefore need to bear these gender differences in mind as they design interventions based on the Developmental model. In another study, Shulman and Ben-Artzi[78] found that the extent to which one attained adult status was highly correlated with ego identity. This finding has important implications for therapeutic programming for younger adults considering that research indicates that due to lengthened adolescent transition in contemporary society, young adults in their twenties tend to be still struggling with adolescent issues such as confusion about personal identity.

As mentioned earlier, some studies have tested Loevinger's[53] hypothesis regarding stabilization of ego development in young adulthood. Morros and colleagues[64] explored the relationship between personality, ego development, and volunteering activities among elders 55–83 years of age. Their hypothesis was that openness to new experiences would be correlated to volunteerism, which in turn would be correlated

with an advanced stage of ego development as measured on Loevinger's nine-stage continuum of development. The level of ego development was measured on the Washington University Sentence Completion Test of Ego Development (WUSCTED),[54] and openness to new experiences on the NEO Five Factor Inventory (NEO-FFI), which is a 60-item Likert-type instrument assessing various domains of personality, with openness to experience being one of them. Volunteerism was assessed by inquiring about the number of hours of involvement in volunteer activities over one's lifetime. Correlational and multiple regression analysis led to the conclusion that volunteer history was correlated with an advanced stage of ego development. Other contributing factors to ego development were found to be education and language fluency. Openness to experience was found to be a strong predictor of development.

In another study, Manners and colleagues[59] investigated whether advanced ego development according to Loevinger's theory could be facilitated through therapeutic intervention. They tested the hypothesis that exposure to what they called *disequilibrating experiences* would lead to transition to higher stages of ego development. Fifty-eight individuals, ages 22 to 53, participated in the study. They were divided into three groups. Group 1 consisted of 21 participants recruited through a University Graduate School Management (GSM) mailing list. Group 2 consisted of 15 participants recruited from a suburban church, and the control group was made up of 22 individuals from both the GSM and the church. Participants in the control group were matched with those in the treatment groups for age, educational level, and gender identification.

A pretest, posttest, and follow-up test 4 months after intervention were conducted using the WUSCTED. Intervention consisted of weekly 90-minute sessions for 10 weeks and focused on didactic input and experiential exercises carefully designed to encourage exploration and reflection on personal emotional discrimination, identity and relationship patterns, and communication skills. Since pretest had indicated that the majority of participants were at the *self-aware* ego developmental stage, intervention was designed to demand a level of functioning at higher stages in order to provide the disequilibrating effect. Data analysis revealed that there was a significant increase in ego functioning for participants in both treatment groups but no change for those in the control group. This finding supported the study's hypothesis.

Both the above studies provide evidence for use of complexity/chaos theoretical approaches while designing therapeutic interventions based on the Developmental conceptual model of practice in occupational therapy, as discussed earlier in the recommendations for reinterpretation of the model. Both studies suggest that therapists should attempt to provide environmental experiences that would act as perturbations (what Manners and colleagues[59] called *disequilibriating experiences*) that push the human system away from a stable stage of performance so that it may reorganize at a higher stage.

Other topics that have been investigated through research include the effectiveness of transcendental meditation in facilitating development of higher levels of consciousness and cognitive functioning,[68] the effect of regrets due to unattained life goals on subjective well-being,[44] turning points (factors that change developmental trajectories) among adults,[72] and the effect of psychological hardiness on ability to cope with life stresses such as involuntary job loss,[24] among others. However, few of these studies have been conducted by occupational therapists to demonstrate clinical effectiveness of the Developmental conceptual model of practice in the treatment of adult psychiatric clients.

In a search conducted using the "OT Search," a major and authoritative database cataloguing sources of occupational therapy literature and maintained by the American Occupational Therapy Association (AOTA), 60 sources were identified that discussed topics somewhat related to adult human development. Of the 60, 15

abstracts dealt with topics that were directly related to adult human development. Out of those 15, 10 were conceptual papers dealing with the following issues:

- Development of guidelines for elderly client education using the lifespan developmental framework[38]
- Changing dynamics of the role of caregiving among women and men[70]
- Factors that contribute to job satisfaction[35]
- Development of a work assessment program for adult long-term psychiatric care[1]
- Facilitation of expression of sexuality by aging adults[33]
- Managing the stress experienced by adolescents with physical disabilities as they try to acquire skills necessary to manage their daily lives[7]
- Preparation of individuals with intellectual disabilities to assume adult worker role responsibilities[84]
- Intervention strategies to help adolescents learn adaptive skills necessary to master developmental tasks[25]
- A therapeutic model to help clients develop hope for the future[80]
- The importance of personally meaningful occupation during points of transition in life[10]

Thus only five published papers were identified that were based on research investigating developmental issues from the perspective of occupational therapy.

Among the five studies identified, Lefkofsky[49] described the development and validation of the Adult Screening Questionnaire (ASQ), a screening tool for developmentally disabled adults. In a dissertation written by Burnell,[15] a clinical frame of reference for intervention was proposed to facilitate cognitive functioning of adults with intellectual disabilities. The video replay method used in the frame of reference was found to be effective for the purpose for which it was designed as indicated by increased participants' eagerness to perform, attentiveness, and perceptual discrimination after intervention. A case study conducted by Webster[86] led to identification of factors affecting occupational role development among young adults with mild intellectual disabilities. In another study, Mitchell and Kemp[62] described the Older Adult Disability Scale (OADS), a self-report instrument designed to assess attitudes toward older adults with disabilities. Validation research indicated that the instrument had good internal consistency, high test-retest reliability, and high subscale intercorrelations, which meant that it was a good instrument to assess attitudes toward older adults with intellectual disabilities.

Finally, Hull[41] conducted a study to investigate the effectiveness and quality of rehabilitation services beyond historical measures of increased independence. The findings indicated that there was a moderate positive correlation between life satisfaction and meaningful role performance among older adults 65 years or older discharged from the hospital to the community under a primary caregiver. This finding suggested that helping older adults resume personally meaningful roles in the community is an important aspect of their rehabilitation that would lead to increased life satisfaction. It is, however, clear that occupational therapists have not conducted much empirical research to clinically validate application of this model in the treatment of adult psychiatric clients. More research is needed in this area.

SUMMARY

In this chapter, we discussed the Developmental conceptual model of practice. We also expounded various conceptual models of human development (biological-linear-hierarchical, stage theory, and the currently evolving dynamic systems perspective). The stage theory of development is perhaps the most prevalently applied framework in the Developmental conceptual model used in the treatment of adult psychiatric clients. Although the dynamic perspective is emerging, especially in the application of the model to pediatrics and

neurological conditions, all indications are that it is not prevalently being applied in psychosocial practice. The model is consistent with the current occupational therapy paradigm and the philosophy of occupational therapy in certain ways.

We made recommendations for reinterpretation of the model so that it is more consistent with the paradigm, the philosophy of pragmatism, and the complexity/chaos theoretical framework. We also discussed research validating clinical usefulness of the model. Although there is much empirical evidence available validating the constructs of the model, there is need for more occupational therapy research to demonstrate the model's usefulness in psychosocial occupational therapy practice.

REFERENCES

1. Alleyne A: Practice watch: things to think about—choosing the components of an occupational therapy work assessment program for a psychiatric hospital, *Occup Ther Health Care* 4:171–182, 1987.
2. Ayres AJ: The development of perceptual-motor abilities: a theoretical basis for treatment of dysfunction, *Am J Occup Ther* 17:221–225, 1963.
3. Ayres AJ: *Southern California Perceptual-Motor Tests,* Los Angeles, 1968, Western Psychological Services.
4. Ayres AJ: *Sensory integration and learning disorders,* Los Angeles, 1972, Western Psychological Services.
5. Ayres AJ: *Southern California sensory integration tests,* Los Angeles, 1972, Western Psychological Services.
6. Ayres AJ: *Southern California postrotary nystagmus test manual,* Los Angeles, 1975, Western Psychological Services.
7. Bell C, Quintal J: A life skills program for physically disabled adolescents, *Canad J Occup Ther* 52:235–239, 1985.
8. Bernstein N: *The coordination and regulation of movements,* London, 1967, Pergamon.
9. Bigsby R: Developmental and neurological perspectives: overview of infant and child developmental models. In Crepeau EB, Cohn ES, Schell BA, eds: *Willard and Spackman's occupational therapy,* ed 10, New York, 2003, Lippincott Williams & Wilkins, pp. 243–245.
10. Blair S: The centrality of occupation during life transitions, *Br J Occup Ther* 63:231–237, 2000.
11. Brennan M: Spirituality and psychosocial development in middle-age and older adults with vision loss, *J Adult Devel* 9:31–46, 2002.

12. Breines E: *Occupational therapy activities from clay to computers: theory and practice*, Philadelphia, 1995, FA Davis.

13. Bruce MA, Borg B: *Psychosocial occupational therapy: frames of reference for intervention*, ed 2, Thorofare, NJ, 1993, Slack.

14. Bruce MA, Borg B: *Psychosocial frames of reference: core for occupation-based practice*, ed 3, Thorofare, NJ, 2002, Slack.

15. Burnell DP: *A cognitive frame of reference for curriculum planning with mentally retarded adults, based on the psychological literature*, unpublished doctoral dissertation, Berkeley, California, 1973, Wright Institute.

16. Bursik K: Adaptation to divorce and ego development in adult women, *J Personality Social Psychol* 60:300–306, 1990.

17. Canadian Association of Occupational Therapists: *Enabling occupation: an occupational therapy perspective*, Ottawa, ON, 1997, CAOT Publications ACE.

18. Clark EN: Build a city: a projective task concept. In Hemphill-Pearson BJ, ed: *Assessments in occupational therapy mental health: an integrative approach*, Thorofare, NJ, 1999, Slack, pp. 155–172.

19. Cole MB: *Group dynamics in occupational therapy: the theoretical basis and practice application of group intervention*, ed 3, Thorofare, NJ, 2005, Slack.

20. Condon VA: Physical systems assessment. In Emlet CA, Crabtree JL, Condon VA, et al, eds: *In-home assessment of older adults: an interdisciplinary approach*, Gaithersburg, MD, 1996, Aspen, pp. 76–106.

21. Coster W, Deeney T, Haltiwanger J, et al: *The school function assessment*, San Antonio, 1998, The Psychological Corporation.

22. Cronin A: Development in the preschool years. In Cronin A, Mandich M, eds: *Human development and performance throughout the lifespan*, Clifton Park, NY, 2005, Thomson Delmar Learning, pp. 176–197.

23. Cronin A: Middle childhood and school. In Cronin A, Mandich M, eds: *Human development and performance throughout the lifespan*, Clifton Park, NY, 2005, Thomson Delmar Learning, pp. 198–214.

24. Crowley BJ, Hayslip B, Hobdy J: Psychological hardiness and adjustment to life events in adulthood, *J Adult Devel* 10:237–248, 2003.

25. David SK: The OT treatment of adolescents in a partial hospitalization program [Abstract], *Conference Abstracts and Resources*, Bethesda, MD, 1997, American Occupational Therapy Association, p. 183.

26. Davis JA, Polatajko H: Occupational development. In Christiansen CH, Townsend EA, eds: *Introduction to occupation: the art and science of living*, Upper Saddle River, NJ, 2004, Prentice Hall, pp. 91–119.

27. Emlet CA: Assessing social function, support, and socioeconomic status. In Emlet CA, Crabtree JL, Condon VA, et al, eds: *In-home assessment of older adults: an interdisciplinary approach*, Gaithersburg, MD, 1996, Aspen, pp. 154–179.

28. Emlet CA, Crabtree JL: Introduction to in-home assessment of older adults. In Emlet CA, Crabtree JL, Condon VA, et al, eds: *In-home assessment of older adults: an interdisciplinary approach*, Gaithersburg, MD, 1996, Aspen, pp. 1–16.

29. Emlet CA, Crabtree JL, Condon VA, et al, eds: *In-home assessment of older adults: an interdisciplinary approach*, Gaithersburg, MD, 1996, Aspen.

30. Erikson EH: *Childhood and society*, New York, 1950, Norton.

31. Erikson EH: *Identity: youth crisis*, New York, 1968, Norton.

32. Erikson EH, Erikson JM: *The life cycle completed*, New York, 1987, W.W. Norton.

33. Fazio L: Sexuality and aging: a community wellness program, *Phys Occup Ther Geriatr* 6:59–69, 1987.

34. Fidler G, Fidler J: *Occupational therapy: a communication process in psychiatry*, New York, 1963, McMillan.

35. Frye S: The work role and middle adult development: a look at the blue-collar worker, *J Occup Ther Students* 5(1):29–40, 1990.

36. Gast HL: The relationship between stages of ego development and developmental stages of health self care operations, *Dissertation Abstracts International* 44:3039B, 1984.

37. Gilfoyle EM, Grady AP, Moore JC: *Children adapt*, Thorofare, NJ, 1981, Slack.

38. Hasselkus BR: Patient education and the elderly, *Phys Occup Ther Geriatr* 2(3):55–70, 1983.

39. Helson R, Roberts BW: Ego development and personality change in adulthood, *J Personality Social Psychol* 66:911–920, 1994.

40. Hemphill-Pearson BJ, ed: *Assessments in occupational therapy mental health: an integrative approach*, Thorofare, NJ, 1999, Slack.

41. Hull JB: *The association of engagement in meaningful roles and life satisfaction in older adults after physical rehabilitation* [Monograph], Philadelphia, 1998, Temple University.

42. Ikiugu MN: Meaningfulness of occupations as an occupational-life-trajectory attractor, *J Occup Sci* 12:102–109, 2005.

43. Ikiugu MN, Rosso HM: Understanding the occupational human being as a complex, dynamical, adaptive system, *Occup Ther Health Care* 19(4):43–65, 2005.

44. Jokisaari M: Regrets and subjective well-being: a life course approach, *J Adult Devel* 11:281–288, 2004.

45. Jung CG: *The unconscious self*, New York, 1958, Mentor Books.

46. Jung CG: *The collected works of C.G. Jung*, Princeton, 1953–1983, Princeton University Press.

47. Jung CG: Integrating anima and animus, *Therapy Weekly* 15, 1985.

48. King LJ: Toward a science of adaptive responses, *Am J Occup Ther* 32:429–437, 1978.

49. Lefkofsky S: On the formative stages of the adult screening questionnaire: a managerial approach for screening adult developmentally disabled clients, *Occup Ther Health Care* 6:107–128, 1989.

50. Levinson DJ: *The seasons of a man's life,* New York, 1978, Knopf.

51. Llorens LA: Facilitating growth and development: the promise of occupational therapy, *Am J Occup Ther* 24:93–101, 1969.

52. Llorens LA: Performance tasks and roles throughout the lifespan. In Christiansen C, Baum C, eds: *Occupational therapy: overcoming human performance deficits,* Thorofare, NJ, 1991, Slack, pp. 45–68.

53. Loevinger J: *Ego development,* San Francisco, 1976, Jossey-Bass.

54. Loevinger J: A revision of the Sentence Completion Test for ego development, *J Personality Social Psychol* 48:420–427, 1985.

55. Ludwig FM: Anne Cronin Mosey. In Miller RJ, Walker KF, eds: *Perspectives on theory for the practice of occupational therapy,* pp. 41–63, Gaithersburg, MD, 1993, Aspen.

56. Mandich M: Theoretical framework for human performance. In Cronin A, Mandich M, eds: *Human development and performance throughout the lifespan,* Clifton Park, NY, 2005, Thomson Delmar Learning, pp. 15–36.

57. Mandich M: The newborn. In Cronin A, Mandich M, eds: *Human development and performance throughout the lifespan,* Clifton Park, NY, 2005, Thomson Delmar Learning, pp. 114–138.

58. Mandich M: Infancy. In Cronin A, Mandich M, eds: *Human development and performance throughout the lifespan,* Clifton Park, NY, 2005, Thomson Delmar Learning, pp. 139–163.

59. Manners J, Durkin K, Nesdale A: Promoting advanced ego development among adults, *J Adult Devel* 11:19–27, 2004.

60. Masagatani GN: The cognitive adaptive skills evaluation. In Hemphill-Pearson BJ, ed: *Assessments in occupational therapy mental health: an integrative approach,* Thorofare, NJ, 1999, Slack, pp. 279–284.

61. Michaelson CB: An exploratory study of the health belief model and ego development in predicting health related actions in the aged, *Dissertation Abstracts International* 46:1694B, 1985.

62. Mitchell JM, Kemp BJ: The older adult disability scale: development and validation, *Rehabil Psychol* 41:187–203, 1996.

63. Morfei MZ, Hooker K, Carpenter J, et al: Agentic and communal generative behavior in four areas of adult life: Implications for psychological well-being, *J Adult Devel* 11:55–58, 2004.

64. Morros M, Pushkar D, Reis M: A study of current, former, and new elderly volunteers: a comparison of developmental and trait models of personality, *J Adult Devel* 5:219–230, 1998.

65. Mosey AC: *Three frames of reference for mental health,* Thorofare, NJ, 1970, Slack.

66. Mosey AC: *Activities therapy,* New York, 1973, Raven Press.

67. Newman BM, Newman PR: *Development through life: a psychosocial approach,* Homewood, IL, 1979, Dorsey.

68. Orme-Johnson DW: An overview of Charles Alexander's contribution to psychology: developing higher states of consciousness in the individual and the society, *J Adult Devel* 7:199–215, 2000.

69. Piaget J: *The origins of intelligence in children,* New York, 1952, International University Press.

70. Porat R, Weinblatt N: Differences in the concept of caregiving between men and women in the course of life, *Israel J Occup Ther* 4(1):E25–E26, 1995.

71. Reynolds P, Cronin A: Aging. In Cronin A, Mandich M, eds: *Human development and performance throughout the lifespan,* Clifton Park, NY, 2005, Thomson Delmar Learning, pp. 306–331.

72. Ronka A, Oravala S, Pulkkinen L: Turning points in adults' lives: the effects of gender and the amount of choice, *J Adult Devel* 10:203–215, 2003.

73. Sames KM: *Documenting occupational therapy practice,* Upper Saddle River, NJ, 2005, Pearson/Prentice-Hall.

74. Schuster EO, Francis-Connolly E, Alford-Trewn P, et al: Conceptualization and development of a course on aging to infancy: a life course perspective, *Educ Gerontol* 29:841–850, 2003.

75. Settersten RA, ed: *Invitation to the life course: toward new understandings of later life,* Amityville, NY, 2002, Baywood.

76. Shaw K, Cronin A: Adulthood. In Cronin A, Mandich M, eds: *Human development and performance throughout the lifespan,* Clifton Park, NY, 2005, Thomson Delmar Learning, pp. 284–305.

77. Shortridge SD, Walker KF: Lera A. Llorens. In Miller RJ, Walker KF, eds: *Perspectives on theory for the practice of occupational therapy,* Gaithersburg, MD, 1993, Aspen, pp. 65–102.

78. Shulman S, Ben-Artzi E: Age related differences in the transition from adolescence to adulthood and links with family relationships, *J Adult Devel* 10:217–226, 2003.

79. Simons DF: Adolescent development. In Cronin A, Mandich M, eds: *Human development and performance throughout the lifespan,* Clifton Park, NY, 2005, Thomson Delmar Learning, pp. 215–245.

80. Spencer J, Davidson H, White V: Helping clients develop hopes for the future, *Am J Occup Ther* 51:191–198, 1997.

81. Treml LA: Accessibility and safety. In Emlet CA, Crabtree JL, Condon VA, et al, eds: *In-home assessment of older adults: an interdisciplinary approach,* Gaithersburg, MD, 1996, Aspen, pp. 17–34.

82. Uhlendorff U: The concept of developmental-tasks and its significance for education and social work, *Social Work Soc* 2(1):54–63, 2004.

83. Vergara ER: Prenatal development. In Cronin A, Mandich M, eds: *Human development and performance throughout the lifespan,* Clifton Park, NY, 2005, Thomson Delmar Learning, pp. 91–113.

84. Vidmark I: How children with mental retardation in Swedish schools are prepared for work in adult life, *Work J Prevention Assess Rehabil* 5:185–190, 1995.

85. Warren M: Sensory and neuromotor remediation. In Christiansen C, Baum C, eds: *Occupational therapy: overcoming human performance deficits,* Thorofare, NJ, 1991, Slack, pp. 633–662.

86. Webster PS: Occupational therapy behavior in pediatrics: occupational role development in the young adult with mild mental retardation, *Am J Occup Ther* 34: 13–18, 1980.

87. Wheeler S, Shaw K: Transitions to adult life. In Cronin A, Mandich M, eds: *Human development and performance throughout the lifespan,* Clifton Park, NY, 2005, Thomson Delmar Learning, pp. 263–283.

15
The Occupational Adaptation Model of Practice

Preview Questions

1. List and discuss the theoretical sources of constructs used in the Occupational Adaptation conceptual model of practice as applied in adult psychosocial occupational therapy.
2. Define the following Occupational Adaptation model constructs: occupational adaptation process, occupational adaptation energy, occupational adaptation response mode, occupational adaptation response behavior, person-systems, and relative mastery.
3. Concisely state the theoretical core of the Occupational Adaptation conceptual model of practice.
4. Explain postulations of the Occupational Adaptation conceptual model of practice about the following:
   a. Function
   b. Dysfunction
   c. Change
5. Outline and explain the Occupational Adaptation model's guidelines for client evaluation and therapeutic intervention.
6. Discuss the consistency of the Occupational Adaptation model of practice with each of the following:
   a. The occupational therapy paradigm
   b. The philosophy of pragmatism
   c. The complexity/chaos theoretical framework
7. Discuss available empirical evidence supporting clinical effectiveness of the Occupational Adaptation conceptual model of practice as a guide to intervention in occupational therapy practice.

The occupational adaptation (OA) conceptual model of practice was developed in the early 1990s at Texas Woman's University as a framework to organize research for faculty and students in the newly created occupational therapy doctoral program.[19,25,28,32] In the process of this endeavor, extensive literature review was completed. The authors identified adaptation and occupation as key constructs that define the identity of occupational therapy as a profession. For example, King stated "that the adaptive process constitutes the core of occupational therapy theory, and that specific attributes of adaptation are also the significant and characteristic attributes of occupational therapy" (p. 432).[12] Among these attributes, King identified the demand of the adaptation process for a positive role by the individual, adaptation as a result of environmental demands, subcortical organization of the adaptation process, and adaptation as a self-reinforcing response to environmental demands.

Those four attributes became core constructs of the occupational adaptation model as we will see later in this chapter. The literature review led Schultz and Schkade to conclude "that adaptation is a concept so fundamental to the field that it is recognized as a universally accepted treatment goal" (p. 460).[27] The constructs of adaptation and occupation (which provides occupational therapy its identity[14,15]) became the two main constructs of the model (OA frame of reference). In this chapter, we will discuss in detail the model's background, assumptions, and theoretical core; guidelines for client evaluation and treatment, and consistency with the current occupational therapy paradigm, the philosophy of pragmatism, and the complexity/chaos theory. Additionally, we will note recommendations for reinterpretation of the model and available empirical evidence supporting the model's clinical efficacy.

Evolution of the Occupational Adaptation Model

Interdisciplinary Basis

Occupational adaptation constructs were derived from occupational therapy literature, cognitive and experimental psychology, Hans Selye's[29] theory of stress and adaptation, and the general systems theory.

Background

The OA model sought to build on the long tradition of the view in occupational therapy that occupation is a means of relating to the environment and therefore regaining health and staying healthy. As discussed in Chapter 1, the moral treatment movement adherents considered ordinary daily occupations to be the best means of reaching the human at the highest level—the intellectual realm. They postulated that participation in occupations helped clients divest themselves from absorption in melancholic thoughts and become more productive citizens of the world. Proponents of the arts and crafts movement considered occupations, especially artistic creations, to be the means of decreasing alienation from the self, one's work, other people, and the environment. During the mental hygiene movement, mental illness was seen as a problem of adaptation.[14] Occupation was proposed as a means of interacting with the environment so as to stay in balance with the natural rhythms of life and therefore to be adaptive.

The themes of occupation and adaptation resurfaced in the 1960s with Mary Reilly's call for a return to the roots of occupational therapy. She proposed that the idea that "man, by use of his own hands, as they are energized by the mind and directed by the will, can influence the state of his own health" (p. 2)[15] was perhaps the greatest idea in twentieth-century medicine. Later, she developed the occupational behavior frame of reference in which play, work, and leisure were all seen as a continuum of occupations through which humans adapt to their environment.[16,17] Other occupational therapy theorists like King[12] responded to Reilly's call by proposing adaptive process as a theoretical frame of reference that would unite all aspects of occupational therapy practice.

Reilly's students carried this theme further. For instance, Shannon[30] argued that occupational therapy had been derailed, and reiterated Reilly's call for the profession to return to its authentic course by emphasizing temporal adaptation (how one effectively lives in the environment by occupying time) and behavioral competency (skills needed to attain temporal adaptation) rather than simplistic focus on stimulus-response, instincts and drives, and neuromuscular functioning. Kielhofner[9] followed Shannon's lead with an elaboration of the temporal adaptation frame of reference where he emphasized the role of habits in the adaptive process. Later, he developed the Model of Human Occupation (MOHO) in which he argued that adaptive thoughts, feelings, and actions emerge from a dynamic interaction between the environment and the three human components: volition, habituation, and performance capacity.[10]

Advancing the twin themes of occupation and adaptation further, Schkade and Schultz[20] and Schultz and Schkade[26] developed the OA model based on the notion of *occupation* and *adaptation* as constituting a single, integrated, idiosyncratic internal process. They saw this process as a nonhierarchical and non-stage–specific explanation of the human adaptive process. A person's desire for mastery and the environmental demand for mastery were conceptualized to result in a "press" for mastery. This press was conceived to propel the individual toward performance of occupational tasks in order to meet environmental challenges and attain "relative mastery." They defined relative mastery as an internal experience of satisfaction with performance, satisfaction by others with one's performance, efficiency (in terms of energy and time expended), and effectiveness (successful completion of a task as desired).

Furthermore, the human organism was understood to have a finite amount of adaptive energy, which had to be used conservatively to avoid premature exhaustion. This idea was borrowed from Selye's[29] theory of stress. In this theory, Selye concluded from his research with laboratory animals that excessive high use of adaptive capacity of the endocrine system led to premature death. He termed this phenomenon "the general adaptation syndrome," which he argued exists in humans as well. Schkade and Schultz[20] and Schultz and Schkade[26] argued that if Selye was correct, then occupation adaptation energy was finite. This meant that humans needed to manage use of their adaptation energy carefully in order to continue functioning. This careful management of the adaptation energy could be attained by following a person's internal occupational adaptation process, which they understood to be based on the following core principles:

- Individuals respond to the demand for adaptation across the life span with varying degrees of adaptiveness.
- Adaptiveness is determined by individual uniqueness and the nature of interaction with the environment (occupation).
- The OA process describes the internal mechanism by which humans experience the demand for adaptation, formulate a unique plan of adaptation, act upon their adaptation with an observable occupational response, evaluate

the results, and integrate the effects into their adaptation repertoire.
- The demand for adaptation is embedded within the context of occupational environments (work, play, and self-maintenance) and interwoven with the performance of occupational roles.
- The satisfying performance of occupational roles is a vital component of successful occupational functioning at each stage of life (p. 111).[13]

The Theoretical Core of the Occupational Adaptation Conceptual Model

Over the years, constructs of the OA conceptual model have been developed and elaborated. The model's theoretical core as it stands today can be summarized as follows[1,22,24]: The OA process is a result of interaction between the individual human, with his or her inner *desire to attain mastery* (sense of competency and control), and the environment, which presents the person with a *demand for mastery* in the form of challenges, creating *press for mastery*. When the individual encounters environmental challenges, he or she generates a response geared toward overcoming those challenges and therefore attains a *sense of mastery*. Ideally, the response is adaptive and masterful and meets the person's internal as well as external (environmental) role expectations (resulting in occupational adaptation).

Interaction between a person and the environment is a dynamic process mediated by three constants: a person's internal desire for mastery, environmental demand for mastery, and press for mastery (result of the person-occupational environment interaction). Once the person is able to satisfy internal desire and meet the external demand for mastery successfully, occupational adaptation is said to have occurred. Occupation is the means by which this adaptation is achieved because it "enables human beings to continually adapt to changing needs and conditions in the environment" (p. 166).[31] Furthermore, it is assumed that occupation is a part of human nature.[22] As such, competence in occupational functioning is the measure of human adaptation and therefore the end goal of occupational therapy.

Therefore the occupational adaptation process is conceptualized to proceed as follows:

1. A person perceives an occupational challenge.
2. He or she generates an adaptive response using the mechanism consisting of
   a. *Adaptive energy* (which is a finite amount of energy and therefore must be used judiciously). The adaptation energy consists of both a primary process (requiring intense, structured, focused attention) and a secondary process (which is unstructured, sophisticated, and creative). Use of the secondary process is more economical, whereas the primary process results in expenditure of much energy and the risk of premature exhaustion of adaptation energy in a person's lifetime.
   b. *Adaptive response modes.* There are three possible adaptive response modes:
      i. Existing mode in which the person draws on existing repertoire of problem-solving approaches that have been successful in the past
      ii. Modified mode in which the person makes changes to the existing problem-solving repertoire when existing modes do not work in the prevailing circumstances
      iii. New adaptive response modes when existing modified modes fail to meet the existing challenges
   c. *Adaptive response behaviors.* These may be
      i. *Primitive* (hyperstable behaviors where the person keeps trying the same approaches to solve a problem even when it is clear that they do not work)
      ii. *Transitional* (hypermobile behaviors where the person lacks the discipline or structure to maintain a course of action

long enough to determine whether it works to meet the prevailing challenges)
      iii. *Mature* (blended mobility and stability, which is the most adaptive response behavior)
   d. *Adaptation gestalt*, which refers to the adaptive response subprocess consisting of a configuration of the selected adaptive response energy level, adaptive response mode, and adaptive response behavior into a holistic, integrated response to an occupational challenge.

In addition to the adaptation energy, adaptation response mode, and adaptation response behavior, the adaptive gestalt also includes a configuration of the three *person-systems* (sensorimotor, cognitive, and psychosocial). The *sensorimotor system* is the neuromusculoskeletal system that the person uses to act physically through coordinated movement in response to an occupational challenge. The *cognitive system* constitutes the planning, decision-making, and problem-solving processes required for occupational performance. The *psychosocial system* consists of the person's internal desires, feelings, and drives as well as external expectations and demands from other people in the person's life. These three systems are "internal to the individual" and "produce responses to the moment-to-moment demands, real or perceived, of occupational environments" p. 10).[19]

When a person is able to choose the appropriate adaptive response energy level, adaptive response mode, and adaptive behavior, and configure these three along with the three person-systems into an effective adaptive response plan and process, occupational adaptation occurs, leading to *relative mastery*. Relative mastery is a response to an occupational challenge with

(1) efficiency (use of time, energy, and resources), (2) effectiveness (extent to which the desired goal was achieved), and (3) satisfaction to self and society (the extent to which the individual engaging in the occupation finds it personally satisfying and the extent to which it is socially well regarded) (p. 185).[22]

It is important to point out that the demand for adaptation varies with a person's stage of development, with transition stages such as adolescence, midlife, and so on, requiring more adaptive response and therefore presenting a greater risk for faulty use of the adaptation gestalt and maladaptation than other periods of life.[31]

Postulations about Function, Dysfunction, and Change

Function

It is evident from the above-stated theoretical core that function, according to the OA conceptual model of practice, refers to adaptive response to occupational challenges. This adaptive response is characterized by efficiency, effectiveness, and satisfaction to self and others with occupational performance. This adaptation is manifested through participation in roles according to one's internal and social expectations.

Dysfunction

According to this model, dysfunction may be conceptualized as maladaptation characterized by configuration of an adaptation gestalt that is inadequate as a response to the prevailing occupational challenges. This ineffective adaptation gestalt may consist of the wrong choice of adaptation energy level, adaptive response mode, and prevalent use of either primitive or transitional response behaviors rather than mature ones. Such a poorly organized adaptation gestalt leads to maladaptation with subsequent inefficient and ineffective occupational performance that is unsatisfactory to the person or other people. Subsequently, the person may be unable to perform roles to meet internal and societal expectations.

Change

According to the OA conceptual model of practice, change constitutes tapping into the client's internal adaptive capacity by identifying his or her unique process of adaptation, determining what impedes effective adaptive response, and intervening to enhance the adaptive process. The objective of therapy is to facilitate adaptiveness that is geared toward improving occupational performance, which in turn is postulated to lead to further enhancement of adaptiveness. The therapist aims at helping the client progress "along a continuum from 'dysfunction' to homeostasis and occupational adaptation" (p. 166).[31]

Guidelines for Client Evaluation and Therapeutic Intervention

Client Evaluation

Within the OA conceptual model of practice, assessment seeks to identify ways in which the client's adaptation gestalt is dysfunctional. This means identifying the client's choice of the adaptive energy level, adaptive response mode, adaptive response behavior, the three person-systems, and configuration of all these elements into one integrated and functionally effective adaptive response gestalt. However, the authors of the model clearly state that it "is not a collection of techniques nor is it technique specific" (p. 209).[22] Rather, it is a way of thinking about therapy. As Schultz[24] argues, many of the occupational therapy interventions aim at helping the client develop functional skills with the rationale that those skills will lead to adaptiveness.

The OA model, on the other hand, reverses this position and posits that developing adaptiveness will lead to emergence of functional skills. It is within that rationale that assessment structured within the framework of the OA model should be viewed. Consequently, the authors of the model did not focus on development of assessment instruments since it is not a technique-oriented conceptual framework, and most assessments tend to seek identification of deficient skills that can be mediated using specific techniques. Rather, they developed a series of questions that were geared toward appraisal of the client's adaptive process, limitations to the ability to adapt, how the therapist may be able to manage the environment to facilitate enhanced adaptive capacity, and relative mastery.

Schultz and Schkade[26] developed the following questions for this kind of general assessment:

- What are the patient's occupational environments and roles?
- Which role is of primary concern to patient and family?
- What occupational performance is expected in the primary occupational environment and role?
- What are the physical, social, and cultural features of the primary occupational environment and role?
- What is the patient's sensorimotor, cognitive, and psychosocial status?
- What is the patient's level of relative mastery in the primary occupational environment and role?
- What is facilitating or limiting relative mastery in the primary occupational environment and role? (cited in Schkade & Schultz,[22] p. 213; see also MacRae and colleagues,[13] p. 113)

During the initial evaluation and also after initiation of therapy, the authors suggested that the therapist use the following questions to assess the client's status and progress in therapy on the basis of the occupational adaptation process:

- How is the program affecting the patient's occupational adaptation process?
- Which energy level is used most often (primary or secondary)?
- What adaptive response mode is used most often (preexisting, modified, or new)?
- What is the most common adaptive response behavior (primitive, transitional, or mature)?

- What outcome does the patient show that reflects change in the occupational adaptation process?
  - Self-initiated adaptation?
  - Enhanced relative mastery?
  - Generalization to novel activities?
- What program changes are needed to provide maximum opportunity for occupational adaptation to occur? (p. 213)[22]

Therapeutic Intervention

To reiterate, the authors of the OA conceptual model emphasize that it is "not a collection of techniques but a way of thinking that guides and organizes the intervention process" (p. 222).[28] The role of the therapist therefore is not to implement defined techniques to facilitate development of specific functional skills but rather "to acknowledge and facilitate the client as the agent of therapeutic change. The practitioner sets the stage for the client to progressively assume the agency role. This is critical in influencing the client's internal adaptation process" (p. 222).[28] In this endeavor, the therapist collaborates with the client in the use of both occupational readiness and occupational activities to facilitate the client's development of an effective adaptive process and subsequent relative mastery.[13,20,22,26,28] In this regard, Schultz and Schkade developed the following guidelines for occupational adaptation programming[26]:

- What combination of occupational readiness and occupational activity is needed to promote the patient's *occupational adaptation process?*
- What help will the patient need to *assess occupational responses* and use the results to affect the *occupational adaptation process?*
- What is the best method to engage the patient in the occupational adaptation program? (cited in MacRae and colleagues,[13] p. 113; Schkade & Schultz,[22] p. 213)

CASE STUDY: EDDY

Eddy was a 17-year-old Caucasian male attending a day treatment center in the afternoons three times a week and on Saturdays. He was referred to the center through a court order due to persistent drug and alcohol abuse and behavioral problems at school. He had been involved in several fights at school resulting in repeated detention in jail. At the time he was referred to the day treatment center, the choice was either commitment to a juvenile institution until the age of 21 or treatment at the day treatment center until he attained the age of 18.

Eddy, the eldest of two children, had a 14-year-old sister. Both his parents drank heavily, used drugs, and often fought with each other and physically abused both Eddy and his sister. His father was sent to prison when Eddy was 6 years old. His mother continued abusing alcohol and drugs and became a prostitute. Eddy and his sister were removed from her care by child services and placed with different foster parents. At the time he was attending the day treatment center, he saw his sister only about once a year, usually on Thanksgiving or during Christmas.

I met Eddy when a colleague and I were offering services at the day treatment center while conducting a research study.[8] He was one of the participants in our research. When I conducted the initial interview with him, he presented as a typical teenager, dressed casually in jeans and a T-shirt. He had a tendency to make jokes when asked personal questions that made him uncomfortable. He had the same approach to tasks. When asked to participate in group activities in which he did not feel competent or comfortable, he tended to detach himself and make jokes about the task and other group members. This was one indication of the reason for his inadequate performance in school as evident from his poor grades. He failed all his tests. His reading and writing skills were at fifth-grade level. He particularly did not like to participate in activities involving reading or writing.

Therapeutic intervention for Eddy was guided using the Instrumentalism in Occupational Therapy (IOT) conceptual model of practice[5-7] (see Chapter 8). It included assisting Eddy in establishing a mission statement, identifying occupational activities that would help him achieve that mission, establishing treatment goals, and working toward the goals through group sessions structured using Cole's[2] seven-step format. However, the OA conceptual model would have been applicable to Eddy as well since he clearly had competency problems that interfered with his ability to participate in age-appropriate roles as desired and as socially expected.

If we had used the OA model to guide Eddy's therapy, we would have begun by bearing in mind that he was in a transition stage (adolescence) that placed even more demand for adaptation on him.[31] The effect of this transition on his adaptive capacity was even more significant since his background in a dysfunctional family with a history of abuse, subsequent placement in foster care, and so on, suggested that he may not have learned skills in previous stages that would have made the transition easier. For example, Eddy did not appropriately develop to age-appropriate levels the school skills that should have been mastered in childhood such as reading, writing, and computational literacy. Therefore he currently had issues of incompetence in multiple areas, which hinted at impaired relative mastery.

Using the *Occupational Adaptation Guide to Practice*,[13,22,26] we would have found that Eddy's occupational environments and roles were not supportive of adaptive performance. His childhood was spent in a dysfunctional family within an abusive environment. He did not receive affirmation for competent performance, and it is possible that adaptive functional performance was not expected of him. Currently, he was in foster care and in school. It was probably expected that his behavior would be problematic rather than

Continued

CASE STUDY: EDDY—CONT'D

positive. At his stage of development, Eddy's socially expected primary role was that of a student. The social expectations for a person his age were that he would study, pass his tests, and probably go to college or some other institution to prepare for a career or some means of earning a living. This is what is typically expected of a young man his age in the American culture. However, clearly, he was not living to expectations in this role.

Further assessment would probably have revealed that although his sensorimotor function was intact, his cognitive development may not have been typical for age as indicated by his poor performance in school. Also, he probably felt inadequate and out of place because of his poor academic skills and past poor environment, which suggested problems in his psychosocial person-system. Eddy's relative mastery in his primary role of a student was therefore low because he was not performing to his or society's expectations. Poor skills (most probably cognitive), negative self-perception (poorly functioning psychosocial system), and an environment that did not support adaptive functioning could have been to blame for limitations in Eddy's relative mastery. Assessment of Eddy's adaptive response modes would probably have indicated that he tended to use an existing mode consisting of detachment and using jokes to avoid facing challenges. His adaptive response behavior was mostly hyperstable (repeated pattern of avoidance). His adaptation gestalt therefore consisted of a dysfunctional adaptive response mode, ineffective adaptive response behavior, and dysfunctional cognitive and psychosocial person-systems.

As we planned intervention for Eddy, we would have kept cognizant of the fact that the focus of therapy should be on his internal adaptation process and subsequent attainment of relative mastery. In order to achieve that overarching goal, we would have needed to assist him in developing necessary academic skills, modify his environment so that it supported adaptive functioning, and pose

occupational challenges that facilitated development of appropriate adaptive response modes and behaviors. With that focus in mind, some of the therapeutic goals for Eddy would have been as follows:

Short-term Goals

1. By the end of 3 weeks, Eddy will demonstrate improved adaptive response modes as indicated by the ability to try two or more approaches to solve a problem (2 times a week) when faced with an occupational challenge during group sessions.
2. By the end of 4 weeks, Eddy will demonstrate mature adaptive response behavior as indicated by the ability to discipline himself to pursue a task to completion while creatively examining two or more alternatives of responding to a challenge (3 times a week) during group interventions.
3. By the end of 8 weeks, Eddy will have developed reading, writing, and computational skills at the sixth grade level.

Long-term Goals

1. By the end of 3 months, Eddy will demonstrate adequate adaptive response process as indicated by ability to function in his primary role as a student with efficiency (using all resources available to him as appropriate and completing all academic assignments in reasonable time), effectiveness (completing all academic tasks successfully and accurately), and with satisfaction to self, his teachers, foster parents, and other people in his environment.

Intervention strategies would have included helping him to articulate a future image of himself that would have provided meaning for successful performance of the student role, so that academic activities became important to him. The therapist would have created an environment, first beginning with the therapeutic group setting, where it was

Consistency of the Occupational Adaptation Conceptual Model with the Current Professional Paradigm

The OA model is based on the basic proposition that the role of the occupational therapist is "to acknowledge and facilitate the *client as the agent of therapeutic change.* The practitioner sets the stage for *the client to progressively assume the agency role*" (p. 222, emphasis mine).[28] In other literature as discussed in this chapter, the authors of the model have emphasized the need for the client to determine tasks and roles that are meaningful to him or her. In other words, in therapy based on the OA model, "(1) the client must be actively involved, (2) the activity must have personal meaning for that client, and (3) the activity must involve a process that ends in a product, whether that product is tangible or intangible" (p. 214).[22] This indicates that a therapist using this model as a guide for intervention needs to collaborate closely with the client in order to determine those roles, tasks, and activities that are important to him or her and therefore can be used to facilitate internal adaptation process and subsequent relative mastery.

Consistent with the current occupational therapy paradigm, the model is client-centered and collaborative. Furthermore, participation in occupation that is meaningful to the client is seen as both the means of intervention and the desired outcome of therapy. Also, in this model, the role of the therapist is conceptualized as to help create an environment that facilitates the client's internal adaptation process, and present opportunities to participate in occupations that pose challenges to the client so that he or she can develop appropriate adaptive responses and attain relative mastery. The model is therefore consistent with the occupational therapy paradigm in which the role of the occupational therapist is seen in part as including environmental modification and presentation of opportunities for participation in meaningful occupations. Therefore the OA model is highly consistent with the current occupational therapy paradigm.

Consistency with the Philosophy of Pragmatism

Although the philosophy of pragmatism is not mentioned explicitly in the model as a basis of its philosophical framework, it is clear the model's constructs are remarkably consistent with those of the philosophy. For example, the model places much value on the role of the environment as a catalyst for development of adaptive responses. It also emphasizes the client's active engagement in meaningful occupations and making choices about what is important and about the desired future (agency). All these constructs (environment, active doing, agency, and adaptation) are also central to the philosophical propositions of pragmatism (see Chapter 4).

Consistency with the Complexity/Chaos Theoretical Framework

Again, the complexity/chaos theoretical framework is not discussed in the OA conceptual model's theoretical core. However, the model's conceptualization of the internal adaptation process and relative mastery may be seen as consistent with the postulations of the complexity/chaos theory. The complexity/chaos theory is based on the core proposition that interaction between subsystems of a complex, dynamic, adaptive system leads to increased self-organization of the system and emergence of more adaptive characteristics (see discussion in Chapter 4). Similarly, in the OA model, the internal adaptation process is thought to emerge from a dynamic interaction between an environment that places demands for adaptation on the individual; the individual's internal desire for mastery; and the sensorimotor, cognitive, and psychosocial person-systems. This emergent internal adaptation process is coupled with emergence of relative mastery. In this sense, the postulations of OA are clearly consistent with those of the complexity/chaos theory.

Recommendations for Reinterpretation of the Model

From the above analysis, it is evident that the OA frame of reference is one of the conceptual models of practice in occupational therapy that is consistent with the profession's newly emerged professional paradigm, the philosophy of pragmatism, and the complexity/chaos theoretical framework. Perhaps making those consistencies clearer would significantly strengthen the conceptual validity of the model as understood by occupational therapists that use it. Also, although the model's authors emphasize that it is not technique-oriented, it may be useful to devote more energy to development of what Kielhofner[11] calls *technology for application,* in the form of development and validation of instruments that can be used to operationalize and measure the model's constructs such

as adaptive response modes, adaptive response energy, adaptive response behaviors, internal adaptation process, and relative mastery. Such instruments would make the model less abstract and therefore more accessible to the majority of occupational therapists, and would facilitate outcome research.

Evidence-Based Practice Using the Occupational Adaptation Conceptual Model

The OA conceptual model is relatively young compared to other more established ones such as the MOHO and the Cognitive Disabilities model. Therefore there is little empirical evidence available to validate clinical use of the model. Much of the research that has been conducted so far in connection with the model has either sought to establish the overall clinical usefulness of the model (outcome studies)[28] or to develop and validate the few available instruments designed to be used with the model.[4] The study performed by George and colleagues[4] needs particular scrutiny because of its unique rigorous attempt to develop an instrument for use with the model, which, as mentioned in the recommendations in earlier sections of this chapter, is very much needed for further development of the model. We will therefore discuss the study in more detail.

George and colleagues sought to develop and validate the Relative Mastery Measurement Scale (RMMS).[4] The instrument, consisting of 27 items to which respondents responded by agreeing or disagreeing with each statement, was initially developed and validated by a panel of occupational therapists considered to be experts in the OA model. Nine items were developed to assess each of the three indicators of the construct of relative mastery as defined by Schkade and Schultz[21]: (1) efficiency (use of energy, resources, and time), (2) effectiveness (ability to achieve defined goals), and (3) satisfaction to self and others regarding performance. Agreement that an item measured the domain it was designed to measure was awarded a score of 1, and disagreement was awarded a score of 0. This meant that the maximum possible total score for each participant was 27. Six experts participated in the initial validation study. After analyzing their responses to the 27 items, 15 items were eliminated. Retention of the 12 items was based on the experts' agreement that they measured the domains they were designed to measure and the item congruence (extent to which they measured each of the domains of relative mastery).

The revised instrument consisting of 12 items was used in a subsequent study involving 150 inpatients from two rehabilitation facilities in central Arkansas. Their ages ranged between 22 and 92 years with a mean age of 69 years. Participants completed the instrument in relation to their performance in two activities: (1) lower-extremity dressing and (2) a task individually chosen by each participant. Rasch analysis was used to determine unidimensionality of the instrument items; correlation between therapists' evaluation of participants' performance in lower-extremity dressing and their scores on the RMMS were used to determine concurrent validity of the instrument; and Chronbach's alpha was used to determine the instrument's internal consistency. The findings indicated that the RMMS had good validity and reliability and therefore could be useful as a clinical tool for measuring clients' attainment of relative mastery.

In another recent ongoing study, Schultz[23] tested the basic concepts of OA as they were applied to therapeutic intervention for children with emotional and behavioral disorders (EBD). Fourth- and sixth-grade students participated in the study for 2 years. Preliminary findings indicated that the environment did not support adaptive response for these students. Consequently, they did not feel that they had any ownership or control of this environment. They were not expected to perform positively in their roles as students. As therapy continued, it was found that a role-shifting experience occurred such that the students began to experience themselves positively in their roles as students. They became more agentic as indicated by correction of each other when mistakes were made. Eventually the group was recognized for its positive transformation as indicated by presentation as a model for a "social studies class" (p. CE-7), which was an indication of an adaptive response resulting in group members' fostering adaptive social skills.

Other studies have indicated that (1) occupational therapists are able to accurately identify important environmental demands for students with special needs and include them in their intervention plans[18] and (2) nursing home residents with a diagnosis of CVA engaged in activities for longer periods of time when they were personally meaningful to them than when engaged in activities that were not meaningful.[3] Overall, the little research available indicates that this model has much potential as an effective guide to occupational therapy interventions that are client-centered, collaborative, and occupation-based.

SUMMARY

In this chapter, we presented the OA conceptual model of practice. The model was developed as an attempt to provide an integrating frame of reference for practice. It built on the tradition gleaned from the occupational therapy literature identifying occupation and adaptation as the core constructs of the profession. The model was based on the notion of the coupling between environmental demands for mastery and the individual internal desire for mastery creating a press for mastery. The press for mastery leads to an adaptive response to occupational challenges presented by the environment, leading to relative mastery, which was defined as a response to occupational challenges with efficiency, effectiveness, and satisfaction to self and society with performance.

We also discussed guidelines for client evaluation and intervention directed toward identification of the client's choice of adaptive energy level, adaptive response modes, adaptive response behaviors, and the three person-systems: sensorimotor, cognitive, and psychosocial. We found that the model is highly consistent with the current occupational therapy paradigm, the philosophy of pragmatism, and the complexity/chaos theoretical framework, although these consistencies could be more explicitly stated. Finally, we found that there is limited empirical evidence to support the model's clinical validity, although the little research available indicates that the model has promise as a guide to occupational therapy interventions that are client-centered, collaborative, and occupation-based.

REFERENCES

1. Casper College OTA Program: *Occupations: occupational adaptation frame of reference,* 1999. Retrieved December 22, 2005, from http://wind.cc.whecn.edu/mwonser/OCTH2000/unit5.html.

2. Cole MB: *Group dynamics in occupational therapy: the theoretical basis and practice application of group intervention,* ed 3, Thorofare, NJ, 2005, Slack.

3. Dolecheck JR, Schkade JK: Effects on dynamic standing endurance when persons with CVA perform personally meaningful activities rather than non-meaningful tasks, *Occup Ther J Res* 19:40–54, 1999.

4. George LA, Schkade J, Ishee JH: Content validity of the Relative Mastery Measurement Scale: a measure of occupational adaptation, *Occup Ther J Res* 24:92–103, 2004.

5. Ikiugu MN: Instrumentalism in occupational therapy: an argument for a pragmatic conceptual model of practice, *Internat J Psychosocial Rehabil* 8:108–117, 2004.

6. Ikiugu MN: Instrumentalism in occupational therapy: a theoretical core for the pragmatic conceptual model of practice, *Internat J Psychosocial Rehabil* 8:150–162, 2004.

7. Ikiugu MN: Instrumentalism in occupational therapy: guidelines for practice, *Internat J Psychosocial Rehabil* 8:165–179, 2004.

8. Ikiugu MN, Ciaravino AE: Assisting adolescents experiencing emotional and behavioral difficulties (EBD) transition to adulthood, *Internat J Psychosocial Rehabil* 10(2):57–78, 2005.

9. Kielhofner G: Temporal adaptation: a conceptual framework for occupational therapy, *Am J Occup Ther* 31:235–242, 1977.

10. Kielhofner G, ed: *Model of human occupation: theory and application,* ed 3, Philadelphia, 2002, Lippincott Williams & Wilkins.

11. Kielhofner G: *Conceptual foundations of occupational therapy,* ed 3, Philadelphia, 2004, F.A. Davis.

12. King LJ: Toward a science of adaptive responses, *Am J Occup Ther* 32:429–437, 1978.

13. MacRae A, Falk-Kessler J, Julin D, et al: Occupational therapy models. In Cara E, MacRae A, eds: *Psychosocial occupational therapy: a clinical practice,* Cincinnati, OH, 1998, Delmar, pp. 97–136.

14. Meyer A: The philosophy of occupational therapy, *Am J Occup Ther* 31:639–642, 1977.

15. Reilly M: Occupational therapy can be one of the great ideas of 20th century medicine, *Am J Occup Ther* 16, 1–9, 1962.

16. Reilly M: Defining a cobweb. In Reilly M, ed: *Play as exploratory learning,* Beverly Hills, CA, 1974, Sage, pp. 57–116.

17. Reilly M: An explanation of play. In Reilly M, ed: *Play as exploratory learning,* Beverly Hills, CA, 1974, Sage, pp. 117–149.

18. Schkade J: The impact of the classroom environment on defining function in school-based practice, *Am J Occup Ther* 51:64–69, 1997.

19. Schkade J, Schultz S: *Occupational adaptation: an integrative frame of reference,* unpublished manuscript, 1990, Texas Woman's University, Denton, Texas.

20. Schkade J, Schultz S: Occupational adaptation: toward a holistic approach to contemporary practice, part 1, *Am J Occup Ther* 46:829–837, 1992.

21. Schkade J, Schultz S: Occupational adaptation: an integrative frame of reference. In Neistadt ME, Crepeau EB, eds: *Willard and Spackman's occupational therapy,* Philadelphia, 1998, J.B. Lippincott, pp. 529–531.

22. Schkade J, Schultz S: Occupational adaptation. In Kramer P, Hinojosa J, Royeen CB, eds: *Perspectives in human occupation: participation in life,* New York, 2003, Lippincott Williams and Wilkins, pp. 181–221.

23. Schultz S: AOTA continuing education article: psychosocial occupational therapy in schools, *OT Practice,* September CE 1-CE 8, 2003.

24. Schultz S: *Theory of occupational adaptation overview,* 2005. Retrieved December 15, 2005, from http://www.twu.edu/ot/doctoral/OA_Basics.PPS.

25. Schultz S, Schkade J: *Occupational adaptation: an integrative frame of reference, part 3: implications for treatment,* unpublished manuscript, 1991, Texas Woman's University, Denton, Texas.

26. Schultz S, Schkade J: Occupational adaptation: toward a holistic approach to contemporary practice, part 2, *Am J Occup Ther* 46:917–926, 1992.

27. Schultz S, Schkade J: Adaptation. In Christiansen C, Baum C, eds: *Occupational therapy: enabling function and well-being,* Thorofare, NJ, 1997, Slack, pp. 458–481.

28. Schultz S, Schkade J: Occupational adaptation. In Crepeau EB, Cohn, ES, Schell BA, eds: *Willard and Spackman's occupational therapy,* New York, 2003, Lippincott Williams & Wilkins, pp. 220–223.

29. Selye H: *The stress of life,* New York, 1956, McGraw-Hill.
30. Shannon P: The derailment of occupational therapy, *Am J Occup Ther* 31:229–234, 1977.
31. Stein F, Cutler S: *Psychosocial occupational therapy: a holistic approach,* ed 2, Albany, NY, 2002, Delmar Thomson Learning.
32. Texas Woman's University, School of Occupational Therapy: *Occupational therapy Ph.D.,* 2005. Retrieved December 22, 2005, from http://www.twu.edu/ot/post_phd.htm.

16
The Canadian Model of Occupational Performance

Preview Questions

1. List and discuss the theoretical sources of constructs used in the Canadian Model of Occupational Performance as applied in adult psychosocial occupational therapy. Specifically, explain the influence of client-centered guidelines in counseling developed by Carl Rogers on the model.

2. Define the following constructs as used in the Canadian Model of Occupational Performance: client-centeredness and the subconstructs of collaboration, enablement, empowerment, and autonomy.

3. Concisely state the theoretical core of the Canadian Model of Occupational Performance.

4. Explain postulations of the Canadian Model of Occupational Performance about the following:
   a. Function
   b. Dysfunction
   c. Change

5. Outline and explain the model's guidelines for client evaluation and therapeutic intervention.

6. Discuss the consistency of the Canadian Model of Occupational Performance with each of the following:
   a. The occupational therapy paradigm
   b. The philosophy of pragmatism
   c. The complexity/chaos theoretical framework

7. Discuss available empirical evidence supporting clinical effectiveness of the Canadian

Model of Occupational Performance as a guide to intervention in occupational therapy practice.

The Canadian Model of Occupational Performance (CMOP) is one of several conceptual theoretical approaches to therapy collectively placed in the category of the Person-Environment-Occupation framework.[3] Other models within this category include the Person-Environment-Occupation-Performance model,[10,11] the Ecology of Human Performance model,[17] the Model of Human Occupation,[23,24] the Person-Environment-Occupation model, and the Occupational Performance Model: Australia.[3] Within this list, one may also add the Occupational Adaptation model discussed in Chapter 15[33,34] and the Instrumentalism in Occupational Therapy (IOT) model discussed in Chapter 8.[19-21]

Common to all these theoretical conceptual frameworks is their emphasis on interaction between the person and the environment through meaningful occupation, or as Baum and Christiansen state, "the complex interaction of biological, psychological, and social phenomena and the importance of a satisfactory match between personal, task, and situational characteristics in order for performance to be supported" (p. 244).[3] Another characteristic common to all these models is that they are client-centered in that they employ "a broad range of purposeful client-centered strategies that engage the individual or the group to develop or use resources that enable successful performance of the necessary and meaningful occupations" (p. 244).[3] Since they are client-centered and seek to focus on what is necessary and meaningful to the client in therapy, the client is actively and inextricably involved in his or her own therapy. Thus intervention based on the models is collaborative, requiring close involvement of both the client and therapist in therapeutic planning and intervention.

Another important factor to point out is that the client-centeredness espoused by all the above models can be traced back to the humanistic "third force" psychology of Carl Rogers[32] and Abraham Maslow.[12,29] Baptiste states that Canadian occupational therapists recognized the importance of Rogers' emphasis on "an open and honest clinical relationship, providing the client with the opportunity of playing an active role in the therapeutic experience, and recognizing the critical importance of cultural values" (p. 265)[1] and developed guidelines for client-centered practice based on those principles. Rogers' guidelines were based on the argument that the client had the capacity to understand best those aspects of his or her life that cause pain, to reorganize himself or herself and his or her relationship to life, so as to make necessary changes to achieve self-actualization and maturity, in the process attaining a greater degree of internal comfort. This was the basis of his "client-centered therapy."[32] Rogers' argument is consistent with the assertion by Baum and Baptiste that

> Client-centered rehabilitation supports an individualized approach to therapy[5] and provides clients with opportunities to learn new strategies in order to perform activities that are essential to them and their families…clients identify therapeutic goals and activities that are pertinent to their unique circumstances and environments (p. 9).[2]

Maslow, on the other hand, developed the theory of motivation in which he saw the human as striving first to survive, and then to attain esteem and mastery leading to self-actualization. Client-centered occupational therapy seeks to operationalize that view for application in clinical practice as indicated in the proposition that "Client-centered care has the capacity to help the person improve self-esteem, mastery, and resourcefulness" (p. 9).[2]

Given that all client-centered models are similar in their emphasis on the interaction between humans and the environment through occupation, and on client active involvement in therapy, one may wonder why the CMOP was chosen for discussion in this chapter rather than any of the others. This is because, in the author's experience (and as evidence from literature indicates), the Canadian Occupational Performance Measure (COPM), the assessment instrument associated with the CMOP, has been gaining international popularity among occupational therapists (see "Evidence-Based Practice using the Canadian Model of Occupational Performance" at the end of this chapter). Therefore the model was chosen for detailed discussion so that the occupational therapy student can have a fair understanding of the rationale behind the use of the COPM. In this chapter, we will discuss the model's background; general theoretical constructs of client-centeredness; the theoretical core of the model; postulations about function, dysfunction, and change; consistency with the current occupational therapy paradigm; and clinical efficacy supported by empirical evidence.

Evolution of the Canadian Model of Occupational Performance

Background

The CMOP was the first systematically developed client-centered theoretical model in occupational therapy. The model originated in Canada.[12] Its development was an attempt to bring occupation back into occupational therapy as a central construct. The model's authors argued that occupation had been absent from the profession between the 1940s and 1980s.[36] In this endeavor, their goal was to develop a model with occupation, occupational performance, and enablement as its central domains of focus. This venture began in the 1980s with publication of three documents outlining what therapists in Canada referred to as the *Guidelines for Client-Centered Practice.*[35] The three documents were later combined into one.[6,8] Later, a related document, *Occupational Therapy Guidelines for Client-Centered Mental Health Practice,* was published.[7]

Interdisciplinary Theoretical Basis

Development of the CMOP and client-centered occupational therapy practice in general was based on constructs borrowed from occupational therapy literature and humanistic psychology, particularly the client-centered therapeutic guidelines developed by Carl Rogers.

General Theoretical Constructs of Client-Centered Practice

The CMOP and client-centered occupational therapy are based on Rogerian therapeutic guidelines, which underscore the need to facilitate clients' development of self-awareness, authenticity and congruence, and staying in the "here-and-now." Therapists do this by motivating clients to progress toward personal growth through unconditional positive regard, empathy, and immediacy. (See Chapter 3 for a discussion of these constructs. The reader is advised to review the relevant sections of that chapter at this point.) Further, as mentioned earlier, development of this approach to therapy was given impetus by the general feeling in Canada that occupation, the mainstay of occupational therapy, had been absent in the profession between 1940s and 1980s and needed to be reintroduced.[36] Therefore while developing guidelines for client-centered practice in occupational therapy, they emphasized the value of occupation as a core construct in the profession.

The roles of the occupational therapist in the perspective of client-centeredness include being an *enabler, facilitator,* and *coach.** As an enabler, the therapist provides input and education, opportunities for learning and engagement,

*References 1,2,6,8,25,26,37.

and ultimately for adaptation. Facilitation means viewing the client as the one who best understands his or her life. Therefore he or she identifies his or her occupational performance issues. The therapist merely facilitates the process. Coaching denotes such things as encouraging, teaching, and providing the client with feedback in order to facilitate performance of occupations perceived to be necessary and meaningful.

The notion that the client is the expert regarding his or her occupational performance issues means respecting the client's uniqueness as an individual. This entails collaboration with the client in identifying occupational performance needs rather than the therapist assuming the role of expert. *Collaboration* means sharing power, which, in the medical model of care, is reserved for the health care professional as the expert. Further, true collaboration means being able to establish mutual trust with the client, which calls for effective use of therapeutic relationship. In client-centered practice, where it is recognized that the therapist is not the expert on occupational performance issues, therapeutic relationship is used to facilitate exploration of occupational performance issues and their resolution as a collaborative endeavor between the client and therapist. Respectful collaboration with the client, on the other hand, means respecting his or her uniqueness, including the client's cultural values and issues, which to a great extent determine occupational performance priorities.

Therefore the emphasis in client-centered practice is on choice and autonomy, partnership, responsibility, enablement, and congruence. The client is viewed as an autonomous individual with a right to make choices according to personal values and priorities. The goal of therapy is conceptualized as empowerment of the client to perform activities valued by self and others in the cultural context. The responsibility of making occupational performance choices rests with the client, and the therapist is a facilitator. Finally, therapeutic intervention has to be congruent with the client's reality in his or her lived world. This means that the therapist adopts an attitude of flexibility in order to accommodate different world views and respects diversity in order to be truly respectful of the individuality of all clients.

In the shift of perspective necessitated by the client-centered approach, how language is used is important. In the medical model, the recipient of occupational therapy services is referred to as the *patient*. The term *patient* reinforces the sick role, in which the person is seen as a dependent, passive recipient of therapeutic services from an expert therapist. In other words, a patient needs and expects to be taken care of by the professional. As Baptiste asserts, in client-centered practice, the term *client* is replacing the term *patient*. The construct of client denotes a focus on the problems of living rather than ideas of pathology and illness. The client is encouraged to take responsibility for personal health and therefore to be an active agent working collaboratively with the therapist in all therapeutic endeavors. As E. Townsend (personal communication, February 14, 2006) argues, client-centered practice

is the essence of occupational therapy. We cannot do things *to* people since we are not a technical application...and we are not a prescriptive profession which hands out standardized exercises, etc. We must engage the client as an active agent and participant who chooses whether or not to do something to bring out changes which have meaning from the client's point of view.

Theoretical Core of the Canadian Model of Occupational Performance

As mentioned earlier, the CMOP was created as an attempt to operationalize the client-centered principles of Carl Rogers for application in occupational therapy. Therefore it shares and indeed is based on the theoretical perspectives of client-centered practice discussed above. The model addresses occupational performance, which is conceptualized as resulting from a dynamic interaction between the person, environmental context, and occupation over a person's lifetime. *Occupational performance* means "the ability to choose, organize, and satisfactorily perform

meaningful occupations that are culturally defined and age appropriate for looking after one's self, enjoying life, and contributing to the social and economic fabric of community" (p. 30).[28]

Dynamic interaction between the person and the environment through occupation is depicted diagrammatically with the person, conceptualized as a spiritual entity, being at the center and connected to the environment and occupation, both of which contribute toward shaping that spirituality (Figure 16-1).

As shown in Figure 16-1, spirituality is at the center. This model is one of the first to explicitly incorporate spirituality as a core construct of occupational therapy. *Spirituality,* as used in this context, does not mean religiousness as commonly may be thought. Rather, it means "the essence of

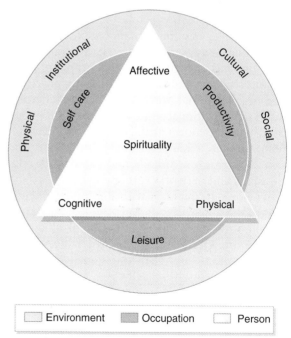

Figure 16-1. Diagrammatic depiction of the Canadian Model of Occupational Performance. (Adapted from Law M, Polatajko H, Baptiste S, et al: Core concepts of occupational therapy. In Townsend E, ed: *Enabling occupation: an occupational therapy perspective,* Ottawa, ON, 2002, Canadian Association of Occupational Therapists, p. 32.)

the self...our truest self, and...something which we attempt to express in all our actions" (p. 42).[28] Given this definition, although spirituality is at the center of the CMOP, it is really the individual person who occupies this position, since humans are essentially spiritual beings in their very essences. Furthermore, spirituality, this essence of self, is expressed and shaped by interaction with the environment through occupational performance.

The spiritual human has affective, cognitive, and physical components through which he or she expresses himself or herself.[8,25] In other words, feelings, information processing through thinking and decision making, choices about what is meaningful, and ability to act physically on those decisions constitute the spiritual core of humans. Surrounding this core is an environmental context with which he or she dynamically interacts. This environmental context consists of the physical environment (e.g., natural and built surroundings, geographical topography), institutions (policy and decision-making processes and organizational procedures such as religious, judicial, educational, and other practices); cultural beliefs; values; artifacts; tool use; ceremonial practices; ethnic and racial affiliations; and social systems (e.g., family and community relationships and networks, groupings).

The human interacts with this environmental context through occupations, which are classified into the categories of self-care, productivity, and leisure. Occupation is defined as everything people do to occupy their time "including looking after themselves (self-care), enjoying life (leisure), and contributing to the social and economic fabric of their communities (productivity)" (p. 30).[28] Further, in this model, occupation is conceptualized as consisting of activities and tasks. Activities are individual discreet actions necessary to complete a task, for example, writing. An activity is therefore the basic unit of a task. A task is "a set of purposeful activities in which a person engages" (p. 33).[28] Thus tasks are made up of activities. For example, writing a paper is a task in which the act of writing is an activity. Tasks are also constituent parts of occupations, which are "groups of activities and tasks of everyday life, named, organized and given value and meaning by individuals and culture" (p. 34).[28] For instance, being a student is an occupation in which writing papers are tasks. In other words, an occupation (whether it is completing the morning self-care routine, shopping for groceries, working as a teacher, or playing golf for pleasure) fulfills a function, meets needs and purposes in life, and is meaningful to self and one's culture.

In the category of self-care are personal care tasks (e.g., grooming, bathing, toileting), functional mobility (ability to make transfers and get from one place to the next effectively and safely), and community management (e.g, use of public transportation, shopping).[8] Productivity includes both paid and unpaid work, including volunteering and homemaking. Within the leisure category are quiet recreation (such as reading), active recreation (for example, participation in sports activities), and socialization. Finally, occupational performance is defined as "the ability to choose, organize, and satisfactorily perform meaningful occupations that are culturally defined and age appropriate for looking after one's self, enjoying life, and contributing to the social and economic fabric of a community" (p. 30).[28] In the model, it is also emphasized that change in any of the tripartite components (person, environment, or occupation) leads to change in other components, occupational performance, and satisfaction with that performance.

Postulations about Function, Dysfunction, and Change

Function

Based on the above statement of the theoretical core, function denotes effective interaction with the environment through occupational performance in self-care, enjoyment, and productivity in a cultural and age-appropriate manner. This means optimum mental, physical, and social functioning that makes it possible for one to choose and organize satisfactory performance of activities that are meaningful and essential to self, family, and community.

Dysfunction

Dysfunction occurs when one is unable to interact with the environment effectively due to inability to perform occupations necessary for self-care, enjoyment, and productivity in an age-appropriate manner according to cultural expectations. The person is unable to choose and organize satisfactory performance of occupations due to mental, physical, institutional, or social deficits. Consequently, there is dissatisfaction with self and others with one's performance.

Change

In the CMOP, it is proposed that the therapist enable clients by collaborating with them in identifying occupations that are meaningful and which they want, are expected, or need to perform; assessing self-perception about performance and satisfaction with that performance; and formulating a plan to improve performance of those occupations more effectively and satisfactorily.[8,25,28] In other words, the model's focus is the client's inability to perform activities/tasks/occupations that are essential to self and family due to mental, physical, institutional, and/or social impairments and/or due to environmental barriers.[2] The overarching goal of this model is to facilitate the client's ability to perform occupations that are meaningful to him or her, are age-appropriate, and are recognized and expected in the culture.

Guidelines for Client Evaluation and Therapeutic Intervention

Client Evaluation

Evaluation is conducted using the COPM.[25,26] This is an individualized semistructured interview that takes about 20 to 30 minutes to complete. The interview is used to guide the client in identifying occupational performance issues (occupations that he or she wants, is expected,

or needs to perform), assessing performance and satisfaction with performance, generating a plan to improve performance, and assessing progress in both performance and satisfaction.[15,16,18,25,26]

The COPM consists of four sections and is completed in five steps. Section I consists of demographic information: name, age, and therapist. In Section II, Step 1 consists of directions that the therapist follows to guide the client in identification of occupational performance issues in self-care, productivity, and leisure. The client is encouraged to think of a typical day and identify activities that he or she needs, is expected, or wants to do every day. In Step 2, he or she is asked to identify those activities that are difficult to do to his or her satisfaction. These activities are listed under the appropriate headings (self-care, productivity, and leisure). In Step 3, the client is asked to identify from the list the five most important problems. In Section III, Step 4, the problems are rated on a scale from 1 to 10 regarding ability to perform and satisfaction with performance. Performance scores are summed up and divided by the number of problems. The same thing is done with the satisfaction scores. This yields a single performance and single satisfaction score, respectively. In Step 5, the client decides on a date for reassessment in collaboration with the therapist. Section IV provides space where notes can be written during assessment and at reassessment. Finally, during reassessment, the client once again rates self-perception of performance and satisfaction with performance, and the performance and satisfaction scores are calculated accordingly. Progress in therapy is indicated by subtraction of satisfaction score 1 from satisfaction score 2, and performance score 1 from performance score 2, respectively.

Therapeutic Intervention

Intervention based on client-centered conceptual models of practice, among which is the CMOP, generally consists of four stages (Box 16-1).[2] Stage I constitutes *biomedical rehabilitation.*

| **Box** 16-1 | Four Stages of Intervention |

Stage I: Biomedical Rehabilitation
Stage II: Client-Centered Rehabilitation
Stage III: Community Rehabilitation
Stage IV: Independent Living

This is a limited phase aimed mainly at enablement of the client to reach optimum mental, physical, and/or social performance potential. This is where specific mental, physical, and/or social-skill deficits that limit occupational performance are addressed. Strategies to address these skill deficits are borrowed from other models (biomechanical and cognitive/psychosocial/behavioral).

Stage II is the *client-centered rehabilitation* phase. This stage aims at helping the client attain improved self-esteem, mastery, and resourcefulness. The client is offered opportunities to engage in occupations that are essential to self, family, and community (occupations that one wants, needs, or is expected to perform). This affords the client an opportunity to become engaged, learn, interact effectively with the environment, and thus adapt. Through relevant occupational tasks and activities, the client learns problem-solving skills and strategies that are necessary for effective and satisfactory performance of occupations that are meaningful to self, are age-appropriate, and are recognized and expected in one's culture.

In Stage III, the focus of therapy is the *community* (environmental context or community rehabilitation). The therapist acts as an advocate and works to facilitate elimination of barriers, whether physical or attitudinal, that may be contributing to disablement of the client. Therapeutic interventions at this stage may include assessment of buildings to ensure accessibility, advocacy for accessibility of facilities and services for people with psychosocial dysfunctions, and so on.

Finally, in Stage IV *(independent living)*, the therapist works with independent living agencies to ensure that clients have access to employment, housing, health care, transportation, education, and so on. The overall goal of therapy is to empower clients so that they have access to all resources and are able to fully participate in society. In all these endeavors, true to the client-centered premise of the model, the therapist collaborates with the client so that the focus of therapy continues to be performance of those occupations that are meaningful to the client; are age-appropriate; contribute to self-care, enjoyment of life, and contribution to society; and are recognized and expected in the client's culture.

Consistency of the Canadian Model of Occupational Performance with the Current Occupational Therapy Paradigm

Guidelines of the CMOP, along with those of other client-centered models, are based on the basic premise that "Through collaborative partnerships, occupational therapists enable persons to achieve satisfactory performance

---

CASE STUDY: SHEREE

Sheree, a 30-year-old Caucasian female, was admitted at the psychiatric facility with an Axis I diagnosis of schizoaffective disorder (bipolar type) and borderline personality disorder with significant antisocial and schizotypal features. Prior to admission, she lived with her 35-year-old boyfriend whom she had met only 2 weeks before.

Her only family, a 34-year-old brother, visited her regularly at the hospital. During clinical evaluation, Sheree presented with flat affect, anxiety, depression, and withdrawal. She was on 500 mg of Depakene, PO t.i.d.; Zyprexa 10 mg, PO b.i.d.; Klonopin, 0.5 mg PO t.i.d.; and Vistral 50 mg, q.i.d.

CASE STUDY: SHEREE—CONT'D

Sheree had a history of poly-substance abuse, with subsequent arrest and commitment to drug treatment about 3 years before admission, and a history of alcohol abuse, sexual promiscuity, and STDs such as herpes. According to the clinical notes, she also had been noncompliant with therapy prior to that admission, although she denied it. However, she admitted that she was not well and that her life was not satisfying to her or her brother, and she needed help so that she could get her life back together.

Sheree had formal education up to tenth grade but later completed her GED. Just before admission, she had been working at Wal-Mart in janitorial services. It was her third week at the job when she was admitted. Her history indicated that she had not been able to hold a job for any significant length of time for many years. Her past jobs had included working in a motel, as a cleaner for a cleaning agency, and as a packer in a mushroom packing company. She also had never been able to live independently. She lived with her brother from the time she quit school until she was 25 years old when she moved out to live with her ex-boyfriend. Since then, she had lived with a variety of boyfriends. No relationship had lasted for more than 1 year.

Sheree's interests included cooking, gardening, drawing, crafts activities such as making ceramics, needlework, photography, visiting friends, and swimming. She also identified having sex as one of her leisure interests. Socially, she was isolated, often engaging in solitary occupations. She did not seem to have any friends. She responded to therapist's inquiries appropriately but did not initiate conversation. She was independent in basic ADLs but totally dependent for all IADLs. For example, she was unable to budget her money, shop for groceries, or keep her own living space clean.

Evaluation

Because Sheree indicated that she and her brother were concerned about her life, and that she felt the need to turn her life around, it was hypothesized that she was at a point in her development where she was ready to grow and change. Consequently, a client-centered, collaborative approach would be an effective approach to therapy. The COPM was used to guide assessment. In the area of self-care, Sheree identified shopping and managing finances as activities that she needed to do. In productivity, she identified volunteering, cleaning, doing laundry, and cooking as activities that she was interested in doing. In leisure, she was interested in doing ceramic crafts and needlework, swimming, and corresponding with friends. She rated the importance of each of the identified activities/tasks/occupations as follows:

Shopping	10
Managing finances	10
Volunteering	6
Household management (cleaning, doing laundry, and so on)	10
Quiet recreation (ceramics and needlework)	7
Socialization (corresponding with friends)	10
Acitve recreation (swimming)	9

Continued

CASE STUDY: SHEREE—CONT'D

From the list on p. 299 Sheree identified the five most important problems as shopping, managing finances, household management, socialization, and active recreation. She rated her self-perception of performance and satisfaction as follows:

Occupational Performance Problem	Performance	Satisfaction
Shopping	7	5
Managing finances	5	4
Household management	8	5
Socialization	6	5
Active recreation (swimming)	7	5

The total scores were 33/5 = 6.6, and 24/5 = 4.8 for performance and satisfaction, respectively. Based on the above evaluation findings, Sheree and the therapist collaboratively established the following therapeutic goals:

Short-term Goals

1. By the end of 3 weeks, Sheree will demonstrate improved house management skills as indicated by independently keeping her room clean, consistently making her bed, and doing her laundry at least once a week.
2. By the end of 3 weeks, Sheree's social skills will have improved significantly as indicated by spontaneously initiating and sustaining conversation with at least one other client during occupational therapy group activities at least 3 times a week.
3. By the end of 3 weeks, Sheree will resume her active recreational interests as indicated by independently and spontaneously going swimming in the hospital pool at least 2 times a week.
4. By the end of 4 weeks, Sheree's self-care skills will have improved significantly as indicated by the ability to make a shopping list for 1 month of nonperishable grocery items and shop for the items from the local grocery store independently.

5. By the end of 4 weeks, Sheree will demonstrate the ability to manage her finances effectively as indicated by establishing a monthly budget that takes care of her basic needs such as rent, food, utilities, and so on, and is within the income she had just before admission to the hospital.

Long-term Goals

1. By the end of 6 weeks, Sheree will be discharged from the hospital with the following:
   a. A regular job under the supervision of a job coach
   b. Her own apartment where she will live under weekly supervision from her brother
   c. A healthy balance between work, self-care, recreation, and socialization

Therapeutic Intervention

Based on the above goals, Sheree's intervention was structured as follows:

- During Phase I (biomedical rehabilitation), individual and group activities were used to help Sheree develop cognitive skills such as prioritizing and choice making necessary for successful completion of activities/tasks such as budgeting, and social interaction skills such as dressing

---

CASE STUDY: SHEREE—CONT'D

appropriately, initiating conversation, and being socially engaged.

- During Phase II (client-centered rehabilitation), Sheree was afforded opportunities for grocery shopping, housekeeping (e.g., cleaning her own hospital room, making her bed, doing laundry), socialization, and recreation. She and her therapist regularly reviewed her experiences in these activities, identifying any problems and formulating solutions to the problems collaboratively.

- During Phase III (community-based rehabilitation), the therapist consulted with Sheree's former employer, Wal-Mart, to help her secure the job she had before admission.

- In Phase IV (independent living), the therapist contacted the independent living agency in the area to help secure an apartment for Sheree. Working with the agency, the therapist explored contingencies for Sheree's transportation, and education so that she could be empowered through opportunities for more secure, better-paying jobs. Sheree made remarkable progress in therapy and was discharged from the hospital after 6 weeks. Her self-perceived performance score at discharge was 9, and the satisfaction score was 8.8.

Sheree's brother indicated that he was impressed with her level of functioning and sense of responsibility. After discharge, she lived in her own apartment with her brother's supervision as planned. She resumed her job at Wal-Mart, and her brother provided her transportation until alternative means of transportation could be arranged. The reader should note that Phases III and IV of therapy may not be practical for some occupational therapists working in inpatient settings. For such therapists, because of institutional bureaucracy, lack of necessary infrastructure, and so on, follow-up and support of the client in his or her endeavor to settle in the community may not be an option. If this is the case, the therapist may consider referring the client to an occupational therapist practicing in a community-based rehabilitation setting for the necessary support during transition from the hospital to the community.

Refer to Lab Manual Exercises 18-1 and 18-2 to enhance your skills in using the CMOP guidelines for client evaluation and treatment planning.

---

in occupations of their choice" (p. 30).[28] Therefore the model is highly consistent with the occupation-based, client-centered, collaborative perspective of the current occupational therapy paradigm. It can even be argued that it has probably contributed significantly to the emergence of the new professional paradigm since it was the first systematic attempt to apply client-centered strategies in occupational therapy. This postulation is supported by the frequency of topics in client-centeredness in occupational therapy literature since 1997,[35] after the *Guidelines for Client-Centered*

Practice were established when the CMOP was published.[6]

Further, according to the guidelines of the model, the role of the therapist is seen as to enable and empower the client by managing the environment to minimize barriers, providing opportunities for performance of meaningful occupations, and educating/counseling the client by assisting him or her to identify occupational performance issues, rate self-perception of performance and satisfaction with performance, prioritize, and establish goals to improve performance and satisfaction with performance. These strategies are consistent with the perceived role of the occupational therapist as facilitator of occupational performance through environmental modification, providing opportunities, and counseling/education. Therefore this model is consistent with the current occupational therapy paradigm.

Consistency with the Philosophy of Pragmatism

The CMOP is highly cognitive. The client identifies activities perceived to be important and essential in his or her life, rates self-perception of performance and satisfaction with performance, and makes decisions about changes to be made based on those assessments. This reliance on perceptions of importance, performance, and satisfaction is consistent with the construct of belief as a rule for action in the philosophy of pragmatism. The client acts on the basis of what is believed to be important, the believed competence in performance, and satisfaction with how one believes that he or she is able to perform. The model also emphasizes the environmental context and occupation as the means by which humans dynamically interact with this context. This is consistent with the constructs of environment as a source of experience, contextualization, and doing (occupational performance) in pragmatism. Finally, human agency is central to both the philosophy of pragmatism and this model. The human chooses and organizes performance in order to do things perceived to be important satisfactorily. Therefore (although it is not explicitly stated in the model's theoretical core) the postulations of the CMOP are consistent with those of the philosophy of pragmatism.

Consistency with the Complexity/ Chaos Theoretical Framework

In the CMOP, the contribution of complexity/ chaos theoretical postulations to its theoretical core is not explicitly identified. However, in their latest formulation of the model, its authors clearly make an argument for a "dynamic interdependence between person, environment, and occupation" (p. 33).[28] Furthermore, it is hypothesized in the model's latest theoretical statements that: "Change in any aspect of the Model would affect all other aspects" (p. 33).[28] The stated dynamic interaction between the person, environment, and occupation (and the hypothesized interdependence between the three such that when one is changed, all the others change) alludes to the model's subscription to the complexity/chaos theoretical postulation of the human as a complex, dynamic adaptive system in dynamic interaction with the environment. To that extent, the model is consistent with complexity/chaos theoretical postulations. The major difference between the CMOP and complexity/chaos theory is that the model does not emphasize self-organization and emergence of qualities as a result of the postulated dynamic interaction between the person, environment, and occupation.

Recommendations for Reinterpretation of the Model

The CMOP, as the above analysis indicates, is one of the models that are highly consistent with the newly emerged occupational therapy paradigm. It presents an innovative approach to application of client-centered strategies developed by Carl Rogers in occupational therapy. However, as mentioned, the model is highly cognitive, which limits its usefulness with clients who may have cognitive deficits. It may help for the authors of the model to clarify guidelines for intervention with such clients. It is important to observe though, that the model can still be useful with such clients. In a video developed to demonstrate assessment using the COPM,[27] a mother is guided to identify occupational performance issues, rate her perception of performance, and rate satisfaction with performance of her son who does not have the cognitive development necessary to be interviewed directly. However, the guidelines regarding how to proceed in such situations (when the therapist is treating individuals who cannot effectively participate in an interview, such as children, elderly clients with dementia, and adults with traumatic brain injuries) can be clarified further.

Also, consistency of the model's postulations with those of the philosophy of pragmatism can be explicated. This would give the model a clearly stated philosophical foundation. This would enhance the ability of therapists using it to make an even stronger argument for its foundational beliefs, values, and assumptions. Finally, explicit identification with the complexity/chaos theoretical framework may add some explanatory value to the model. One useful approach in this regard might be to develop and explicate the hypothesis that the outcome of therapy (performance of occupations the person wants, needs, or is expected to perform, which are recognized by one's culture, with satisfaction to self and others) is an emergent phenomenon resulting from the dynamic interaction between the person, environment, and occupation.

Evidence-Based Practice Using the Canadian Model of Occupational Performance

The COPM, which is the assessment instrument associated with the CMOP, is one of the most internationally used and researched instruments in occupational therapy. Dedding and colleagues state that it "has received international attention because it is an important method of assessment for directing occupational therapy interventions and measuring client-centered outcomes" (p. 661).[15] Many of the studies that have been carried out in relationship to the CMOP have been designed to evaluate the COPM's validity and reliability[15,18,30] and its use as an outcome assessment instrument.* We will discuss two of these studies in detail.

*References 4,9,13,14,16,31,38–40.

Eyssen and colleagues[18] conducted a study to investigate the interrater agreement of occupational performance problems prioritized by clients interviewed using the COPM. They also sought to determine the test-retest reliability of both individual problem as well as mean performance and satisfaction scores. The sample consisted of 105 outpatients who had volunteered from a variety of University medical centers in Amsterdam. Out of the 105 volunteers, 95 completed the study, and data gathered from them were used in the analysis. The COPM was administered twice, 2 weeks apart, by two different evaluators who were occupational therapists and experienced in conducting the interview.

Comparison of retest with pretest scores using a variety of statistical methods indicated fair to moderate interrater reliability of prioritization of problems, and good reproducibility of mean performance and satisfaction scores. The researchers concluded that the reliability of individual problem rating was weak considering poor reproducibility. This seems to be an inherent problem with this kind of instrument as found by Ikiugu and Ciaravino,[22] because the client's perception of occupational performance issues that are considered important changes with time due to a variety of reasons. However, they concluded that mean performance and satisfaction scores were reliable and should be used in clinical decision making rather than individual problem scores.

In another study,[15] researchers investigated convergent and divergent validity of the COPM as compared with the Disability Impact Profile (DIP), a standardized 39-item self-administered instrument assessing the impact of disability on a client's life, and the short version (68-item) Sickness Impact Profile (SIP), which assesses the impact of illness on functioning and behavior. All data were collected in about 2 weeks. The study sample consisted of 160 clients from two University medical facilities in Amsterdam who volunteered to participate. Out of the 160, 105 clients met the criteria for inclusion in the study. Data were missing for

6 of the 105 clients, leaving only 99 participants in the study.

Analysis of data revealed that the correlation between the total SIP and COPM scores was weak. This was hypothesized to be the anticipated result because all domains of the SIP except the physical domain do not seek to identify performance problems that are perceived by the client to be important in the same way as the COPM. There was significant correlation between scores in the physical domain of the SIP and the COPM performance scores as predicted. Also, the occupational performance issues identified using the COPM were consistent with items in the DIP and the SIP as hypothesized. The researchers concluded that the COPM had good convergent and divergent validity, indicating that it is a valid tool that can help elicit client information that may not be identified using other standardized instruments. Furthermore, qualitative data indicated that clients liked collaborating with the therapist in determining the direction of their own therapy, which use of the COPM required. This was consistent with the finding by Wressle and colleagues[39] that use of the COPM leads to enhancement of client participation in the rehabilitation process.

The above findings were confirmed by another study involving 141 Taiwanese clients with psychiatric disorders, where it was found that the COPM had excellent test-retest reliability ($r = .842$), indicating its applicability in that culture.[30] In this study, it was similarly found that the instrument was useful in helping identify occupational performance problems that could not be explicated using other standardized instruments. Cup and colleagues[14] also found that the instrument had good performance and satisfaction score test-retest reliability. All the above studies indicate that generally the COPM has fair to good reliability and validity, and measures occupational performance issues in a different way than other available standardized instruments.

In another study, Persson and colleagues[31] investigated change in self-perception of performance and satisfaction with performance by clients with chronic pain after going through a multidisciplinary rehabilitation process. This study also aimed at exploring the correlation between the changes mentioned above and changes in clients' sense of psychological well-being and other factors. One hundred eighty-eight clients from a rehabilitation unit in Sweden were involved. Data were gathered before and after a 5-week multidisciplinary rehabilitation program. Data analysis using the one-sample *t*-test revealed that there were significant changes in COPM performance and satisfaction scores following participation in the rehabilitation program. Furthermore, changes in the scores were correlated with those in pain severity and general activity levels as measured on the Multiphasic Pain Inventory (MPI), indicating concurrent validity of the COPM. The researchers concluded that the instrument is useful for measuring outcome of chronic pain rehabilitation.

Usefulness of the COPM as an outcome measure has also been established in rehabilitation of clients with rheumatoid arthritis,[40] as a measure of the effectiveness of a day service in meeting the occupational performance needs of clients with stroke,[13] rehabilitation of mental health clients,[38] and a community living skills (CLS) group in meeting the needs of clients with enduring mental health problems,[4] among others. It is evident from all the above-cited studies that the COPM is a good instrument for clinical use in client-centered occupational therapy. Since the instrument directly operationalizes constructs of the CMOP,[25] one can argue that there is ample research evidence validating clinical usefulness of the model.

SUMMARY

In this chapter, we presented the Canadian Model of Occupational Performance. It was found that the CMOP is one of a group of models that are categorized in the Person-Environment-Occupation and client-centered theoretical framework. The

CMOP was probably the first model to systematically incorporate client-centered principles developed by Carl Rogers in its guidelines for application in occupational therapy. It was also the first model to place spirituality at the forefront of occupational therapy practice.

We also examined the background and constructs of the CMOP. The human, in his or her essence (spirituality), is conceptualized to be at the core of intervention. This spiritual human essence has physical, cognitive, and affective components, through which one dynamically interacts with the environmental context consisting of physical, institutional, cultural, and social aspects. The interaction between the person and environment occurs through occupational performance consisting of self-care, productivity, and leisure. It was found that the overarching goal of therapy based on this model is to facilitate choice, organization, and performance of occupations that one wants, needs, or is expected to perform, are age-appropriate, and are recognized in one's culture.

Lastly, we examined guidelines for client evaluation and intervention using the model. We then discussed the COPM (the assessment instrument associated with this model). Analysis revealed that the model is consistent with the current occupational therapy paradigm, the philosophy of pragmatism, and the complexity/chaos theoretical framework, although these consistencies could be made more apparent. Finally, review of available research revealed that the COPM has fair to good validity and reliability, and has been found to be a good outcome measure in clinical practice.

REFERENCES

1. Baptiste SE: Client-centered practice: Implications for our professional approach, behaviors, and lexicon. In Kramer P, Hinojosa J, Royeen CB, eds: *Perspectives in human occupation: participation in life,* New York, 2003, Lippincott Williams & Wilkins, pp. 264–277.
2. Baum CM, Baptiste S: Reframing occupational therapy practice. In Law M, Baum CM, Baptiste S, eds: *Occupation-based practice: fostering performance and participation,* Thorofare, NJ, 2002, Slack, pp. 3–15.
3. Baum CM, Christiansen CH: Person-environment-occupation-performance: an occupation-based framework for practice. In Christiansen CH, Baum CM, eds: *Occupational therapy: performance, participation, and well-being,* Thorofare, NJ, 2005, Slack, pp. 243–255.
4. Brown F, Shiels M, Hall C: A pilot community living skills group: an evaluation, *Br J Occup Ther* 64:144–150, 2001.
5. Brown SJ: Tailoring nursing care to the individual client: empirical challenge of a theoretical concept, *Research Nurs Health* 15:39–46, 1992.
6. Canadian Association of Occupational Therapists: *Occupational therapy guidelines for client-centered practice,* Toronto, Canada, 1991, CAOT.
7. Canadian Association of Occupational Therapists: *Occupational therapy guidelines for client-centered mental health practice,* Toronto, ON, 1993, CAOT Publications ACE.
8. Canadian Association of Occupational Therapists: *Enabling occupation: a Canadian perspective,* Toronto, Canada, 1997, CAOT.
9. Chesworth C, Duffy R, Hodnett J, et al: Measuring clinical effectiveness in mental health: is the Canadian occupational performance an appropriate measure? *Br J Occup Ther* 65:30–34, 2002.
10. Christiansen CM, Baum CM, eds: *Occupational therapy: overcoming human performance deficits,* Thorofare, NJ, 1991, Slack.
11. Christiansen CM, Baum CM, eds: *Occupational therapy: enabling function and well-being,* ed 2, Thorofare, NJ, 1997, Slack.
12. Cole MB: *Group dynamics in occupational therapy: the theoretical basis and practice application of group intervention,* ed 3, Thorofare, NJ, 2005, Slack.
13. Corr S, Phillips CJ, Walker M: Evaluation of a pilot service designed to provide support following stroke: a randomized cross-over design study, *Clin Rehabil* 18:69–75, 2004.
14. Cup EH, Scholte op Reimer WJ, Thijssen MC, et al: Reliability and validity of the Canadian Occupational Performance Measure in stroke patients, *Clin Rehabil* 17:402–409, 2003.
15. Dedding C, Cardol M, Eyssen IC, et al: Validity of the Canadian Occupational Performance Measure: a client-centered outcome measurement, *Clin Rehabil* 18:660–667, 2004.
16. Dekkers MK, Soballe K: Activities and impairments in the early stage of rehabilitation after Colle's fracture, *Disabil Rehabil* 26:662–668, 2004.
17. Dunn W, Brown C, McGuigan A: Ecology of human performance: a framework for considering the effect of context, *Am J Occup Ther* 48:595–607, 1994.
18. Eyssen IC, Beelen A, Dedding C, et al: The reproducibility of the Canadian Occupational Performance Measure, *Clin Rehabil* 19:888–894, 2005.

19. Ikiugu MN: Instrumentalism in occupational therapy: an argument for a pragmatic conceptual model of practice, *Internat J Psychosocial Rehabil* 8:108–117, 2004.

20. Ikiugu MN: Instrumentalism in occupational therapy: a theoretical core for the pragmatic conceptual model of practice, *Internat J Psychosocial Rehabil* 8:150–162, 2004.

21. Ikiugu MN: Instrumentalism in occupational therapy: guidelines for practice, *Internat J Psychosocial Rehabil* 8:165–179, 2004.

22. Ikiugu MN, Ciaravino AE: Assisting adolescents experiencing emotional and behavioral difficulties (EBD) transition to adulthood, *Internat J Psychosocial Rehabil* 10(2):57–78, 2006.

23. Kielhofner G: *A model of human occupation: theory and application*, ed 2, Baltimore, 1995, Williams & Wilkins.

24. Kielhofner G, ed: *Model of human occupation: theory and application*, ed 3, Philadelphia, 2002, Lippincott Williams & Wilkins.

25. Law M, Baptiste S, Carswell A, et al: *Canadian Occupational Performance Measure*, ed 3, Ottawa, ON, 1998, CAOT Publications ACE.

26. Law M, Baptiste S, Carswell A, et al: *Canadian Occupational Performance Measure*, Ottawa, ON, 2000, CAOT Publications ACE.

27. Law M, Baptiste S, Pollock N, et al: *Canadian Occupational Performance Measure* [Video], Ottawa, ON, 1996, CAOT. (Available from the Canadian Association of Occupational Therapists, Carlton Technology and Training Center, Suite 3400, 1125 Colonel By Drive, Ottawa, ON K1S 5R1.)

28. Law M, Polatajko H, Baptiste S, et al: Core concepts of occupational therapy. In Townsend E, ed: *Enabling occupation: an occupational therapy perspective*, Ottawa, ON, 2002, Canadian Association of Occupational Therapists, pp. 29–56.

29. Maslow AH: *Motivation and personality*, ed 2, New York, 1970, Harper and Row.

30. Pan AW, Chung L, Hsni-Hwei G: Reliability and validity of the Canadian Occupational Performance Measure for clients with psychiatric disorders in Taiwan, *Occup Ther Internat* 10:269–277, 2003.

31. Persson E, Rivano-Fischer M, Eklund M: Evaluation of changes in occupational performance among patients in a pain management program, *J Rehabil Med* 36:85–91, 2004.

32. Rogers CR: A current formulation of client-centered therapy, *Soc Service Rev* 24:442–450, 1950.

33. Schkade JK, Schultz S: Occupational adaptation: toward a holistic approach to contemporary practice, part I, *Am J Occup Ther* 46:829–837, 1992.

34. Schultz S, Schkade J: Occupational adaptation: toward a holistic approach to contemporary practice, part 2, *Am J Occup Ther* 46:917–926, 1992.

35. Townsend E: Introduction. In Townsend E, ed: *Enabling occupation: an occupational therapy perspective*, Ottawa, ON, 2002, Canadian Association of Occupational Therapists, pp. 1–8.

36. Townsend E, ed: *Enabling occupation: an occupational therapy perspective*, Ottawa, ON, 2002, Canadian Association of Occupational Therapists.

37. Townsend E, Brintnell S: Context of occupational therapy. In Townsend E, ed: *Enabling occupational therapy perspective*, Ottawa, ON, 2002, Canadian Association of Occupational Therapists, pp. 9–25.

38. Warren A: An evaluation of the Canadian Model of Occupational Performance measure in mental health practice, *Br J Occup Ther* 65:515–522, 2002.

39. Wressle E, Eeg-Olofsson A, Marcusson J, et al: Improved client participation in the rehabilitation process using a client-centered goal formulation structure, *J Rehabilitative Med* 34:5–11, 2002.

40. Wressle E, Lindstrand J, Neher M, et al: The Canadian Occupational Performance Measure as an outcome measure and team tool in a day treatment programme, *Disabil Rehabil* 25:497–506, 2003.

Chapter 17

Integrating Conceptual Models of Practice

Preview Questions

1. Why is it necessary to integrate theoretical conceptual models in psychosocial occupational therapy practice?
2. Explain the difference between eclecticism and integrationism.
3. Discuss strategic eclecticism.
4. Discuss the proposed framework for conceptual model integration in occupational therapy practice.
5. Explain how you will integrate conceptual models in your own practice.

In this section of the book, we have discussed nine conceptual models of practice that may be used in psychosocial occupational therapy. We will conclude the section by cautioning the reader that the models are not meant to be used individually in clinical practice. Feixas and Botella state the following about psychotherapy theory:

> The historical development of psychotherapy can be described as a sequence of proposals of theoretical approaches that entail differing constructions of human problems and of how to address them psychologically.[5] Attending to the content of most of these competing discourses, one could end up believing that each one is *unique,* markedly *different,* and supposedly *better.* In fact, each one has developed its own terminology, rendering dialogue among them confusing, if not impossible (p. 192).[4]

Similar sentiments can be expressed in regard to conceptual models used in occupational therapy. Each of the models, as the reader can see from Chapters 8 through 16, is presented as different from the others, approaching occupational performance issues in a unique way. However, the reality is that no single model is adequate to fully address the scope of client problems that each of our clients present to us. What Guterman and Rudes state about psychotherapy, that "no single clinical theory is adequate to account for all types of problems and clients" (p. 1),[9] holds true for occupational therapy. Therefore there is a need to integrate several conceptual models of practice in clinical practice in order to reasonably cover the wide scope of each of our client's occupational performance issues.

In this chapter, we will briefly discuss integration of models in clinical practice by presenting guiding principles, suggesting a framework for integration, and then illustrating with an example. It is important to point out explicitly that no claim is being made to an exhaustive examination of the topic in such a brief discourse. The intention in this chapter is to stimulate thinking of how and why occupational therapists use conceptual models in clinical practice. It is hoped that this conscientization will spark thought and research in the topic among fellow occupational therapists.

Guiding Principles

A review of occupational therapy literature indicates a general recognition that many therapists tend to be eclectic in practice. MacRae and colleagues state that "Some occupational therapists choose to develop an eclectic approach to practice, based on several models and theories. An eclectic approach may at times best meet the needs of clients or patients" (p. 125).[17] This is consistent with the finding in psychotherapeutic literature that a single model is limited and therefore "commitment to a single model is difficult once one recognizes its limitations and relative value" (p. 194).[4] This recognition necessitates a search for "more inclusive and well-developed solutions, trying to integrate aspects from different approaches in an attempt to extend current models" (p. 194).[4] Therefore there has been increasing tendency in psychotherapy to desist from identification with any one theoretical school of thought. Many psychotherapists identify themselves as eclectics.[21] Thus eclecticism, by definition, is nonadherence to a specific theoretical view.

However, there has been criticism that eclecticism is an excuse for mediocrity. Markowitz, for instance, advances the generally held view that "adherence to one specific model yields better results than a muddled, mixed (read 'eclectic') approach" (p. 612).[16] He continues to argue that "Moreover, no one is really 'knowledgeable' about how best to combine differing treatments" (p. 612).[16] This argument supports the caution given by MacRae and colleagues that "therapists should understand the specific borrowed elements of the approaches before attempting to create their own framework for practice" (p. 125).[17] The present author agrees with those who argue that a single model is limited; therefore it is necessary to integrate several models in order to address a client's problems effectively. Furthermore, the author disagrees with the assertion by Markowitz that no one is knowledgeable about how to combine treatment strategies from a variety of theoretical models. Literature is available discussing systematic ways of combining theories for application in practice.[9] These ways are referred to as *eclectic models*.[6-8,15,18]

It is important to remember that there is a difference between eclecticism and integrationism.[4] Whereas eclecticism denotes nonad-

herence to a specific theoretical perspective, integrationism

> implies a transition from eclectic stances to what is presently known as the *integrationist movement* in psychotherapy. Such a movement includes ways of selecting theories and psychotherapeutic techniques and contributing to the growth and qualitative development of the psychotherapeutic field in a collaborative climate of integrative exploration (p. 194).[4]

There are three sources of integrationism: technical eclecticism, theoretical integration, and common factors. Technical eclecticism refers to selection of applicable techniques and procedures irrespective of the theory from which they are derived. In other words, it is an emphasis on techniques rather than theoretical arguments. This type of integration is pragmatic in the sense that techniques that work are applied without so much regard for theoretical consistencies. In theoretical integration, an attempt is made to develop a hybrid theory by combining principles from two or more theories. A good example is development of an approach in psychotherapy combining principles from psychodynamic and behavioral theories.[1] Integrationism based on common factors refers to a search for commonalities between theoretical models rather than differences.

Eclecticism was at its height in the 1970s and gave way to integrationism in the 1980s.[4] This effort originated from a proliferation of theories in psychotherapy (there are about 400 different theories in that profession). Of course, we do not have that problem in occupational therapy, and integrationism (referring to combination of theoretical models in practice) has not yet been discussed in any significant manner in the professional literature. Nevertheless, considering recent development of a variety of conceptual models of practice, it is necessary to begin thinking of how we integrate them to address clients' occupational performance issues.

The discourse in this chapter tends to lean more toward eclecticism rather than theoretical integrationism. The author does not think there are so many conceptual models of practice in the profession at the moment to warrant consideration of hybrid theory creation. Furthermore, creation of such hybrid theories may be complicated and take a long time, which may not be immediately useful to practicing therapists who want ideas that they can apply immediately. There is one specific type of eclecticism that may offer occupational therapists useful guidelines for combining conceptual models. This is *strategic eclecticism.*[2,3,9–11,13] This is a process-oriented approach that guides assembly of strategies dynamically in the process of solving problems. In other words, strategic eclecticism "allows for the systematic selection of disparate theories and techniques within a process-oriented model that emphasizes a theory of change rather than the content to be changed" (p. 2), or "the systematic, compatible, and effective application of diverse theories and techniques within a metamodel" (p. 5).[9]

In strategic eclecticism, it is suggested that a metatheory such as narrative therapy, which focuses on constructive (cultural) story making and its effects on an individual client,[23,24] be used to organize the overall framework of therapy. Techniques can be borrowed from other compatible theories in the dynamic process of problem solving in collaboration with the client. This idea is consistent with the client-centered, collaborative framework of the current occupational therapy paradigm emphasized throughout this book. However, it will further be argued in this chapter that instead of using a metatheory (e.g., client-centeredness) and then simply integrating therapeutic techniques from a variety of conceptual models, the occupational therapist may choose a theoretical model that best fits the client's occupational performance issues. This model is used as a lens through which the therapeutic process is generally viewed.

Consistent with the dictates of the current occupational therapy paradigm, the theoretical

model in question needs to be client-centered and collaborative. It forms what Held referred to as *content framework,*[10] to guide the process of evaluation and therapeutic goal setting and planning. Strategies from other compatible models are then used to effect change so that the established goals are achieved through clinical reasoning (what Held referred to as *process*). We will now discuss the proposed framework for integration of conceptual models in occupational therapy.

A Framework for Integrating Conceptual Models of Practice in Occupational Therapy

The proposed framework for conceptual model integration is depicted in Figure 17-1. If we were to use the principles of strategic eclecticism as described above, we would consider client-centeredness to be the metatheory (because it is a core principle of the current occupational therapy paradigm) and borrow strategies from the conceptual models depending on the specific needs of the client and the treatment strategies and techniques that make sense to him or her. In other words, given the newly emerged occupational therapy paradigm, the client-centered collaborative perspective should generally guide how we conduct therapy. That is why in the proposed framework as depicted in Figure 17-1, the entire space represents the context of therapy that is conceptualized to be client-centeredness and collaboration.

In addition, it is proposed that a therapist choose a conceptual model of practice that most resonates with the client's occupational performance issue(s), because it best explains them. For example, for a client whose primary issue is generating appropriate adaptive response behaviors because his or her typical response to challenges tends to be hyperstability, the Occupational Adaptation (OA) conceptual model may be the best to illuminate the issue (see discussion of the OA model in Chapter 15). If the client has difficulty completing a task and

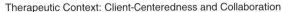

Therapeutic Context: Client-Centeredness and Collaboration

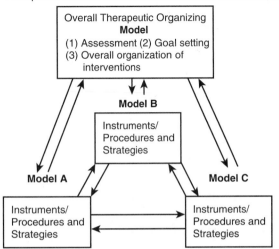

Figure 17-1.   A framework for integration of conceptual models in psychosocial occupational therapy.

mastering skills necessary to transition to the next developmental stage, for example a teenager who is unable to master the social skills necessary for dating, the developmental conceptual model might be the best to explain therapeutic concerns. Also, note that some conceptual models such as OA[19,20] or Instrumentalism in Occupational Therapy (IOT)[14] are specifically designed to be used in combination with other models.

As illustrated in Figure 17-1, the chosen model becomes an overall momentary organizing framework for the client's therapy (momentary because therapy is a dynamic process, and issues and needs may change with time). It guides assessment, goal setting, treatment planning, and overall organization of intervention. If we adopt the terminology by Held, it becomes the "content" model. *Content*, as used in strategic eclecticism, means "explanatory concepts that must be addressed across cases to solve problems" (p. 27).[12] In other words, the principles of the model provide a general understanding of the client's occupational performance issues and a framework for addressing them, within a client-centered, collaborative perspective. This

approach would be consistent with the contention by Duncan, Parks, and Rusk that "Should [a client's worldview] (one may also add the client's occupational performance issues) appear congruent with a particular theoretical orientation, the therapist may utilize that content to structure intervention" (p. 172).[2]

Within the framework of this "content" model, instruments, procedures, strategies, and techniques are chosen from a variety of models, through clinical reasoning, for use in specific interventions. For instance, for a client whose primary adaptive response behavior is hyperstability (as conceptualized within the framework of OA theory), modeling and vicarious learning strategies from the Behavioral/Cognitive-Behavioral model may be used to help him or her develop a habit of "shifting set"[19,20] so as to develop more mature adaptive response behaviors. This is similar to the notion of *process* in strategic eclecticism, which means choosing interventions, methods, and techniques to be used to bring about change.[9,12]

This concept is illustrated in Figure 17-1, where three models (A, B, and C) are presented as providing complementary intervention instruments and strategies for therapy provided within the framework of an overall organizing conceptual model. This does not mean that a therapist can integrate only four models at a time (one organizing model and three models to provide treatment strategies). The four are used only for illustration. A therapist can integrate as many conceptual models as is indicated by the client's occupational performance issues and needs.

The reader should also note in Figure 17-1 that arrows go back and forth connecting all the models being integrated. These arrows indicate that therapy is a dynamic process. Within this process, the overall organizing model, which structures assessment, treatment planning, and overall intervention, informs the choice of models to provide specific intervention strategies. The chosen strategies in turn determine how the models are combined and how constructs of the organizing model are operationalized at any specific therapeutic instance. In other words, the framework that is visualized is heterarchical, where all models are used together in a dynamic manner, rather than hierarchical, where one model would be seen as superior and directing how other models are used. We will use the case study of Sheree introduced in Chapter 16 to illustrate the proposed conceptual framework for model integration.

The reader may recall that Sheree was concerned about the need to turn her life around. She indicated dissatisfaction with her ability to perform occupations that she needed to perform in order to live independently according to age-appropriate, cultural expectations. She also expressed concern that her brother was not satisfied with her performance. Because of her expressed issues with regard to performance and satisfaction with performance, the Canadian Model of Occupational Performance (CMOP) was seen as having the best explanatory value for her concerns. It was chosen to provide an overall organizing framework for Sheree's therapy. It was used to guide her assessment (using the COPM), treatment planning, and overall determination of the focus of therapy.

However, during intervention, techniques and methods were borrowed from other models. For instance, the Behavioral/Cognitive-Behavioral model provided intervention strategies in group activities designed to help Sheree and others learn to successfully choose, prioritize, and perform activities such as budgeting and social interaction. Borrowing strategies from the OA

model, activities were provided to challenge Sheree to develop adaptive responses leading to relative mastery. This enhanced her performance and satisfaction with performance as targeted by the CMOP.

Tasks that were used in therapy were also chosen on the basis of age-appropriateness and bearing in mind skills that Sheree needed to develop in order to transition to young adulthood, including being able to take care of herself, social skills so that she could date as appropriate, get married (if she wanted to) when time was appropriate, and so on. Choice of these activities was therefore based on the Developmental conceptual model of practice. Constructs were also borrowed from the Model of Human Occupation (MOHO) to inform patterning of learned skills into habits that supported effective choice, organization, and satisfactory participation in meaningful occupations that she wanted, needed, or was expected to perform; were age-appropriate; and were recognized by culture.

In other words, within the therapeutic context of client-centeredness and collaboration, the CMOP provided overall organization of Sheree's therapy. Intervention methods and strategies were borrowed from the Behavioral/Cognitive-Behavioral, OA, and Developmental models, as well as from the MOHO, among others. These strategies were incorporated through clinical reasoning that the therapist used in collaboration with Sheree, to deduce what was useful for her at each moment of therapy. The case of Joel provides further illustration.

CASE STUDY: JOEL

Joel was a 62-year-old Caucasian male with an Axis I diagnosis of paranoid schizophrenia. Prior to meeting the therapist, he had been admitted to a state hospital for 180 days through a court order. Before the admission, he had been incarcerated at a county corrections facility for 2 months after con-viction for disorderly conduct. While in incarceration, Joel assaulted a corrections officer. He also had several incidences of violence involving other inmates. He was transferred to the local veterans' affairs (VA) hospital where he was referred to the occupational therapy department for rehabilitation.

Continued

Before being arrested and incarcerated, Joel had been homeless. He informed the therapist that he had never been able to hold a job for more than 1 month. Currently, his only income was from the Social Security fund and pension from the VA.

Review of Joel's case history indicated that he graduated high school in 1960 and then was at a state university for 2 years where he studied electronic engineering. At the time of the interview, he was single and had never been married. During the interview, Joel indicated that before his arrest, his typical day consisted of waking up at 6:00 A.M. and going to a soup kitchen where he volunteered his services. He was able to eat at the kitchen. He would then spend his evenings at his older brother's house, where he would eat dinner. Joel would then sleep either at his brother's house or at a homeless shelter. However, there were many nights when he ended up sleeping in the streets. He stated that although his brother did not mind him staying at his house, he was not comfortable doing it because he did not want to burden him and wanted to be "independent." Joel liked to write music and play the piano. He thought that he was going to establish a career as a musician and use money earned from that career to support himself and live independently in the community after discharge from the hospital.

Some of Joel's clinical features included delusions. He believed that electromagnetic fields associated with electricity allowed other people to read his mind and control his thoughts. Thus he was very suspicious and as a result was socially withdrawn due to paranoia. His medications included Lithium (450 mg, b.i.d.), Cogentin (1 mg, b.i.d.), Laxitane (50 mg, b.i.d.), and Zyprexa (20 mg). Because of his unstructured daily routine associated with homelessness, he often forgot to take his medication. Joel's ADL performance was also poor as indicated by dirty clothes and an offensive body odor, suggesting that he did not bathe regularly. His hair, hands, and nails were dirty. Joel indicated

to the therapist that he would like to have his own apartment and live there independently after discharge from the hospital.

It was immediately apparent from the above-described information that Joel believed that his thoughts were controlled by other people. He was also involved in violent acts indicating that, apart from the belief that he did not have control of his mind, he had problems controlling his impulses. These features pointed toward a deficient volition component of the human system as conceptualized in the Model of Human Occupation (MOHO) (see Chapter 12). Furthermore, he was homeless, his routine was dysfunctional, and he had never been able to hold a job (apart from maybe when he was in the military). This indicated that his habits and routines were dysfunctional to the point of affecting his role performance and making him maladaptive.

Based on the above observations, the therapist decided to use the MOHO to provide a general framework to structure therapy for Joel. The Occupational Circumstances Assessment-Interview and Rating Scale (OCAIRS), the Role Checklist, and the Interest Checklist were used to evaluate his volition, habituation, and performance capacity. Subsequently, the therapist established short-term and long-term goals in collaboration with Joel using the MOHO guidelines described in Chapter 12 to help him become more adaptive. In addition, Joel indicated that he wanted to obtain his own apartment and to live independently. His motivation to be independent indicated that the Canadian Occupational Performance Measure (COPM) could be useful in helping him identify occupations/tasks/activities that he needed, wanted, or was expected to perform; assess his performance of those occupations/tasks/activities; and assess his satisfaction with that performance.

However, it was also observed that some of Joel's aspirations may not be realistic. He was a 62-year-old man who thought that he could begin

CASE STUDY: JOEL—CONT'D

a music career and use his earnings from that career to support his independence. The therapist decided that it would be useful to help Joel determine what legacy he really wanted to establish for himself so that he could be more realistic in his choice of occupations. The Assessment and Intervention Instrument for Instrumentalism in Occupational Therapy (AIIIOT) (see Chapter 8) was used to help Joel establish a personal mission statement and identify occupations/tasks/activities in which regular participation would lead him to achieve that mission. These occupations/tasks/activities were then used as a basis for the COPM assessment. Based on the COPM assessment, his goals were adjusted accordingly.

Based on the above discussion, it is clear that the therapist used the MOHO to provide a general framework for understanding Joel's occupational performance issues (primarily resulting from deficits in the volition and habituation components of his person-system). Complementary evaluation tools (the COPM and the AIIIOT) were borrowed from the Canadian Model of Occupational Performance (CMOP) and the Instrumentalism in Occupational Therapy (IOT) model, respectively. Furthermore, during therapy, in recognition of the fact that schizophrenic symptoms are exacerbated by stress, Joel was taught progressive relaxation techniques that he could use in order to increase his level of relaxation under stressful circumstances.[22]

Psychoeducation techniques were also used to help him identify the difference between his delusions and reality so that he could consciously choose to ignore the delusions when they interfered with his occupational performance. This was meant to help him manage his paranoia and increase his social interaction, which in turn would lead to role resumption (including participation in the worker role). Both progressive relaxation and psychoeducation strategies were derived from the Behavioral/Cognitive-Behavioral Conceptual Model of practice (see Chapter 10). Therefore in Joel's therapy, assessments and therapeutic strategies were derived from the Behavioral/Cognitive-Behavioral conceptual model, the CMOP, and the IOT conceptual models to address deficits in the volition, habituation, and performance capacity components of his human system that were determined (using the MOHO as the overall lens through which his occupational performance issues were understood) to impend adaptive functioning.

Refer to Lab Manual Exercise 19-1 to facilitate development of clinical reasoning skills necessary for rational, effective, and dynamic integration of conceptual models of practice in clinical practice.

SUMMARY

In this chapter, we suggested a framework for integrating conceptual models in clinical practice. We advanced an argument that integration is necessary because no single conceptual model of practice is adequate to address effectively the entire scope of every client's occupational performance issues that we see in practice. The issue of integration has been discussed in psychotherapy literature since at least the 1970s. While combination of models in occupational therapy practice has been referred to as eclecticism, it was found that in psychotherapy literature, a distinction is made between eclecticism and integrationism. In this regard, *eclecticism* means nonadherence to a single theoretical model, preferring use of techniques from a variety of models for intervention as client issues dictate. Integrationism, on the other hand, refers to an attempt to transcend eclecticism and calls for creation of hybrid theories by combining compatible theoretical principles from a variety of models.

In this chapter, we advocated strategic eclecticism as a guide to development of a framework to help therapists integrate conceptual models of practice more consciously and systematically. We argued that while client-centeredness and collaboration forms the context of therapy, a therapist may choose one conceptual model of practice that best explains the client's presenting occupational performance issues to provide general organization of therapy. Strategies, instruments, procedures, and so on are then borrowed from a variety of other conceptual models and combined dynamically as therapeutic intervention proceeds. The strategies, instruments, procedures, and so on that are borrowed from other conceptual models are determined by the therapist through clinical reasoning. Thus it is a dynamic process that unfolds as therapy progresses. As mentioned in the introduction to this chapter, the suggested framework is by no means based on rigorous exploration of the issue of integration. It is just a thought meant to stimulate discussion and hopefully research on the issue for those who believe that it is important for therapists to be guided by clear principles as they endeavor to use a combination of conceptual models in clinical practice.

REFERENCES

1. Dollard J, Miller N: *Personality and psychotherapy*, New York, 1950, McGraw-Hill.
2. Duncan BL, Parks MB, Rusk GS: Eclectic strategic practice: a process constructive perspective, *J Marital Fam Ther* 16:165–178, 1990.
3. Duncan BL, Parks MB, Rusk GS: Strategic eclecticism: a technical alternative for eclectic psychotherapy, *Psychotherapy: Theory, Research, Practice, Training* 27:568–577, 1990.
4. Feixas G, Botella L: Psychotherapy integration: reflections and contributions from a constructivist epistemology, *J Psychotherapy Integration* 14:192–222, 2004.
5. Feixas G, Miro MT: *Aproximaciones a la psicoterapia: una introduction a los tratamientos psicologicos* [Approaches to psychotherapy: an introduction to psychological treatments], Barcelona, Spain, 1993, Paidos.
6. Fraser JS: Process level integration: corrective vision for a binocular view, *J Strategic Systematic Therapies* 4(3):43–57, 1984.
7. Guterman JT: Developing a hybrid model of rational-emotive therapy and systematic family therapy: a response to Russell and Morrill, *J Mental Health Couns* 13:410–413, 1991.
8. Guterman JT: Disputation and reframing: constructing cognitive-change methods, *J Mental Health Couns* 14:440–456, 1992.
9. Guterman JT, Rudes J: A narrative approach to strategic eclecticism, *J Mental Health Couns* 27(1), 1–12, 2005.
10. Held BS: Toward a strategic eclecticism: a proposal, *Psychotherapy* 21:232–241, 1984.
11. Held BS: The process/content distinction in psychotherapy revisited, *Psychotherapy* 28:207–217, 1991.
12. Held BS: The problem of strategy within the systematic therapies, *J Marital Ther Fam Ther* 18:25–35, 1992.
13. Held B, Bowdoin C: Toward a strategic eclecticism: a proposal, *Psychotherapy: Theory, Research, Practice, Training* 21:232–241, 1984.
14. Ikiugu MN: Instrumentalism in occupational therapy: guidelines for practice, *Internat J Psychosocial Rehabil* 8:164–177, 2004.
15. Liddle HS: On the problem of eclecticism: a call for epistemologic clarification and human-scale theories, *Fam Proces* 21:243–250, 1982.
16. Markowitz JC: Psychotherapy and eclecticism, *Psychiatric Services* 56:612, 2005.
17. MacRae A, Falk-Kessler J, Julin D, et al: Occupational therapy models. In Cara E, MacRae A, eds: *Psychosocial occupational therapy: a clinical practice,* Albany, NY, 1998, Delmar, pp. 97–136.
18. McBride MC, Martin GE: A framework for eclecticism: the importance of theory to mental health counseling, *J Mental Health Couns* 12:495–505, 1990.
19. Schkade J, Schultz S: Occupational adaptation: toward a holistic approach to contemporary practice, part 1, *Am J Occup Ther* 46:829–837, 1992.
20. Schultz S, Schkade J: Occupational adaptation: toward a holistic approach to contemporary practice, part 2, *Am J Occup Ther* 46:917–926, 1992.
21. Smith D: Trends in counseling and psychotherapy, *Am Psychologist* 37:802–809, 1982.
22. Stein F, Cutler SK: *Psychosocial occupational therapy: a holistic approach,* ed 2, Albany, NY, 2002, Delmar.
23. White M: *Re-authoring lives: interview and essays,* Adelaide, South Australia, 1995, Dulwich Center.
24. White M: *Reflections on narrative practice,* Adelaide, South Australia, 2000, Dulwich Center.

PART V

Application of Psychosocial Occupational Therapy Across the Continuum of Care

In Parts I through IV of the book, the foundations of occupational therapy were articulated, general practice considerations outlined, and specific intervention guidelines presented. In Chapters 1 and 2, the historical and philosophical foundations of occupational therapy were explored. Chapter 3 presented a discourse on psychological theories underlying the practice of psychosocial occupational therapy. With those 3 chapters, the background of the profession was established, completing Part I of the book.

Part II consisted of Chapter 4, in which the contemporary conceptual foundation of the profession was laid out. This foundation consisted of a newly emerged paradigm of the profession. The philosophical foundation of this paradigm was proposed to be the philosophy of pragmatism, and the chaos/complexity theory was postulated to be the scientific framework best placed to provide constructs that could explain occupation and occupational therapy in all their complexity. Therefore, in Parts I and II of the book, a foundation of the profession as understood from reviewed literature was established.

In Part III, general practice considerations were briefly outlined in three chapters. In Chapter 5, client assessment was discussed. In Chapter 6, a clinical reasoning process was stated and a model for assisting students to acquire basic clinical reasoning skills was proposed. In Chapter 7, intervention was presented generally through a discussion of ethical principles used in occupational therapy practice and ethical reasoning as a part of the clinical reasoning process. The use of self, use of meaningful occupations, and use of groups and group processes as media for thera-

peutic intervention were briefly discussed. Cross-cultural considerations in therapeutic practice were also briefly examined. The objective of the chapter was to present a general outline of strategies and approaches that underlie all occupational therapy, irrespective of the specific area of practice.

Part IV consisted of 10 chapters, nine of which presented specific conceptual models of practice used in psychosocial occupational therapy. The background for each model was explored; the theoretical core of the model and its postulations about function, dysfunction, and change were articulated; guidelines for client evaluation and clinical intervention were outlined; and a case example was presented to help ground theory through illustration of application. The connection between this part of the book and the foundations established in Parts I and II was maintained by discussing the model's consistency with the paradigm of occupational therapy, the philosophy of pragmatism, and the chaos/complexity theoretical framework. To provide the reader with information that may be useful in evidence-based practice, research findings supporting clinical usefulness and effectiveness of the model and its tools were also presented.

In Chapter 17, a model for integration of conceptual models in practice was proposed. It is hoped that an occupational therapist who reads Parts I through IV of this textbook—and completes the corresponding exercises suggested in the accompanying laboratory manual—will have an enhanced awareness of the conceptual foundations of occupational therapy, and further skills to facilitate systematic theory-based practice in a client-centered, collaborative context. In Part V, ideas about occupational therapy practice across the continuum of care will be discussed, including a general discussion of occupational therapy interventions for client populations in various age groups, conditions such as substance abuse, community-based practice, and interventions to address psychosocial issues associated with physical illnesses. This content is meant to facilitate critical reflection among occupational therapists regarding how psychosocial occupational therapy in nontraditional settings (traditional referring mostly to institution based settings) may be systematized and strengthened. Furthermore, it is meant to help the therapist consider the possibility that psychosocial skills are applicable in all areas of occupational therapy practice and not only in traditional psychiatric settings.

Chapter 18

Psychosocial Occupational Therapy Across Ages

Preview Questions

1. Describe the Lifespan Developmental Framework.
2. What is the difference between human lifespan development and human development as traditionally understood in developmental theory?
3. Why is it important for occupational therapists to understand human Lifespan Development theory?
4. Discuss the developmental tasks in each of the following:
   a. Childhood
   b. Adolescence
   c. Emerging adulthood
   d. Adulthood
   e. Older adulthood
5. Discuss the psychosocial issues affecting mastery of developmental tasks in the stages listed in item 4.
6. Explain the focus, with examples, of occupational therapy intervention in each of the developmental stages listed in item 4.

The role of occupational therapy in therapeutic intervention for client populations at different age groups is best understood within the Lifespan Developmental framework. The construct *development* in part means "unfolding."[7,52] Therefore *lifespan development* may be understood to mean a dynamic unfolding of human capacities and complexities throughout life, from birth to death. Consequently, the Lifespan Developmental framework refers to focused attention to "the depth and breadth of the human experience over a life time" (p. 842).[60] The theory of human growth and development on the other hand has traditionally emphasized the first half of life.[60]

To highlight the contribution that occupational therapy has made to the enhancement of human participation in meaningful occupations at every stage of life, it is essential that occupational therapists understand Human Lifespan Development theory. As mentioned in Chapter 3, Human Development theory in general is a source of some of the principles that tend to be used by occupational therapists in all areas of practice, irrespective of the conceptual models of practice that they adopt. In order for intervention strategies and media to be client-centered and consistent with the current professional paradigm, they have to be of interest and relevant to the client. Age-appropriateness according to cultural expectations is one of the factors that determine that interest and relevance.

One way to broach the subject of occupational therapists' contribution to enhancement of participation in meaningful occupations at various human developmental stages is to consider the developmental tasks associated with each stage. This would allow distinction between typical and atypical occupational functioning of individuals in those stages. In this regard, developmental theories of Jung,[37] Erikson and Erikson,[19] Piaget,[53] Havighurst,[26] Levinson and colleagues,[44] and Levinson[43] discussed in Chapter 3 can be illuminating. Havighurst's theory is particularly important because of his pioneering work on developmental tasks.[68]

A *developmental task* is defined as an internal desire to master certain skills, achievements, and adjustments based on maturation (physically, cognitively, emotionally, and socially), cultural demands and expectations, and personal interests.[26,27,41,55,67] Note that cultural demands and expectations are emphasized in this definition. Therefore it is important to consider the cultural context when contemplating developmental tasks of individuals.[50] Given the foregoing definition, *developmental tasks* are defined in this chapter as skills (e.g., study, socialization, self-care skills) and events (e.g., graduating high school, getting a job, getting married), according to an individual's cultural expectations, that may be the focus of occupational therapists as they intervene to facilitate participation in meaningful occupations by individuals at various developmental stages. For this purpose, human lifespan will be divided into four developmental stages: *childhood, adolescence, adulthood,* and *late adulthood.* This division seems to be typical in life course theory literature.[*] For each stage, we will discuss developmental tasks as identified from literature.

We will also explain functional issues interfering with performance of those tasks as outlined in the *Diagnostic and Statistical Manual of Mental Disorders—Text Revision (DSM IV-TR)* and other psychopathology literature. We will then present general occupational therapy interventions to address these issues. At the end of the chapter, we will analyze the case examples presented in Chapters 5 to 16 to illustrate how they fit in the Lifespan Developmental perspective.

[*]References 16,25,29,30,56,61,62.

Childhood

Developmental Tasks

Childhood covers the period between before birth (prenatal) to middle childhood.[16] This period can be divided into prenatal, newborn, infancy, preschool, and middle to late childhood stages.[*] The psychosocial developmental tasks of this stage include establishing a healthy attachment to a caregiver,[57] developing a conscience, attitudes toward oneself, ability to get along with peers, masculine and feminine social roles, attitudes toward social groups and institutions, morality and values, and a measure of personal independence.[26] Other tasks are listed in Box 18-1.

Effective accomplishment of the above tasks leads to the ability to competently perform childhood occupations such as "physical and

---

Box 18-1	Psychosocial Development Tasks of Childhood

Being accepted by adults
Dressing in ways that are pleasing to adults
Being accepted by a significant adult (e.g., teacher) outside of the home
Seeing himself or herself as a contributing member of the class (e.g., helping other children)
Developing reading and writing skills
Speaking before a class
Developing relationships with peers/classmates
Developing socially acceptable ways of expressing emotions rather than crying
Developing self-evaluation skills in relation to academics
Feeling a desire to be loved
Intending to improve his or her skills
Needing to have successful and rewarding school experiences
Developing appropriate coping mechanisms
Being able to tell people when he or she is hurting
Developing a relationship with his or her parents
Gaining acceptance of peers

Adapted from Gay JE, Williams RB, Flagg-Williams JB: Identifying and assisting schoolchildren with developmental tasks, *Educ* 117:571, 1997.

[*]References 11,12,39,46,47,69.

imaginary play, self-care activities, school, and family chores and responsibilities" (p. 48).[16]

Issues Interfering with Accomplishment of Childhood Developmental Tasks

According to the American Psychiatric Association (APA),[1] typical psychosocial disorders of infancy, childhood, and adolescence are mental retardation; learning disorders; motor skills disorder; communication disorders; pervasive developmental disorders; attention deficit and disruptive behavior disorders; feeding and eating disorders of infancy or early childhood; tic disorders; elimination disorders; and other disorders of infancy, childhood, or adolescence, including separation anxiety disorder. These disorders lead to impairment of skills in communication; self-care; taking care of personal effects; social/interpersonal interaction; attending to tasks; using community resources; self direction; academic, work, and leisure performance; health; and safety.

Manifestations of these skill deficits may be observed in inability to form peer relationships, to be successful in school/academic activities, and to separate from significant others and become independent. For example, aggressive and disruptive behaviors of children early in life have been found to be indicative of antisocial behaviors, which predict the tendency to engage in delinquency and violence later in life, as well as academic and social incompetence.[14] Lack of quality infant-caregiver attachment has also been found to be related to lack of competent peer affiliations in later childhood and adolescence.[57] There are many other examples in literature of how impairments in childhood affect emotional, social, and occupational performance. The overall effect is impaired self-care ability, and social and academic (occupational) functioning. In some conditions such as eating disorders, serious physical impairment or even death may occur.

Focus of Occupational Therapy Intervention

Occupational therapists treating children with psychosocial dysfunctions rely on occupations/tasks/activities that are appropriate for the child's

age and that can be broken down into steps that a child can easily understand.[42] In addition, the steps should be "age-appropriate for a child to carry out independently" (p. 274).[42] The therapist should communicate that the child needs to carry out the activity on his or her own or by asking for help.[42] Many of the interventions can be carried out in group sessions. While planning groups and activities to use for intervention, the therapist needs to provide structure and consistency through interpretation of the child's behaviors, disciplining the child through use of strategies such as time out, setting limits, and so on. These strategies are used to facilitate learning of skills such as understanding social behaviors and cues from other people and appropriate expression of emotions,[14] which tend to be lacking for these children. Ultimately, the role of the occupational therapist is to use meaningful, age-appropriate occupations/tasks/activities and therapeutic relationship to help provide an environment that best facilitates learning of skills needed to accomplish age-specific developmental tasks.

Adolescence

Developmental Tasks

There is wide agreement in literature that adolescence is a stage of transition from childhood to adulthood.[5,16,54,60,64] Many adolescents make this transition without serious difficulties.[24] Even for such individuals, however, there is usually uncertainty and therefore some turbulence experienced at this stage. Many of these anxieties result from the fact that adolescents are treated as children while at the same time being expected to behave like adults.[24,63] This turbulence "manifests as confusion, insecurity, indecision, disorganization, moodiness, and alienation" (p. 2).[32] For those who have emotional or behavioral disturbance, the transition is even more treacherous, and it is necessary to develop ways of helping them make the transition successfully. That is why "In recent years, there has been an increased interest in late adolescence and the transition to adulthood" (p. 217).[64]

Tasks of this stage of life include development of an individual identity, emotional independence from family, an individual set of values to guide behavior, peer relationships, intimacy skills, preparing for future education and transition to worker role, and preparing for marriage and family life.[22,57,59,64] Of particular importance for successful transition is academic success "and occupational achievement, financial and residential independence, independence from parental influence, and the establishment of romantic relationships" (p. 218).[64] Graduating from high school is a particularly important event for this transition,[2] which is probably comparable to initiation that takes place at this age in some cultures.[7]

Issues Interfering with Accomplishment of Adolescent Developmental Tasks

According to the *DSM-IV-TR,* some of the psychosocial disorders associated with this age include attention-deficit/hyperactivity disorder (ADHD), major depressive disorder (MDD), schizophrenia, generalized anxiety disorder (GAD), conduct disorder, separation anxiety disorder (SAD), and eating disorders. All these and other psychosocial disturbances cause disruptions that lead to inadequate mastery of age-appropriate skills and accomplishment of developmental tasks. For example, the hyper-impulsiveness and inattention associated with ADHD[4] may lead to difficulty completing academic-related tasks successfully.

The symptoms of schizophrenia include "marked social or occupational dysfunction and difficulty with independent self-care. Educational advancement becomes disrupted...and relationships and social contacts are limited" (p. 76).[65] One of the possible symptoms of SAD is "persistent unwillingness to attend school" (p. 95).[49] This leads to poor accomplishment of school-related tasks and possible academic failure. Ultimately, the effect of these disruptions is that the adolescent is unable to master developmental tasks typical of the age, such as successful completion of school, choice and preparation

for a career, establishment of peer relationships, development of skills needed for intimacy, emotional independence, establishment of an individual identity, and so on. This failure endangers successful transition to adulthood according to socio-cultural expectations.

Focus of Occupational Therapy Intervention

The focus of occupational therapy when working with adolescents depends largely on the issues for which they are being treated. For example, some therapists who work with adolescents with eating disorders perceive their role as to facilitate development of coping skills and manage symptoms using client-centered, occupation-based approaches, among other things.[38] In all cases, because adolescence is a time of transition, which is associated with uncertainty and turbulence, therapists strive to provide "structure and consistency, limit setting, therapeutic relationship, and a team approach" (p. 302)[24] in their interventions. The type of intervention used also depends on the cultural context.[54] For instance, in cultures in which initiation marks social acceptance of adolescents as adults, limit setting is done differently, with the therapist communicating the expectation of more adult behavior. This is different in the Western culture, where it is clearly socially recognized that clients in this stage are not yet adults. In some of these cultures, adolescents may even be expected to contribute economically to the family.

Therapy, at least in the Western cultural setting, aims at providing adolescents with a safe environment where they can test behaviors, decrease acting-out behavior, and act out their conflicts associated with this developmental stage. The therapeutic environment, often a group setting, should offer "an immediate peer group in which the members can express themselves, find a listening audience, and share in their struggles to understanding" (p. 78).[54] Therapy should also focus on helping adolescents acquire the specific family, school, work, community participation, and peer relationship skills that they need in order to transition more successfully into adulthood.[24,31,32] One useful approach to achieve those objectives would be to keep clients focused on preparation for their future roles as adults by helping them articulate a vision of that future and a philosophy to guide their transition to it.

Adulthood

According to developmental theorists such as Jung,[35–37] Erikson and Erikson,[19] Levinson,[44] and Loevinger,[45] adulthood emerges after the transition stage of adolescence. The individual develops a sense of identity, carving a place for himself or herself among peers as an individual in his or her own right, working, and establishing a family. However, many researchers in human lifespan development now point out that because of the long years of education required to prepare for a career in the Western industrialized world, there has been a tendency to postpone assumption of adult responsibility until later years.[16] Many theorists now postulate that there is a new developmental stage in the Western culture that they call *emerging adulthood,* "characterized by a period of prolonged exploration among 18- to 25-year-olds before they settle down into stable adult roles and responsibilities" (p. 124).[57]

This new developmental stage has resulted in a corresponding shift in cultural expectations of an individual during these years. For example, many 20- to 25-year-old young adults who are in college are still expected to be living with their parents and to be economically dependent, whereas in the past, they would have been expected to be married with their own families and economically independent. It has been suggested that in the Western world today, individuals do not assume full adult responsibilities until about 28 years of age.[59] This shift has necessitated a change in developmental tasks of adulthood as defined by culture. Therefore it is more appropriate to examine these tasks in two categories: those of emerging adulthood (18 to about 30 years of age) and adulthood (30 to about 40 years of age).

Developmental Tasks of Emerging Adulthood

As implied in the above discussion, the tasks of emerging adulthood include exploration of career and relationship options while the individual acquires the education necessary for settlement into a satisfactory life characterized by an enjoyable occupation and moral reasoning. Emerging work and relationship skills around age 20 mark the beginning of this self-exploration and preparation.[57] At this stage, individuals may be conceptualized to be in Loevinger's[45] self-awareness stage of ego development,[48] which explains their preoccupation with exploration and reflection focusing on emotional discrimination, identity, relationship patterns, and communication skills. It is important to point out, however, that this prolonged stage of self-exploration and choice making is not typical of all young adults. It happens mostly for those who decide to go to college and pursue further education in preparation for a career. Some individuals get married and settle down to work and establish a family soon after high school.

Developmental Tasks of Adulthood

The self-reflection and choice making of emerging adulthood culminates in consolidation at around age 28. At this time, individuals become "established in occupations and have families, and many will be involved in wider societal concerns and community activities. It is during this decade that individuals form their first template of adult life" (p. 239).[59] Intimacy and commitment to a career have been suggested to be very important for satisfaction with life during this stage. Ego identity is presumed by some developmental theorists to be stabilized at this time.[45]

Issues Interfering with Accomplishment of Emerging Adulthood Tasks

Failure to attain emotional autonomy, attain behavioral consistency, and learn to take responsibility for one's behavior, which are tasks to be mastered as one transitions through adolescence to adulthood,[64] leads to lack of attainment of identity and self-responsibility typical for emerging adulthood. Transition through adolescence may be affected by any number of factors, including psychosocial illnesses (e.g., schizophrenia, MDD) and emotional disturbances such as SAD. For example, schizophrenia is associated with dissolution of identity, social isolation, and ultimately lack of exploration in areas of "occupational choice, relationships, sexual orientation, political beliefs, religion, and a myriad of other areas representing individuation" (p. 76).[65] Other psychosocial disturbances affect the ability to master tasks typical of this age in a similar manner, but perhaps to a lesser extent depending on the condition.

Issues Interfering with Accomplishment of Adulthood Tasks

Similarly, any condition affecting ability to complete the task of self-exploration during emerging adulthood leading to choice of occupation, establishment of relationships and intimacy, formation of political and religious beliefs, and so on, affects the ability to settle down with a family and career, and participate in wider social activities as is expected in adulthood.

Focus of Occupational Therapy Intervention in Emerging Adulthood

Based on the developmental tasks of emerging adulthood as described above, the occupational therapist may use a variety of meaningful occupations/tasks/activities to help young adults (ages 18–27) accomplish the self-exploration task of emerging adulthood. Some of the issues addressed in therapy may include career choice, characteristics of successful intimate relationships, the effect of one's behavior on establishment of desired intimacy and peer relationships, participation in the wider social activities through politics, and volunteering. Occupational tasks, such as creative leisure activities, may also be used to facilitate exploration of one's individual identity.

Focus of Occupational Therapy Intervention in Adulthood

Adults who have severe disabilities and who are unable to take care of themselves may be treated by the occupational therapist in daycare centers or other institutions. For such individuals, therapeutic activities should be aimed at helping them to

develop their self-esteem and self-worth, establish support systems, engage in socialization, and become involved in purposeful activity. Activities programming is a medium for creating community among the clients and a means of replacing the occupational and social involvements no longer existent in the client's lives" (p. 205).[51]

For those who do not have severe disabilities but have psychosocial disturbances, there may be some problems accomplishing the adult tasks of maintaining a career, earning a livelihood to support a family, and maintaining an intimate relationship necessary for family life. Such issues may need to be addressed in occupational therapy. Even typically developing adults may need help, especially in this era when job maintenance is becoming increasingly difficult and job skills no longer last a lifetime. This problem is evident in the number of websites available that offer advice regarding how to keep a job.[66,70] According to the U.S. Department of Labor, Bureau of Labor Statistics, in 2000, 1,094,211 individuals were laid off from their jobs.[70]

According to Sowers, even academia is not immune to this job insecurity.[66] Downsizing and subsequent loss of jobs is a common phenomenon in all job markets. This increasing job insecurity creates anxiety for adults because many people define themselves by their careers and their ability to earn a livelihood for their family. Occupational therapists may need to find ways of assisting these individuals to learn how to keep their skills current to ensure job security. In addition, occupational therapists may assist individuals at this developmental stage to integrate other meaningful occupations in their lives to create a healthy, meaningful, and balanced lifestyle, which can take the edge off the anxiety associated with the possibility of losing a means of earning a livelihood.

Middle Adulthood

Developmental Tasks

According to developmental theorists,[19,35–37,44] the adult stage of development extends to about 35 years of age, after which one enters a midlife transitional stage (approximately 35 to 45 years of age). This is a period of self-reappraisal when an individual reevaluates his or her previous values, beliefs, commitments, and life structure. There is a tendency to respond to inner calling for a deeper self-understanding rather than adherence to societal expectations. The individual tends to respond more to spiritual values and is preoccupied with philosophy and belief systems rather than materialism. The inner drive is toward what Jung called the *ultimate selfhood* (transcendence). This tendency is consistent with the proposal by Lifespan Developmental theorists that "individuality increases with age as reflected by a move towards more self-reflection or interiority, inner direction, and individuation" (p. 227).[15] This self-reappraisal culminates in middle adulthood and extends to the beginning of older adulthood in the late fifties to early sixties.

Issues Interfering with Accomplishment of Middle Adulthood Tasks

Because midlife is a time of reevaluation of one's life, there are some inevitable changes that lead to some turbulence, somewhat akin to what happens in adolescence. As a result, midlife has often been associated with crisis, although the term *crisis* denotes a dramatic event that is not really a common phenomenon. Many individuals go through the transition without notable stress.[16] However, by the very nature of this stage, even those who make the transition uneventfully experience change, both physically and emotionally. Like all transitions, some values, beliefs, and habits have to be given up and new ones adopted. This is experienced almost like a kind

of death.[7] There is a sense of loss that may lead to inability to enjoy previously valued activities, depression, and social isolation.[23] There may also be other health issues, such as diabetes, which affect other areas of life (e.g., sexual functioning), exacerbating the sense of inadequacy and depression. The problems of midlife may therefore be summarized as including depression, sense of inadequacy, fear, anxiety, indecision, fear of being trapped in a job or relationship, obsession with old age, illness, and death.[20] Some of the manifestations of these psychosocial dynamics may include irrational job changes, infidelity, divorce, alcoholism, resentment, and forsaking of responsibility.

Focus of Occupational Therapy Intervention

According to Figler, resolving issues of midlife include taking charge of an individual's life and making the best of it. It is also important to remember that this stage potentially offers "a special kind of opportunity to break with the social conditioning that has carried us successfully this far and to do something really new and different. It is a season more in tune than the earlier ones with the deeper promptings of the spirit" (p. 52).[7]

Bearing this in mind, the role of the occupational therapist may be to facilitate self-exploration that would lead to reestablishment of a healthy lifestyle, relationships, and participation in previously enjoyed activities.[23] Meaningful occupations/tasks/activities that are creative, such as fine art, sculpture, painting, and poetry, may be appropriate media to facilitate this self-exploration and self-discovery, and the onset of new beginnings consistent with the needs of this developmental stage.

Older Adulthood

Developmental Tasks

According to the Department of Health,[13] old age begins at 50 years of age. However, in human lifespan development literature, it seems that the term *older adults* refers to individuals who are 65 years of age or older, while practicing psychotherapists consider old age to begin at 60 years of age.[3] For the purpose of this book, old age will be considered to begin somewhere between ages 50 and 65, maybe around age 60. According to Jung,[34] while the "morning of life" consisted of preoccupation with nature, instincts, propagation of life, and self-entrenchment in this world, the second half (old age) was characterized by increased focus on culture, spirituality, and self (what he referred to as *individuation,* manifested through self-illumination). He conceptualized this change in focus to begin at midlife and to continue into old age.

Erikson,[17,18] on the other hand, postulated that the task of old age was to negotiate between ego integrity and despair. To him, successful aging meant accepting one's life as lived and one's position, experiences, successes, and failures in the world. If one was unable to accept life as lived, the result was despair, experience of death as being too close, fear of the eventuality of death, and regret due to a sense of not having accomplished what he or she hoped to do in life. This fear and regret is manifested and expressed through rage, contempt, disgust, and general difficulty getting along with people. The description of tasks indicative of successful aging by Erikson, that is, the ability to accept one's life without regrets, seems consistent with the notion of harmonization of the "ideal self" with the "real self" proposed by Rosenberg.[58] The *ideal self* refers to the person that one aspires to be. The *actual self* refers to the person that one actually is. The goal in life is to make the actual self match the ideal self by either completing tasks necessary in order to be the person that one aspires to be, or revising one's goals or adjusting the conceptualized ideal self so that it is closer to the actual self.

According to Heidrich and Powwattana, successful aging in part consists of adjustment to losses (e.g., loss of strength and other capabilities) and reconstruction of one's goals so that there is "greater congruence between aspects of the ideal and actual self due to lowered ratings of ideal self-assessments" (p. 252).[28] In other words, successful aging consists of reappraisal

of the ideal self to make it more congruent with the actual self, among other things. Erikson, and Heidrich and Powwattana[28] seem to be in agreement with Edwards and Christiansen in their assertion that "Late adulthood is often a time of accommodation of changing physical, emotional, and social status" (p. 49).[16]

Issues Interfering with Accomplishment of Older Adulthood Tasks

One of the prevailing themes in older adulthood is loss.[3,16,21,40] There is a decline in physical health and increasing frailty; loss of participation in productive occupation after retirement; and loss of friends, home, and sometimes even spouse. As a result, many older adults experience depression, anxiety, and fear of even more losses. More specifically "A pessimistic appraisal of their own present and future peculiar to the old people redoubles due to the development of the psychopathological depression" (p. 59).[40]

Focus of Occupational Therapy Intervention

Based on the tasks of older adulthood, which include reconciliation of the ideal with the actual self and adjustment to loss, one of the goals of intervention is to help older individuals readjust their life goals and adapt to loss. It has been found in research that those with ideal and actual selves that were more in harmony "had higher levels of purpose in life and positive relations with others and lower levels of depression" (p. 252).[28] Articulating one's purpose in life, establishing positive relationships, and having lower levels of depression leads to "achievement of comfortable psychological and social condition" (p. 59).[40] Subsequently, a better quality of life is realized. Reminiscence is an intervention strategy, often used with older adults, to assist them in achieving the harmonization of ideal and actual selves, and adapting to changes associated with the aging process. This is because "Reminiscence is a naturally occurring process of recalling the past, that is hypothesized to resolve conflicts from the past and make up the balance of once [sic] life" (p. 1088).[6]

Occupational therapists are highly involved in interventions aimed at alleviating psychosocial issues of older adults. They work with them in long-term care facilities, daycare centers, psychiatric institutions, and even in the community. A model for working with the elderly living in the community was developed by Clark and colleagues.[9] In their well-known "Lifestyle Re-Design" study involving well-elderly participants conducted between 1994 and 1996, they developed a preventive occupational therapy intervention protocol aimed at helping elderly individuals living in the community in Los Angeles develop an appreciation of the relationship between participation in meaningful occupations and health. During the intervention, the elders learned how to select suitable activities and perform them in order to remain healthy and establish a satisfying lifestyle. In this well-designed randomized control trial, it was found that preventive occupational therapy was effective in mitigating "against the health risks of older adulthood" (p. 197).[10]

Even more instructive was the choice of activities used in their intervention protocol. They included tasks, exercises, and reflection on the power of occupation in the maintenance of a healthy lifestyle; the relationship between aging, occupation, and health; the effect of transportation, occupation, and health; safety; the importance of maintaining social relationships; cultural awareness; and managing finances.[33] This protocol indicates areas of focus for occupational therapists as they try to address issues associated with the developmental tasks of this client population, which include adjustment to changes associated with the process of aging as discussed earlier.

In an adult daycare program developed at St. Mary's Hospital Medical Center in Madison, Wisconsin,[51] the certified occupational therapy assistant (COTA) ran a program for the elderly that consisted of activities similar to those used by Clark and colleagues.[9] The aim of the program was to help enhance the elders' self-esteem, establish a support system, engage in socialization, and participate in meaningful occupations. A variety of leisure and self-care activities were used. They included cognitive tasks such as card games, storytelling, and other educational programs, as well as self-care, work, and homemaking. Reminiscing activities were also used.

A more comprehensive program involving clients with a wide variety of cognitive abilities ranging from dementia to highly functioning elderly individuals was developed at the New York Hospital.[8] For all the clients, irrespective of the level of functioning, interventions were aimed at enhancing optimal performance in cognitive tasks, interpersonal relationships, self-care, leisure, work, and use of community resources. The above three are just a few of the examples illustrating how occupational therapists are involved in psychosocial rehabilitation of older adults. Considering that one of the tasks of this age is to harmonize the ideal and actual selves,[28,58] and reminiscence has been found to be effective in achieving this harmonization by resolving "conflicts from the past" (p. 1088),[6] it may be beneficial for occupational therapists to examine further how to use meaningful occupational tasks that encourage reminiscence as a central part of intervention with this client population.

Focus of Occupational Therapy Across Ages

As mentioned in the introduction to this chapter, Lifespan Developmental constructs are some of the theoretical notions that are used by occupational therapists irrespective of area of practice and the conceptual model of practice that they use. This is because, as illustrated in the above discussion, all clients fall in certain developmental stages. By extension, every client that we see in therapy is dealing with developmental tasks associated with the developmental stage in which he or she is. In this section, we will use case studies from earlier chapters to demonstrate this argument. Table 18-1 shows case examples used for illustration in Chapters 5 to 16. Each case example shows the client's developmental stage, developmental tasks associated with that stage, and issues addressed in therapy.

Table 18-1. ILLUSTRATION OF HOW OCCUPATIONAL THERAPY FOCUSES ON DEVELOPMENTAL TASKS IRRESPECTIVE OF CONCEPTUAL MODEL OF PRACTICE USED

Chapter	Client	Age (in yrs)	Model Used in Therapy	Developmental Tasks	Issues Addressed in Therapy
Childhood					
9	Karanja	14	Psychodynamic	**Acceptance by parents and other significant adults**[*] **Development of reading and writing skills** **Speaking in class** Development of relationships with peers Learning how to express emotions appropriately Successful performance in play, self-care, and **school activities**	Forgetfulness Poor performance in school Fear of disappointing his family
Adolescence					
5	Francine[†]	17		Development of identity Emotional independence **Development of values to guide behavior** **Establishing peer relationships** **Developing intimacy skills** Graduation from high school	Loss of interest in activities Blaming others for all her problems Her boyfriend broke up with her Feeling of rejection by her boyfriend and best friend
14	Ken	18	Developmental	See above	Poor performance in school Withdrawal from peer relationships Anxiety about his life
15	Eddy	17	Instrumentalism in Occupational Therapy and Occupational Adaptation	See above	Substance abuse Emotional and behavioral disturbances (physical aggressiveness) Poor performance in school
Emerging Adulthood (No Examples)					
Adulthood					
8	Henry	38	Instrumentalism in Occupational Therapy	**Commitment to career/job** **Establishment of family (Intimacy)**	Divorced twice Drinking heavily

*Throughout this table, developmental tasks in bold print are some of the issues identified in clients and addressed in occupational therapy intervention.

†The case of Francine was used to illustrate the relevance of the *DSM-IV-TR* diagnosis as part of the clinical data-gathering process in occupational therapy. Therefore no conceptual model of practice was identified to guide therapeutic intervention with her.

‡Strained marital relationship was interpreted to be indicative of a manifestation of Drake's reevaluation of his commitments.

Table 18-1. Illustration of how Occupational Therapy Focuses on Developmental Tasks Irrespective of Conceptual Model of Practice Used—Cont'd

Chapter	Client	Age (in yrs)	Model Used in Therapy	Developmental Tasks	Issues Addressed in Therapy
				Stabilization of ego identity **Involvement in social concerns and community activities**	
13	Leo	31	Sensory Processing/ Motor Learning	See above	Auditory hallucinations Social isolation Needs assistance in self-care Works only 8–10 hours a week Dependent in community mobility
16	Sheree	30	Canadian Model of Occupational Performance	See above	Substance abuse Sexual promiscuity Has only tenth grade level of education Dependent in instrumental activities of daily living
Middle Adulthood					
6 and 10	Drake	46	Behavioral	**Reevaluation of values, beliefs, commitments, life structure, and so on‡** Inward focus through reflective activities Tendency toward more spiritual or philosophical preoccupations	Strained marital relationship Substance abuse
12	Jay	48	Model of Human Occupation	See above	Substance abuse Strained marital relationship Unemployed Difficulty making decisions and using complex problem solving
Older Adulthood					
11	Sara	76	Cognitive Disabilities	Harmonization of ideal self with actual self **Adjustment to loss (of strength, economic independence,**	Living in long-term care Decreased cognitive functioning

Continued

Table 18-1. Illustration of how Occupational Therapy Focuses on Developmental Tasks Irrespective of Conceptual Model of Practice Used—Cont'd

Chapter	Client	Age (in yrs)	Model Used in Therapy	Developmental Tasks	Issues Addressed in Therapy
				home, relationships, spouse, health, and so on)	Decreased sitting tolerance, balance, and totally dependent in all self-care activities

As shown in Table 18-1, irrespective of the conceptual model of practice used, every client demonstrated developmental issues that the therapist had to assist him or her to negotiate (while taking into consideration the client's cultural context and expectations). This is what is meant by the notion of occupational therapy across ages.

Refer to Lab Manual Exercises 20-1 and 20-2 to improve your skills in identifying pertinent developmental tasks and planning treatment for your clients.

SUMMARY

In this chapter, we used the Lifespan Developmental framework to demonstrate how occupational therapy is applied across all ages. Developmental constructs are useful irrespective of the area of practice or the conceptual model of practice chosen by an occupational therapist. Thus it is important that occupational therapists have a good understanding of the Lifespan Developmental framework.

One of the constructs that may be useful in this framework is the idea of developmental tasks. These are the tasks that an individual has to master at every developmental stage in order to develop and adapt to the social/cultural context successfully. We examined the developmental stages of childhood, adolescence, emerging adulthood, adulthood, middle life, and older adulthood. In each developmental stage, we identified developmental tasks that are typically mastered, particularly in Western cultures. We then explored psychosocial issues affecting the ability to master these tasks. We also discussed the role of occupational therapy in addressing these issues. We used case studies from Chapters 5 to 16 to illustrate how essential it is for a therapist to address developmental tasks of a client irrespective of the conceptual model of practice used.

REFERENCES

1. American Psychiatric Association: *Diagnostic criteria from DSM-IV-TR,* Washington, DC, 2000, APA.
2. Asetline RH, Gore S: Biological maturation in adolescence and the development of drinking habits and alcohol abuse among young males: a prospective longitudinal study, *J Youth Adolescence* 19:33–41, 1993.
3. Atkins D, Loewenthal D: The lived experience of psychotherapists working with older clients: an heuristic study, *Br J Guidance Couns* 32:493–509, 2004.
4. Biederman J, Faraone SV: Attention-deficit hyperactivity disorder, *Lancet* 366:237–248, 2005.
5. Bogin B: *Patterns of human growth,* ed 2, New York, 1999, Cambridge University Press.
6. Bohlmeijer E, Smit F, Cuijpers P: Effects of reminiscence and life review on late-life depression: a meta-analysis, *Internat J Geriatr Psychiatr* 18:1088–1094, 2003.
7. Bridges W: *Transitions: making sense of life's changes: strategies for coping with the difficult, painful, and confusing times in your life,* Menlo Park, California, 1980, Addison-Wesley.
8. Butin DN, Heaney C: Program planning in geriatric psychiatry: a model for psychosocial rehabilitation. In Cottrell RP, ed: *Proactive approaches in psychosocial occupational therapy,* Thorofare, NJ, 2000, Slack, pp. 211–217.
9. Clark F, Azen SP, Zemke R, et al: Occupational therapy for independent-living older adults: a randomized controlled trial, *J Am Med Assoc* 278:1321–1326, 1997.

10. Clark F, Azen SP, Zemke R, et al: Occupational therapy for independent-living older adults: a randomized controlled trial. In Cottrell RP, ed: *Proactive approaches in psychosocial occupational therapy*, Thorofare, NJ, 2000, Slack, pp. 193–201.

11. Cronin A: Development in the preschool years. In Cronin A, Mandich M, eds: *Human development and performance throughout the lifespan*, Clifton Park, NY, 2005, Thomson Delmar Learning, pp. 176–197.

12. Cronin A: Middle childhood and school. In Cronin A, Mandich M, eds: *Human development and performance throughout the lifespan*, Clifton Park, NY, 2005, Thomson Delmar Learning, pp. 198–214.

13. Department of Health: *National service framework for older people*, London, 2001, Department of Health.

14. Diken IH, Rutherford RB: First step to success early intervention program: a study of effectiveness with Native-American children, *Educ Treatment Children* 28:444–465, 2005.

15. Dollinger SJ, Clancy-Dollinger SM: Individuality in young and middle adulthood: an autophotographic study, *J Adult Devel* 10:227–236, 2003.

16. Edwards D, Christiansen CH: Occupational development. In Christiansen CH, Baum CM, Bass-Haugen J, eds: *Occupational therapy: performance, participation, and well-being*, Thorofare, NJ, 2005, Slack, pp. 43–60.

17. Erikson EH: Identity and the life cycle, *Psychological issues monograph,* New York, 1959, International Universities Press, p. 1.

18. Erikson EH: Eight ages of man, *Internat J Psychiatr* 11:291–300, 1966.

19. Erikson EH, Erikson JM: *The life cycle completed,* New York, 1987, W.W. Norton.

20. Figler HR: *Overcoming executive midlife crisis,* New York, 1978, John Wiley & Sons.

21. Garner J: Psychotherapies and older adults, *Austr New Zealand J Psychiatr* 37:537–548, 2003.

22. Gay JE, Williams RB, Flagg-Williams JB: Identifying and assisting schoolchildren with developmental tasks, *Educ* 117:569–578, 1997.

23. Gwinnell E: Risk factors for the development of Internet adultery, *J Sex Educ Ther* 26:45–49, 2001.

24. Haiman S, Lambert WL, Rodriques BJ: Mental health of adolescents. In Cara E, MacRae A, eds: *Psychosocial occupational therapy: a clinical practice,* Clifton Park, NY, 2005, Thomson Delmar Learning, pp. 298–333.

25. Hatch LR: *Beyond gender differences: adaptation to aging in life course perspective,* Amityville, NY, 2000, Baywood.

26. Havighurst RJ: *Human development and education,* London, 1972, Longmans, Greene.

27. Havighurst RJ, Prescott DA, Redl F: Scientific study of developing boys and girls has set up guideposts. In Johnson BL, ed: *General education in the American high school,* Chicago, 1942, Scott Foresman, pp. 105–135.

28. Heidrich SM, Powwattana A: Self-discrepancy and mental health in older women with chronic illnesses, *J Adult Devel* 11:251–259, 2004.

29. Hendricks J: *Perspectives on aging and human development,* Amityville, NY, 1993, Baywood.

30. Hendricks J: It's about time. In McFadden SH, Atchley RC, eds: *Aging and the meaning of time: a multidisciplinary exploration,* New York, 2001, Springer, pp. 21–50.

31. Ikiugu MN, Ciaravino EA: *Assisting adolescents experiencing emotional and behavioral difficulties (EBD) transition to adulthood,* Workshop presented at the American Occupational Therapy Association's 86th Annual Conference & Expo, 2006, Charlotte, NC.

32. Ikiugu MN, Ciaravino EA: Assisting adolescents experiencing emotional and behavioral difficulties (EBD) transition to adulthood, *Internat J Psychosocial Rehabil* 10(2):57–78, 2006.

33. Jackson J, Carlson M, Mandel D, et al: Occupation in lifestyle redesign: the well elderly study occupational therapy program, *Am J Occup Ther* 52:326–336, 1998.

34. Jung CG: Aims of psychotherapy. In Read H, Fordham M, Adler G, eds: *Collected works of C.G. Jung, volume 16,* London, 1929, Routledge, pp. 36–52.

35. Jung CG: *The unconscious self,* New York, 1958, Mentor.

36. Jung CG: *The collected works of C.G. Jung: Volume 8—The structure and dynamics of the psyche,* Princeton, NJ, 1960, Princeton University Press.

37. Jung CG: Integrating anima and animus, *Therapy Weekly* 15, November 8, 1985.

38. Kloczko E, Ikiugu MN: The role of occupational therapy in the treatment of adolescents with eating disorders as perceived by mental health therapists, *Occup Ther Mental Health* 22(1):63–83, 2006.

39. Koontz-Lowman D: Family and disability issues through infancy. In Cronin A, Mandich M, eds: *Human development and performance throughout the lifespan,* Clifton Park, NY, 2005, Thomson Delmar Learning, pp. 164–175.

40. Kotova LA, Bondarev RP, Semyonova NV: The role and place of psychotherapy in the complex treatment of elderly patients and its significance for improvement in their quality of life, *Internat J Mental Health* 33(3): 58–62, 2004.

41. Kurtz J: *Developmental tasks of children and youth—record analysis,* Unpublished manuscript, 1973.

42. Lambert WL: Mental health of children. In Cara E, MacRae A, eds: *Psychosocial occupational therapy: a clinical practice,* Clifton Park, NY, 2005, Thomson Delmar Learning, pp. 265–297.

43. Levinson DJ: *The seasons of a woman's life,* New York, 1996, Alfred A. Knopf.

44. Levinson DJ, Darrow CN, Klein EB, et al: *The seasons of a man's life,* New York, 1978, Ballantine Books.

45. Loevinger J: *Ego development: conceptions and theories,* San Francisco, 1976, Jossey-Bass.

46. Mandich M: The newborn. In Cronin A, Mandich M, eds: *Human development and performance throughout the lifespan,* Clifton Park, NY, 2005, Thomson Delmar Learning, pp. 114–138.

47. Mandich M: Infancy. In Cronin A, Mandich M, eds: *Human development and performance throughout the lifespan,* Clifton Park, NY, 2005, Thomson Delmar Learning, pp. 139–163.

48. Manners J, Durkin K, Nesdale A: Promoting advanced ego development among adults, *J Adult Devel* 11:19–27, 2004.

49. Masi G, Mucci M, Millepiedi S: Separation anxiety disorder in children and adolescents, *CNS Drugs* 15(2):93–104, 2001.

50. Melendez L: Parental beliefs and practices around early self-regulation: the impact of culture and immigration, *Infants Young Children* 18(2):136–146, 2005.

51. Neustadt LE: Adult day care: a model for changing times. In Cottrell RP, ed: *Proactive approaches in psychosocial occupational therapy,* Thorofare, NJ, 2000, Slack, pp. 203–208.

52. Ottenheimer Publishers, Inc: *New Webster's dictionary and Roget's thesaurus,* New York, 1992, Book Essentials.

53. Piaget J: *The origins of intelligence in children,* New York, 1963, W.W. Norton.

54. Posthuma BW: *Small groups in counseling and therapy: process and leadership,* ed 4, Boston, 2002, Allyn & Bacon.

55. Prescott DA: Communicating knowledge of children to teachers, *Child Devel* 19:15–24, 1948.

56. Quadagno JS: *Aging and the life course,* ed 2, Boston, 2002, McGraw-Hill.

57. Roisman GI, Masten AS, Coatsworth JD, et al: Salient and emerging developmental tasks in the transition to adulthood, *Child Devel* 75:123–133, 2004.

58. Rosenberg M: *Conceiving the self,* Malabar, FL, 1979, Robert E. Krieger.

59. Schiller RA: The relationship of developmental tasks to life satisfaction, moral reasoning, and occupational attainment at age 28, *J Adult Devel* 5:239–254, 1998.

60. Schuster EO, Francis-Connolly E, Alford-Trewn P, et al: Conceptualization and development of a course on aging to infancy: a life course retrospective, *Educ Gerontol* 29:841–850, 2003.

61. Settersten RA: *Lives in time and place: the problem and promises of developmental science,* Amityville, NY, 1999, Baywood.

62. Settersten RA, ed: *Invitation to the life course: toward new understandings of later life,* Amityville, NY, 2002, Baywood.

63. Shannon PD: The adolescent experience, *Am J Occup Ther* 26:284–287, 1972.

64. Shulman S, Ben-Artzi EB: Age-related differences in the transition from adolescence to adulthood and links with family relationships, *J Adult Devel* 10:217–226, 2003.

65. Sisun JB, Eskedal GA: Schizophrenia and the developmental moratorium, *J Adult Devel* 12:75–84, 2005.

66. Sowers AE: *Contemporary problems in science jobs,* 1996. Retrieved January 25, 2006, from http://www.his.com/_gaene/cpsj.html.

67. Tryon C, Lilienthal JW: Guideposts in child growth and development, *NEA J* 39(3):188–189, 1950.

68. Uhlendorff U: The concept of developmental-tasks and its significance for education and social work (electronic version), *Social Work Soc* 2(1):54–63, 2004.

69. Vergara ER: Prenatal development. In Cronin A, Mandich M, eds: *Human development and performance throughout the lifespan,* Clifton Park, NY, 2005, Thomson Delmar Learning, pp. 91–113.

70. Weir Associates, Inc: *Searching for job security,* 2002. Retrieved January 25, 2006. from http://members.bellatlantic.net/_billfish/.

Chapter 19

Expanded Psychosocial Occupational Therapy Practice

Preview Questions

1. Discuss the argument that every occupational therapist, irrespective of area of specialization, is a psychosocial therapist.
2. Outline and discuss psychosocial skills that occupational therapists can use in order to realize better outcomes in physical disabilities rehabilitation.
3. State and discuss psychosocial issues associated with each of the following:
   a. Physical disabilities perceived to be non-terminal
   b. Physical disabilities perceived to be terminal
   c. HIV/AIDS
4. Discuss psychosocial occupational therapy interventions that may be used to address psychosocial issues associated with each of the following:
   a. Physical disabilities perceived to be non-terminal
   b. Physical disabilities perceived to be terminal
   c. HIV/AIDS

According to Pendleton and Schultz-Krohn, "It has been charged by many occupational therapists (OTs) that those therapists who are working with persons with physical disabilities seldom address...psychosocial issues directly or adequately" (p. 360).[31] This statement is troubling, considering that it can be argued that every physical disability has corresponding

psychosocial issues. For example, if you have a simple injury, such as a sprained ankle it affects your physical functioning. You become slow and clumsy at times, and this may affect your social life. For example, if you are walking with a group of friends, you may feel that you are holding them back because you are too slow. Their attempts to help you in any way may be interpreted as inadequacy on your part, depending on your psychological makeup and past experiences. Your experiences dealing with this injury may trigger past memories of insecurity or dependence. All these are psychological outcomes of a simple ankle sprain.

The World Health Organization (WHO) recognizes this interaction between physical disabilities and psychosocial issues in the newly developed International Classification of Function (ICF).[41] In this document, body functions refer to both physical and psychological functions, indicating recognition of the interaction between the physical and psychosocial domains of a human. Since the 1990s, the American Occupational Therapy Association (AOTA) has also recognized the psychosocial core of occupational therapy, and that every physical condition affects psychosocial well-being, and every psychosocial problem affects physical functioning.[12]

There is ample support in literature of the fact that physical disabilities have psychosocial effects that need to be addressed by the therapist. Furthermore, "psychosocial issues confronting people with disabilities are complex, need to be explicitly recognized by the individual as well as those working with him or her, and must be addressed directly with appropriate occupational therapy psychosocial intervention" (p. 360).[31] We will discuss these effects in this chapter as follows: (1) psychosocial skills applicable to all occupational therapy clients irrespective of issues being addressed, (2) psychosocial issues associated with physical disabilities perceived to be nonterminal, (3) psychosocial issues associated with physical disabilities perceived to be terminal, and (4) psychosocial issues associated with HIV/AIDS. HIV/AIDS will be presented as a separate topic because of the specific way in which victims of the condition experience stigmatization and shame due to the attitude of society toward affected individuals. We will argue that every occupational therapist working with clients affected by any condition(s) in the above three categories needs to use psychosocial skills in order to address their rehabilitation concerns adequately.

Psychosocial Skills Applicable to all Occupational Therapy Clients

Research indicates that the extent to which clients with physical disabilities are satisfied with care received from medical establishments depends on the personal attention that they receive. They value the physician's or medical practitioner's expression of interest in their circumstances, engagement, friendliness, and warmth.[29,39,43] These qualities are the characteristics of therapeutic use of relationship discussed in Chapter 7. The medical practitioner's interest is a characteristic of attention, which is the first step in establishing intersubjectivity that is necessary for communication of empathy.[10,13,37] Empathy is an important part of active listening that encourages self-exploration and self-expression on the part of the client. Friendliness and warmth are attending skills, which precede response to the

client's concerns drawing him or her to engage in the therapeutic process.

It seems therefore that occupational therapists (as well as physicians and other health care professionals) must have psychosocial skills such as attending, active listening, and responding, which are all aspects of a therapeutic relationship, in order to provide interventions that are satisfying to clients with physical disabilities. These skills increase the client's satisfaction with care received, which in turn increases chances of compliance with therapeutic regimens and the psychological adjustment necessary to cope with the physical manifestations of the disease.[39] Increased compliance with therapy and better psychological coping in turn result in better therapeutic outcomes.

Psychosocial Issues Associated with Physical Disabilities Perceived to be Nonterminal

Clients receiving rehabilitation services often have either an acquired disability or exacerbation of an existing disability. Individuals in these circumstances experience loss, fear, and anticipation of future loss.[11,25,27] This is especially true for disabilities acquired in adulthood. Psychosocial issues associated with adult-onset disabilities include depression, stress, social isolation, loss of control, dependency, guilt, anger, refusal of help, and decreased self-esteem.[25,27,31]

Since physical disability is experienced as loss, reaction to the disability may be compared to a response to death or anticipation of death.[25] Therefore onset of a physical disability activates a grieving process similar to the grief experienced in the event of death. Occupational therapists need to bear in mind this grieving process in order to help their clients adjust to the disability, which is a necessary step for effective rehabilitation. One of the models that explain this grieving process is the well-known five-stage grief process by Elisabeth Kubler-Ross.[21] The five stages are denial, anger, bargaining, depression, and acceptance. We will briefly describe these stages.

Denial

According to Kubler-Ross, the first step in the grieving process is denial. A person grieving the loss of a loved one acts as if that person is still alive. For instance, a widow or widower may continue to set a place at the dinner table for the dead spouse, refusing to accept the fact that the loved one is gone. People with disability respond to the loss due to disability in the same manner. They begin by denying the loss, including the fact that they have a disability and need to change the way they function. Literature suggests that denial hinders healing, and therapists should challenge clients to accept their condition.[11] However, during times of stress, denial, also known as the reality negotiation process,[38] seems to serve a useful purpose, especially in the early stages of disability. It helps maintain the optimism necessary to maintain the integrity needed in order to move toward healing.

One may think that denial refers to the client's refusal to accept existence of the disabling condition. However, according to Lazarus,[23] there are two types of denial: *denial of facts* and *denial of implications*. Sometimes, a client may manifest denial of implications by acting as if the disability or handicap does not exist,[42] such as a person with a spinal cord injury insisting on trying to stand up and get out of the wheelchair. A client may also manifest this denial of implications by denying that the physical disfigurement due to a disabling condition is important.[16] This lack of concern about physical looks may very well be a true characteristic of a certain client, but it is not the case for most people. Therefore when a client maintains that physical disfigurement is not a matter of concern to him or her, the therapist may want to investigate further the extent to which this lack of concern may be a manifestation of denial. Following is an illustration of the above-described phenomenon.

CASE STUDY: ABE

Abe was a 28-year-old Caucasian male admitted to the hospital's orthopedic unit after a severe accident. He was working on his father's farm when he slipped off a moving tractor, and his right leg was caught under the plough. His right femur was crushed, necessitating an above-knee amputation of the right lower extremity. After 2 weeks in the hospital, Abe was discharged with a referral to continue outpatient rehabilitation focusing on pre-prosthesis training.

Abe was the youngest child in a family of three sons. His two older brothers, 30 and 34 years old, worked as a physician assistant and civil engineer, respectively. None of them were married. Abe did not go to college. He dropped out of high school and joined a group of motor bikers with whom he rode across the country. After a while, he came back home and started working on his father's farm. Both his father and mother lived with him on the farm. Prior to the injury, he enjoyed working on cars, riding the bull in the local rodeo, riding his bike, and running the local marathon. He had many friends, many of whom were either bikers or rodeo riders. Just before the accident, he had broken up with his girlfriend, whom he had dated since high school, after she caught him cheating on her with her best friend.

Abe's brother brought him to therapy. During the first meeting with the therapist, he was in a wheelchair. He also had a pair of crutches and an *initial prosthesis* made of plaster of Paris for prosthetic training. He was scheduled to see the surgeon and his prosthetist in about 2 weeks to be fitted with a *prep prosthesis*. During this meeting, Abe was rather quiet, did not look at the therapist, and answered questions with "yes" or "no" or short phrases. Abe was requested to wear his initial prosthesis so that his dynamic balance and ability to complete ADLs in sitting and standing positions while wearing the prosthesis could be evaluated.

Continued

He responded by telling the therapist that he did not want to wear the prosthesis because he did not think that he would need it.

The therapist commented that he understood that the prosthesis was not cosmetically appealing but it was necessary for this phase of training. Besides, in time, he would be fitted with a better-looking prosthesis. Abe said that he did not care about how the prosthesis looked. He did not care much about looks. He simply did not want to wear the contraption because he did not think he needed it. Further discussion indicated that Abe thought that he would resume his former activities such as rodeo riding and running the marathon, although it was not clear how he would do this without the prosthesis.

In the above vignette, it is clear that Abe was in denial of both the reality of his disability and its implications. He continued to insist that he would not need to wear the prosthesis although it was clear that he did. He also insisted that he would resume all his physically demanding activities, including rodeo riding and running the marathon. This was an indication that Abe was in denial of the limitations that his amputation may impose on his physical activities. Finally, Abe stated that he did not care about looks. Although it is true that some people are not so much concerned about physical looks, this statement should have signaled to the therapist the possibility that Abe was in denial about the implications of his amputation on how he looked. For a young single man without a girlfriend, who enjoyed participating in attention-attracting activities such as biking, rodeo riding, and running the marathon, it was unlikely (although not impossible) that Abe was totally unconcerned that the amputation significantly affected his physical looks. Disability emanating from an amputation was likely to affect the chances of Abe getting married or having an intimate relationship as well as having a career,[27] and he probably realized it.

As mentioned earlier, although many rehabilitation professionals assume that their role is to help the client accept his or her condition so as to achieve physical and psychological integrity,[27] denial during these early stages is normal and actually serves a psychologically protective purpose.[11] Furthermore, changes in function, mobility, employability, and so on, that result from a physical disability such as an amputation lead to a discrepancy between the ideal and actual self as described by Rosenberg.[36] The individual must adjust personal goals so that the ideal self is closer to the actual self. To help Abe transition through denial successfully so as to achieve this harmony between his ideal and actual selves, one might have helped him engage in self-enhancing evaluation through personal goal setting, taking into account the realities of changes resulting from the amputation.[11,18]

The reason that individuals with newly acquired disabilities respond with denial is probably because disability requires a significant change of identity. According to Clark,[5] childhood occupations are the foundation upon which adult character is formed. An individual spends a lifetime cultivating this identity. It is therefore very scary to anticipate having to give it up and reconstitute oneself as a new person—a disabled individual. Thus Clark likens the experience of disability and rehabilitation to a rite of passage, consisting of three stages: *separation* (one separates from former identity and life), *transition* (one is reduced to his or her lowest common denominator, where all trappings of former life are given up), and *reentering* the world as a new person. This experience is not unlike the transition through critical life stages such as adolescence to adulthood. Like all transitions,[3] disability is experienced as death and rebirth to a new beginning. Although this presents an opportunity for new beginnings, it is also a journey to the unknown, and the unknown is frightening to most people. Denial may be a resistance to separation from the known self and the prospects of the coming journey toward the future unknown self.

According to Clark,[5] one way to help individuals through this transition may be by occupational storytelling and story making. Exploring the client's occupational history (storytelling) reconnects the individual with his or her former identity and illuminates values and strengths that can be used to reconstitute a new identity. This occupational storytelling is a form of reminiscence that could help reconcile the ideal self with the actual self.[18] Occupational story making begins when the individual comes to terms with the need to reconstitute oneself, realistically assesses what he or she can expect to be able to do (what Charmaz calls experience and definition of impairment; meshing of commitments and responsibilities to changed physical capabilities; and acceptance of physical changes and incorporating these changes to self-redefinition[4]), establishes goals, and begins acting so as to realize a newly reconstituted self.

In the case of Abe, the therapist did not use occupational story making or storytelling. If it had been used, occupational storytelling could have been facilitated using instruments such as the Occupational Performance History Interview, version 2 (OPHI-II)[20] to help Abe examine his occupational history and how this history has defined him as a person up to the point of the accident. This would have been a basis for appraisal of changes that had occurred as a result of the accident, which had to be faced realistically. Assessment of current capabilities could have been accomplished using instruments such as the Occupational Circumstances Assessment Interview and Rating Scale (OCAIRS)[17] or the Role Checklist,[28] which would have helped him to examine how his habits, routines, and roles had changed and the implications of these

changes for future functioning and lifestyle. Occupational storytelling facilitated using the above-mentioned instruments would have led Abe to face the physical and occupational changes as a result of his newly acquired disability, leading to acceptance so that the journey toward reconstitution of self could begin.

Anger

According to Kubler-Ross,[21] once the realities of loss cannot be denied anymore, the grieving individual enters the anger phase. The person is angry at everyone, such as the deceased loved one for his or her perceived betrayal and at other people for not going through the same grief. It is suggested in literature that individuals with an acquired disability go through the same process.[25] For these individuals, anger may be manifested by such behavior as lashing out or refusing help. A person going through this stage is the typical "difficult" client.[26] He or she is noncompliant, is complaining, and may be perceived by caretakers as being abusive. This anger may be, and often is, mixed with guilt.[25] The client may feel guilty because he or she blames himself or herself for what happened (e.g., the client may feel responsible for causing the accident that resulted in the disability or for not eating responsibly, which led to the stroke or heart attack).

In the case of Abe, his anger started manifesting during the pre-prosthetic training as it became clear to him that he could not ignore the fact that his life had changed drastically. He was no longer the former adventurous, bike- and rodeo-riding, virile man that he had perceived himself to be. At this time, he started expressing anger and self-pity. When the therapist tried to instruct him in procedures to complete basic ADLs while wearing the prosthesis, Abe removed the device and threw it at him. He made snide remarks about the stupidity of therapy and commented to the therapist that he should not think that he was so smart because he was a therapist. Then, he sobbed uncontrollably saying that he was useless and a cripple.

It is very difficult to persist in trying to help a client who throws things at you, calls you names, and is generally uncooperative. In this author's experience in long-term care, the typical practice may be to leave such a client alone and document that he or she has refused therapy. According to medical insurance guidelines, after three such refusals, the therapist is required to discharge the client based on the rationale, dictated by the insurance companies, that he or she is not likely to benefit from therapeutic services. Contrary to such practice, however, during this phase, it is crucial that the therapist continue to be available and supportive to the client. Failure to do so would lead the client to feel that he or she has been abandoned.[5] The occupational therapist should continue to support the client by "empathic attunement" in order to help him or her "become aware of the range of feelings about the illness" (p. 124).[14]

The occupational therapist can achieve this by responding to what the client says without judging, and then paraphrasing, interpreting, or summarizing it to help him or her clearly articulate his or her feelings. For example, when Abe stated that therapeutic activities were stupid, the therapist could have responded as follows: "You feel angry because you think you are being asked to do things that you do not see as relevant to your life?" Such a response could have led to self-exploration and possible recognition that he was not really angry at the therapeutic activities but at the inconvenience of having to turn his life upside down as a result of the acquired disability.

Bargaining

During this stage, the client clings to the hope that there is still a way to make his or her condition normal again.[21,30] Maybe some miraculous medical technology will be discovered that will make it possible to fix everything that is wrong. Maybe if he or she does all the right things, his or her condition will be normalized. For example, as Abe's therapy continued, he started expressing the belief that if he had been a nice person, obedient to his parents, and had listened to both his parents and his brothers and had attended college, he would have been spared his misfortune. During one session, he told the therapist that if he had a second chance, he would give up risky ventures such as biking and rodeo riding, and he would be a perfect son, committing all his energy to running the farm as his father desired.

During this stage, the therapist should continue to use the therapeutic relationship to support the client by validating his or her feelings, anxieties, fears, and hopes. Apart from validation, the client can be encouraged to start thinking about self-reorganization in order "to live a normal life amidst abnormal conditions" (p. 125).[14] The Canadian Occupational Performance Measure (COPM)[22] and other client-centered semistructured interview instruments such as the Assessment and Intervention Instrument for Instrumentalism in Occupational Therapy (AIIIOT)[19] may be used during this stage to facilitate the process of beginning to think about the kind of life the client wants to live.

Depression

As reality of the permanence of the disabling condition sinks in, the client slips into depression. He or she feels that he or she cannot live like this, and that there is no longer anything worth living for.[21,30] The client may state that he or she does not care and is not interested in anything. Helping the client to share these feelings with someone may be a good way to provide the needed support during this stage. Introducing the client to a peer support group may be a good intervention. Indeed, a peer group consisting of individuals with a similar disability, in various stages of recovery, can be used to provide a support system through the entire grieving process. For example, Abe could have been introduced to a group of amputation survivors so that he could have a source of support as he adapted to his own amputation and accompanying functional limitations. Such a group would be an invaluable source of support, especially during the depression stage.

Acceptance

Only after the individual has fully accepted the reality of the disability is it possible to commit fully to the self-reorganization necessary to function optimally in spite of the disability. That is why rehabilitation professionals aim at facilitating acceptance[25] as a means to full adaptation to disability. Once acceptance is reached, the client is able to surrender to the changed body, allowing "a new construction of self with routines and habits that support the new self" (p. 370).[31] This process of self-reconstruction begins with a revision of personal goals to incorporate a new image as a person with a disability.[5,31] This is similar to the process of self-reappraisal or revision of personal goals in order to harmonize the ideal and actual selves.[18,36] Using client-centered instruments such as the COPM and AIIIOT, the therapist can guide the client to establish personal goals consistent with the changed body, and make occupational choices accordingly. This leads to the individual finally working toward becoming an optimally functioning person, and therefore living a full and satisfying life.

It is important to point out that the grieving process should not be construed to be always as linear as described above. For instance, when Abe met the therapist for the first time, he was in a stage of denial. However, he was also depressed as indicated by downcast eyes, and monosyllabic responses to the therapist's attempts to carry on a conversation. Therefore stages occurring later in Kubler-Ross's model may be experienced earlier in the client's grieving process, and sometimes stages may be revisited over and over again. For instance, even after acceptance, the client may still continue to experience bouts of depression or even bargaining once in a while.

Also, the grieving process for degenerative conditions such as multiple sclerosis or Parkinson's disease is different from that of nonprogressive disabling conditions. This is because the course of progressive conditions is unpredictable and uncertain, which introduces a new complexity to the psychosocial sequence.[14] As the condition progresses, more and more physical functional capabilities continue to be lost. With each loss, the sense of self is compromised afresh,[31] and the grieving process begins again. For such conditions, it is essential that occupational therapists be aware of the need to provide continued psychosocial support with each exacerbation of the progressively degenerative condition.

Psychosocial Issues Associated with Conditions Perceived as Terminal

Clients with chronic conditions experienced as terminal have the same psychosocial issues as those with debilitating conditions perceived to be nonterminal: depression, fear, anxiety, sexual performance difficulties, isolation, and so on.[6,35,40] They go through the grieving process as described earlier, consisting of denial, anger, bargaining, depression, and acceptance. In addition, because a terminal condition is incurable and its course waxes and wanes in unpredictable ways, the client experiences a sense of uncertainty about the future. This heightens fear (particularly fear of recurrence) and anxiety. For such clients, quality of life (QOL) in the remaining days of their lives becomes particularly important. Although QOL is an important issue for all clients with chronic, debilitating conditions, it is even more paramount for those whose conditions are terminal because they face a continually deteriorating situation that is ultimately expected to end in termination of life. For some conditions, such as ovarian cancer,[40] sexuality is also a significant issue.

Therapeutic intervention for clients with terminal conditions addresses not only their physical needs but also their QOL needs.[35] This means that occupational therapists should seek to understand the client's perception of QOL. Pratheepawanit and colleagues insist that therapists should be aware of and incorporate QOL issues in their clinical decisions. They assert that since in terminal illnesses "interviews are usually unsystematic, having QOL information routinely available to clinicians should enhance their clinical decision making and perhaps improve the patient-clinician partnership in this process" (p. 333).[35] In this case, QOL means the perceived relationship between present experience of reality and one's hopes and expectations. It consists of physical, psychosocial, existential, and support domains. The physical domain pertains to issues of physical symptoms and physical well-being. The psychosocial domain consists of both psychological and social issues, including anxiety, depression, sense of social connectedness, and so on. The existential domain has to do with the fear and anxiety of the uncertainty associated with end of life, and the support domain pertains to the available support system to help the client negotiate the grieving process.

Two instruments have been found to be useful in helping health care professionals assess clients' perception of their QOL. These are the McGill Quality of Life Questionnaire (MQOL) and the Patient Evaluated Problem Scores (PEPS).[7-9,35] The occupational therapist can use these instruments in addition to client-centered occupational therapy assessments such

as the COPM to facilitate collaboration with clients in the process of addressing QOL issues. Spirituality has also been found to be a very good resource for clients with terminal illnesses.[6,35] The Canadian Model of Occupational Performance (CMOP) may be useful in guiding occupational therapy interventions that emphasize spiritual support because spirituality is one of the central constructs of the model. In addition to facilitating engagement in occupations that make the last days of the client's life meaningful, the therapist can help him or her explore and engage in meaningful occupations related to spiritual practices, such as meditation, rituals, or religious observances.

Having a social support system, including family support, and preparation of family for the client's death are also important considerations in the treatment of clients with terminal illness.[6] In short, occupational therapy intervention for clients with conditions perceived to be terminal should address issues of QOL, including the client's satisfaction with life.[31] Satisfaction with life is dependent on the client's satisfaction with family life, participation in leisure activities, continued engagement in productive endeavors, self-care, and a satisfying sexual life.

CASE STUDY: MRS. DODGE

Flo was an occupational therapist working for a respite care agency. Mrs. Dodge, a 49-year-old Caucasian woman, was one of her clients. Mrs. Dodge had been diagnosed with breast cancer about 4 years before meeting Flo. At the time, she had a modified radical mastectomy followed by a course of radiotherapy. However, 4 years later, her cancer had recurred and spread into her lungs and ovaries. Ovarian surgery followed by chemotherapy was recommended. Although such treatment would probably have lengthened her life, her prognosis was generally poor. The oncologists

were not certain how long she was likely to live. They estimated that it would be anywhere between 6 months to a few years.

Mrs. Dodge opted to forgo treatment and instead spend the last few days or years of her life with family as meaningfully as possible. On occupational therapy assessment using the COPM, Mrs. Dodge identified her priorities as having a satisfying intimate and sexual life with her husband, and spending quality time with her three daughters, who were 23, 25, and 27 years old. She was concerned that due to the physical side-effects of cancer, such as her hair falling out, her husband of 27 years (who was 53 years old) would no longer find her sexually attractive.

Based on the above information, Flo decided to involve the entire family in Mrs. Dodge's treatment. First, she had Mr. and Mrs. Dodge explore interesting and meaningful leisure activities in which they could participate together to enhance their level of intimacy based on sharing deeply meaningful and enjoyable activities. Both of them liked cooking, throwing parties, dining out, and visiting art and science museums. With the assistance of the therapist, they made it one of their goals to cook an innovative meal that would require and utilize their creativity at least once every 2 weeks, throw a party at least once a month, and go out together either to an art or science museum at least once a week.

Flo then invited Mrs. Dodge's three daughters to therapy. As a family, they explored how the daughters might be able to spend more time engaging in meaningful activities with their mother. They decided to make a scrapbook depicting the lives of the three daughters and their parents. This proved to be a very meaningful and rewarding reminiscing activity. The five of them were able to connect deeply and share valuable memories through this activity. Mrs. Dodge later commented that this activity made her feel that her impending death was a celebration of a deeply meaningful family life rather than a loss. The event also served to prepare the daughters for the anticipated loss of their mother and Mr. Dodge for the loss of his loved spouse. After therapy, Mrs. Dodge lived for 5 more years, long enough to see all her daughters through college, and two of them married with their own families. The 5 years were very satisfying to Mrs. Dodge according to her family.

Psychosocial Issues Associated with HIV/AIDS

The human immunodeficiency virus (HIV) causes acquired immunodeficiency syndrome (AIDS). Infection with HIV is often associated with substance abuse and/or sexual indiscretions.[1,2,34] As such, affected individuals are often viewed as having brought the problem on themselves and therefore as undeserving of sympathy or treatment. Furthermore, in the United States, the majority of those infected are minorities (African-American and Hispanic females).[1,24,34] All these factors lead to a "spoiled identity" among those infected with HIV, because the condition is perceived to be "morally as well as physically contagious" (p. 171).[1] The condition is therefore associated with much social stigma, perhaps more so than other chronic debilitating conditions. There is evidence that even health care professionals discriminate against individuals with HIV, especially if the individuals are also substance abusers.[24] Because this extreme stigmatization poses special psychosocial issues for this group of clients, we will discuss the condition separately from the other chronic debilitating conditions.

HIV infection can be categorized in one of four stages: acute infection, asymptomatic disease, symptomatic phase, and advanced AIDS disease.[34] During the acute phase, the person experiences flulike symptoms, but the symptoms disappear. There is then an asymptomatic phase that can last for up to 10 years after infection. During this phase, there is no indication that the individual has the disease. After enough white blood cells (T4 cells) have been destroyed, the individual's immune system begins to be significantly compromised. The symptomatic phase begins when opportunistic infections begin to set in. During the advanced stage of infection, the immune system is severely compromised and the person has full-blown AIDS. At this stage, opportunistic diseases and physical changes as a result of the disease lead to functional impairments such as shortness of breath, visual impairments, physical disfigurement with consequent postural deficits, fatigue, and so on.

Physical disfigurement, when combined with stigmatization, severely affects self-image. Other psychosocial issues associated with HIV/AIDS include fear (especially of a painful and lonely death), the feeling that one has been given a death sentence, depression, shame and guilt, denial, and anger.[2,24] In later stages of the disease, the person might experience disorientation and confusion.[34] Many victims of HIV/AIDS lose income and become financially dependent, and many of them become homeless. It is also important to point out that with the introduction of retroviral drugs, life expectancy for those with HIV infection, at least in industrialized nations such as the United States, has increased significantly.[2] However, occupational therapists need to understand the side effects of these drugs, such as toxicity and resistance, because these side effects affect occupational functioning.[34]

Given that homelessness, substance abuse, and social isolation seem to be the major issues associated with HIV/AIDS, areas of focus for therapeutic intervention include money management, management of drug and alcohol abuse, and enhancement of social relationships.[2] Because of possible disorientation and confusion associated with dementia in the advanced stages of AIDS, safety and subsequent limitation in occupational performance choices may also be important therapeutic issues of focus, particularly for occupational therapists.[34]

Occupational therapy intervention for clients with HIV/AIDS is guided by the themes of "Symbolism, control, temporal rhythms, occupation, and occupational role and environment" (p. 823).[34] Such an intervention is aimed at enhancing wellness (which is part of good QOL discussed in other sections of literature[6,35,40]), empowerment, and health promotion for clients.[15,34] Pizzi described an assessment developed around those five themes, which he called the Pizzi Holistic Wellness Assessment (PHWA). He defined wellness as "a state of optimized health satisfying to the individual" (p. 53).[33]

The assessment "emphasizes self-perceptions of health and strategies for self-responsibility facilitated by therapists" (p. 56).[33] It is based on the following: (1) self-rating by the client in a variety of areas on a 10-point scale with anchors at 0 (poor health) and 10 (excellent health), (2) identifying factors in his or her life that influence the self-rating, (3) articulating problems experienced as a consequence of the factors identified in item 2 above, (4) identifying how these problems affect performance of daily activities, and (5) describing ways of overcoming the problems. The gathered data is integrated, and wellness goals are formulated collaboratively by the client and therapist. A plan of intervention to achieve these goals is established accordingly.

The PHWA has been used to empower clients with HIV/AIDS to change their lives so that they are able to live according to their beliefs and in that way contribute to their own health. The overall objective of intervention is to create within clients an increased self-understanding and a sense of meaning in their lives so as "to enhance competent performance of self-chosen occupations that contribute to valued roles" (p. 824).[34] Many clients with HIV/AIDS may be in denial,[14,24] and there is need for acceptance before meaningful changes in lifestyle can be achieved.[25] However, the therapist also needs to be aware not to push clients into acceptance too quickly because denial may be serving a psychologically protective role for the client, at least in the early stages of adaptation to the disease.[11] The PHWA can be used to initiate conversation between the therapist and client regarding any problems associated with the condition and what the client can do to overcome these problems. This would be the first step toward the client's acceptance of his or her condition.

CASE STUDY: ANDY

Andy was a 48-year-old African-American male who was a Gulf War marine veteran. About 6 months before meeting the therapist, he started experiencing increased affliction with persistent flulike colds, and then started developing skin lesions. He also started becoming short of breath and experiencing fatigue very quickly with minimal exertion. Andy went to the Veterans Affairs hospital and was diagnosed with the early stages of AIDS. Andy was married and had two daughters, 17 and 15 years old.

Antiretroviral drugs were prescribed for Andy to lengthen his life, but he was not following the treatment regimen as prescribed. The social worker was working with Andy to get him to agree to have his wife informed of his HIV status so that she could also be tested. In the meantime, he was referred to the occupational therapist for assessment with the goal of providing adaptations so that he could continue to effectively perform ADLs given his decreasing endurance and shortness of breath. During the initial interview with the therapist, Andy seemed unwilling to acknowledge that he had AIDS and told the therapist that his problems really originated from sleeping in the cold and inhaling sand when he was in Kuwait during the Gulf War. This was what he was telling his family and friends as well. Andy drank and smoked heavily, and he had a history of repeated extramarital affairs.

Many issues became apparent, including the ethical problem of what to do to protect Andy's wife as well as his other sexual partners. As can be seen, the social worker was trying to deal with these ethical issues. It was also clear that Andy needed to take responsibility and commit to the treatment regimen and to changing his lifestyle, including cutting down on unhealthy behaviors such as drinking and smoking, and abstaining from unprotected sex with his wife and other women.

However, these changes were not likely to occur as long as Andy denied that he had a health problem that affected not only him but other people, and that he had a responsibility to initiate changes to protect himself and others close to him. Administering the PWHA might have been one way to help Andy begin this process of acceptance, self-understanding, and taking of responsibility. As the therapist administered the assessment, it would have been important to pay attention to how he or she used the therapeutic relationship in order to support Andy through this difficult process. This would have entailed assuming a nonjudgmental attitude, conveying acceptance and empathy, and not blaming him for endangering other people through his denial.

The therapist initially might have followed Andy's cue and gone along with the story that his health problems were a result of sleeping out in the cold and inhaling sand several years before. Irrespective of the story about the cause of his problems, the therapist could have helped him rate his perceived health; identify factors that influenced this self-rating; identify experienced problems such as decreased endurance, shortness of breath, and fatigue; identify how these problems affected his ability to perform ADLs; and identify how he could overcome these problems (e.g., by stopping drinking and smoking, not engaging in unprotected sex). This could have been the beginning of the process of getting Andy to acknowledge the reality of his problems and his responsibility in alleviating these problems.

Once the process of self-exploration was initiated, the Pizzi Assessment of Productive Living (PAPL)[32] could have been used to explore more specifically what Andy could have done in order to take control of his life and develop a healthy, meaningful lifestyle. The PAPL could have been used to guide Andy to assess his performance in ADLs and leisure activities, his physical limitations (such as decreased activity tolerance and endurance and how they affected his ability to

Continued

CASE STUDY: ANDY—CONT'D

perform activities perceived as important), his judgment in regard to sexual functioning, his perceived body image, social and physical environments that affected his functioning, stressors in his life, his coping skills, and occupations that he perceived to be important. (Refer to Chapter

21 of your Lab Manual to view a copy of the PAPL.) Andy could have used this information in collaboration with the therapist to establish long-term and short-term goals to enable him to change his routines, habits, and lifestyle so as to live a more healthy meaningful life.

Occupational therapy intervention for individuals with HIV/AIDS may be conceptualized to occur through the following steps[34]: (1) help the client to maintain a lifestyle that is consistent with adherence to the medical treatment regimen, (2) help the client to find ways of continuing participation in occupations perceived to be important and meaningful with the changing physical capabilities as the disease progresses, (3) help the client to discover meaning through continued performance of life roles according to social expectations, (4) facilitate the client's transition through the grieving process, and (5) educate caregivers to alleviate their fears and help them assist the client to continue living a healthy, meaningful lifestyle to the extent possible.

Complete Lab Manual Exercise 21-1 to practice using psychosocial skills for intervention when working with clients with primary diagnoses of physical dysfunctions.

SUMMARY

Occupational therapy intervention for clients with physical disabilities necessarily needs to include addressing psychosocial issues associated with the conditions. Every physical condition has psychosocial consequences that need to be addressed for effective outcomes to be realized. Occupational therapists need psychosocial skills in order to address clients' issues holistically. These skills include therapeutic use of self, including effectively attending to the client, being accepting and nonjudgmental, and being

empathic. Use of these skills increases clients' compliance with therapeutic interventions in addition to addressing pertinent psychosocial issues, leading to overall better therapeutic outcomes.

It is necessary to separate terminal from nonterminal conditions because contemplation of end of life poses psychosocial issues that are uniquely different from those associated with living a long life with disability. Some of these issues include anxiety and fear due to the uncertainty that comes with the knowledge that there is a likelihood of sudden exacerbations of the condition leading to further losses of function and eventually death.

We explored HIV/AIDS separately because the stigma associated with the condition poses unique psychosocial issues that are not quite similar to the experiences of those with other forms of physical disabilities. It was found that some of the objectives of occupational therapists working with these clients include facilitating clients' transition through the grieving process necessitated by the loss associated with the conditions and empowering them to change their lifestyles and engage in meaningful occupations that enable them to live healthy, meaningful lives.

REFERENCES

1. Abrahamson M: Keeping secrets: social workers and AIDS, *Social Work* March, 169–173, 1990.
2. Arns PG, Martin DJ, Chernoff RA: Psychosocial needs of HIV-positive individuals seeking workforce re-entry, *AIDS Care* 16:377–386, 2004.

3. Bridges W: *Transitions—making sense of life's changes: strategies for coping with the difficult, painful, and confusing times in your life*, New York, 1980, Addison-Wesley.

4. Charmaz K: The body, identity, and self: adapting to impairment, *Sociological Quarterly* 36:657–680, 1995.

5. Clark F: Occupation embedded in a real life: Interweaving occupational science and occupational therapy, *Am J Occup Ther* 47:1067–1078, 1993.

6. Cohen SR, Boston P, Mount BM, et al: Changes in quality of life following admission to palliative care units, *Palliative Med* 15:363–371, 2001.

7. Cohen SR, Mount BM, Bruera E, et al: Validity of the McGill Quality of Life Questionnaire in the palliative care setting: a multi-center Canadian study demonstrating the importance of the existential domain, *Palliative Med* 11:3–20, 1997.

8. Cohen SR, Mount BM, Strobel MG, et al: The McGill Quality of Life Questionnaire: a measure of quality of life appropriate for people with advanced disease. A preliminary study of validity and acceptability, *Palliative Med* 9:207–219, 1995.

9. Cohen SR, Mount BM, Tomas JJ, et al: Existential well-being is an important determinant of quality of life. Evidence from the McGill Quality of Life Questionnaire, *Cancer* 77:576–586, 1996.

10. Crepeau EB: Achieving intersubjective understanding: examples from an occupational therapy treatment session, *Am J Occup Ther* 45:1016–1025, 1991.

11. Elliott TR, Richards JS: Living with the facts, negotiating the terms: unrealistic beliefs, denial, and adjustment in the first year of acquired physical disability, *J Personal Interpersonal Loss* 4:361–381, 1999.

12. Fidler GS: Position paper: the psychosocial core of occupational therapy, *Am J Occup Ther* 49:1021–1022, 1991.

13. Flaskas C: Thinking about the therapeutic relationship: emerging themes in family therapy, *Austr New Zealand J Fam Ther* 25(1):13–20, 2004.

14. Garrett C, Weisman MG: A self-psychological perspective on chronic illness, *Clinical Social Work J* 29(2):119–132, 2001.

15. Gutterman L: A day treatment program for persons with AIDS, *Am J Occup Ther* 44:234–237, 1990.

16. Haan N: Coping and defense mechanisms related to personality inventories, *J Consulting Psychol* 29:373–378, 1965.

17. Haglund L, Henriksson C, Crisp M, et al: *The Occupational Circumstances Assessment Interview and Rating Scale (OCAIRS) (version 2.0)*, Chicago, 2001, Model of Human Occupation Clearinghouse, Department of Occupational Therapy, College of Applied Health Sciences, University of Illinois at Chicago.

18. Heidrich SM, Powwattana A: Self-discrepancy and mental health in older women with chronic illnesses, *J Adult Devel* 11:251–259, 2004.

19. Ikiugu MN: Instrumentalism in occupational therapy: guidelines for practice, *Internat J Psychosocial Rehabil* 8:164–177, 2004.

20. Kielhofner G, Mallinson T, Forsyth K, et al: Psychometric properties of the second version of the Occupational Performance History Interview (OPHI-II), *Am J Occup Ther* 55:260–267, 2001.

21. Kubler-Ross E: *On death and dying*, New York, 1969, Macmillan.

22. Law M, Baptiste S, Carswell A, et al: *Canadian Occupational Performance Measure*, ed 3, Ottawa, ON, 2000, CAOT Publications ACE.

23. Lazarus RS: The costs and benefits of denial. In Breznitz S, ed: *The denial of stress*, New York, 1983, International Universities Press, pp. 1–80.

24. Moser KM, Sowell RL, Phillips KD: Issues of women dually diagnosed with HIV infection and substance use problems in the Carolinas, *Issues Mental Health Nurs* 22:23–49, 2001.

25. Moulton PJ: Chronic illness, grief, and the family, *J Community Health Nurs* 1(2):75–88, 1984.

26. Napier-Tibere B, Haroun L: *Occupational therapy fieldwork survival guide: a student planner*, Philadelphia, 2004, F.A. Davis.

27. Nosek MA, Hughes RB: Psychosocial issues of women with physical disabilities: the continuing gender debate, *Rehabil Counseling Bull* 46:224–233, 2003.

28. Oakley F, Kielhofner G, Barris R: An occupational therapy approach to assessing psychiatric patients' adaptive functioning, *Am J Occup Ther* 39:147–154, 1985.

29. Ong LM, Visser MR, Lammes FB, et al: Doctor-patient communication and cancer patients' quality of life and satisfaction, *Patient Educ Couns* 41(2):145–156, 2000.

30. Pangrazio P: Surviving disability is a journey [electronic version]. In Christenson D, Bonn E, Harrington T, et al, eds: *Disability survival manual for persons adapting to disability by persons living with disability*, Phoenix, AZ, 2004, ABIL. Retrieved February 8, 2002, from www.abil.org.

31. Pendleton HM, Schultz-Krohn W: Psychosocial issues in physical disability. In Cara E, MacRae A, eds: *Psychosocial occupational therapy: a clinical practice*, Clifton Park: New York, 2005, Thomson Delmar Learning, pp. 359–393.

32. Pizzi M: HIV infection and occupational therapy. In Mukand J, ed: *Rehabilitation for patients with HIV disease*, New York, 1991, McGraw-Hill, pp. 283–326.

33. Pizzi M: The Pizzi Holistic Wellness Assessment, *Occup Ther Health Care* 13(3/4):51–66, 2001.

34. Pizzi M, Burkhardt A: Occupational therapy for adults with immunological diseases: AIDS and cancer. In Crepeau EB, Cohn ES, Schell BA, eds: *Willard and Spackman's occupational therapy*, New York, 2003, Lippincott Williams & Wilkins, pp. 821–834.

35. Pratheepawanit N, Salek MS, Finlay IG: The applicability of quality-of-life assessment in palliative care: comparing two quality-of-life measures, *Palliative Med* 13:325–334, 1999.

36. Rosenberg M: *Conceiving the self*, Malabar, FL, 1979, Robert E. Krieger.

37. Smith SA, Thomas SA, Jackson AC: An exploration of the therapeutic relationship and counseling outcomes in a problem gambling counseling service, *J Social Work Pract* 18:99–112, 2004.

38. Snyder CR: Reality negotiation: from excuses to hope and beyond, *J Social Clin Psychol* 8:130–157, 1989.

39. Walker MS, Ristvedt SL, Haughey BH: Patient care in multidisciplinary cancer clinics: does attention to psychosocial needs predict patient satisfaction? *Psycho-Oncol* 12:291–300, 2003.

40. Wenzel LB, Donnelly JP, Fowler JM, et al: Resilience, reflection, and residual stress in ovarian cancer survivorship: a gynecologic oncology group study, *Psycho-Oncol* 11:142–153, 2002.

41. World Health Organization: *International classification of functioning, disability and health (ICF)*, Geneva, 2001, WHO.

42. Wright GN, Remmers HH: *Manual for the handicap problems inventory*, Indianapolis, IN, 1960, Purdue Research Foundation.

43. Young GJ, Meterko M, Desai KR: Patient satisfaction with hospital care: effects of demographic and institutional characteristics, *Med Care* 38:325–334, 2000.

20

Occupational Therapy for Clients with Substance Abuse Disorders

Elizabeth A. Ciaravino

Preview Questions

1. Define the following terms as they are used in substance abuse literature: *dependence, tolerance, withdrawal,* and *abuse.*
2. Explain the historical roots of current substance abuse rehabilitation programs.
3. Describe the currently available treatment programs for clients suffering from substance abuse problems.
4. Explain the role of occupational therapy in the treatment of clients suffering from substance abuse problems.
5. Explain the implications of medication currently used to treat substance abuse to occupational therapy intervention.

The purpose of this chapter is to provide the reader with a comprehensive analysis of the clinical features of individuals who fit the criteria for any of the substance abuse disorders as listed in the fourth edition of the *Diagnostic and Statistical Manual of Mental Disorders (DSM-IV-TR).*[4] Of particular interest is the development and refinement of the description of disorders throughout the past few decades, informing the reader of concomitant changes in the delivery of treatment services. Finally, the reader should have a clear sense of the role of occupational therapy in the treatment of clients who meet the criteria for substance abuse disorders.

DEFINITIONS

Before considering the specific disorders that comprise the diagnoses in the section on substance-related disorders,[4] it is important to clarify some essential terms that are associated with this group of disorders. First is the issue of *dependence* versus *abuse.*

Dependence on a substance implies that there is repeated ingestion of the drug and/or alcohol that results in tolerance, withdrawal, and compulsive ingestion behaviors. The client who meets criteria for a diagnosis that has the qualifier dependence attached to it, such as cocaine dependence, has experienced cognitive, behavioral, and physiological symptoms related to ongoing substance use. *Tolerance,* as the name implies, is manifested in the need for increasing amounts of the substance for the same effect. An individual who is dependent on a drug and/or alcohol becomes aware that he or she now requires increasing amounts in order to experience the same effect from the substance. *Withdrawal* is the term that describes very specific behavioral, cognitive, and physiological responses to decrease or cessation of the substance. The withdrawal syndrome also affects the individual's ability to carry out daily routines and may be associated eventually with high-risk and illegal activities in order to obtain more of the particular substance. An example is the individual who is withdrawing from heroin abuse. The individual experiences extreme physiological changes, uses poor judgment, and engages in behaviors that are dangerous in order to obtain more heroin.

Abuse in relation to a particular substance implies a propensity for its repeated use, despite the general disruption in all areas of daily living for the individual. However, there is no evidence of tolerance or withdrawal symptoms. This is usually associated with individuals in their earlier stages of substance/alcohol involvement, many times preceding substance dependence.[4]

Classification of Substance Abuse Disorders

The *DSM-IV-TR* classifies various substance-related disorders according to groups of substances.[4] These include alcohol, amphetamines, caffeine, cannabis, cocaine, hallucinogens, inhalants, nicotine, opioids, phencyclidine, and sedatives. In addition, two other diagnoses are for polysubstance abuse disorders or disorders of other or unknown substances.

Historical Context

Roots from People Helping People

In the 1930s, two men, Bill W. and Doctor Bob, determined that they could help each other with their addictions by gathering people together who had similar problems with alcohol. People have the potential to be helped when they reach out to others. This became the basic premise of Alcoholics Anonymous (AA).[1,16] At that same time, two public health hospitals were funded through the U.S. government following acknowledgement that many heroin addicts were being admitted to hospitals for treatment. The facilities in Lexington, Kentucky, and Fort Worth, Texas, used a variety of experimental treatments for heroin addiction.[16] While many modalities were not unlike what one might

observe in inpatient facilities today (e.g., individual counseling, group therapy, activities, and experimental medications), there was limited success for individuals once they left inpatient treatment. With the growth of AA, individuals with heroin and other drug addictions first began to attend the program, but a movement arose that recognized the need for a specific format for individuals with drug addictions. Groups began to form in New York and Los Angeles that eventually became known as Narcotics Anonymous (NA).[16]

Spotlight on Female Substance Abusers

A pivotal work that shed light on the harsh reality and the need for specific interventions, and the benevolence of one man, was a work entitled *The Junkie Priest, Father Daniel Egan, S.A.*, written by John Harris.[8] The book describes the work done by Father Egan in the area of drug prevention and education. Most specifically, it highlights the necessity for treatment involving use of purposeful activity, and it underlines the powerful positive outcome of people interacting meaningfully with others, even when there are observable differences between them. Such was the case with Father Egan, who noted that female substance abusers were in dire need of treatment, especially those who had served time in prison for prostitution and were discharged to the streets. His interactions with them certainly highlighted the value of client-centered treatment emphasized by occupational therapy today. His empathy and insight led him to establish halfway houses for women, from which they might turn their lives around through meaningful goal setting and lifestyle changes.

Father Egan took this as a mission for his daily work. He was a member of the first White House Conference on Drugs and the White House Conference on Youth. He was the founder of a treatment program in Greenwich Village, and New Hope Manor in Barryville, New York. New Hope Manor continues to be a residential treatment community for women who are chemically dependent. The facility credits Father Egan and his work with female substance abusers in Greenwich Village in the 1960s as the springboard for the current comprehensive treatment program (http://newhope manor.org). Within the perspective of the current occupational therapy practice framework,[3] Father Egan can be viewed as a promoter for healthier choice of occupations for these young women who prostituted themselves for money in order to afford drugs.

Therapeutic Communities

Early programs established in the United States in the 1950s were labeled *therapeutic communities*. Established as long-term treatment centers, the basic premise for treatment was relearning of skills necessary for a drug-free life. Residents were expected to acquire new skills for living, earning privileges as they took on more responsibilities. Their daily schedules included chores, classes designed to help them resume formal education, and verbal groups. One early program, Synanon, however, gained a great deal of notoriety for becoming a cult and exercising strict control over the residents. Current treatment programs are now based upon specific treatment models that are not limited to behavior management, but also include reality therapy, psychodynamic approaches, and social/cognitive frames of reference.

Currently there are over 500 substance abuse and mental health treatment programs that provide a variety of services for persons with substance abuse disorders. Services include assessment, detoxification, residential treatment, transitional housing and treatment, educational and vocational services, and continuing care. In a 2003 survey of therapeutic communities, there were over 19,000 beds and almost 11,000 slots reported to be available for outpatient treatment. This translated into a total of 55,910 individuals treated residentially, and 28,245 treated on an outpatient basis in the year 2002. This study did not account for the beds and outpatient slots that are part of general hospitals.[18]

Current Treatment Settings

Referral Sources

It is important to recognize that a significant proportion of individuals with substance abuse disorders may first come to the attention of helping professionals in settings other than substance abuse treatment facilities. As examples, soup kitchens[15] and homeless shelters[11] are often places where individuals with significant substance abuse issues frequent. As such, they are places where pertinent information regarding treatment may be distributed. They are also places where occupational therapy assessments may be administered.

The criminal justice system serves as a significant referral source, both in terms of inmates who require treatment and for those not incarcerated but in need of treatment following an infraction of the law. It is not unusual for individuals to be referred for treatment from the court system or following an application for public assistance. In the latter case, there may be an admission of drug use as the reason for needing public assistance funds or through a medical examination that is part of the application process.

Settings

Treatment settings for substance abuse are detoxification inpatient units characterized by a relatively short stay; inpatient and partial-day programs; intensive outpatient programs; residential programs (therapeutic communities) that could result in a 12- to 18-month stay; and outpatient aftercare. Whatever the setting, the typical program includes services from an interdisciplinary team consisting of professionals from the disciplines of psychiatry, nursing, social work, drug counseling, and occupational therapy. Occupational therapy's contributions are in the areas of life skills training, stress management, leisure skills, and prevocational/vocational issues. Most programs encourage clients to utilize AA and/or NA in addition to treatment within the facility, and may even make available twelve-step meetings in facilities for clients.

Drug treatment courts are becoming more popular for the coordination of treatment for offenders with substance abuse problems. The function of drug treatment courts is to monitor nonviolent offenders. Once someone is arrested, and if they are considered to be nonviolent, they can enroll in the treatment court as an alternative to regular courts. Once they are involved in the treatment court, they appear weekly in front of a judge and undergo random drug testing. The court commissions different people in the community to treat these individuals. In one study, participants who were successful in drug courts tended to be employed at the time of their initial arrest and to have not used drugs intravenously.[14] An example of how occupational therapy may contribute in this setting is the implementation of a life skills group that assists individuals in setting realistic goals toward independent living that does not include illegal substances or alcohol use.[6]

Medications

Methadone is a synthetic narcotic that has a dual purpose in the field of substance abuse treatment. It is the primary drug used for detoxification from heroin and other opioids for individuals with a substance dependence disorder. It is also used in methadone maintenance programs. The medication is administered to individuals who have not demonstrated the ability to remain drug free. The use of methadone in this manner provides the individual with relief from withdrawal symptoms and therefore reduces cravings. About 20% of the estimated heroin addicts in the United States receive this latter form of treatment.[2] The implications for occupational therapy interventions are varied, and we will discuss them later in this chapter.

Drug Treatment in the Criminal Justice System

Aside from the fact that it is a crime to use, possess, manufacture, and/or distribute drugs, the effects of drug-related behaviors are far-reaching and extremely negative. According to the Bureau of Justice Statistics,[7] approximately 21% of the state prison population and 59% of the federal inmate population consists of individuals incarcerated for drug-related offenses. Both represent an increase from previous years. In 1999, approximately 6.3 million adults were under correctional supervision to some degree.[7] Additionally, 98,913 juveniles (9% of who were drug offenders) were incarcerated in public or private juvenile facilities for nonstatus offenses. The Federal Bureau of Prisons (BOP) provides drug treatment to all eligible inmates, prior to their release from custody, in accordance with the requirements of the Violent Crime Control and Law Enforcement Act of 1994. The BOP operates several types of drug abuse programs: residential programs, transitional programs, nonresidential programs, and drug education programs. Prison populations have been instrumental in testing the effectiveness of screening instruments for substance abuse.[13]

Developmental Concerns

Based on the Substance Abuse and Mental Health Services Administration's (SAMHSA) National Survey on Drug Use and Health among youths aged 12 to 17, there is a somber indication that those who used an illicit drug in the past year were almost twice as likely as those who had not to engage in violent behavior (26.6% to 49.8%).[17] The rates of past-year violent behaviors for youths aged 13, 14, and 15 were noteworthy for being distinctly higher than those either younger or older. In addition, it was noted in the survey that the likelihood of engaging in violent behavior increased with increase in the reported number of drugs used in the previous year.[17] These statistics call attention to the necessity for education, psycho-education, and treatment that is tailored to this particular age group. Occupational therapy has much to contribute in terms of teaching these youths interpersonal skills, problem-solving skills, coping skills, and identity formation to decrease their propensity for drug use and violence.

Occupational Needs of Individuals with Substance Abuse Disorders

Whether it is illegal substance or alcohol abuse, people whose lives are disrupted by any of these substances have specific needs that can be addressed by occupational therapists. Following a comprehensive occupational therapy evaluation that reviews ADLs, educational and work history, and health care issues, a suitable plan of treatment should include activities that enhance skills in the above areas. Clients who have relied upon drugs and/or alcohol have compromised their ability to profit from daily challenges and experiences, may have neglected basic self-care, and may have used illegal means to obtain employment.

A common analogy is that the individual who has a dependency on drugs and/or alcohol has stopped developing emotionally, interpersonally, and intrapersonally at the age that the substance abuse began. For example, a client who is now 28 but began abusing drugs and/or alcohol around the age of 15 will need extra help in problem solving, relationship issues, and assuming adult responsibilities, since the point of reference (or performance skills, interests, and occupations) is generally in the range of what would be seen in a 15-year-old individual.

Assessments

Occupational therapists have at their disposal a number of evaluation tools for clients with substance abuse disorders. The Occupational Performance History Interview, version 2 (OPHI-II)[9] is an example of a comprehensive assessment instrument that can shed light on the extent to which substance/alcohol abuse has affected the client's overall occupational performance. It is also an important initial instrument to use in order to help establish rapport, and to assist the individual in telling his or her life story. The Canadian Occupational Performance Measure (COPM)[10] is an assessment that allows the client to discuss openly those occupations in the areas of leisure, self-care, and productivity that

are important and in need of improvement. It is also an assessment that can be used repeatedly to track progress.

The Role Checklist[12] is a self-report instrument that is also used to educate the client about the various performance roles one might typically have, and identify roles that have been compromised by the substance abuse. There may be individually designed assessments within a facility that an occupational therapist might use. As an example, one's use of time during a typical week is an area that is useful to explore as an individual enters a treatment program. Additionally, psychiatric assessments such as the Beck Depression Inventory[5] help to further delineate symptoms that coexist with the substance abuse.

 Complete Lab Manual Exercise 22-1 to facilitate development of your skills in assessing female drug abusers.

Treatment Interventions

Occupational therapy's unique contribution to the treatment of substance abuse disorders covers a broad spectrum. Assessments that further define current occupational performance difficulties and provide insight into the individual reasons for the progression of the disorder pave the way for planning for engagement in activities that facilitate learning new skills, relearning prior skills, and/or learning compensatory skills. An example of the latter could be a client in his or her late thirties or forties who makes the decision to enter a shorter training program, rather than attempt to return to school to complete a college degree. His or her treatment plan would include short-term objectives that lead to entrance into a vocational training program, rather than the client whose overall skills as a student during adolescence were not disrupted by the substance abuse. The occupational therapist has the expertise to help each client plan for specific life skill changes.

There is a specific need to be addressed in this area of treatment for females with substance abuse disorders. In many cases, females have relied upon men for financial support, have been taken advantage of, or have compromised their own dignity through activities such as prostitu-tion. As such, they may require a more detailed plan for intervention aimed at improving performance in self-care, leisure, and productive living pursuits.

CASE STUDY: CLAUDIA

Claudia is a 24-year-old Caucasian female who currently resides in a transitional housing program in which she was placed through the correctional system. She arrived 3 months ago following release from prison for a "receiving stolen property" charge. She has also had prior arrests for possession of heroin. Claudia's early history is noteworthy for being raised by her mother and her maternal grandmother. She stated that her father left when she was 4 years old. Her mother had significant psychiatric issues including numerous hospitalizations and periods at home when she would express suicidal thoughts.

Claudia has a 22-year-old brother who is presently an active alcoholic. She describes her early education as being difficult because of her extreme shyness and lack of interaction with peers. She stated that she attended school regularly and came home immediately after school to help out at home. She stated that she also had a great deal of difficulty with reading and with paying attention to the teacher, stating that she often daydreamed.

Claudia described her high school years as difficult because of the continued anxiety, her mother's mental health issues, and her brother's excessive drinking. Her grandmother passed away when she was 15, which was a significant loss. In the eleventh grade, she began dating a 19-year-old man who was abusing drugs. She began to drink with him and eventually began using heroin. At that time, she dropped out of school and began working as a waitress in a local diner.

The relationship between Claudia and her boyfriend ended, but she continues using heroin intermittently. She obtained a job at a local bar as a topless dancer, primarily because a friend was doing it, but she did not feel comfortable doing it. Instead, she began shoplifting at large department stores. Her method included stealing expensive clothing, returning it to the store for a store credit, and then selling the credit certificates for one-half of what they were worth. Eventually she was arrested and served 3 months in jail before being released to the transitional housing program.

When interviewed by the occupational therapist using the COPM as a guide, Claudia acknowledged that areas of basic self-care were lacking. She also stated that she had no particular leisure interests, had doubts about her ability to complete her education, and was worried about getting involved in relationships with men who were bad for her. She stated that her doctor had advised her to take Paxil to help with depression and anxiety; she stated that since going to prison she had been clean and sober.

Based on the assessment using the COPM, the main goal for Claudia was to attend AA meetings and to obtain a sponsor. In addition, she agreed to have a conversation with at least one female at each meeting that she attends (minimal expectation was to introduce herself and tell the individual that she was new to AA), to explore at least one leisure interest that she might like to pursue, and to attend at least one activity in the program related to vocational planning. Claudia's work in individual sessions was in the area of gaining insight into the extent to which her family experiences compromised her development and developing assertiveness skills necessary to help her begin to seek help from others. Other aspects of occupational therapy treatment included enhancing coping skills, continued focus on vocational planning, and improvement in leisure and basic self-care activi-

CASE STUDY: CLAUDIA—CONT'D

ties. She was encouraged to produce a spending plan (budget) based on her limited finances from public assistance and to make appointments with a gynecologist, psychiatrist, and dentist.

At the end of 6 months, Claudia had successfully completed a life skills group program and was enrolled in GED classes. She had successfully detached from her mother and brother, except for their occa-

sional attendance at a family therapy meeting. She continued to experience episodes of extreme anxiety and self-doubt, but had managed to call friends from AA to help her through these times.

 Complete Lab Manual Exercise 22-2 to develop your skills in planning therapeutic interventions for clients with substance abuse problems.

Twelve-Step Programs

An important aspect of successful treatment for many people who are addicted to substances is programs such as AA, NA, and related chapters for family members, children, and spouses (such as Adult Children of Alcoholics, and Naranon). While extremely integral to many individuals for their relapse prevention as well as ongoing personal growth, the effectiveness of twelve-step programs is not well-established through research. This may be in large part due to the anonymous nature of its structure and the tradition of attraction, rather than promotion or publicity of services. However, from an occupational therapy perspective, involvement in a fellowship such as AA or NA should not be viewed as ancillary, but as integral to recovery. It is a primary, life-affirming, and positive occupation for many who are involved.

SUMMARY

Clients with substance abuse disorders are given a diagnosis based on a variety of possible addiction to substances, including alcohol, amphetamines, caffeine, cannabis, cocaine, hallucinogens, inhalants, nicotine, opioids, phencyclidine, and sedatives. One condition for the diagnosis is a major disruption in one's daily functioning and occupational performance. The history of people helping people with substance abuse disorders is rich, and

continues to unfold as occupational therapists continue to look for ways to offer their expertise to help individuals with substance abuse disorders.

REFERENCES

1. Alcoholics Anonymous: *Alcoholics Anonymous: the story of how many thousands of men and women have recovered from alcoholism,* ed 4, New York, 2001, Alcoholics Anonymous World Services.
2. American Methadone Treatment Association: *News Report,* pp. 1–14, 1998.
3. American Occupational Therapy Association: Occupational therapy practice framework: domain and process, *Am J Occup Ther* 56(6):609–639, 2002.
4. American Psychiatric Association: *Diagnostic and statistical manual of mental disorders: DSM-IV-TR,* ed 4, text revision, Washington DC, 2000, APA.
5. Beck AT, Ward CH, Mendelson M, et al: An inventory for measuring depression, *Arch General Psychiatr* 4:561–571, 1961.
6. Brachtesende A: Lessons from drug court, *OT Practice,* September, pp. 9–10, 2004.
7. Bureau of Justice Statistics: *Correctional Populations in the United States, 1992,* Washington, DC, 2000, U.S. Department of Justice.
8. Harris J: *The junkie priest, Father Daniel Egan, SA,* 1965, Pocket Books.
9. Kielhofner G, Mallinson T, Crawford C, et al: A user's manual for the Occupational Performance History Interview (version 2) (OPHI-II), Chicago, 1998, Model of Human Occupation Clearinghouse, University of Illinois at Chicago.
10. Law M, Baptiste S, Carswell A, et al: Canadian Occupational Performance Measure, ed 2, Toronto, Ontario, 2000, CAOT.

11. McCracken L, Black M: Psychiatric treatment of the homeless in a group-based therapeutic community: a preliminary field investigation, *Internat J Group Psychother* 55(4):595–605, 2005.
12. Oakley F, Kielhofner G, Barris R, et al: The Role Checklist: development and empirical assessment of reliability, *Occup Ther J Res* 6:157–170, 1986.
13. Peters J, Greenbaum P, Steinberg M, et al: Effectiveness of screening instruments in detecting substance use disorders among prisoners, *J Substance Abuse Treatment* 18:349–358, 2000.
14. Roll J, Prendergast M, Richardson K, et al: Identifying predictors of treatment outcome in a drug court program, *Am J Drug Alcohol Abuse* 31:641–656, 2005.
15. Rosenblum A, Magura S, Kayman D, et al: Motivationally enhanced group counseling for substance users in a soup kitchen: a randomized clinical trial, *Drug Alcohol Dependence* 80:91–103, 2005.
16. Stone R: *My years with Narcotics Anonymous: A history of NA,* Joplin, MO, 1997, Hulon Pendleton.
17. Substance Abuse and Mental Health Services Administration: *Research findings from the SAMHSA 2002, 2003, and 2004 National Surveys on Drug Use and Health,* Rockville, MD, 2006, Office of Applied Studies, The NDSUH Report, Issue 5.
18. Therapeutic Communities of America: TCA News, Fall 2005. Retrieved January 8, 2006, from http://www.therapeuticcommunitiesofamerica.org/.

21

Integration of Caregiver Issues in Psychosocial Occupational Therapy Intervention

Preview Questions

1. Define caregiving as a family role.
2. Describe the basic socio-emotional needs that are primarily met within the family unit according to the Fundamental Interpersonal Relations Orientation model.
3. Discuss the relationship between the psychological well-being of family caregivers and their ability to be allies in occupational therapy intervention for a client with psychosocial illness.
4. Explain how occupational therapists may involve family caregivers in treatment planning and interventions so that they are allies in psychosocial client rehabilitation.
5. Discuss the construct of the family as an occupational therapy client and the occupational therapist's role in addressing psychosocial needs of family caregivers so that they are more effective as allies in therapeutic interventions for the client.
6. Explain how the occupational therapist may identify signs of client abuse by caregivers and how he or she would respond to such suspected abuse.

Although caregivers of individuals with psychosocial illness may be individuals outside the family, in most cases they tend to be family members.[30] This is logical since according to the Fundamental Interpersonal Relations Orientation (FIRO) model, which has been applied to family-oriented interventions, the family is the primary context within which the client's needs for inclusion, control, and affection are met.[24,26] In other words, the family is the initial venue in which one feels a sense of belonging, control over one's life, and cared for. Therefore it is necessary for family caregivers to assist a client with psychosocial illness to meet these needs.

The ability of family caregivers to meet the client's needs for inclusion, control, and affection depends on their own psychological health. There is ample evidence from research indicating that the emotional status of family caregivers significantly affects a client's sense of well-being and quality of life (QOL).[16,17,27] It is important that occupational therapists develop effective interventions aimed at supporting family members of clients with psychosocial illnesses in order for clients' therapeutic goals to be met effectively so that their QOL is enhanced. In this chapter, we will discuss the role of occupational therapy in supporting caregivers so that they can be effective allies in the client's therapeutic process as follows: (1) the role of family caregivers as allies in the rehabilitation of clients with psychosocial illnesses, (2) the idea of the family as an occupational therapy client, and (3) issues of abuse in the context of caregiving and the therapist's responsibility in addressing these issues.

Caregivers as Allies in Psychosocial Rehabilitation

As mentioned earlier, the family is an important source of fulfillment of a client's need for inclusion, control, and affection. We also mentioned that the family is charged with the responsibility of meeting these needs because they are the primary caregivers. The term *caregiver* means "a person (they may be a relation or not) who invests time and effort in giving care" (p. 344).[30] A primary caregiver has also been defined as "the relative who the patient considered to be most helpful to them and/or the relative who was most involved in the support/advocacy group" (p. 3).[3]

Even though the caregiver as defined above does not have to be a family member, there is a tendency for the family to assume this responsibility. For example, in Finland, Stengard asserts that due to increasingly limited resources for professional caregiving within the community, families are increasingly being called upon to assume the responsibility of caregiving for their loved ones with psychosocial illness.[27] If the family constitutes the primary caregiver, it means that they have to be allies in the rehabilitation endeavors for the client. The family is the source of crucial information regarding what medication works best for the client, and they are the eyes and ears of rehabilitation professionals in helping monitor the side effects of medication. They also provide information about decompensation behaviors (where *decompensation* means changes in a client's behavior and mood as manifested in the clinical symptoms, such as poor concentration, disruption of usual routine, or assaultive or destructive behavior), since they live with the client on a daily basis.[21] There is also evidence that when rehabilitation professionals maintain contact with family members and involve them in therapeutic endeavors, clinical outcomes are more positive.[11]

From the above argument, it is evident that involvement of the family is crucial to successful client rehabilitation and therefore they are an invaluable ally to the rehabilitation process.

In addition, there is evidence indicating that family caregivers are willing to be involved in the treatment of their loved ones with psychosocial illness.[17] Thus it is essential that occupational therapists develop therapeutic models for involvement of family caregivers in the treatment of clients with psychosocial illnesses for more effective therapeutic interventions. Involvement of family caregivers in the occupational therapy process may involve working with families to explore ways of helping clients resume expected roles (including the worker role), as well as enhancing social functioning, which seem to be issues of primary concern for families with loved ones who have psychosocial illness.[11] More specifically, some of the ways in which the family may be involved in occupational therapy interventions for their loved ones with psychosocial illness may be by collaborating with the therapist to supervise the client in order to limit abuse of drugs and alcohol, prevent the client's hazardous behavior, convey concern for the client's well-being, and monitor the care received by the client from the entire rehabilitation team.[27]

In addition, the family may be a source of information regarding change of the client's symptoms, history of the illness that may influence occupational therapy goals, client's source of physical support, including providing him or her with housing, food, and supervision to ensure compliance with the treatment regimen, and the primary social support network.[21,30] A fully involved family, in collaboration with the occupational therapist, would (1) evaluate the client's occupational performance (the therapist may use formal assessments, such as the COPM to guide the family in this process), (2) assess the extent to which his or her occupational performance facilitates his or her sense of inclusion, control, and affection, (3) identify ways in which various family members may help the client enhance occupational performance so as to meet the needs of inclusion, control, and affection, (4) establish goals to facilitate client's occupational performance, and (5) assign family members homework to help achieve established goals.[5]

CASE STUDY: PRISCILLA

Priscilla is a 30-year-old Caucasian woman with a diagnosis of schizophrenia. Priscilla was the second child born in a family of three (two daughters and a son) raised by a single mother. Her older sister is 33 years old, and her younger brother is 28 years old. Priscilla started displaying what the family referred to as "strange behaviors," including withdrawal, talking to herself, and so on, when she was in high school. Consequently, she dropped out of school and ran away from home. After several days living in the streets, Priscilla was brought home by the police. She was taken to the hospital and diagnosed with schizophrenia. Since then, she has been in and out of the hospital nine times. During exacerbations of her illness, Priscilla neglects her personal hygiene and is dependent in all self-care activities. She has occasionally had odd jobs such as working as a cleaner in a local grocery store, but does not have a history of sustained employment. For the most part, Priscilla stays at home, sleeping most of the time. She does not assist in any of the chores in the house, does not pursue any leisure activities, and has no friends.

Interview with the family members indicates that they feel helpless because treatment does not seem to be improving Priscilla's condition. For them, her illness is like a merry-go-round where she has relapses, is taken to the hospital, gets medication, takes it for a while, stops taking it, gradually deteriorates, has another relapse, and so on. They do not feel that the health care system has been beneficial in getting Priscilla out of this vicious cycle. Also, during Priscilla's relapses, her mother, a secretary for a city power company, has to miss work, since Priscilla cannot be left home alone.

Both Priscilla's older sister, who works for a telephone company, and her brother, a mechanic in the maintenance unit of the local community college, have to miss work at times in order to assist with Priscilla's care. Further interview reveals that her brother does not often bring friends home

during Priscilla's relapses for fear that they may learn of her illness. The family has tried to keep her condition secret, which they acknowledge takes enormous emotional energy. As a result, they do not socialize much.

It is obvious that there is a sense of shame and fear of stigmatization in the family, leading to social isolation. The family members' routines have been significantly disrupted, and their roles, including work and socialization, have been adversely affected. They have no social support system. Also, the rehabilitation does not seem to be working, with Priscilla, stuck in a vicious cycle of flare-ups of the disease, hospitalization, control of symptoms through hospitalization, discharge, and then relapse. Compliance with the treatment regimen is obviously poor as indicated by the history of stopping medication, which subsequently leads to exacerbation of the symptoms.

Intervention that incorporates the family as an ally in therapy may involve the occupational therapist meeting with Priscilla, her mother, and her two siblings. The family could then be requested to monitor the side effects of the medication that Priscilla is taking. The severity of side effects may be one reason that Priscilla finds it difficult to comply with the medication regimen. For example, typical antipsychotic drugs such as Haldol, a dopamine receptor antagonist,[23] may induce movement side effects such as tardive dyskinesia (involuntary choreiform rhythmic athetoid movements involving the jaw, tongue, upper extremities, and trunk), which are extremely uncomfortable at best and in severe cases may constitute medical emergency.[15]

Careful documentation of such side effects may be crucial in Priscilla's treatment. The therapist may give the feedback to the psychiatrist who could then prescribe alternative antipsychotic drugs, increasing Priscilla's likelihood to comply with treatment. Other side effects of medication, such as drowsiness, dizziness, irregular heartbeat,

Continued

CASE STUDY: PRISCILLA—CONT'D

and blurred vision, directly affect occupational performance and therefore need to be taken into consideration during occupational therapy treatment planning. Other interventions during the family meeting may include the following:

1. Exploring Priscilla's occupational functioning, including her routines and habits
2. Determining the extent to which Priscilla's occupational performance enhances her sense of inclusion, control, and affect. For instance, how does the fact that she does not contribute to completion of chores in the family make her feel with regard to her sense of belonging in the family? Do the other family members resent the extra burden she poses to them due to her need to be taken care of, and how do they communicate that resentment? What does the fact that she is dependent in self-care mean in regard to her sense of control?
3. Once Priscilla's current occupational performance is established, the family may explore ways of enhancing her participation in order to increase her sense of inclusion, control, and affection. For instance, instead of doing laundry

for her, the mother might be advised to supervise Priscilla while she does her own laundry. While she may not be able to cook, she may be asked to assist with doing the dishes after meals. Her siblings may be asked to include her in their leisure activities so that she is more involved in all family transactions. Her participation in these activities would need to be planned carefully so that they are not overwhelming to her or the family members.

4. Once ways in which family members may help facilitate Priscilla's occupational performance are established, therapeutic goals would then be established.
5. Homework would be given to family members accordingly to ensure that the goals are met. Priscilla's mother and the two siblings would be aware of their specific tasks, agreed upon by the family with the therapist's facilitation, to help enhance her occupational performance.

 Refer to Lab Manual Exercise 23-1 to help you develop skills in incorporating family caregivers as allies in a client's therapy.

Caregivers as Occupational Therapy Clients

In order for family members to be effective allies in the client's therapy as described above, their psychosocial needs have to be addressed as well. Research indicates that the emotional status of the family caregivers affects a client's well-being and QOL significantly.[16,17] For example, high emotionality in the family, when combined with severe client problems, results in significantly low QOL for the client. The emotional status of caregivers is in turn affected by the client's illness. This effect may be positive or negative.

Negative effects include psychological distress due to the client's behaviors such as moodiness and unpredictability, and negative symptoms such as withdrawal, stigmatization by society,

and perceived lack of support by healthcare professionals.[30] Family members experience a sense of loss of the person that their loved one was before the illness, and loss of dreams of what he or she might have become. As a result, they experience the grieving process described in Chapter 19 consisting of denial, guilt (blaming themselves with assumptions that somehow they caused the illness), and fear (e.g., siblings fear that they or their children may develop the illness).[21] The client's disruptive symptoms (which interfere with family routines), lack of social support, disrupted family relationships, and social isolation due to stigmatization are other factors contributing to the family caregivers' psychological distress.[16,27]

In some sections of literature, addition of the caregiving role to the family has been described as *caregiver burden*.[4,25] Objectively, this burden manifests as disruption of family routines, relationships, and so on. Subjectively, it manifests as psychological distress in the form of anxiety, stress, anger, helplessness, and despair. However, in other literature, it is argued that characterizing caregiving as a burden is misleading since there are positive experiences associated with the role, including acceptance, hope, and support for a loved one with psychosocial illness.[30]

However, it is clear that there is a need to find ways of addressing the negative experiences of caregivers as a way of enhancing their effectiveness in being allies to the rehabilitation of clients and thus improving their QOL.[17,30] The necessity of addressing caregivers' needs is recognized in the recommendations by the Department of Health.[8] Occupational therapists, like other psychosocial rehabilitation professionals, need to establish a framework for these needs to be addressed. In as far as the said framework focuses on interventions meant to support family caregivers, they may be considered to be occupational therapy clients.

Caregiver-Centered Occupational Therapy Interventions

As mentioned earlier, some of the needs of family caregivers include coping with the client's changed mood and behavior, and dealing with loss, anger, anxiety, and depression. One of the ways in which these needs may be addressed may include developing "Interventions aimed to target these needs, such as caregivers support groups and family work" (p. 346).[30] Furthermore, dissatisfaction with the caregiving role has been found to be correlated with living with the client, poor functioning of the client (such as the client not working and being dependent in self-care), poor compliance with treatment, and social isolation of the family.[11,13,27] These, among others, are the family caregiver issues that need to be addressed.

The need for family-centered, collaborative models of health care that attend to the physical and psychosocial challenges for the entire fam-

ily has been recognized in the last 25 years.[20] Interdisciplinary training programs specializing in family systems approaches in health care have been developed. Many of these models aim at developing interventions attuned to family needs by appraising the demands of the client's illness on the family, challenges accompanying the illness, and family system variables impacting on and impacted by the illness. The training often takes a few weeks to several years, depending on the type of certification that the professional is seeking. Occupational therapists seeking to enhance their family systems skills may consider attending this type of training (see Berman and Heru,[2] Rolland and Walsh,[20] and Welter-Enderlin[31] for a description of various types of such interdisciplinary training programs).

The training programs focus on helping healthcare professionals develop relevant family systems knowledge, skills, and attitudes.[2] Trainees acquire knowledge about how to apply systems theory to families, family development over the life cycle, family resilience, strengths, vulnerability and adaptation, types of families, effect of psychosocial illness on the family, and relationship between the family and larger social systems. They develop skills that enable them to identify family members involved in the client's care, foster a therapeutic alliance with the family using therapeutic relationship, elicit each family member's perspective on challenges posed by the family member's illness, assess the emotional climate of the family, and make decisions about therapy that include family members.

Attempt is made in the training to facilitate development of attitudes that allow the professional to collaborate effectively with the family in therapeutic planning and intervention, such as allowing each family member to describe what he or she sees as the presenting problem, identifying and acknowledging the family's prior problem-solving abilities in order to affirm the family, openly acknowledging limitations while maintaining hopefulness within the family unit, demonstrating a balanced concern for the welfare of each family member, and working collaboratively with family members as allies.

Using the above-delineated knowledge, skills, and attitudes, the occupational therapist may then apply a family caregiving model referred to as the "Stress-Appraisal-Coping Paradigm," which has been proposed as one way of addressing family caregiver issues.[28,29] The model consists of six 1-hour sessions with the following content:

1. Engagement: Employing the attending and active listening skills described in Chapters 3 and 7, the therapist uses the therapeutic relationship to relate to and get the family involved in discussing the challenges that they are facing as a family.
2. Education of the family caregivers: The family is educated about their loved one's psychosocial illness, including its etiology, course, clinical features and their manifestations (how they affect the client's functioning and relationship with family members), available treatment and its documented effectiveness, other services available to both the client and family members, and so on.
3. Identification of challenges: The family identifies challenges posed by the client's illness and their implications for each family member (e.g., the need for some family members to miss work, the need for each family member to reorganize daily routines).
4. Development of coping strategies: The therapist facilitates a family discussion of strategies to resolve identified challenges using a systematic problem-solving process.

In Priscilla's case, intervention would entail meeting with her, her mother, and the two siblings, educating them about Priscilla's condition and what is to be expected given what is known about the course of schizophrenia (e.g., that most probably, Priscilla will be dependent on medication for the rest of her life, but that she can learn to distinguish between reality and her hallucinations, thus being able to live a reasonably normal life), and available treatment for Priscilla (e.g., alternative forms of medication and therapy). The family can then discuss the meaning of Priscilla's illness to each of them. For instance, what does it mean to each family member when Priscilla has to be supervised throughout the day? Each of them might have to sacrifice by missing a day of work each week to assist in her care.

The family then explores the challenges posed by Priscilla's illness and how to resolve them. For instance, what other services are available for Priscilla that may provide some relief for the family? Is there an adult day care center offering a variety of occupations that may be beneficial to Priscilla where she may be dropped in the morning and picked up in the evening until she is able to function independently?[6,14,19] This would enable family members to continue working so that their financial well-being is not adversely jeopardized. Each family caregiver–oriented session should begin by reviewing the homework given in the previous week to family members to facilitate Priscilla's occupational functioning.[5] The session should then end "with an outcome, which serves as an occupational intervention for the family to try out during the following week" (p. 97).[5]

In addition to addressing family caregiver issues directly, enhancing the client's functional status also indirectly impacts the family's psychosocial well-being. Studies indicate that appraisal of the burden of care by caregivers determines their psychological well-being.[11,13] This appraisal depends on the severity of the client's symptoms and his or her behavioral disturbances, age, employment status, and social functioning. In a study by Harvey and colleagues,[11] it was found that for a client who was young, had severe symptoms, was unemployed, and had poor social functioning, family members tended to appraise their caregiver role more negatively and therefore were more psychologically distressed. This finding implies that when the occupational therapist enhances the client's performance of expected roles, including worker and social functioning roles, family members feel supported and their psychosocial status is affected positively.

In the study by Harvey and colleagues, it was also found that overinvolvement of family caregivers in the care of the client increases their psychological distress and subsequently affects the client's QOL negatively. It was concluded from this finding that it may be beneficial to help family caregivers balance their commitment to caregiving with detachment. It has been suggested that this balance may be achieved through counseling "that helps relatives to focus on their own needs rather than the patient's illness" (p. 460).[11] Occupational therapists may help achieve this objective by assisting family caregivers to identify and pursue personally meaningful and gratifying occupations, such as leisure pursuits, giving them a break from the caregiving role. Family caregiver–oriented occupational therapy intervention is summarized in Box 21-1.

Finally, while designing interventions, the therapist should be aware of the implications of the idea of a family as a system. If one accepts the argument that the family may be considered to be a complex, dynamic adaptive system, the therapist's interventions, whether they include giving information to the family, using homework, and so on, may be considered to constitute perturbations that are designed and timed to push the entire family system toward higher levels of self-organization and therefore adaptation (see discussion of interventions based on complexity/chaos theory in Chapter 4).

The Occupational Therapist's Responsibility in Issues of Abuse

Client abuse has been reported in psychiatric and physical rehabilitation settings in the United States since the early 1990s. For example, in Texas, investigations in psychiatric and rehabilitation units verified allegations of exploitation, in which kickbacks were paid to health care professionals so as to receive client referrals, clients were kept in therapy longer than needed,

---

Box 21-1 Family Caregiver-Oriented Occupational Therapy Intervention

- Engage the family in collaborative problem identification and treatment planning.
- Provide the family with information about the client's illness and available treatment.
- Collaboratively identify challenges posed by the client's illness and how they affect each family member's share of caregiver burden and occupational functioning.
- Discuss how those challenges may be addressed using a problem-solving framework.
- Explore ways in which family caregivers may facilitate the client's occupational performance in such a way as to enhance his or her feelings of inclusion, control, and affection.
- Establish treatment goals consistent with identified challenges.
- Use "homework" to help family members participate collectively in addressing the challenges and facilitating the client's occupational performance so as to meet established goals.
- Find ways of enhancing the client's performance of expected roles (work, self-care, and social functioning) as a way of indirectly affecting the psychosocial well-being of family caregivers and therefore affecting the client's QOL positively.

---

and so on.[22] In another case, investigation of a long-term care facility in New York revealed that there were incidences of sexual abuse and assault of residents by other residents.[9] Such reports continue to appear in the news. For instance, three individuals were recently arrested in a variety of facilities in Louisiana on charges of physically hitting elderly clients in their charge due to refusal to leave the dining room when required to, or barricading them in their rooms because they wandered in the facility halls at night.[10]

A study by the National Center on Elder Abuse (NCEA) revealed that "approximately 450,000 elderly persons in domestic settings were abused and/or neglected during 1996" (p. 1).[18] In the study, it was found that elders who were abused were likely to experience confusion.

Furthermore, female elders were more likely to experience abuse, and this chance increased if they were minorities (African American or Hispanic). Other studies have indicated that abuse, especially to elderly individuals, is even more extensive than reported in the study by the NCEA with about 1 million elders being abused each year.[12] The situation might have changed since 1996 with increased awareness prompted by such studies. However, it is likely that issues of abuse of vulnerable clients may come to the attention of an occupational therapist in the course of his or her practice.

In the study by the NCEA, it was revealed that state laws distinguished between abuse, neglect, and exploitation. *Physical abuse* was defined as use of physical force likely to cause physical bodily injury, pain, or impairment. *Sexual abuse* was defined as any form of nonconsensual sexual contact, and *emotional* or *psychological abuse* was defined as infliction of emotional pain or anguish. *Neglect* was defined as failure or refusal to fulfill one's obligations to an elderly person, jeopardizing his or her health or safety. The neglect could be by a caregiver or self-neglect by the elderly person. *Financial* or *material exploitation* was defined as "the illegal or improper use of an elder's funds, property, or assets" (p. 12).[18] For other vulnerable individuals, such as those incarcerated in penal institutions, exploitation may include illegal or improper use of the incarcerated as a source of labor for the caregiver's personal gain. Finally "Abandonment was defined as the desertion of an elderly person by an individual who had physical custody or otherwise had assumed responsibility for providing care for an elder or by a person with physical custody of an elder" (p. 12).[18] Although the above definitions pertain to elderly individuals, they are applicable to other categories of clients who are vulnerable due to mental or physical illness or handicap.

The principles of ethics that guide occupational therapy practice are *beneficence, nonmalficence, autonomy,* and *justice* (see a detailed discussion of these principles in Chapter 7).[1]

Examination of the above definitions reveals that, at the very least, abuse, neglect, and exploitation violate the principles of beneficence and justice. For example, failure to protect the client from physical abuse and subsequent injury violates the principle of beneficence, which mandates that it is not enough that the occupational therapist desist from causing harm. He or she must actively prevent harm from happening to clients for whom he or she is responsible. Improper use or misappropriation of a client's financial or material resources or improper use of clients as laborers violates the ethical principle of justice, which states that the therapist is obligated to do everything possible to ensure equitable distribution of resources and fair treatment of all clients. The dictates of the ethical principles make the occupational therapist obligated to act if issues of abuse, neglect, or exploitation of clients by caregivers, either within an institution or at home, come to his or her attention.

In order to address these issues effectively, the occupational therapist needs to understand their nature. For example, why does abuse, neglect, or exploitation occur? What puts clients at risk? In order to understand these issues, it is important to bear in mind that dependency and social isolation are major contributing factors to abuse, neglect, and exploitation.[7] When an individual is dependent for self-care, food, shelter, medical care, clothes, and so on, he or she is extremely vulnerable and chances of abuse increase significantly. That explains why women, children, and individuals with disabilities are the most likely to experience domestic abuse.[12] They constitute the most dependent and therefore the most vulnerable groups. Also, social isolation increases that vulnerability because chances of outsiders to the family knowing about the abuse and reporting it are decreased. By definition, "A person is considered to be isolated when she is excluded or kept away from family, friends or regular activity" (p. 13).[12] Therefore the therapist needs to be increasingly attentive to possible abuse when the client is dependent for personal care, especially when he or she is cognitively not able to report the abuse verbally, and when the person is socially isolated.

Much of client abuse is perpetrated by caregivers, whether they are family members, hired help, or employees of institutions. Sometimes, the abuse may be unintentional. It may result from the caregiver feeling overwhelmed and frustrated. For instance, a caregiver who does not get much sleep because he or she has to attend to the needs of the client may lash out when the client becomes "difficult" by refusing to comply with instructions. Sometimes, neglect may be caused by lack of resources to take care of the client. This is so, especially among clients from the lower social economic class. However, in some cases, abuse occurs simply because the caregiver is an unmitigated sociopath. This is particularly true in cases of exploitation in which the caregiver uses the client's financial and material resources for personal gain.

The occupational therapist should be cognizant of any subtle signs of abuse, such as the client being overly anxious in the presence of certain individuals, evidence of domination of the client by the caregiver, unexplained traumatic injuries, cuts, gastrointestinal problems, sleep disturbances, or depression.[7,12] If abuse is suspected, it should be reported to the relevant protective agency according to the rules and procedures of the state in which one is practicing. If there is no legal mechanism for reporting suspected abuse within the state, the therapist may refer clients to areas where community resources can be obtained, such as crisis lines, domestic violence shelters, victim advocacy programs, and individual counseling services.

Apart from reporting abuse, the occupational therapist may intervene in other ways. Bearing in mind that chances of abuse increase when a client is dependent and both the client and family are isolated, interventions may include (1) helping the client become more independent so as to decrease vulnerability, (2) teaching the client social interaction skills so that he or she can inter-

act with other people and decrease isolation, (3) introducing caregivers and the family as a whole to support groups to help develop social support networks, decreasing family and caregiver isolation, (4) training the client in assertiveness skills so that he or she is able to report abuse, and (5) educating caregivers to help them develop effective caregiving skills. Adequate skills increase caregiving effectiveness. As a result, caregivers are empowered, less overwhelmed, and less frustrated. This decreases their tendency to physically abuse clients unintentionally.

SUMMARY

In this chapter, we discussed collaboration between occupational therapists and caregivers as allies in therapy for clients with psychosocial illness. Caregivers are often family members. Their collaboration with the therapist in the client's therapeutic planning and intervention is important, considering that the family is the primary venue where needs for inclusion, control, and affection are met. However, the extent to which family caregivers are able to be allies in therapeutic interventions for clients is dependent on their own psychological well-being. This psychological well-being is often dependent on their appraisal of the caregiving role. If the client is young, unemployed, dependent, and socially low-functioning, their appraisal of the caregiving role is more negative.

We also discussed the need for occupational therapists to intervene to help improve the psychological well-being of caregivers as a way of indirectly affecting the QOL and well-being of clients. We then described intervention strategies to address caregiver issues. These include direct intervention in which the entire family examines the challenges posed by the client's condition and finds ways of addressing those challenges. Indirect intervention includes working with the client to increase the level of independence and function so as to help decrease caregiver burden. We also suggested referral to day care centers as a way of providing respite to family members. Finally, we explored abuse issues in the context of caregiving and the responsibility of the therapist when abuse, neglect, or exploitation is suspected. We underscored that the client's dependence and social isolation of both the client and family are factors contributing to client vulnerability and risk of abuse. Suggested ways of addressing abuse issues by the occupational therapist therefore include facilitating client independence, educating family caregivers, assertiveness training, teaching social skills, and facilitating client and family social integration.

REFERENCES

1. American Occupational Therapy Association: *Occupational therapy code of ethics, 2005.* Retrieved February 22, 2006, from http://www.org/general/docs/ethicscode05.pdf.
2. Berman E, Heru AM: Family systems training in psychiatric residences, *Family Process* 44:321–335, 2005.
3. Brady C, Goldman C: Similarities and differences in caregiver adaptation: focus on mental illness and brain injury [electronic version], *Psychosocial Rehabil J* 18(1):1–12, 1994.
4. Bulger MW, Wandersman A, Goldman CR: Burdens and gratifications of caregiving: appraisal of parental care of adults with schizophrenia, *Am J Orthopsychiatry* 63:255–265, 1993.
5. Cole MB: *Group dynamics in occupational therapy,* ed 3, Thorofare, NJ, 2005, Slack.
6. Coviensky M, Buckley V: Day activities programming: serving the severely impaired chronic client. In Cottrell RP, ed: *Proactive approaches in psychosocial occupational therapy,* Thorofare, NJ, 2000, Slack, pp. 165–169.
7. Davidson DA: Protecting vulnerable clients. In Crepeau EB, Cohn ES, Schell BA, eds: *Willard and Spackman's occupational therapy,* New York, 2003, Lippincott Williams & Wilkins, pp. 919–922.
8. Department of Health: *National service framework for mental health,* London, 2000, Department of Health.
9. Fisher I: Patients abuse other patients at nursing home, report says, *The New York Times,* B4, August 25, 1995.
10. Foti CC: Attorney General's Medicaid Fraud Control Unit makes arrests in alleged patient abuse cases across the state [electronic version], *US Fed News Service, Including US State News,* 1–2, April 5, 2006.
11. Harvey K, Burns T, Fahy T, et al: Relatives of patients with severe psychotic illness: factors that influence appraisal of caregiving and psychological distress, *Social Psychiatry Psychiatric Epidemiol* 36:456–461, 2001.
12. Helfrich CA, Lafata MJ, MacDonald SL, et al: Domestic abuse across the lifespan: definitions, identification and risk factors for occupational therapists, *Occup Ther Mental Health* 16(3/4):5–34, 2001.
13. Joyce J, Leese M, Kuipers E, et al: Evaluating a model of caregiving for people with psychosis, *Social Psychiatry Psychiatric Epidemiol* 38:189–195, 2003.
14. Linroth R, Zander S, Forde S, et al: Ramsey county day treatment services: day treatment to extended day treatment centers to focus groups. In Cottrell RP, ed: *Proactive approaches in psychosocial occupational therapy,* Thorofare, NJ, 2000, Slack, pp. 157–161.
15. MacRae A: Demonstrating effectiveness in occupational therapy. In Cara E, MacRae A, eds: *Psychosocial occupational therapy: a clinical practice,* Clifton Park, NY, 2005, Thomson Delmar Learning, pp. 687–709.
16. Martens L, Addington J: The psychological well-being of family members of individuals with schizophrenia, *Social Psychiatry Psychiatric Epidemiol* 36:128–133, 2001.
17. Mubarak AR, Barber JG: Emotional expressiveness and the quality of life of patients with schizophrenia, *Social Psychiatry Psychiatric Epidemiol* 38:380–384, 2003.
18. National Center on Elder Abuse: *The national elder abuse incidence study,* 1998. Retrieved February 22, 2006, from www.aoa.dhhs.gov/abuse/report.
19. Neustadt LE: Adult day care: a model for changing times. In Cottrell RP, ed: *Proactive approaches in psychosocial occupational therapy,* Thorofare, NJ, 2000, Slack, pp. 203–208.
20. Rolland JS, Walsh F: Systemic training for healthcare professionals: the Chicago Center for Family Health Approach, *Family Process* 44:283–301, 2005.
21. Roth S, McCune CC: The client and family experience of mental illness. In Cara E, MacRae A, eds: *Psychosocial occupational therapy: a clinical practice,* Clifton Park, NY, 2005, Thomson Delmar Learning, pp. 3–25.
22. Rundle RL: Rehabilitation facilities brace for Texas investigation: industry fears replay of panel's fraud inquiry into psychiatric hospitals, *Wall Street Journal,* B.4, June 16, 1992.
23. Sadock BJ, Sadock VA: *Synopses of psychiatry: behavioral sciences/clinical psychiatry,* ed 9, Philadelphia, 2003, Lippincott Williams & Wilkins.
24. Schaber P: FIRO model: a framework for family-centered care, *Phys Occup Ther Geriatr* 20(4):1–18, 2002.
25. Schene AH: Objective and subjective dimensions of family burden: towards an integrative framework for research, *Social Psychiatry Psychiatric Epidemiol* 25:289–297, 1990.
26. Schutz W: The interpersonal underworld, *Harvard Business Review* 36(4):123–135, 1958.

27. Stengard E: Caregiving types and psychosocial well-being of caregivers of people with mental illness, *Psychiatric Rehabil J* 26(2):154–164, 2002.

28. Szmukler GI, Burgess P, Herrman H, et al: Caring for relatives with serious mental illness: the development of the experience of caregiving inventory, *Social Psychiatry Psychiatric Epidemiol* 31:137–148, 1996.

29. Szmukler GI, Kuipers E, Joyce J, et al: An exploratory randomized controlled trial of a support programme for careers of patients with a psychosis, *Social Psychiatry Psychiatric Epidemiol* 38:411–418, 2003.

30. Treasurer J, Murphy T, Szmukler G, et al: The experience of caregiving for severe mental illness: a comparison between anorexia nervosa and psychosis, *Social Psychiatry Psychiatric Epidemiol* 36:343–347, 2001.

31. Welter-Enderlin R: The state of the art of training in systemic family therapy in Switzerland, *Family Process* 44:303–320, 2005.

Chapter 22
Community-Based Occupational Therapy Intervention

Preview Questions

1. Explain the influence of the community support and the independent living movements on the trend toward development of community-based rehabilitation services for clients with psychosocial illnesses.
2. Define the concept *community* as used in community-based rehabilitation.
3. Define *community-based practice*.
4. Describe at least two models of community-based occupational therapy practice.
5. Describe the framework of community-based occupational therapy practice and the role of the occupational therapist.
6. Explain the role of the occupational therapist in the rehabilitation and integration of clients with psychosocial illnesses who are homeless and those who have been newly released from penal institutions into the community.

According to the U.S. Surgeon General,[14] the latest development in mental health has been the community support movement. This movement focuses on the need for social welfare of clients discharged from psychiatric institutions, by making community resources accessible to them, facilitating their integration as full participants in community life. It is closely allied to the independent living movement, which is based on the premise that environmental barriers, not individual client factors, are the cause of disability.[10] The principles of both the community support and the independent living movements are consistent with the basic tenet of the new occupational therapy paradigm, which proposes that the ultimate objective of occupational therapy intervention is to facilitate participation in life through engagement in personally meaningful occupations.[1]

Furthermore, these principles are given credence by research findings that indicate that institutionalization in psychiatric hospitals has negative side effects such as loss of skills due to inactivity.[15] As a result of these movements and subsequent research findings there has been a tendency toward establishment of community mental health programs. Subsequently, "many persons suffering from a chronic mental illness are now being treated in their communities, rather than institutions" (p. 52).[3] The momentum toward community mental health is consistent with the legal mandate to treat clients in the least restrictive environments.[15] The community is evidently much less restrictive than institutional care.

With this tendency toward community mental health, it is imperative that occupational therapists be cognizant of their role in the rehabilitation of clients with psychosocial needs within the community. This chapter aims to (1) present and define some models and programs of community-based rehabilitation in which occupational therapy may be involved, (2) outline a framework for occupational therapy intervention within those programs, and (3) suggest ways in which occupational therapists may be involved in a variety of community-based rehabilitation programs for clients with psychosocial illnesses, including working within agencies that cater to the homeless and individuals released from penal institutions.

This chapter is not meant to be an authoritative directive about how to do community-based occupational therapy. Rather, it is meant to heighten the occupational therapist's awareness of the important role of occupational therapy in this area of practice. It is hoped that students and therapists reading this chapter will think of ways in which they can make community contacts and initiate occupational therapy services in various community agencies that cater to clients with psychosocial disorders but in which there are no occupational therapy services.

Models of Intervention in Community-Based Rehabilitation Programs

Community-based rehabilitation program models range from halfway group homes to day care centers. They include group home models such as transitional facilities, personal care homes, independent living facilities, quarterway houses, and hostels.[15] One of the difficulties involved in providing services within these settings is that they have not been very well-defined. One way of understanding them may be by defining community-based rehabilitation in general, then examining how the models fit within the framework of community-based practice.

According to Wittman and Velde, a *community* may be defined as a "person's natural environment, that is, where the person works, plays and performs other daily activities" (p. 2).[16] This definition identifies community with individual performance (of work, play, and other activities) and participation. Consequently, Wittman and Velde define community-based practice as "skilled services delivered by health practitioners using an interactive model with clients," and what they call community-built practice as consisting of skilled services "delivered by health

practitioners using a collaborative and interactive model with clients" (p. 3).[16]

The emphasis on collaboration and interaction in these definitions denote that community-based practice is necessarily client-centered. Furthermore, Wilberding[15] suggests that all group home types of community-based rehabilitation programs seem to refer to a form of psychosocial milieu therapy involving 8 to 15 clients with mild to moderate disability. This is reminiscent of milieu therapy programs emphasized by Pinel[11] and Tuke[13] during the moral treatment era as discussed in Chapter 1. Many of the programs are run on a 24-hour basis by a qualified team of professionals. The quarterway program described by Wilberding[15] will be described in detail as an example of a group home model of rehabilitation.

According to Wilberding, the quarterway house model is a bit different from other group home models. It provides a higher staff-to-client ratio, thus making it possible to cater to more severely disabled clients. It is defined as "a group home, transitional in nature and the first step after hospitalization in preparation for community placement" (p. 137).[15] It consists of a daily structured program designed to develop community functioning skills in the areas of work, self-care, and leisure pursuits. Consistent with the arguments in literature about the ultimate goal of community-based rehabilitation,[2,3,17] the primary objective of the quarterway program, according to Wilberding, is integration of the client into the community.

The Mt. Airy House quarterway program in Baltimore, Maryland, described by Wilberding, is conducted as follows:

1. The client is evaluated using the "Resident Assessment Form" (Figure 22-1). As shown in Figure 22-1, the assessment is comprehensive. It covers not only the areas of work, self-care, and leisure, but also interpersonal skills and the client's ability to maintain general health. Further, the authors define what they mean by problem or excessive behaviors (Box 22-1).

**Mt. Airy House
RESIDENT ASSESSMENT**

Resident's Name: Date:
Person Filling Out Form:

SCALE: 1. Good functioning or not a behavior problem
2. Mildly impaired functioning or mild/infrequent behavior problem
3. Moderately impaired functioning or moderate behavior problem
4. Seriously impaired functioning or serious/frequent behavior problem
Content areas below contain both functional behaviors and problem behaviors

	1	2	3	4	
I. EATING					
1. Eats and drinks neatly					
2. Chooses a well-balanced diet					
3. Eats or drinks too much					
4. Eats or drinks too fast					
5. Refuses regular meals					
6. Takes food or drink that has been discarded or that belongs to another					
II. HYGIENE					
7. Bathes or showers using soap daily					
8. Brushes or combs hair daily					
9. For males, shaves as needed or keeps beard neat					
10. Takes care of nails					
11. Brushes teeth at least once a day					
12. Changes clothes daily					
13. Wears appropriate clothing					
14. Has noticeable body odor					
15. For females, wears excessive or bizarre makeup					
16. Changes clothes excessively					
17. Disrobes publicly or exposes self					
III. PERSONAL DOMESTIC ACTIVITIES					
18. Gets up in a.m. on time					
19. Makes bed daily					
20. Keeps room neat and clean					
21. Changes bed linens as needed					
22. Stores soiled clothing for washing					
23. Does personal laundry					
24. Puts clean clothes away					
25. Prepares lunch and snack food for self safely					
26. Uses smoking materials safely and smokes only in designated areas					
27. Weeps excessively					
28. Bedroom has noticeable odor					
29. Is incontinent					

Figure 22-1.   Formal Assessment.
(Adapted from Wilberding D: The quarterway house: More than an alternative of care. In Cottrell RP, ed: *Proactive approaches in psychosocial occupational therapy,* Thorofare, NJ, 2000, Slack, pp. 139–140.)

IV. HOUSEHOLD DOMESTIC ACTIVITIES AND JOB READINESS

30. Follows requests and directions
31. Follows through on tasks started
32. Starts and completes tasks promptly, neither too fast nor too slow
33. Able to work independently
34. Cooperative with others in completing tasks
35. Consistent in work performance
36. Has adequate duration of attention and ability to focus on tasks
37. Maintains own schedule throughout day without being reminded
38. Participates in shopping for, and stocking, house supplies
39. Performs household clearing tasks
40. Prepares meals adequately and safely for house
41. Cleans up after house meals
42. Performs other household chores as assigned or needed

V. INTERPERSONAL SKILLS

43. Speaks up in community meetings appropriately
44. Initiates conversation with others
45. Establishes relationship with resident advisor
46. Maintains relationship with family/significant others
47. Able to express positive feelings
48. Able to express negative feelings
49. Able to respond constructively to anger and/or criticism
50. Goes on staff-accompanied group outings
51. Uses telephone appropriately
52. Threatens others
53. Makes hostile, vulgar, rude comments
54. Shouts or yells
55. Talks too much
56. Intrudes on others
57. Talks to self
58. Engages in inappropriate sexual behavior
59. Is uncommunicative or withdrawn
60. Hits others or throws things
61. Steals or takes things from others

VI. HEALTH

62. Able to identify psychiatric problems/symptoms
63. Understands nature of psychiatric illness and need for treatment
64. Reports physical problems appropriately to house staff and/or doctor
65. Follows through on advice from doctor or nurse
66. Treats own minor physical problems appropriately
67. Cooperates with person who dispenses medication
68. Can reliably self-administer medication

Figure 22-1.   Cont'd.

Continued

VII.	**MONEY MANAGEMENT**					
	69. Buys own clothes					
	70. Purchases own personal items					
	71. Budgets money for the week					
	72. Makes deposits/withdrawals at bank as needed					
	73. Counts change in store					
	74. Behaves inappropriately at store					
VIII.	**TRANSPORTATION**					
	75. Cooperative on van trips					
	76. Walks to places on grounds and in Towson					
	77. Follows pedestrian rules					
IX.	**LEISURE**					
	78. Works regularly on a hobby					
	79. Takes walks outside					
	80. Works in the garden or yard					
	81. Listens to the radio or watches TV appropriately					
	82. Goes to the movies or sporting events					
	83. Plays sports or table games					
	84. Reads the newspaper, books, or magazines					
X.	**COMMENTS**					

Figure 22-1.   Cont'd

2. The client is introduced to community resources such as the doctor's and dentist's offices, the grocery store, and the library. An account is opened at the local bank for the client, and he or she is introduced to the bank staff. Before this is done, community resource providers and managers, such as grocery store and bank managers, the doctor, dentist, and so on, are requested to participate in the program. Their participation is completely voluntary.

3. Short- and long-term goals are established, and a rehabilitation program is established focusing on problems identified through the assessment in step 1. Rehabilitation goals generally focus on helping the client: observe the treatment regimen (e.g., comply with the medication schedule), develop and maintain daily living skills (in self-care, work, and leisure), and find a place to live.

The program described above is designed to support the client's transition from the hospital to the community and eventual integration into the community. As mentioned earlier, it is behaviorally based and the assessment reflects that focus because it identifies clearly defined behaviors that are seen as problematic so that they can be addressed in therapeutic intervention. However, psychoeducation techniques[4] may also be used to achieve the goals of intervention. Pyschoeducation refers to a model of therapy in which the therapist becomes a teacher and the clients are students. The therapist (teacher) uses educational modules complete with learning objectives, class activities, homework, quizzes, and examinations, to facilitate learning and behavioral change in the client. Just as an instructor would carefully plan the syllabus for a course, the psychoeducational program is carefully planned, with the content chosen to achieve the desired outcome.

Wollenberg described another model program, which was initiated by University of Kansas Medical Center occupational therapy students who were on level II fieldwork.[17] This

---

Box 22-1   Excessive Behavior List

1. Impulsivity
   - Money
   - Massive consumption of anything
   - Splitting (running away)
   - Shoplifting
   - Substance abuse
   - Self-destruction
   - Threatening others
   - Destruction of property
2. Poor boundaries
   - Asking for things beyond what is reasonable
   - Acting in an intrusive manner toward others
   - Wandering off
3. Socially inappropriate behavior*
   - Vulgar and rude comments to others
   - Talking and/or laughing to yourself while out and about
   - Dressing in bizarre ways
   - Poor hygiene
   - Inappropriate sexual behavior
4. Angry outbursts
5. Dangerous smoking
6. Inability or unwillingness to respond to limits or requests

---

*This means behaving in ways that would embarrass someone else, make someone else nervous, or make people look at you funny.
Adapted from Wilberding D: The quarterway house: More than an alternative of care. In Cottrell RP, ed: *Proactive approaches in psychosocial occupational therapy*, Thorofare, NJ, 2000, Slack, p. 141.

program used a recovery model whose objective was to help clients attending a community mental health center achieve their life dreams. It combined the principles of community-based rehabilitation and family caregiver integration discussed in Chapter 21, as indicated by the statement: "For example, classes are provided in which consumers [clients] can bring their family members or significant others to learn about mental illness in the framework of recovery" (p. 99).[17] This approach obviously facilitates family caregiver participation as allies to client rehabilitation.

The program was client-centered, consistent with the core principles of the new occupational therapy paradigm (see Chapter 4). It emphasized involvement of the client as a central decision maker in determining and prioritizing services and interventions. Clients, therefore, set their own therapy goals. The program also used a holistic perspective addressing both the clients' physical and psychosocial concerns. The process of intervention consisted of 7 steps: referral, screening, evaluation, intervention planning, intervention implementation, reevaluation, and termination.

During the *referral* stage, clients, case managers, other professionals, and the community at large were educated about the value and scope of occupational therapy for clients. This stage is similar to what Ikiugu and Ciaravino did in a program for adolescents with emotional and behavioral disorders.[8,9] They contacted the director of a day treatment center in the community catering to the needs of these adolescents. They talked to the staff and clients regarding a possible role of occupational therapy at the center. Once everybody understood what occupational therapy could offer, they were very cooperative in ensuring that the proposed program was successful. In the Kansas program, a referral form that was easy to use and quickly identified areas of concern was developed (Figure 22-2). As is apparent in the referral form, the referral source was asked to predict anticipated level of recovery expected as a result of occupational therapy intervention, as well as suggested areas needing specific skill development. The client could refer himself or herself to occupational therapy, in which case he or she would identify an expected level of recovery and areas needing skill development.

During *screening*, the appropriateness of occupational therapy services was determined. Further information was gathered through a chart review and through interviews with the client and the case manager. Assessment instruments were chosen. If occupational therapy services were not deemed appropriate, the client was referred to

Occupational Therapy Referral

Consumer Name: _____   ID Number_____

Address: _____   Telephone_____

_____

Case Manager: _____

Reason for Referral: _____

_____

_____

_____

Please provide a goal from the Individual Service Plan that corresponds to the requested service.

Domain: _____

Goal: _____

_____

Overcoming Stuckness	Returning to Basic Functioning	Discovering Self-empowerment	Learning and Self-redefinition	Improving Quality of Life
• Acknowledging and accepting illness • Desire and motivation to change • Finding/having source of hope/inspiration	• Taking care of basic needs: eating, hygiene, basic physical health • Being active: exercising, leisure activities • Connecting with others	• Taking responsibility for own recovery • Taking responsibility for behaviors • Determined and hard working • Courage to challenge self and take risks	• Recapturing parts of old self and discovering new aspects of self • Learning there is more to self than illness	• Striving to attain overall sense of well-being • Striving for ideals often associated with stable mental health • Serving as a recovery role model for others

Areas of Specific Skill Development (Please check all that apply)

Self-Management	Household Management	Community Participation
☐ Grooming/hygiene (bathing, dressing, oral hygiene, etc...)	☐ Cleaning	☐ Interpersonal relationships (conflict resolution, communication)
☐ Health maintenance (nutrition, fitness socialization, etc...)	☐ Laundry	
	☐ Shopping	☐ Vocational participation
☐ Life/Stress management	☐ Money management	☐ Educational preparation
☐ Personal and community safety	☐ Child/elder care	☐ Leisure/recreational participation
☐ Community mobility	☐ Meal preparation	☐ Community responsibility
☐ Other _____	☐ Other _____	☐ Other _____

Additional comments: _____

_____

_____

_____

_____

Referred by: _____   Date: _____

Figure 22-2.   Occupational Therapy Referral.
(Adapted from Wollenberg JL: Recovery and occupational therapy in the community mental health setting, *Occup Ther Mental Health* 17[3/4]:103, 2001.)

other professionals as indicated. Based on information gathered from the screening, *evaluation* was completed using chosen assessment instruments. All attempts were made to complete evaluation in the client's natural environment (e.g., cooking skills would be assessed in the kitchen of the client's apartment). After evaluation, *intervention* was planned collaboratively by the therapist and the client. Intervention planning took into account the client's goals and dreams. Short- and long-term goals were established accordingly. This is similar to what occurred in the program for adolescents conducted by Ikiugu and Ciaravino,[8,9] where each adolescent was guided to articulate a desired adult future that he or she aspired to attain. Activities likely to lead to achieving that future were identified. Goals were established using the adolescent's own language. They were written in first-person language as stated by the client.

After collaborative treatment planning, *intervention* designed to achieve established goals was implemented. Similar to the quarterway house model described earlier, "interventions typically take place in the consumer's home, at a local grocery store, or other community settings" (p. 108).[15] Similar to the evaluation, interventions are provided as much as practicable within the client's natural environment in order to make it easier for carryover of learned skills. For example, skills related to making a shopping list would be learned by cuing the client to identify needed items in the apartment and making a list accordingly; skills related to shopping for groceries would be learned by visiting the grocery store and actually shopping for groceries from the shopping list. This is similar to the intervention used in the program by Ikiugu and Ciaravino in which, for instance, career identification skills were learned by taking the adolescents to a university career center and having them search for information on the Internet with the help of the career development staff. Interpersonal relationship skills needed for successful completion of academic activities were learned by working with students in the classroom to identify non-productive interaction behaviors and address them as they occurred.

As therapeutic intervention continued, outcomes were *reevaluated* regularly, in collaboration with the client, to determine progress toward established goals; then the treatment plan was continually modified as necessary. Finally, occupational therapy services were *discontinued* once the goals were achieved, or the client transitioned to other services if it was determined that occupational therapy intervention would not lead to further positive outcomes. The therapist was responsible for ensuring that proper supports were in place before therapy was terminated. For instance, if therapy was discontinued because the client had achieved goals, the therapist ensured that community resources were available to facilitate the client's continued optimal performance. If referral to another professional was indicated, the therapist did the referral and introduced the client to the professional so that the transition was coordinated and less anxiety-provoking.

In both the quarterway model and the community mental health program described above, it is evident that a framework for community occupational therapy practice may consist of a process summarized as consisting of the following steps:

1. Educating clients, case managers, other professionals, and the public at large regarding the role and scope of occupational therapy in community mental health
2. Establishing a client referral system
3. Identifying appropriate assessment instruments and completing client evaluation
4. Integrating family caregivers and other key persons controlling community resources in the therapeutic process
5. Implementing individualized interventions as much as possible within the client's natural environment
6. Supporting the client as he or she attempts to reintegrate into the community, for instance by introducing him or her to key individuals within the community

Other roles of occupational therapy as suggested in reviewed literature include home assessment to identify risks and recommend home modifications to facilitate safe optimal functioning[7] and addressing "community re-integration issues through a variety of interventions including training in daily living skills, assertiveness, behavior management, coping skills, self awareness skills, social skills, and time management" (p. 52)[3] using psychoeducation and functional tasks to facilitate development of required skills. Functional activities such as arts, crafts, and ADLs such as money management are used as media for intervention. The ultimate goal for these programs is to facilitate functioning and reintegration into the community.

Working with Varieties of Clients Within the Community

The six-stage framework for community occupational therapy practice as described above can be applied to a variety of community day treatment and respite programs found everywhere in the United States and other parts of the world. Such programs include shelters for the homeless and soup kitchens. It has been argued that deinstitutionalization based on untested theories of rehabilitation has resulted in undesirable consequences such as homelessness.[5] Deinstitutionalized individuals with mental illness lack stable housing, financial resources, and often have legal problems.[6] These are the kinds of individuals likely to frequent homeless shelters and soup kitchens.

In some of the facilities set up for the homeless and run mostly by religious organizations, clients attend during the day, participate in a variety of activities, and leave in the evening. Occupational therapists may be instrumental in providing services for clients attending such facilities to help initiate the process of reintegration in the community. The six-step framework described earlier in this chapter may be used by the occupational therapist to initiate programs to provide such services. The process would involve educating

professionals running the agencies about the role of occupational therapy, establishing a referral system for clients and educating the staff about the system, evaluating clients, planning and implementing intervention, and continually reevaluating and modifying the intervention plan as appropriate.

Finally, community-based practice means that occupational therapists are likely to work with clients with psychosocial illnesses who have been released from jails and prisons, or those released under alternative sentencing with mandated involvement in educational activities, mental health, or drug/substance abuse treatment.[12] Occupational therapists have been working in the area of forensic psychiatry for some time. Many of the services in this area of practice are provided within forensic state hospitals where clients are referred by the court after they have been determined to be incompetent to stand trial, not guilty by reason of insanity, or guilty but mentally ill. Depending on the needs of clients, therapeutic media may be crafts, arts, role play, psychoeducation, and so on. For instance, clients referred to therapy after being determined to be incompetent to stand trial may be engaged in tasks designed to help them develop an understanding of the legal charges against them; the roles of the judge, defense attorney, and other officers of the court; and how to respond to questions during court proceedings. Once competency to stand trial is attained, they are taken back to jail for reinstatement of court proceedings.

In the community, the occupational therapist is part of an interdisciplinary team in a release program whose interventions are designed to assist individuals newly released from penal institutions develop skills that they need in order to reintegrate successfully in the community. The therapist provides:

...living and job skills training and activities that focus on self-confidence, accomplishment, goal setting, taking responsibility, and problem solving. They also have the very important function of focusing on skill development to facilitate compliance with release requirements and court ordered conditions (p. 577).[12]

The six-step framework described in this chapter may be applied in these types of release programs as well.

 Refer to Lab Manual Exercise 24-1 to help you explore further how you can develop occupational therapy services in community-based agencies that serve clients with psychosocial disorders.

SUMMARY

With the advent of the community support movement and the independent living movement, many clients with mental illness are increasingly being treated within the community, consistent with the legal mandate to provide treatment to individuals in least restrictive environments. We noted that a variety of group home models have been established within which community-based rehabilitation may be provided. Based on the two models discussed in this chapter and the other roles of community-based occupational therapy practitioners as gleaned from literature, a framework of community occupational therapy practice emerges.

The role of occupational therapy within this framework consists of the following steps: education of clients, other professionals, and the community about how occupational therapy may contribute to the reintegration of clients into the community; establishment of a client referral system; choice of assessment instruments; intervention planning and implementation; re-evaluation of the outcome of treatment and modification of the treatment plan as indicated; termination of therapy; and support of the client in the process of reintegration in the community. The above framework may be applied to facilities that cater to homeless mentally ill individuals such as homeless shelters and soup kitchens, as well as to individuals newly released from the penal systems and attending release programs. It is hoped that this chapter sensitized the reader to the variety of practice opportunities available to occupational therapists within the community.

REFERENCES

1. American Occupational Therapy Association: Occupational therapy practice framework: domain and process, *Am J Occup Ther* 56:609–639, 2002.
2. Baxley S: Options for community practice: the Springfield Hospital model. In Cottrell RP, ed: *Proactive approaches in psychosocial occupational therapy*, Thorofare, NJ, 2000, Slack, pp. 129–132.
3. Bickens MB, DeLoache SN, Dicer JR, et al: Effectiveness of experiential and verbal occupational therapy groups in a community mental health setting, *Occup Ther Mental Health* 17(1):51–72, 2001.
4. Crist PH: Community living skills: a psychoeducational community-based program. In Cottrell RP, ed: *Proactive approaches in psychosocial occupational therapy*, Thorofare, NJ, 2000, Slack, pp. 147–154.
5. Doyle R: Deinstitutionalization, *Scientific Am* 287(6):38, 2002.
6. Drebing CE, Rosenheck R, Schutt R, et al: Patterns in referral and admission to vocational rehabilitation associated with coexisting psychiatric and substance-use disorders, *Rehabil Counseling Bull* 47(1):15–23, 2003.
7. Horowitz BP: Occupational therapy home assessments: supporting community living through client-centered practice, *Occup Ther Mental Health* 18(1):1–17, 2002.
8. Ikiugu MN, Ciaravino EA: Assisting adolescents experiencing emotional and behavioral difficulties (EBD) transition to adulthood, *Internat J Psychosocial Rehabil* 10(2):57–78, 2006.
9. Ikiugu MN, Ciaravino EA: *Assisting adolescents experiencing emotional and behavioral difficulties (EBD) transition to adulthood*, Charlotte, NC, 2006, workshop presented at the American Occupational Therapy Association's 86th Annual Conference & Expo.
10. McColl MA: The concept of occupation 1975 to 2000. In McColl MA, Law M, Stewart D, et al, eds: *Theoretical basis of occupational therapy*, Thorofare, NJ, 2003, Slack, pp. 39–61.
11. Pinel P: *A treatise on insanity*, New York, 1962, Hafner.
12. Snively F, Dressler J: Occupational therapy in the criminal justice system. In Cara E, MacRae A, eds: *Psychosocial occupational therapy: a clinical practice*, Clifton Park, NY, 2005, Thomson Delmar Learning, pp. 567–590.
13. Tuke S: *Description of the retreat: an institution near York for insane persons of the Society of Friends containing an account of its origins and progress, the mode of treatment, and a statement of cases*, London, 1964, Dawsons of Pall Mall.

14. United States Surgeon General: *Mental health: a report of the Surgeon General,* 2005. Retrieved May 13, 2005, from http://www.surgeongeneral.gov/library/mental-health/home.html.

15. Wilberding D: The quarterway house: More than an alternative of care. In Cottrell RP, ed: *Proactive approaches in psychosocial occupational therapy,* Thorofare, NJ, 2000, Slack, pp. 135–145.

16. Wittman PP, Velde BP: Occupational therapy in the community: what, why, and how, *Occup Ther Health Care* 13(3/4):1–5, 2001.

17. Wollenberg JL: Recovery and occupational therapy in the community mental health setting, *Occup Ther Mental Health* 17(3/4):97–114, 2001.

Lab Manual

Chapter *1*

Introduction

The idea of a psychosocial rehabilitation laboratory manual is not common. Therefore we will explain the concept in this chapter. We will then present the organization of the manual and provide instructions regarding how to use it.

What is a Psychosocial Laboratory Manual?

In the basic sciences, laboratory manuals are used to provide procedural instructions to students and researchers so that they can carry out laboratory experiments accurately. In medical practice, manuals help laboratory clinicians to carry out investigations necessary for diagnosing disease or monitoring patients who are under treatment. Borrowing the concept of a laboratory manual from basic sciences and clinical laboratory practice, this manual is envisioned as a means of providing instructions to occupational therapy instructors, students, and clinicians so that they are able to apply psychosocial clinical techniques accurately and efficiently. Even though the analogy with basic sciences is useful, one must remember that psychosocial problems are complex. It is not possible to reduce the functioning of the human mind to linear procedural operations. Many times, cookbook instructions do not work under such complex conditions. Therefore instructions in this manual must be seen only as suggestions providing general direction to clinicians. Occupational therapists using the manual must use their initiative, attention to what is happening in each clinical situation, imagination, and interpersonal skills so they can formulate therapeutic strategies that meet the individual needs of each client.

Why the Manual is Necessary

Kielhofner states that "Many practitioners bemoan that theory does not always keep pace with the changing demands of practice environments or speak to all the situations and problems encountered in practice. Consequently, in place of using theory to guide practice, therapists often rely on experience and common sense" (p. 7).[4]

It is conceivable that this seemingly hostile attitude toward theory by clinicians originates from difficulties encountered in attempting to apply it in complex, fast-paced clinical contexts. Furthermore, it is not clear to me that occupational therapy students are systematically taught how to translate theory into practice. As a psychosocial rehabilitation instructor, one of my frustrations has been the inability to find textbooks that make it easy to teach students this transition from theory to practice. Many textbooks that are popular in psychosocial occupational therapy, such as those written by Bruce and Borg,[1] Stein and Cutler,[5] and Cara and McRae,[2] provide good background in theoretical concepts used in psychosocial occupational therapy. However, the assumption seems to be made that the occupational therapist will intuitively make the transition to application of theoretical concepts in clinical practice. Although this may be the case, this manual is based on the argument that a systematic approach to learning how to apply theoretical concepts may facilitate the ability of a therapist to bridge theory and practice.

So far, the book that I have found to be most suited to teaching practical clinical skills is *Mental Health Concepts and Techniques for the Occupational Therapy Assistant* by Early.[3] Although this textbook is written for occupational therapy assistants, I have found it the most effective in providing direction about application of theory in practice. This scarcity of available systematic guidelines to help instructors teach practical application of theoretical concepts led me to think that it is necessary to write this manual. Therefore the purpose of the manual is to provide guidelines, exercises, and laboratory activities to help students and clinicians bridge theory and clinical practice more effectively.

Organization of the Manual

The vision used to develop this manual is that of a therapist receiving referral from a psychiatrist to treat a client. The manual provides exercises that will help the occupational therapy student or clinician to practice clinical decision making from the moment the order to treat is received to the time of discharge from therapy. With this vision in mind, Part I of the manual, consisting of Chapters 2 to 9, provides exercises designed to help the reader appreciate the identity of occupational therapy as a profession and develop general clinical skills that will be the foundation for all psychosocial occupational therapy practice.

By completing the exercise in Chapter 2, you will become fully grounded in the history and rich heritage of the profession. This will provide a sound foundation for subsequent occupation-based, client-centered practice. Chapters 3 to 6 provide exercises designed to help you learn how to (1) conduct a medical chart review upon receipt of the physician's order to treat, (2) interview the client, (3) interpret clinical information gathered through the chart review and client interview, and (4) use the therapeutic relationship based on concepts derived from a variety of psychological theories to interact with the client and family members effectively.

Chapters 7 to 9 present exercises that help the reader to build on skills developed through activities in earlier chapters by providing guidelines for (1) learning and applying clinical reasoning skills, (2) translating clinical data guided by the professional paradigm into meaningful treatment goals, (3) learning ethical decision-making skills, (4) using groups and group techniques as therapeutic media to meet established treatment objectives, (5) developing cultural competency in clinical practice, and (6) keeping clinical records and discharge planning. Part II of the manual, consisting of Chapters 10 to 18, presents exercises to help you learn how to apply theoretical constructs from each conceptual practice model of psychosocial occupational therapy in client evaluation, treatment planning, and intervention. In Chapter 19, you will participate in an exercise to facilitate development of skills necessary to integrate a variety of conceptual models of practice to address a client's specific occupational performance issues.

In Part III, you will participate in exercises that help you develop an awareness of how occupational therapy may be provided across the continuum of care. The exercise in Chapter 20 will help you develop enhanced appreciation of the need to take into account the human lifespan developmental perspective when planning intervention. Chapter 21 provides exercises to help demonstrate how psychosocial occupational therapy may be applied to clients with a variety of conditions, including physical disabilities and HIV and AIDS. Exercises in Chapters 22 and 23 present an opportunity to reflect on the occupational therapist's role in providing occupational therapy to clients with substance abuse problems and integration of caregiver issues in therapy, respectively.

How to use the Manual

This manual is designed to be used in conjunction with the textbook by the same title. In most cases, each chapter in the manual corresponds to a chapter in the textbook presenting theoretical basis of the lab exercises. For instance, Chapter 6, "Clinical Application of Psychological Constructs" provides clinical operationalization of constructs in Chapter 3 of the textbook, which discusses psychological theories that have contributed to development of concepts used in psychosocial occupational therapy. The student or clinician should therefore read the relevant chapter in the textbook before completing the exercises in the manual. While doing the exercises, the student or clinician is encouraged to work with a colleague to help facilitate self-exploration in the case of exercises that are based on personal experiences and to use role play for exercises based on case vignettes. Specific instructions are provided as appropriate for each exercise.

It is my hope that educators, students, and clinicians will find this manual useful in help-ing bridge the gap between theory and practice. Above all, have fun as you practice and work at developing skills that will make it easier for you to do occupation-based, theory-based, and evidence-based practice.

REFERENCES

1. Bruce M, Borg B: *Psychosocial frames of reference: core for occupation based practice,* ed 3, Thorofare, NJ, 2000, Slack.
2. Cara E, McRae A: *Psychosocial occupational therapy in clinical practice,* Albany, NY, 2005, Delmar Thompson Learning.
3. Early MB: *Mental health concepts and techniques for the occupational therapy assistant,* New York, 2000, Lippincott Williams & Wilkins.
4. Kielhofner G: *Conceptual foundations of occupational therapy,* ed 3, Philadelphia, 2004, F.A. Davis.
5. Stein F, Cutler SK: *Psychosocial occupational therapy: a holistic approach,* ed 2, Albany, NY, 2002, Delmar Thompson Learning.

Application of the Occupational Therapy Paradigm: Gathering and Interpreting Information, and Using Clinical Reasoning Skills to Identify Occupational Performance Issues and Plan Intervention

In this part of the manual, you will engage in a series of exercises to help you learn to apply constructs of the newly evolved occupational therapy paradigm described in Chapter 4 of the textbook. Exercise 2-1 in Chapter 2 will help you connect with the professional heritage (return to the roots consistent with Reilly's[2] call; see also Peloquin[1]) by deepening your understanding of the profession's important historical events and the intellectual and social circumstances surrounding these events. In Chapters 3 to 9, we provide exercises corresponding to Chapters 3 to 7 of the textbook. Through these exercises, the reader will enhance his or her general skills necessary to operationalize the professional paradigm's constructs so that they are applicable in clinical practice.

REFERENCES

1. Peloquin SM: 2005 Eleanor Clarke Slagle lecture: embracing our ethos, reclaiming our heart, *Am J Occup Ther* 59:611–625, 2005.
2. Reilly M: Occupational therapy can be one of the great ideas of 20th century medicine, *Am J Occup Ther* 16:1–9, 1962.

Chapter 2
Getting Grounded on the Rich Occupational Therapy Heritage

After reading Chapters 1 and 2 of your textbook, you are now aware of the origin of occupational therapy and its rich heritage, particularly in psychosocial rehabilitation. In this chapter, you will deepen this knowledge even further by engaging in an exercise that will help you to identify significant events in the profession's genealogy and the intellectual constructs associated with these events, and then trace these constructs to current occupational therapy practice.

EXERCISE 2-1: HISTORY OF OCCUPATIONAL THERAPY: FROM THE MORAL TREATMENT TO THE PRESENT

This exercise is designed to be a fun activity for the class. It is modeled on American Jeopardy (an activity that may be a meaningful leisure occupation for many students and clinicians in the United States).[*] To complete the exercise, the class is divided into two or more groups that compete against each other. The examiner reads an answer to a question, and a group member asks the question to which the answer was read. A correct response earns the group the amount of money corresponding to the question in that category (Table 2-1). The group that asks the correct question chooses the category from which the next answer will be derived. As the

[*] I am indebted to the occupational therapy class of 2007 at the University of South Dakota for introducing me to this fun way of learning content that could otherwise be dreary and daunting.

exercise continues, the examiner chooses two questions at random from any category. These questions are awarded Double Jeopardy status. Correct response to any of these questions earns the group double the amount of money listed. The exercise is conducted in this way until all questions have been answered. For the Final Jeopardy question, group members stake any amount of money that they wish to bet. If their answer is correct, they are awarded that amount of money. If it is wrong, they lose the money.

The questions in this exercise are meant for students who are being introduced to the history of the profession for the first time. An instructor may formulate questions of increasing difficulty using the content in Chapters 1 and 2 of the textbook depending on the level and background of students in class. Also, instructors may modify the exercise as indicated to make it relevant and meaningful to students from other cultures. The questions whose answers are provided here are listed at the end of the chapter.

Jeopardy Answers

Category 1: The Moral Treatment Movement

1. He was appointed the director of Asylum de Becetre in Paris in 1792, where he initiated mental health reform known as the moral treatment movement.
2. This school of philosophy was founded by a British philosopher John Locke and helped change attitudes toward mental illness.

Table 2-1. THE OCCUPATIONAL THERAPY JEOPARDY WINNINGS MATRIX

Category 1	Category 2	Category 3	Category 4	Category 5
100	100	100	100	100
200	200	200	200	200
300	300	300	300	300
400	400	400	400	400
500	500	500	500	500

Note: The amounts of money written in the cells are in U.S. dollars. If an instructor is working with students from another culture and decides to use this exercise, the amounts can be in whatever currency is used by people in that culture.

3. This era in Europe was characterized by an integration of John Locke's philosophy, Descartes' rationalism, and Newtonian scientific world view to generate ideas that were used to support the moral treatment movement in France and England.
4. He is referred to as the father of American psychiatry, signed the Declaration of Independence, and spearheaded the construction of the first mental health institution where moral treatment principles were used in the United States.
5. She was one of the leaders in the moral treatment movement in the United States who was treated at the York Retreat in England where she experienced the clinical application of moral treatment principles firsthand.

Category 2: The Arts and Crafts Movement

1. This physician used principles from the arts and crafts movement to treat clients suffering from neurasthenia at a hospital in Marblehead, Massachusetts. He engaged them in crafts activities instead of the "rest cure" commonly prescribed for the condition by many physicians at the time.
2. John Ruskin, the British philosopher whose philosophy was the intellectual foundation of the arts and crafts movement, borrowed constructs from this European political philosopher whose philosophy suggested evolution of societies through class struggle, leading to a classless society.

3. This construct, which was used to describe a worker's separation from his or her work, other workers, and the product of his or her labor, was the cornerstone of the philosophy that provided intellectual principles for the arts and crafts movement.
4. He used John Ruskin's philosophical ideas to found the arts and crafts movement.
5. Arts and crafts were used in this house to help poor immigrants from Europe reconnect with their cultural roots and to ease their transition into the American culture. The program run in the house provided a model for application of arts and crafts in occupational therapy.

Category 3: The Mental Hygiene Movement

1. This psychiatrist suggested that the relationship between mental hygiene and psychiatry was comparable to that between public health and medicine in general.
2. A book by this mental health client who was a former Yale University graduate provided impetus to the development of the mental hygiene movement.
3. There is evidence that Adolph Meyer's constructs about habits, which were used by Slagle in her habit-training program, were borrowed from the philosophy and psychology of this famous American philosopher.
4. These two American pragmatic philosophers worked with Jane Addams and Julia Lanthrop at the Hull House in Chicago,

where they interacted with important personalities in occupational therapy such as Eleanor Clarke Slagle; this provides evidence that ideas from the philosophy of pragmatism influenced the development of occupational therapy.

5. Instrumentalism, a construct borrowed from his philosophy, could be particularly useful in occupational therapy because it is based on the idea that the human mind is an instrument for adaptation to the environment.

Category 4: The Founding of Occupational Therapy

1. The formal founders of occupational therapy met at this house in this city.
2. This was the name of the new professional society founded in this year.
3. This founder of the profession was the secretary when the six founders met, and she later became George Edward Barton's wife.
4. The nine first principles of the newly founded profession were written by this psychiatrist.
5. Intellectual propositions from these four sources formed the character of the newly founded profession as is evident in an analysis of the first nine principles of the discipline.

Category 5: Development of Occupational Therapy: 1900s to the Present

1. During World War I, the Orthopedic Department of the Armed Forces sought to train workers known as these to help in the reeducation of soldiers injured at war so that they could either return to active duty or integrate successfully into civilian life.
2. The name of this professional society changed to the American Occupational Therapy Association (AOTA) during this year, and the first essentials for professional education were established jointly by the association and the American Medical Association (AMA) during this year.
3. After the stock market crash in 1929, the AOTA had difficulty implementing the new professional standards. Occupational therapy strived for recognition as a legiti-

mate medical discipline so that it could survive. At this point, the profession formally became this.

4. After joining the rehabilitation movement following World War II, occupational therapy lost its original holistic perspective and adopted this approach based on the medical model.
5. Activities in the profession following the call by this scholar for occupational therapists to return to professional roots led to the recent emergence of a new professional paradigm focusing on these four core unifying concepts and themes.

Final Jeopardy

Within the newly emerged professional paradigm, the role of the occupational therapist is conceived as consisting of these four functions.

Jeopardy Questions

Category 1
1. Who was Philippe Pinel?
2. What is empiricism?
3. What was the enlightenment?
4. Who was Benjamin Rush?
5. Who was Dorothea Linde Dix?

Category 2
1. Who was Herbert J. Hall?
2. Who was Karl Marx?
3. What is alienation?
4. Who was William Morris?
5. What was the Hull House?

Category 3
1. Who was Dr. Gray?
2. Who was Clifford Beers?
3. Who was William James?
4. Who were John Dewey and George Herbert Mead?
5. Who was John Dewey?

Category 4
1. What was Consolation House in Clifton Park, New York?

2. What was the National Society for the Promotion of Occupational Therapy (NSPOT) founded in 1917?
3. Who was Isabel Newton?
4. Who was William Rush Dunton Jr.?
5. What were the moral treatment movement, the arts and crafts movement, the philosophy of pragmatism, and medicine?

Category 5

1. Who were reconstruction aides?
2. What was the NSPOT, which became the AOTA in 1921 and facilitated development of the essentials of professional education in 1923?

3. What is a medical ancillary?
4. What is reductionism?
5. Who was Mary Reilly, and what is a focus on occupation, a holistic viewpoint, the environment, and an integrating scientific framework based on dynamic systems theory?

Final Jeopardy

What are (1) providing clients with an opportunity to engage in meaningful occupations, (2) modifying the environment to facilitate occupational performance, (3) providing assistive/technical devices to facilitate occupational performance, and (4) providing education/counseling to facilitate occupational performance?

Chapter **3**
Reviewing the Client's Medical Chart

Complete Exercise 3-1 after reading Chapter 5 in the textbook. It is necessary to point out that this exercise is relevant only for therapists who are working or anticipate practicing in custodial-type health care institutions, where the medical model is used to guide treatment. For those working in the community, school system, or other similar settings in which the medical model is not prevalent, clients may not have medical charts. You should, however, be aware that a physician referral might be a legal requirement depending on the state in which you are practicing. Therefore you should make yourself familiar with your state's licensure laws related to the practice of occupational therapy so that you know whether and under what circumstances a physician referral is required.

Even for those working within the medical model, however, it is important to remember that, as Bonder argues, the focus of occupational therapy is always to enhance function or occupational performance.[3] Therefore, interpretation of the medical data, consistent with the professional paradigm, should be individualized and done on the basis of how the medical condition or symptoms/clinical features affect occupational performance and participation in life.[1]

EXERCISE 3-1: MEDICAL CHART REVIEW

Physician/Psychiatrist Order to Treat

An order to treat is really a referral from a physician. Legally, an occupational therapist does not need a physician order or referral to treat a client,[4] although as mentioned above, the therapist should check with the state licensure laws to make sure. In most cases, a physician referral is legally needed only when the client has a condition requiring medical oversight. Also, most insurance companies and third-party payers do not typically pay for services provided to clients without physician orders. That is why physician referrals are required for clients whose services are paid for by insurance before commencing treatment. Once an order to treat is received, the therapist begins by reviewing the chart to become familiar with the client's condition, any precautions, history of the illness, and so on. A physician order to treat a client may read as follows: "Occupational therapy to evaluate and treat as indicated," "patient to receive occupational therapy services for ADLs and social-skill training," "patient to receive occupational therapy services BID 5 times a week for 4 weeks for training in ADLs," "occupational therapy to evaluate patient for safety and need for care at home," and so on. Some physicians can be very specific, while others give the therapist much leeway regarding what is to be done with the client in therapy.

Following is a chart review guide with suggestions regarding information to be noted by the therapist upon receipt of the order.

Chart Review Guide

1. Client particulars, such as address, age, referral source, current medication, and so on
2. Medical insurance information

3. Client's diagnosis: Axis I diagnosis (see the *DMS IV-TR*[2] for a description of the multi-axial diagnostic system)
4. Other diagnoses: Axis II to V diagnoses
5. History: presenting complaint, history of present illness, past illnesses, family history, personal history (prenatal to adult-hood), sexual history, fantasies and dreams, and values
6. Physician notes on the results of medical examination

Lab Exercise

For this exercise, refer to D.M.'s case below.

CASE STUDY: D.M.

D.M.[*] is a 52-year-old married Caucasian male with a diagnosis of post-traumatic stress disorder (PTSD) and mood disorder, not otherwise specified (NOS), secondary to combat experience in Vietnam. He voluntarily presented himself to the hospital for admission about 1 week ago following an event in which he hit his 21-year-old son for the first time in his life. He became very upset because he was afraid that he would hurt his family. He has a history of diabetes mellitus, obstructive sleep apnea, back pain, and hypertension. His current medications include antidepressants (trazodone, lorazepam [a tranquilizer], and sertraline [Zoloft]), alpha blockers for treatment of hypertension (terazosin, lisinopril), sleep aids, analgesics (acetaminophen [Tylenol]), hypoglycemic medications, anti-rheumatics, magnesium hydroxide (antacid), glyburide (for treatment of diabetes), and albuterol inhaler (a bronchodilator for a suspected asthmatic condition).

D.M.'s presenting problem is depression with suicidal ideation. He complains of difficulty sleeping due to frequent flashbacks of his Vietnam combat experience, where he lost many friends who died in his arms from enemy fire. Since he came back from Vietnam about 25 years ago, he has been treated on and off as an outpatient, but he finally stopped coming for therapy because he claimed that "nothing seemed to help." The onset of his depressive episodes frequently seems to coincide with major holidays. The current admission occurred just around Christmas. In the past, D.M. has attempted suicide by overdose on Zoloft.

D.M. completed high school and enlisted in the army when he was 18 years old. He was shipped to Vietnam for combat soon after basic training. After leaving service at the age of 27, he started working as a construction worker. He has been a construction worker since then, except when he has episodes of depression. He stopped working about 6 months ago due to increasing back pain, which resulted from a work-related accident about 5 years ago.

D.M. lives with his wife and 21-year-old son. His wife reports that he does not socialize much with friends or family, and he is often isolated. He spends most of his time watching television and playing computer games alone. Because of his poorly controlled diabetes mellitus, his doctor has prescribed a weight loss diet of 1000 calories or fewer per day. This was necessary because in the last 2 years, he has significantly gained weight and has experienced problems with his vision. He also experiences coughing and wheezing, which is indicative of a possibility of asthma. He also reports chest pain, and has edema in the lower extremities, probably related to his hypertension. He also has a history of substance abuse, particularly alcohol and cocaine.

---

[*] Refer to D.M.'s case description throughout Part I of the manual.

CASE STUDY: D.M.—CONT'D

During psychiatric evaluation, D.M. reported worsening memory over the last 3 months or so, and has difficulty making decisions. His clinical features include dysphoria, anhedonia, and a sense of hopelessness. His interests include mechanics, building, playing cards, and writing. Previous occupational therapy evaluation indicated a cognitive level of 5.8 on the Allen Cognitive Level Screening (ACLS) test. He is independent in basic ADLs. D.M. was referred to occupational therapy for intervention to increase his social skills and level of engagement in meaningful occupations, which the psychiatrist felt are lacking in his life at the moment.

After reading D.M.'s case description, in groups of three, discuss and answer the following questions:

1. How would you use the chart review guide to tease out important information about D.M.?
2. How would you use identified information in occupational therapy intervention?

REFERENCES

1. American Occupational Therapy Association: Occupational therapy practice framework: domain and process, *Am J Occup Ther* 56:609–639, 2002.
2. American Psychiatric Association: *The diagnostic and statistical manual for mental disorders*, ed 4, Washington, D.C., 2000, APA.
3. Bonder B: *Psychopathology and function*, ed 3, Thorofare, NJ, 2004, Slack.
4. Sames KM: Documenting occupational therapy practice, Upper Saddle River, NJ, 2005, Pearson/Prentice-Hall.

Chapter 4

Meeting the Client and Conducting an Initial Interview

Once the therapist reviews the medical chart, he or she forms a hypothesis regarding the occupational performance needs of the client. At this point, it is hoped that you are already forming a hypothesis about D.M.'s occupational performance needs after completing Exercise 3-1 in Chapter 3. After reading the section discussing the initial interview in Chapter 5 of your textbook, complete Exercise 4-1. This exercise will provide you with an opportunity to prepare for initial contact with a client. This initial contact constitutes the beginning of the initial interview, when the therapist begins establishing rapport and developing a therapeutic relationship necessary for a successful therapeutic intervention.

Also, note that this chapter is meant to provide a general overview of the areas of occupational performance that should be of interest during the initial interview. We will provide specific and more detailed assessment instruments in later chapters, where we present exercises designed to practice using various conceptual models of practice. Note also that, consistent with the occupational therapy paradigm as discussed in Chapter 4 of your textbook, the focus of the initial interview is performance of meaningful occupations by the client in the past and present, and anticipated performance in the future. The exercise also provides an opportunity for you to explore personal occupational performance over time as a way to enhance your experiential grasp of the impact of an occupation-based, client-centered initial interview on the individual client.

EXERCISE 4-1: INITIAL INTERVIEW

Screening and Acknowledging Order to Treat

After chart review, the therapist visits and speaks to the client briefly to introduce himself or herself and assess the need for occupational therapy services. However, therapists should be careful not to let information obtained from the chart influence their first impression of clients. It is important to be open-minded so that you can make an objective, unbiased assessment. Now, in a small group of three to four students, answer the following questions:

1. What kind of questions would you ask D.M. during this brief meeting to determine the need for therapy?
2. What quick observations would be relevant at this time?

Now, in pairs, take turns interviewing each other for about 10 minutes each. When you interview your colleague, try to determine his or her values and interests, occupational and role performance before the junior year of college (or some other important transition in his or her life), current occupational and role perfor-

Clue: Your interview and observations should be aimed at identifying the client's values and interests, premorbid occupational functioning and role performance, current occupational functioning and role performance concerns, and desire regarding future occupational and role performance.

mance status, and desire for future occupational and role performance. After interviewing the client briefly, note in the chart that you have received order to treat and made contact with the client. The note may read as follows:

Order to treat received. Contact made with the client. Evaluation and treatment planning will be completed within the next 48 hours.

Chapter **5**

Interpreting Gathered Information

This chapter is meant to provide you with the preliminary skills for cue identification, pattern recognition, and hypothesis generation necessary for beginning clinical reasoning capability. It may be helpful to read the "Clinical Reasoning Skills Used in Occupational Therapy" section in Chapter 6 of the textbook before completing Exercise 5-1 in this chapter. In Chapter 7 of this manual, we will provide more exercises to facilitate the development of clinical reasoning skills. For the moment, in this chapter you will practice beginning interpretation and piecing together information gathered from the chart review and brief initial interview in order to start recognizing patterns and generating hypotheses about the client's occupational performance needs. As you reflect on the information, bear in mind that your main focus as an occupational therapist is the occupational functioning of clients, as it is affected by the clinical condition and its features.[1] Now, look at the information that you have gathered about D.M. so far. Answer the questions in the following exercise in your small lab groups.

EXERCISE 5-1: BEGINNING TO MAKE SENSE OF GATHERED INFORMATION

1. Make a hypothesis about the occupational performance challenges that D.M. may have. Your hypothesis should be supported by evidence from the information you have gathered, including the following:
   * His multi-axial diagnoses
   * His occupational and role performance history
2. In groups of two, let one person role play D.M., and let the other role play his therapist. The person playing D.M. should try to demonstrate occupational performance challenges that D.M. would be expected to have, and the therapist should try to help resolve these challenges. Have fun with the activity!

REFERENCE

1. Bonder B: *Psychopathology and function,* ed 3, Thorofare, NJ, 2004, Slack.

Chapter **6**
Clinical Application of Psychological Constructs

Exercises 6-1 to 6-5 in this chapter will help you practice the application of psychological constructs discussed in Chapter 3 of the textbook in clinical practice. These psychological skills constitute the building blocks of clinical practice in psychosocial occupational therapy (and possibly in other specialties). These exercises are presented in this chapter rather than earlier chapters because it is necessary to introduce you to preliminary clinical procedures such as chart review and data interpretation in preparation for application of psychological constructs in clinical practice. It is recommended that you review Chapter 3 of the textbook before completing exercises in this chapter.

The exercises in this chapter are meant to cater to varying levels of clinical preparedness. For example, for entry-level students without a strong background in psychology and psychotherapy, exercises such as active imagination may be beyond their scope. For those in postprofessional programs and practicing occupational therapists, such exercises may be a way of enhancing clinical competency by developing deeper insights regarding various psychologically derived therapeutic approaches. It is recommended that the instructor make a judgment regarding the level of student preparedness and structure the exercises accordingly. Now, working in pairs, use the following exercises to practice various psychological intervention skills. In each case, one person should play the client, and the other should play the therapist. After 10 minutes, switch roles.

EXERCISE 6-1: FREUDIAN AND NEO-FREUDIAN TECHNIQUES

Exercise 6-1, A: Free Association

For about 2 minutes, the person playing the client should verbalize at will whatever comes to mind. Do not try to evaluate what you are saying or to make sense of it. The person playing the therapist should write down these statements without commenting. Take 2 minutes to brainstorm together regarding what these statements mean until you come up with an explanation that really "clicks" (makes sense) for the "client." Switch roles and do the same for the other person in the pair.

Exercise 6-1, B: Active Imagination

The person playing the client should try to remember a recent dream. Write this dream down in detail. If you cannot remember a dream, take a few moments to breathe in and out deeply (about 10 times) and relax as much as possible. Now try to fantasize about something. Make your fantasy as detailed and vivid as possible. Write down the fantasy in all its detail. Whether it is a dream or fantasy, identify the actors and other objects in the story. With the assistance of the "therapist," make a dialogue with each of the actors or objects until you feel satisfied that you understand its message as completely as possible. Now try to write a summary of any insights you have gained about yourself through this exercise.

EXERCISE 6-2: BEHAVIORAL TECHNIQUES

Think of a goal that you want to achieve (e.g., to be more physically fit, keep current with your course readings, get a part-time job, and so on). Identify activities in which you would need to engage so as to achieve these goals. Now break down the activities into their components. For example, in order to keep current with course readings, you may identify reading regularly as the activity. Define the activity more concretely. For instance, you will need to read for 2 hours every evening. Then identify what you will be reading each evening. Now, identify a reinforcer. This should be something you really like. It could be a bowl of ice cream, going out to the movies, socializing with friends on the phone, and so on. Now, make a reinforcement schedule for yourself. For example, you may state that every time you read for 2 hours every evening for three consecutive evenings, you will allow yourself to go to a movie. In small lab groups, discuss how you may use similar techniques to help D.M. achieve his goal to participate in meaningful occupations with his family upon discharge from the hospital. Try this intervention for yourself, and after a few weeks, if you like, report to the class how well it has worked for you.

EXERCISE 6-3: COGNITIVE/ BEHAVIORAL TECHNIQUES

Take a few moments to think about something that may be causing you anxiety now. It might be a forthcoming examination that you are a little anxious about, a relationship that you are afraid might not work, or a job situation. Whatever it is, think about some of the thoughts that are associated with your situation that make you feel anxious. These are automatic thoughts about how you tell yourself that you should be performing in the situation. For example, you may be telling yourself, "I must get an A in this test." "I should never get less than an A in any test." "I ought not to get less than an A in any test." Once you identify

the *musts, shoulds,* and *oughts* that occur in your mind automatically, think about them and try to ask yourself whether they are rational. Challenge the rationality of your thoughts candidly and honestly. For example, is it really rational that you must get an A in all your tests? Now, try to change the statements. Instead of telling yourself that you *must* obtain some kind of an outcome, such as "I *must* obtain an A in the forthcoming test," change it to a *preference* such as, "I would *prefer* to get an A in the forthcoming test (or whatever the issue is), but I do not have to." How does it feel when you change the statement? Share any insights that you have gained from the exercise with the class.

EXERCISE 6-4: SOCIAL LEARNING THEORY

This exercise is based on Albert Bandura's Cognitive Social Learning Theory.

If you are a student enrolled in a course, think about how you imagine it will feel to attain an A in the course. If you are a therapist, think about how it would feel to be recognized professionally for your clinical expertise. Why do you think you would feel that way? How did you learn to feel good about doing well in your classes or at work? For example, did your parents reward you in some way when you did well? Do you still need to be rewarded externally for doing well, or do you now like to do well for the sake of it? If you answered yes to the above questions, it means that initially, you were rewarded for doing well. Eventually, you internalized the value of doing well, and now, when you perform satisfactorily, you feel good even though there may not be any external rewards.

Now, think about your chosen career. How did you become attracted to occupational therapy? Did you for instance see occupational therapists or some other helping professionals being rewarded in some way for what they do (e.g., by being awarded prestige)? Did you think: "That is great. I would like to do that so that I can get similar attention"? If you answered yes to the above questions, you probably learned vicariously the value of being an occupational therapist by noticing the positive social consequences experienced by those who do similar work. Now look at D.M.'s case description. In a small lab group (three to four students), discuss and answer the following question: How would you use vicarious learning to help D.M. learn to enjoy engaging in meaningful occupations and performing his social roles satisfactorily?

EXERCISE 6-5: CLIENT-CENTERED TECHNIQUES

This exercise is based on Carl Rogers' client-centered therapy.

Working in pairs, practice attending and responding skills by completing the following exercise. One person should play the client, and the other should play the therapist. The "client" identifies an issue of concern and begins talking to the "therapist" about it. When you play the role of the therapist, pay attention to what you are doing to make your client comfortable. For example, how are you using your posture, facial expression, verbal tone, and so on? Through all these communication signals, do you communicate acceptance, interest, respect, and understanding to your client? Now begin responding to what the client says, using the general response form: You feel _____ because _____. For instance, "You feel frustrated because you do not understand the course material?" (See the Appendix for "feeling vocabulary" that you can use in your responses.) Keep responding and encouraging the client to do self-exploration until you collaboratively arrive at the action phase (see the phases of Rogerian therapy in Chapter 3 of the textbook).

Chapter 7

Clinical Reasoning

In this chapter, you will participate in an exercise to help you develop your clinical reasoning skills. You will use a tool known as the M-A-P-P (Figure 7-1) to help you develop these skills (refer to Figure 6-2 in Chapter 6 of your textbook for an example of how to proceed). As you engage in the exercise, remember that clinical reasoning, like any other skill, is perfected through practice and experience. Therefore, you should take the following case only as a beginning. You will need to practice, applying the process that you will learn here, to a variety of cases in order to master the requisite skills. As an instructor using this manual, you should work the case ahead of time and let students compare their conclusions with yours. Before you begin working the case, answer the following question: From where do the contents of my cognitive structure (schema)

that help me interpret clinical data and arrive at decisions about intervention come (e.g., my courses in abnormal psychology, occupational therapy theory, psychology, sociology)?

EXERCISE 7-1: CLINICAL REASONING PROCESS IN THE CASE OF D.M.

Now, work through D.M.'s case using the M-A-P-P process, and formulate short-term and long-term goals for him (print and use the blank M-A-P-P form in Figure 7-1). How do your conclusions about D.M.'s occupational performance issues compare with your earlier hypothesis (in Chapter 5)? Did you have any extra insights that you did not have when you answered the questions in Chapter 5? Now compare your conclusions with those of your instructor.

The M-A-P-P Process of Assessment

MANIFESTATION (What is Observed)	ASSESSMENT (Clinical Interpretation of Observations)	REASON FOR SUGGESTED ASSESSMENTS	PRIORITY (Importance to Client's Treatment)
			Strengths 1. 2. 3. 4. 5. 6. 7. 8. Limitations 1. 2. 3. 4. 5. 6. 7. 8.

Figure 7-1.   The M-A-P-P: An instrument to facilitate development of clinical reasoning skills.

Continued

PLAN
Proposed Treatment Plan to Facilitate Change by Building on Existing Strengths

CONCLUSIONS (What are your conclusions given the manifestations, assessments, and priorities)	GOALS (What, Where, When, Why)	METHODS (Who, How)
	What Where When Why	Who How

Figure 7-1.　Cont'd.

PLAN
Summary of Intervention Plan

Problem	Goals	Interventions	Frequency	Target Date

Figure 7-1. Cont'd.

Continued

Concise Statement of D.M.'s Treatment Goals

Short-Term Goals (STGs)

1.

2.

3.

4.

5.

Long-Term Goals (LTGs)

1.

2.

Figure 7-1. Cont'd.

PART II

General Intervention Skills

By now, having read Chapters 1 to 6 of your textbook and completed various exercises in Part I of this manual, you are well-acquainted with the conceptual foundations of occupational therapy, including its history and professional paradigm. You have also practiced the use of psychological constructs that underlie psychosocial occupational therapy; client interviewing and other forms of data gathering; and the clinical reasoning process used to arrive at appropriate goals that address the client's occupational performance issues.

To help you complete building basic skills needed in psychosocial occupational therapy, Part II of this manual presents a variety of exercises to help you develop skills in attending to your client and building rapport; establishing a therapeutic relationship; and using the therapeutic relationship, groups and group processes, and meaningful occupations as media for therapeutic intervention. You will also participate in exercises to help you develop awareness of how cultural factors influence therapeutic discourse.

Chapter **8**

General Intervention Skills in Psychosocial Occupational Therapy

After reading Chapter 7 of your textbook, you are now aware that ethical decision making is a cognitive process. In Chapter 7, we also discussed therapeutic media used in occupational therapy (therapeutic use of relationship, use of groups and group techniques, and use of meaningful occupations). You also read and hopefully reflected on how cultural perspectives affect therapeutic discourse. The exercises in this chapter will help you apply what you read in Chapter 7 in clinical practice.

EXERCISE 8-1: ETHICAL DECISION MAKING

This exercise is in two parts: Exercise 8-1A will help increase your awareness of experiences that have contributed to your ethical cognitive schema (see discussion of the construct in Chapter 7 of your textbook) that helps you interpret and make sense of ethically related data, and make ethical decisions. This awareness will enhance your ethical decision-making abilities. Exercise 8-1B will give you an opportunity to practice ethical decision making in a clinical context.

Exercise 8-1, A: Developing Insight Regarding Your Ethical Cognitive Schema

Reflect and answer the following questions:

1. What ethical conceptual model do you subscribe to (deontological, teleological, or other)? Explain.
2. How does the view derived from that ethical conceptual model influence the way you make ethical decisions (e.g., decisions about right and wrong, what should or should not be done)?
3. Identify the values you acquired from:
   a. Your family
   b. Your Sunday school/Hebrew school (or other organized institutional setting for teaching values in your culture)
   c. Your school
   d. Friends
   e. College/professional education
   f. The media (e.g., television, radio, newspapers, Internet, movies)
   g. Other sources
4. How did the values identified above influence the development of your ethical perspective (whether deontological, teleological, or other)?

Exercise 8-1, B: Ethical Clinical Reasoning

For this exercise, refer to Mukangu's case below.

CASE STUDY: MUKANGU

Mukangu is a 14-year-old African male who migrated to the United States with his family 3 years ago. His mother is a graduate student pursuing a Master of Arts degree in psychology, and his father works as a checkout clerk at a Wal-Mart Super Center. Mukangu was referred for occupational therapy services following an accident in which he was hit by a car while riding his bike. He sustained mild closed head injuries. He presented to occupational therapy with complaints of forgetfulness, stating that he could not remember how to spell even the simplest words. Mukangu was very distressed about this. His family values education, and he was preparing to take the SAT and go to college when the accident occurred. His dream was to become a medical doctor.

Evaluation indicates that Mukangu needs occupational therapy to provide him with opportunities to engage in occupations that would afford him experiences through which he can learn skills to help him identify and pursue realistic goals and interests, and lead a meaningful life by compensating for his cognitive deficits. However, his family does not have medical insurance and is unable to pay for occupational therapy services. Your clinical supervisor gives you directions to discharge Mukangu from occupational therapy since according to the rules at the facility for which you work you cannot provide services to a client who is unable to pay. *Now, answer the following questions:*

1. What is the ethical issue in Mukangu's case?
2. How would you address the identified ethical issue?
3. Refer to the six-step model of ethical decision making outlined in Chapter 7 of your textbook. Explain how you would apply these steps in order to arrive at a decision regarding how to address Mukangu's issue. Does following the six steps lead to a different decision from the one you arrived at in item 2 above?
4. Explain how your ethical cognitive schema informs your decision.

EXERCISE 8-2: USE OF THERAPEUTIC RELATIONSHIP

In this exercise, you will practice your attending skills as part of learning how to establish a therapeutic relationship. The exercise is in three parts: Exercise 8-2, A, will help you develop attending skills in order to get the client involved. In Exercise 8-2, B, you will practice further the responding skills that you learned in Chapter 6 when you completed Exercise 6-5. These responding skills will help you convey empathy to your client, which will help you establish rapport quickly and build a viable therapeutic relationship. Finally, Exercise 8-2, C, will facilitate development of skills needed for engagement in a client-centered occupational therapy process based on Rogerian guidelines.

Exercise 8-2, A: Attending to the Client

Working in pairs, take about 20 minutes to interview each other (one student acting as the "therapist" and the other as the "client"). Each person will take 10 minutes to play each role. If you are the client, identify an issue of concern in your life (e.g., a challenge related to a course you are taking, a work situation, or a family situation). Begin talking to the therapist about the issue. As you talk, pay attention to how the following affect your willingness or ease to disclose the issue to the therapist:

1. Ambience in the room (physical factors such as space, temperature, décor, furnishings, and seating arrangement)
2. Therapist-related factors (therapist's attire, posture, facial expression, gestures, verbal expression, nonverbal responses, and the general attitude and feeling tone)

After 10 minutes, give the therapist feedback regarding how the above-listed factors affected your ability to express yourself freely and honestly. Now switch roles. Compare the feedback given by the client in each case with the recommendations in the next section.

Recommendations for Creating a Welcoming Therapeutic Atmosphere[2]

1. Ambience (if the session is in the client's room, the therapist may not have control of the physical setting of the room):
   a. Space: The room should not be too big or too small. The size should be such that you do not feel cramped, but at the same time you feel a sense of intimacy. The room should have windows and enough lighting to convey a feeling of openness. If possible, the room should be located in a place where there is no noise interruption. Try to avoid rooms in which windows are facing streets where cars and people may be constantly passing by. Take the phone off the hook or turn off the ringer to avoid interruptions.
   b. Temperature: The temperature should be comfortable for the client.
   c. Décor: The décor should give a homelike feeling. For instance, the colors should be light but not overwhelmingly bright.
   d. Furnishings: The furnishings should similarly convey a homey ambience.
   e. Seating arrangements: Both you and the client should preferably be sitting on high-backed chairs that are supportive and comfortable. The chairs should be arranged such that the therapist and client are seated at an angle of approximately 45 degrees to each other so that eye contact is maintained but the therapist is not staring at the client. There should be no obstacles, such as a table, between the therapist and client. If the session is in the client's room, the client may be lying in bed. In this case, the therapist should sit on a chair beside the bed, making sure that he or she is in full view of the client.

2. Therapist-related factors:
   a. Attire: Your attire should be professional and appropriate. Avoid clothes that may have sexual connotation or that convey sensuality. If part of the initial interview will include engagement in an activity, dress appropriately. For instance, if the activity will involve sitting on the floor, wear pants rather than a short, tight skirt.
   b. Posture: Your posture should be comfortable and open. Crossed legs and arms may convey the attitude of being closed to the client.
   c. Facial expression: Your facial expression should convey warmth and caring (for example, smiling rather than frowning).
   d. Verbal and nonverbal communication: Nonverbal signals (e.g., hand gestures, nodding) and verbal expressions (e.g., "mm," "uh") should convey interest and encouragement to the client to express himself or herself.

All the above factors encourage the client to talk and get involved in the therapeutic process.

Exercise 8-2, B: Responding

Still working in pairs, as the client begins talking about the issue of concern, the therapist should respond to both the content and feeling of what is expressed as practiced in Chapter 6 of the manual, using the general form: You feel _____ because _____ . After about 10 minutes, switch roles.

Exercise 8-2, C: Exploration, Personalization, and Action

The instructor will now demonstrate how the client could be facilitated through self-exploration and personalization of the issue of concern, leading to action (Figure 8-1). After the demonstration, practice facilitating each other's progress through the stages shown in Figure 8-1 (40 minutes). For details of this model of therapeutic discourse, refer to the discussion of Rogerian client-centered therapy in Chapter 3 of your textbook.

EXERCISE 8-3: USE OF GROUPS AND GROUP TECHNIQUES

In this exercise, you will practice developing a group protocol to address therapeutic goals for clients who are members of an occupational therapy group. Following are therapeutic goals of six clients that were established collaboratively by the client and therapist. They are stated in first person using actual language used by clients (corrected for grammatical errors). The six clients are going to be in an occupational therapy group that you are planning. They are all adolescents with emotional and behavioral disorders (EBD) referred to occupational therapy by the court system or teachers. In small groups of three, use the listed goals to establish a group protocol using Cole's[1] seven-step group format (refer to Figure 7-1 of your textbook for an example of a group protocol).

Client A

1. By the end of 3 weeks, I will demonstrate increased closeness and respect to my family as indicated by talking to each family member at least two times a week without using curse words.
2. By the end of 3 weeks, I will show increased socialization as indicated by going to the mall with a friend at least two times a week.

Client B

1. By the end of 2 weeks, I will show increased initiative about preparing for my future as indicated by gathering information about how to pursue a career as a social worker and sharing it with my therapist.

2. By the end of 2 weeks, I will show increased ability to pay attention to other people close to me as indicated by expressing love and affection to my boyfriend without his prompt at least three times a week.
3. By the end of 3 weeks, my performance in class will have improved to be consistent with my goal to be a social worker as indicated by attaining an average grade of B+ or better in all tests and class assignments.

Client C

1. By the end of 3 weeks, my behavior in school will have improved significantly as indicated by being placed in detention no more than two times a week.
2. By the end of 3 weeks, I will demonstrate a sense of responsibility for my future as indicated by gathering information about how to prepare for a career as an actor and sharing it with the therapist.

Client D

1. By the end of 4 weeks, I will demonstrate better self-care ability as indicated by improved cooking skills to be able to make scrambled eggs and other simple meals independently.
2. By the end of 3 weeks, my study skills will have improved significantly as indicated by attaining an average grade of C+ or better in all tests and class assignments.

Client E

1. By the end of 1 month, I will demonstrate increasingly responsible behavior as indicated by not being arrested or placed in detention at school more than once every 2 weeks.

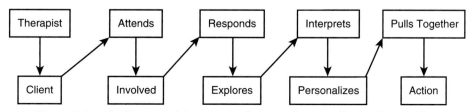

Figure 8-1. Facilitation of therapeutic discourse by attending and responding.

2. By the end of 3 weeks, I will demonstrate improved sense of responsibility over my health as indicated by stopping smoking and drinking.

Client F

1. By the end of 3 weeks, I will demonstrate improved sense of trustworthiness to my friends, teachers, and family as indicated by following through with my responsibilities every time I promise to do something.
2. By the end of 3 weeks, I will demonstrate improved study habits as indicated by maintaining an average grade of *B+* or better in all tests.

Once you have established your protocols in small groups, come back together and discuss your plans as a class. Choose one protocol to guide a 1-hour group process in class. If the class is larger than 15 students, divide it into small groups of no less than six and no more than eight students and use the group protocols to run independent group processes for each of the small groups.

EXERCISE 8-4: DEVELOPING CULTURAL COMPETENCY

Now, refer to Mukangu's case introduced at the beginning of the chapter. After reviewing the section on cultural issues in occupational therapy in Chapter 7 of your textbook, answer the following questions:

1. What are some of the cultural factors that may influence the therapeutic relationship between you, Mukangu, and his family?
2. How would you address these factors in therapy?

Discuss your answers to the above questions in small groups of three students, and then share your insights with the class.

REFERENCES

1. Cole MB: *Group dynamics in occupational therapy,* ed 3, Thorofare, NJ, 2005, Slack.
2. Posthuma BW: *Small groups in counseling and therapy: process and leadership,* Boston, 2002, Allyn & Bacon.

Chapter *9*

Documentation, Progress Notes, and Discharge Planning

Diligent record keeping is crucial in therapy so that the therapist is able to document therapeutic actions and keep track of the client's progress.[1,2] This allows accountability on the part of the therapist. Progress in most rehabilitation settings is documented using the *SOAP* format. *SOAP* is an acronym that stands for *Subjective, Objective, Assessment,* and *Plan.*

Subjective refers to the feeling component where the client's statements about how he or she feels are recorded. Such statements may include the following: The client states, "I feel awful today," or "I am exhilarated today." The therapist's observation of the feeling status of the client may also go here. This would include statements such as "Mrs. B seems to be in low spirits this morning." The *Objective* part of the note includes statements describing observable behavior noted by the therapist. This may include activities used in therapy and the client's specific responses to interventions. Evaluation results are also included here. This part should be written in such a way that the client's current status of functioning can easily be compared to the previous status (see example in Drake's case in Chapter 10 of your textbook). This allows easy assessment of progress or lack thereof. The *Assessment* part contains a summary of the client's progress in therapy and identification of goals that need to continue to be addressed and new problems on which therapeutic interventions need to focus. The therapist makes an appraisal of the treatment plan and decides whether therapy is working or the plan needs

to be modified. The *Plan* section contains the therapist's statement of planned response to issues identified in the assessment.

Now, based on your readings in Chapter 6 of your textbook, and the example of a progress note for Drake in Chapter 10, write two SOAP notes and a discharge summary for D.M. (introduced in Exercise 3-1) following the outline below:

Progress Note 1

S:

O:

STG	Previous Status	Current Status

A:

P:

Progress Note 2

S:

O:

STG	Previous Status	Current Status

A:

P:

Discharge Summary:

S:

O:

LTG	Status at the Beginning of Therapy	Current Status

A:

Recommendation(s)

S, Subjective; *O*, objective; *STG*, short-term goal; *LTG*, long-term goal; *A*, assessment; *P*, plan.

REFERENCES

1. Early MB: *Mental health concepts and techniques for occupational therapy assistants*, ed 3, New York, 2000, Lippincott Williams & Wilkins.
2. Sames KM: Documenting occupational therapy practice, Upper Saddle River, NJ, 2005, Pearson/Prentice-Hall.

PART III

Specific Interventions: Application of Conceptual Models of Practice

By completing various exercises in Parts I and II of this manual, you have hopefully developed the general foundational skills necessary for effective psychosocial occupational therapy interventions. With this foundation, you are now ready to explore in greater depth the link between theory and practice. According to Kielhofner,[1] conceptual models of practice (*frames of reference* according to Mosey[2]), are the means by which theory and practice are bridged.

In Part III of this manual, you will participate in a variety of exercises to help you build this bridge by exploring experientially ways of operationalizing constructs from conceptual models of practice for application in clinical practice. It is hoped that completing these exercises will help you develop the expertise necessary for theory-based, client-centered, and occupation-based practice.

REFERENCES

1. Kielhofner G: *Conceptual foundations of occupational therapy,* ed 3, Philadelphia, 2004, F.A. Davis.
2. Mosey AC: *Applied scientific inquiry in the health professions: an epistemological orientation,* ed 2, Bethesda, MD, 1996, American Occupational Therapy Association.

Chapter **10**

The Instrumentalism in Occupational Therapy Conceptual Model of Practice

The following exercise will help you develop experiential insight in how to apply the Instrumentalism in Occupational Therapy (IOT) conceptual model of practice. You will develop insight in how to administer assessment and intervention to your clients based on the model. It is suggested that you read Chapter 8 of your textbook before completing the following exercises.

EXERCISE 10-1: ARTICULATING A MISSION STATEMENT AND IDENTIFYING OCCUPATIONAL PERFORMANCE NEEDS

Before beginning the exercise, find a compact disk containing soothing music, preferably instrumental. Classical music usually works well. Find a quiet place where you can concentrate for about 30 to 45 minutes without interruption. Start playing the music and lie down so that you are as comfortable as possible. Clear your mind by breathing in and out slowly and deeply about 10 times. Here is how you know you are breathing in deeply. Place your hand on your abdomen. As you breathe in, your abdomen should rise. Use a word with each breath to help you relax. For instance, every time you breathe in, say to yourself, "serenity in." Every time you breathe out, say "tension out." Focus on the music as you breathe in and out, and feel the tension drain out of every muscle.

Now, begin visualizing your eulogy following the directions on the Assessment and Intervention Instrument for Instrumentalism in Occupational Therapy (AIIIOT) (Figure 10-1). Note the warning in Chapter 8 of your textbook. Eulogy visualization is not suitable for clients who are likely to experience decompensation due to decreased reality testing[4] or severe emotional disturbances. It could particularly be contraindicated for clients who have hallucinations or delusions, or those who are homicidal, depressed/suicidal, or terminally ill. For such clients, skip the eulogy visualization exercise and directly ask them to develop a personal mission statement. The IOT conceptual model is also not suitable for use with children who may not have the maturity necessary to think about an overview of their life extending far into the future.

After the eulogy visualization, write your personal mission statement, identify occupations in which regular engagement would help you achieve the mission, and rate yourself on four scales (frequency, adequacy, satisfaction, and belief in ability to engage in the identified occupations). Calculate an aggregate score for each of the four scales. For all identified occupations whose satisfaction with performance is rated less than 4, set short-term goals whose achievement will lead to engagement in the occupations with desired frequency and adequacy.

Note that findings from the pilot study by Ikiugu and Ciaravino[3] have been incorporated into the instrument. The revised AIIIOT allows the client to rate himself or herself on

Assessment and Intervention Instrument for Instrumentalism in Occupational Therapy (AIIIOT)

When using this instrument, the therapist should find a quiet place where the client can concentrate and respond in detail to all items without interruption. The client should be given as much time as necessary to respond to all the items in this instrument exhaustively. The instrument consists of four sections. Section I is designed to lead the client to formulate a personal mission statement to create a purpose toward which to strive. Section II involves identification of some of the occupations in which to engage so as to attain the stated mission. Section III provides scales for evaluation of the frequency and perceived adequacy of engagement in the occupations, satisfaction with that engagement, and the beliefs about ability to engage in the occupations adequately. Finally, in section IV, ratings are added together to give an index of frequency, adequacy, satisfaction, and beliefs about ability to engage in the listed occupations.

I.   Personal Mission Statement

The therapist should read the following directions loudly and guide the client to complete the exercise (see Covey[2]).

Imagine that you are attending your own funeral. It is now time to read the eulogy. Write down in detail what you would like each of the following to say about you:
- Family (father, mother, spouse, son/daughter, sister/brother, cousin, any other family member that you feel close to)
- Friends (one or two close friends)
- Work/professional associate
- A member of the church, temple, or other community organization to which you are affiliated.

Now go over what you have written and take a few moments to think about what you imagine each of the people is saying about you. These statements represent the kind of person that you would like to be and that you can be. Summarize the statements in a few sentences, stating what you consider to be your personal mission statement. Your mission statement will provide direction toward which you will strive from now on. The statement should consist of four aspects as identified in the eulogy: family, friends, work/professional life, and engagement in religious/community organizations.

II.   Identification of Occupations

For each of the four areas, identify two concrete occupations in which you will need to engage on a regular basis in order to achieve your mission in life.

A. Family

1.
2.

Figure 10-1.   Assessment and Intervention Instrument for Instrumentalism in Occupational Therapy, revised (AIIIOT, revised).
(Adapted from Ikiugu MN: Instrumentalism in occupational therapy: guidelines for practice, *Internat J Psychosocial Rehabil* 8:176–177, 2004.)

Continued

the basis of occupations perceived to contribute toward achievement of personal mission in life at the time of reassessment. Also, the language in the instrument has been revised to emphasize constructs such as "occupations" and "engagement" consistent with the occupational therapy paradigm as articulated in the new *Occupational Therapy Practice Framework*.[1]

EXERCISE 10-2: IDENTIFYING YOUR OCCUPATIONAL PERFORMANCE PATTERNS

After completing the AIIIOT, complete the Daily Occupational Inventories (DOIs) (Form IOT 2) shown in Figure 10-2 by entering occupations in which you have participated on an hourly basis from 6:00 A.M. to midnight for the last 4

B. Social (Friendship)

1.
2.

C. Work/Profession

1.
2.

D. Affiliation to Religious/Community Organizations

1.
2.

III.   Evaluation

For each of the identified occupations, rate yourself on a scale of one (1) to four (4) regarding the (a) frequency, (b) adequacy, (c) satisfaction, and (d) beliefs regarding your ability to engage in the occupation.

Descriptors

Frequency

1 = does not engage in the occupation; 2 = rarely engages in the occupation; 3 = regularly engages in the occupation; 4 = frequently engages in the occupation.

Adequacy

1 = I am not able to engage in the occupation; 2 = I engage in the occupation with difficulty and the outcome is inadequate; 3 = I engage in the occupation with difficulty but the outcome is good if I complete it; 4 = I engage in the occupation easily, am always able to complete it, and the outcome is always adequate.

Satisfaction

1 = I am disappointed with my engagement in the occupation; 2 = I am somewhat satisfied with my engagement; 3 = I am satisfied with my engagement but would like to improve; 4 = I am happy with my engagement as it is.

Figure 10-1.   Cont'd.

days. Try to be as accurate as possible in your entries.

After completing the DOIs, do the following:
1. Make a list of all occupations in which you engaged in the last 4 days. The occupations are organized in the list by the following categories as defined in the *Occupational Therapy Practice Framework* (AOTA, 2002)[1]: Activities of Daily Living (ADLs), Instrumental Activities of Daily Living (IADLs), Education, Work, Play, Leisure, and Social Participation.

2. Rank the occupations in the list in order of their perceived importance in helping you achieve your stated mission in life.
3. For each occupation, indicate the frequency with which you entered it in the inventory (same as frequency of participation).

EXERCISE 10-3: CALCULATING YOUR OCCUPATIONAL PERFORMANCE SCORE

Now, list the top five ranked occupations on Form IOT 3 (Occupational Performance Calculation

Text continued on p. 416.

Belief

1 = I do not believe that I am capable of engaging in the occupation; 2 = I believe that I can engage in the occupation but with much help; 3 = I believe I can engage in the occupation with some help; 4 = I believe I can engage in the occupation adequately and independently.

	Frequency 1 2 3 4	Adequacy 1 2 3 4	Satisfaction 1 2 3 4	Belief 1 2 3 4

A. Family

1. — — — —   — — — —   — — — —   — — — —
2. — — — —   — — — —   — — — —   — — — —

B. Social (Friendship)

1. — — — —   — — — —   — — — —   — — — —
2. — — — —   — — — —   — — — —   — — — —

C. Work/profession

1. — — — —   — — — —   — — — —   — — — —
2. — — — —   — — — —   — — — —   — — — —

D. Affiliation to religious/community organization

1. — — — —   — — — —   — — — —   — — — —
2. — — — —   — — — —   — — — —   — — — —

Scores (x11, x12, x13, x14)

_____   _____   _____   _____
Frequency   Adequacy   Satisfaction   Belief

Scores (x21, x22, x23, x24)

_____   _____   _____   _____

To obtain total scores, add the ratings for each column and place the aggregate score at the bottom of the column. These scores are denoted x11, x12, x13, and x14 for frequency, adequacy, satisfaction, and beliefs respectively.

To obtain the scores at the end of the therapy week, have the client rate himself or herself again and add the scores under each column. Denote the scores x21, x22, x23, and x24. Progress made in therapy during the week is indicated by x21-x11, x22-x12, x23-x13, and x24-x14 respectively.

Comments:

Figure 10-1. Cont'd.

FORM IOT 2: Daily Occupational Inventory (DOI)

Enter each occupation in which you participate next to the indicated time on the inventory. For example:

6:00 am - Woke up, got out of bed, exercised, meditated, had breakfast.

7:00 am - Drove to work, listened to the news over the radio.

8:00 am - Got into the office, checked voicemail, checked email messages, answered emails, made a list of activities for the day.

Make sure to indicate the date (MM/DD/YY) for which you are logging in occupations. Bring the completed inventory with you when you come for therapy.

_____

1st Day

Client's Name _____   Date _____

    6:00 am -

    7:00 am -

    8:00 am -

    9:00 am -

  10:00 am -

  11:00 am -

  12:00 pm -

    1:00 pm -

    2:00 pm -

    3:00 pm -

    4:00 pm -

    5:00 pm -

    6:00 pm -

    7:00 pm -

    8:00 pm -

    9:00 pm -

  10:00 pm -

  11:00 pm -

  12:00 am -

Figure 10-2. Daily Occupational Inventories.

2nd Day

Client's Name_____ Date _____

  6:00 am -

  7:00 am -

  8:00 am -

  9:00 am -

10:00 am -

11:00 am -

12:00 pm -

  1:00 pm -

  2:00 pm -

  3:00 pm -

  4:00 pm -

  5:00 pm -

  6:00 pm -

  7:00 pm -

  8:00 pm -

  9:00 pm -

10:00 pm -

11:00 pm -

12:00 am -

Figure 10-2.   Cont'd.

Continued

3rd Day

Client's Name_____ Date _____

6:00 am -

7:00 am -

8:00 am -

9:00 am -

10:00 am -

11:00 am -

12:00 pm -

1:00 pm -

2:00 pm -

3:00 pm -

4:00 pm -

5:00 pm -

6:00 pm -

7:00 pm -

8:00 pm -

9:00 pm -

10:00 pm -

11:00 pm -

12:00 am -

Figure 10-2. Cont'd.

4th Day

Client's Name_____ Date _____

6:00 am -

7:00 am -

8:00 am -

9:00 am -

10:00 am -

11:00 am -

12:00 pm -

1:00 pm -

2:00 pm -

3:00 pm -

4:00 pm -

5:00 pm -

6:00 pm -

7:00 pm -

8:00 pm -

9:00 pm -

10:00 pm -

11:00 pm -

12:00 am -

Figure 10-2. Cont'd.

FORM IOT 3: Occupational Performance Calculation Guide (OPCG)

Occupation	Participation Index (PI)	Frequency (F)	Score (P$_i$)
1. _____	(5 points/entry)	_____	_____
2. _____	(4 points/entry)	_____	_____
3. _____	(3 points/entry)	_____	_____
4. _____	(2 points/entry)	_____	_____
5. _____	(1 point/entry)	_____	_____

Total participation score (P$_t$)   _____

Daily participation score (P$_t$) = Σ(P$_i$), P$_i$ = F $\times$ PI, where P$_i$ = Performance score for each of the five occupations, F = Frequency of participation in the occupation as indicated by the number of entries in FORM IOT 2, and PI = Performance index of the occupation according to ranking by the client (I = 5 points for occupation ranked number 1, 4 points for number 2, 3 points for number 3, 2 points for number 4, and 1 point for number 5). Therefore, P$_t$ = Σ(P$_i$) = Σ(F $\times$ PI).

Figure 10-3.   The Occupational Performance Calculation Guide (OPCG).
(Adapted from Ikiugu MN, Rosso HM: Understanding the occupational human being as a complex, dynamical, adaptive system, *Occup Ther Health Care* 19(4):65, 2005.)

Continued

Guide) (OPCG), shown in Figure 10-3. Calculate your occupational performance score (P$_t$) using the algorithm provided at the bottom of the form.

Participation scores can be calculated again during reassessment. Progress in therapy is indicated by P$_{t2}$ − P$_{t1}$, where P$_{t1}$ is the score at the beginning of therapy and P$_{t2}$ is the score at reassessment.

REFERENCES

1. American Occupational Therapy Association: Occupational therapy practice framework: domain and process, *Am J Occup Ther* 56:609–639, 2002.
2. Covey SR: *The seven habits of highly effective people,* New York, 1990, Simon & Schuster.
3. Ikiugu MN, Ciaravino AE: Assisting adolescents experiencing emotional and behavioral difficulties (EBD) transition to adulthood, *Internat J Psychosocial Rehabil* 10(2):57–78, 2006.
4. Roth S, McCune CC: The client and family experience of mental illness. In Cara E, MacRae A, eds: *Psychosocial occupational therapy: a clinical practice,* Clifton Park, NY, 2005, Thomson Delmar Learning, pp. 3–25.

Chapter **11**
The Psychodynamic Conceptual Model of Practice

In this chapter, you will learn to administer the three most commonly used psychodynamic occupational therapy assessments: the Lerner Magazine Picture Collage (LMPC),[4] the Azima battery, and the Barbara Hemphill (BH) battery.[2,3] Before you get to the lab, your instructor will have all the materials necessary to complete the assessments. He or she will instruct and guide you to complete the activities. You will follow the instructions for each assessment as outlined in Chapter 9 of your textbook. Familiarize yourself with the instructions before completing the exercise.

EXERCISE 11-1: SELF EVALUATION USING EXPRESSIVE MEDIA ASSESSMENTS

After completing the assessments, answer the following questions:

- Why did you select the pictures that you selected for your LMPC?
- What is the meaning of the content of your finger painting?

- Overall, what have you learned about yourself through these tasks?

Based on what you have learned from the assessments, make at least three short-term goals for yourself, to be achieved by the end of the semester. Now, discuss your responses in class. Using the individual goals, make a seven-step group intervention protocol following the guidelines by Cole[1] (see Exercise 8-3). Choose one of the following activities to develop an intervention that addresses the goal shared by most class members: baking, cooking, games, gardening, relaxation exercise, sewing, decorating, dancing, clay work, finger painting, painting with water colors, poetry, building models, or using a computer. Complete a 1-hour group process with the chosen activity as the group task.

EXERCISE 11-2: CLIENT EVALUATION USING EXPRESSIVE MEDIA ASSESSMENTS

For this exercise, refer to Albert's case below.

CASE STUDY: ALBERT

Albert was a 19-year-old African-American male who was brought to the occupational therapy clinic by his mother secondary to excessive drinking. During evaluation, he stated that he was also experiencing impotence but he did not want his mother to know. Albert had been visiting prostitutes for sex since he was 14 years old. At age 16, he contracted a sexually transmitted disease (STD), after which he started drinking heavily and became impotent. He stated that when a doctor confirmed

Continued

CASE STUDY: ALBERT—CONT'D

that he was impotent, he lost interest in everything and dropped out of school.

Albert was second in a family of three siblings (all boys). His older brother was at the university. He felt that this brother was better than he was. He described his life at home as "tense," stating that "everybody's attention is focused on me."

What occupational therapy assessments derived from the Psychodynamic conceptual model of practice could you use to evaluate Albert? In groups of two, complete the following:

1. Demonstrate how you would administer the assessments, with one student playing the "client" and the other playing the "therapist."
2. Make a treatment plan for Albert based on the intervention guidelines provided in the Psychodynamic conceptual model.
3. Choose an occupation that you would use as a medium in therapy to help Albert achieve his therapeutic psychodynamic goals. Explain the reason for your choice of the occupation.
4. Discuss your treatment plan for Albert in class.

REFERENCES

1. Cole MB: *Group dynamics in occupational therapy,* ed 3, Thorofare, NJ, 2005, Slack.
2. Drake M: The use of expressive media as an assessment tool in mental health. In Hemphill-Pearson BJ, ed: *Assessment in occupational therapy mental health: an integrative approach,* Thorofare, NJ, 1999, Slack, pp. 129–137.
3. Hemphill-Pearson BJ: How to use the BH battery. In Hemphill-Pearson BJ, ed: *Assessment in occupational therapy mental health: an integrative approach,* Thorofare, NJ, 1999, Slack, pp. 139–152.
4. Lerner CJ: Magazine Picture Collage. In Hemphill B, ed: *The evaluative process in psychiatric occupational therapy,* Thorofare, NJ, 1982, Slack, pp. 139–154, 361–362.

Chapter **12**

The Behavioral/Cognitive-Behavioral Conceptual Model of Practice

After reading Chapter 10 of your textbook, you are now aware that therapists using the Behavioral/Cognitive-Behavioral conceptual model of practice aim at helping clients remain functional by learning skills and performance capabilities that help them counteract stressful circumstances in their lives. More specifically, the objective of a therapist using this model is to assist the client to identify and modify maladaptive behaviors, learn information-processing skills to facilitate adaptive occupational performance, and identify self-defeating cognitive distortions that impede adaptive functioning and replace them with those that support adaptive functioning. In this chapter, you will engage in an exercise to facilitate beginning mastery of intervention strategies used in this model to help clients achieve the above-mentioned objectives (you may also want to revisit Exercises 6-2 to 6-4 at this time). Please read Chapter 10 of your textbook before completing this exercise.

EXERCISE 12-1: USING BEHAVIORAL/ COGNITIVE-BEHAVIORAL STRATEGIES IN THERAPY

For this exercise, refer to Kuria's case below.

CASE STUDY: KURIA

Kuria was a 12-year-old Kenyan primary school student who was brought to the counseling center after he was suspended from school for behavioral problems. He was the second child in a family of four children (three boys and one girl). Both his parents were poor farmers in their small, 3-acre piece of land in a small village in the central province of Kenya. His uncle worked as a clerk with the Ministry of Health in Nairobi. He was brought to therapy by his uncle who was asked by his parents to help. He had been caught smoking (which was against school rules), and refused to do the punishment that he was given (cleaning staff toilets). When confronted about his punishment, he became belligerent, shouting at the teacher and threatening to hit her. At home, he had become unruly and threatening to his brothers and his sister.

Kuria had always been a weak student. Often, he came last in his class in examinations. He often turned in work late, and many times his assignments were incomplete. He was withdrawn and did not associate with other students. At one time, he had beaten another boy in his class very badly for making a comment about his dirty school uniform. At 8 years of age, he was caught smoking for the first time. Since then, he had problems with school authorities for smoking and other behavioral problems. He was described as being disruptive in

Continued

CASE STUDY: KURIA—CONT'D

class, bullying other students, and smoking. He had been suspended from school several times. However, this time, the school headmaster informed the parents that Kuria would not be accepted back in school unless he received therapy and significantly changed his attitude and behavior.

On the first meeting with Kuria, the therapist observed that his hair was unkempt, and his clothes were dirty. He emitted a body odor, indicating that he had not taken a bath for a while. He seemed unconcerned and angry. When asked why he refused to do his punishment and threatened to beat up his teacher, he said that he was dumb and did not want to go to school anyway. At some point during the initial interview, Kuria was asked to tell time by the clock on the therapist's office wall. He

was unable to read the clock. The therapist decided to consult a psychologist to have Kuria tested for dyslexia. The tests revealed that indeed, he was dyslexic and could not process both verbal and numeric information appropriately. He expressed his concern that people, including his teachers and other students, would really know how dumb he was. The therapist surmised that this fear was the source of his behavioral problems. Apparently, he would rather be perceived as a tough miscreant rather than a stupid kid. Further interview revealed that Kuria enjoyed sports and particularly liked to play soccer and ping pong. However, because of his behavioral problems, he was not included in the school soccer team and could not find a partner with whom to play ping pong.

Using Ellis' *G, ABC, D* model as a guide (see Chapters 3 and 10 of your textbook):

1. Identify the following:
   a. Dysfunctional behavior that interferes with Kuria's adaptive occupational participation, including events that precede that behavior.
   b. Possible information-processing problems that may interfere with his ability to engage in occupations that he wants, is expected to do, or needs to do.
   c. Automatic cognitive distortions that may be interfering with his adaptive occupational performance.
2. Identify behaviors, information-processing skills, and thought patterns that Kuria may need to develop in order to complete occupations that he wants, is expected to do, or needs to do successfully and function more adaptively in his life.
3. State the behavior, skills, and thought patterns identified in item 2 above as behavioral goals that are observable, measurable, and

stated in action words expressing what would be readily seen, heard, read, and so on, once the goal is achieved.
4. Describe and demonstrate instruments that you would use to observe and measure the above-stated behaviors, skills, and thought patterns, in order to establish a baseline of Kuria's performance. Describe how you would record the assessment information.
5. Identify and describe in detail intervention strategies including activities, procedures, and techniques that you would use to address the goals stated in item 3 above, including activities that you would use as "experiments" and other procedures that you would use to "dispute" his cognitive distortions.
6. Identify appropriate reinforcers for Kuria, and establish a reinforcement schedule that will be used in therapy.
7. Describe ongoing evaluation of Kuria, including how you would demonstrate progress or lack thereof.
8. In small groups (not exceeding 10 students), choose an activity that may be used as an

intervention medium to address Kuria's goals and those of other clients who may have similar problems. Using Cole's seven-step group format,[1] develop a group protocol. Run a group session in the small lab group based on the protocol.

REFERENCE

1. Cole MB: *Group dynamics in occupational therapy,* ed 3, Thorofare, NJ, 2005, Slack.

Chapter **13**
The Cognitive Disabilities Conceptual Model of Practice

Read Chapter 11 of your textbook before completing the exercises in this chapter. To complete the exercises, you will need: the Allen Cognitive Level Screen (ACLS) testing kit, a copy of the Routine Task Inventory (RTI), and the Allen Diagnostic Module (ADM). Your lab instructor will demonstrate how to administer the three evaluation tools. At a minimum, you will be shown how to administer the ACLS so that you are proficient with this screening test, even if there is not enough time to demonstrate the RTI and the ADM.

EXERCISE 13-1: EVALUATION OF COGNITIVE DISABILITY

After your lab instructor demonstrates how to administer the ACLS, RTI, and ADM, students will group into pairs and practice administering the evaluation tools to each other. By the end of this exercise, each student should ensure that he or she has mastered all three stitches of the ACLS and the administration of the test. After the exercise, the class should reconvene

and the instructor facilitate a discussion using the following questions:

1. Discuss your experiences administering each of the three evaluation tools to your colleague and having them administered to you.
   a. What did you like about each of the tests?
   b. What did you dislike about them?
   c. How will your experience learning the three tools affect your clinical practice in future as an occupational therapist?
2. How do the three tools operationalize the theoretical constructs of the Cognitive Disabilities model (CDM)?
3. How do you think clients of different age groups and cultural backgrounds would react to each of the three tools (positively, negatively, or other reactions)? Explain.

EXERCISE 13-2: USING THE CDM TO GUIDE OCCUPATIONAL THERAPY INTERVENTION

For this exercise, refer to Florence' case below.

CASE STUDY: FLORENCE

Florence is a 73-year-old Caucasian female who was admitted to the subacute rehabilitation center where you work, with a diagnosis of Pick's disease, left shoulder fracture, and contusions to the head. Prior to admission 3 days ago, Florence lived in a

group home with assistance from a certified nurse's aide who came everyday to help her with ADLs. She had been living at the group home for the last 6 months. Her husband passed away about 2 years ago, and before moving to the group home, she

CASE STUDY: FLORENCE—CONT'D

lived at their home where they had lived for 50 years. Florence has one daughter who visits her regularly. Her daughter decided to take her to the group home after she noticed that Florence was getting increasingly forgetful and was unsafe living at home alone. She sustained a shoulder fracture due to a fall when she tripped over a throw rug while going to the bathroom.

Observation of Florence while doing ADLs indicated that she has difficulty motor planning and sequencing activities to complete simple ADLs such as grooming, bathing, dressing, and toileting. During one instance while she was combing her hair, Florence became distracted when a nurse's aide came into the room to get her roommate. She placed the comb on the sink counter behind a bottle of shampoo and seemed

to forget what she was doing. When the therapist redirected her back to the task, Florence could not find her comb. She did not seem to think about looking behind objects such as the shampoo bottle in order to find it.

Therefore, Florence requires constant verbal cueing to stay on task. Her topographical orientation is impaired, and she often gets lost and agitated because she cannot find her room. She is oriented to her name as indicated by responding when called by the therapist. However, it was not possible to test her orientation to time and place during initial evaluation because she is aphasic. On administration of the ACLS, Florence fiddled with the leather, pushing the needle through the holes at random. She eventually lost interest (after less than a minute) and pushed it away.

Answer the following questions based on the above case history, your reading in Chapter 11 of the textbook, and the description of responses to stimuli in Table 13-1:
1. What is Florence' cognitive level?
2. According to the CDM, what is her predicted ability to complete ADLs independently and safely?

3. Would intervention for Florence based on the CDM be expectant, supportive (palliative), or compensational? Explain.
4. Make a treatment plan for Florence, consisting of short-term and long-term goals, based on guidelines from the CDM. Be sure to include discharge recommendations in your treatment plan, and provide a rationale for them.

Table 13-1.   OBSERVABLE BEHAVIORS INDICATIVE OF CHARACTERISTICS TYPICAL OF VARIOUS ALLEN COGNITIVE LEVELS

Allen Cognitive Level (ACL)	Behavior Descriptive of the ACL
1.0	Withdraws from noxious stimuli
	Is passive and dependent
	Moans or cries out
1.2	Responds to stimuli by facial expression
	Uses nonverbal communication
1.4	Tracks a moving cue by turning head
	Swallows
	Expresses pleasure and displeasure by grunting and smiling
1.6	Moves spontaneously in bed
	Sits with support for short periods of time
	Drinks from a cup
	Cries out to express discomfort

Continued

Table 13-1. OBSERVABLE BEHAVIORS INDICATIVE OF CHARACTERISTICS TYPICAL OF VARIOUS
ALLEN COGNITIVE LEVELS—CONT'D

Allen Cognitive Level (ACL)	Behavior Descriptive of the ACL
1.8	Assists with bed mobility
	Raises buttocks and extremities with cues
	Strikes out to protect self
	Communicates through incomprehensible vocalizations and facial expressions
2.0	Overcomes gravity to sit up, lean forward, or pivot-transfer
	May shower and use the toilet with assistance
	Imitates counting to 3
	Responds to inquiries with yes or no
	Uses gestures to communicate
2.2	Spontaneously stands and stretches out arms to protect self when there is risk of fall
	Names touched body parts
	States name
	Speaks primary language
	Stands and sits on command
2.4	Wanders aimlessly until tired
	Bends at waist for ADLs (e.g., spits toothpaste)
	Uses one word to initiate conversation
	Climbs over bedrails
	Voices needs
2.6	Walks to familiar locations
	Catches, bounces, and pulls objects
	Steps over things and walks sideways to avoid obstacles
	Walks independently but needs assistance for safety
	Sings and names destinations
2.8	Uses railings and grab-bars for support
	Clings to things for support until feels safe
	Drinks and eats finger foods independently (with verbal cues)
	May burn self or spill food, and does not observe table manners
	Grips toilet paper or pants but needs assistance to complete toileting
	Learns songs with actions
	Expresses comfort or discomfort using short phrases
3.0	Grasps objects placed in front of him or her
	When dining, misses foods too far from the perimeter of the plate
	States name on request
	Names objects, and may state what to do with them
	Answers questions related to comfort
3.2	Distinguishes between objects
	Realizes that objects (such as faucets) can be moved
	Utters short phrases
	Sorts out objects by color, size, and shape
	Sustains actions only for few seconds at a time
	Writes name with dominant hand

Table 13-1. OBSERVABLE BEHAVIORS INDICATIVE OF CHARACTERISTICS TYPICAL OF VARIOUS ALLEN COGNITIVE LEVELS—CONT'D

Allen Cognitive Level (ACL)	Behavior Descriptive of the ACL
3.4	Sustains action, such as washing table, for up to 1 minute
	May follow right-to-left sequences
	Names objects
	Notices and recalls familiar objects
	Answers questions related to comfort, but does not initiate actions
	Independently locates bathroom or bedroom
	Requires cues for next step to complete ADLs
3.6	Notices effect of actions on objects
	Sorts objects by name, shape, and color, and names them
	Needs verbal cues for sequencing of every step
	Is concerned about privacy
	May put things in drawers
	Correctly uses pronouns
3.8	Uses all objects to complete an activity
	Recalls three-step sequences
	Puts clothes on
	Has initial understanding of what is to be done, but gets lost as activity progresses
	Follows verbal directions to keep working
	Communicates needs
	Cannot solve problems
	Does not realize physical limitations
	Does not wash hands without supervision
4.0	Follows a sequence independently to complete a short-term task
	Performs familiar self-care routine
	Is aware of personal possessions
	Reads but cannot follow written directions
	Is aware of friendly social interactions
	Is aware of gross time parameters such as morning, noon, and night
	Follows simple directions without cues
	Washes hands after toileting
4.2	Differentiates parts of an activity
	Asks for information
	Uses objects that are in plain sight
	Learns his or her way around a building
	Asks for help when needed
4.4	Completes goals
	Notices and uses objects that are in plain sight
	Recognizes errors
	Is aware of social norms
4.6	Scans the environment
	May live alone with daily assistance
	Sees objects in plain sight at a distance

Continued

Table 13-1. OBSERVABLE BEHAVIORS INDICATIVE OF CHARACTERISTICS TYPICAL OF VARIOUS ALLEN COGNITIVE LEVELS—CONT'D

Allen Cognitive Level (ACL)	Behavior Descriptive of the ACL
4.8	Engages in rote learning, using lists
	Asks for verification
	Reads and follows a schedule independently
	Requires assistance for safety hazards
	May attend regularly scheduled activities independently
	Believes that there is nothing wrong with him or her
5.0	Learns independently
	Follows simple written instructions with verbal cues
	Questions the need for activities
	Toilets independently
	Does not see crumbs or spills, and disposes of trash
5.2	Attends to details of actions
	Needs weekly checks to ensure safe ADL performance
	Uses aids such as a clock to orient self to time
	Notices hazards at the surface
5.4	Engages in self-directed learning
	Initiates cleanup
	Adjusts pace
	Is independent in routine bathing
5.6	Is aware of social standards
	Is independent in ADLs, can drive, and can provide child care
	Follows safety precautions
	Has insight in disability and safety hazards
5.8	Consults with others to seek their opinions
	Observes social manners
	Anticipates and takes action to prevent problems
	May live and work independently
6.0	Plans actions
	Independently takes medications as prescribed

Data from Aegis Therapies: *Cognitive checklist,* unpublished document, Fort Smith, Arkansas.

Chapter **14**
The Model of Human Occupation

Read Chapter 12 of your textbook before completing the exercises in this chapter. In Chapter 12, you found that therapists whose therapeutic interventions are guided by the Model of Human Occupation (MOHO) conceptualize the occupational human as a system consisting of four components: volition, habituation, performance capacity, and the environment.[3,4] The four components interact dynamically and heterarchically, leading to emergence of thoughts, feelings, and actions, which could be either adaptive or maladaptive. When emergent thoughts, feelings, and actions are maladaptive, the therapist intervenes by altering one or more (or all four) components. The alteration leads to a shift in the dynamic interaction between the four components, leading to emergence of new thoughts, feelings, and actions that are hopefully more adaptive.

In this chapter, you will practice administering at least three MOHO assessment instruments (one each observation-based, self-report, and interview-based, respectively). Learning how to administer these assessments will provide you with a foundation for treatment planning based on the MOHO. The following instruments are recommended:

- Observation-based—The Assessment of Communication and Interaction Skills (ACIS)[1]: This instrument is recommended over the Assessment of Motor and Process Skills (AMPS) because specialized training and a computer program are required for the latter, which is not realistic for initial education of entry-level occupational therapy students.

- Self-report—The Role Checklist[6]: This instrument is recommended over the Interest Checklist because it assesses past, present, and anticipated future involvement in roles that are socially accepted and meaningful to clients. The assessment is therefore broader, more meaningful, and relevant to goals of therapy (to facilitate client adaptive capacity) than an inventory of interests.

- Interview-based—Occupational Circumstances Assessment-Interview and Rating Scale (OCAIRS)[2]: This instrument is recommended over the Occupational History Interview, version 2 (OPHI-II) because it takes less time than the latter to administer and is therefore more realistic for a lab session with time limitations.

For these lab sessions, provide copies of the ACIS, the Role Checklist, and the OCAIRS to students. If there is time in the lab, students can practice the Modified Interest Checklist,[5] since it is readily available. A copy of the Modified Interest Checklist is shown in Figure 14-1.

EXERCISE 14-1: ADMINISTERING THE MOHO ASSESSMENTS

Your lab instructor will demonstrate how to administer each of the three MOHO assessments: the ACIS, the Role Checklist, and the OCAIRS. After the demonstration, group into pairs and take turns administering the instruments to each other. After each student has had a chance to experience administering the assessments, reconvene in class

INTEREST CHECKLIST

| Activity | What has been your level of interest? | | | | | | Do you currently participate in this activity? | | Would you like to pursue this in the future? | |
| | In the past 10 years | | | In the past year | | | | | | |
	Strong	Some	No	Strong	Some	No	Yes	No	Yes	No
Gardening/Yardwork										
Sewing/Needlework										
Playing cards										
Foreign languages										
Church activities										
Radio										
Walking										
Car repair										
Writing										
Dancing										
Golf										
Football										
Listening to popular music										
Puzzles										
Holiday activities										
Pets/Livestock										
Movies										
Listening to classical music										
Speeches/Lectures										
Swimming										
Bowling										
Visiting										
Mending										
Checkers/Chess										
Barbecues										
Reading										
Traveling										
Parties										
Wrestling										
Housecleaning										
Model building										
Television										
Concerts										
Pottery										

Figure 14-1. The Modified Interest Checklist.
(From The Model of Human Occupation website. Retrieved November 14, 2005, from http://www.moho.uic.edu/images/Modified%20Interest%20Checklist.pdf.)

INTEREST CHECKLIST

| Activity | What has been your level of interest? | | | | | | Do you currently participate in this activity? | | Would you like to pursue this in the future? | |
| | In the past 10 years | | | In the past year | | | | | | |
	Strong	Some	No	Strong	Some	No	Yes	No	Yes	No
Camping										
Laundry/Ironing										
Politics										
Table games										
Home decorating										
Clubs/Lodge										
Singing										
Scouting										
Clothes										
Handicrafts										
Hairstyling										
Cycling										
Attending plays										
Bird watching										
Dating										
Auto-racing										
Home repairs										
Exercise										
Hunting										
Woodworking										
Pool										
Driving										
Child care										
Tennis										
Cooking/Baking										
Basketball										
History										
Collecting										
Fishing										
Science										
Leatherwork										
Shopping										
Photography										
Painting/Drawing										

Figure 14-1.   Cont'd.

and discuss your experiences, using the following questions as a guide:

1. What is your level of confidence administering each of the three instruments?
2. What did you like most about each assessment?
3. What did you like least about each assessment?

4. How do these instruments compare with other assessments that you have learned so far?
5. Do you have any other comments?

EXERCISE 14-2: INTERVENTION USING THE MOHO

For this exercise, refer to Grant's case below.

CASE STUDY: GRANT

Grant is a 35-year-old Caucasian male diagnosed with major depressive disorder (MDD). He has a history of poly-substance abuse, including use of cannabis and amphetamines. He has been admitted several times at the state psychiatric hospital. The last admission was 6 months ago, and he has been in the hospital since then. The psychiatrist referred Grant to occupational therapy this week due to his short attention span, disheveled appearance, poor anger management, and deficient coping strategies. He is now being evaluated by the occupational therapist.

Grant was born and raised in Canton, Ohio. He has a younger sister who visits him at the hospital regularly. His father is in his late sixties and lives in Iowa, and his mother is deceased. The relationship between Grant and his father is strained, and they do not see much of each other. He started abusing substances when he was 13 years old. After receiving his high school diploma, he went to college to pursue a bachelor's degree in music. At that time, he had a busy schedule, and although he was occasionally abusing substances, it was not a significant problem in his life. After graduating college, Grant started playing piano at a nightclub. While employed there, he started abusing alcohol, cannabis, and amphetamines heavily. This became

disruptive to his occupational performance. He received several DUI citations and lost his driver's license as a result.

During his depressive episodes, Grant tends to become angry quickly. He expresses this anger through disruptive behavior and eventually withdrawing. The facility where he is admitted uses token economy, where earned tokens are used to purchase privileges and enjoyed activities. Grant enjoys listening to music and playing piano. He also likes watching sports. However, because of his disruptive behavior due to anger, he has been losing privileges and is not able to participate in the above activities at the present time.

Working in groups of three, choose MOHO instruments that you can use to evaluate Grant's role performance and occupational adaptation. In about 1 hour and 15 minutes, while one student plays the role of the "client," the other two students should administer the chosen assessments. After completing the evaluation, make a treatment plan for Grant (see examples of how to make treatment goals consistent with MOHO constructs in the case of Jay in Chapter 12 of your textbook). Now, reconvene the class and discuss the treatment plans established in the small groups.

REFERENCES

1. Forsyth K, Salamy M, Simon S, et al: *The assessment of communication and interaction skills (version 4.0),* Chicago, 1998, Model of Human Occupation Clearinghouse, Department of Occupational Therapy, College of Allied Health Sciences, University of Illinois at Chicago.

2. Haglund L, Henriksson C, Crisp M, et al: *The occupational circumstances assessment interview and rating scale (OCAIRS), version 2.0,* Chicago, 2001, Model of Human Occupation Clearinghouse, Department of Occupational Therapy, College of Allied Health Sciences, University of Illinois at Chicago.

3. Kielhofner G: Dynamics of human occupation. In Kielhofner G, ed: *Model of human occupation: theory and application,* Philadelphia, 2002, Lippincott Williams & Wilkins, pp. 28–43.

4. Kielhofner G: Volition. In Kielhofner G, ed: *Model of human occupation: theory and application,* Philadelphia, 2002, Lippincott Williams & Wilkins, pp. 44–62.

5. Kielhofner G, Neville A: *The modified interest checklist,* Chicago, 1983, unpublished manuscript, University of Illinois at Chicago. Retrieved from http://www.moho.uic.edu/images/Modified%20Interest%20Checklist.pdf.

6. Oakley F, Kielhofner G, Barris R: An occupational therapy approach to assessing psychiatric patients' adaptive functioning, *Am J Occup Ther* 39:147–154, 1985.

Chapter **15**

The Sensory Processing/Motor Learning Conceptual Model of Practice

In Chapter 13 of your textbook, we introduced the Sensory Processing/Motor Learning (SP/ML) conceptual model of practice. According to this model, *dysfunction* is conceptualized as the inability to access sensory information from the environment, modulate it, and produce coordinated, smooth movements necessary for appropriate occupational functioning. Therapeutic intervention for clients with this problem consists of controlled sensory input to help the client learn to modulate sensations and facilitate smooth, coordinated motor functioning through use of activities designed to provide vestibular and proprioceptive stimulation. After reading Chapter 13 of your textbook, complete Exercise 15-1 below. For students to benefit optimally from the lab experience, instructors should complete the exercise before the lab so they can compare their evaluation findings and treatment plan with those of the students.

CASE STUDY: SAM

Sam is a 26-year-old African-American male who was admitted to the state hospital with an Axis I diagnosis of schizophrenia (nonparanoid type), posttraumatic stress disorder (PTSD), and alcohol dependence. There are no Axis II or III diagnoses, and Axis IV and V diagnoses have been deferred to the psychologist. This is Sam's ninth admission to the state hospital. His first admission was 6 years ago, soon after he was honorably discharged from the U.S. Marine Corps.

Sam is one of four children. None of the other family members has a history of mental illness. Sam presents with general disorganization and inactivity. Prior to the recent admission, it was reported that he spent most of his days sleeping and was unable to take care of basic self-care needs. Since admission, Sam has been observed to be withdrawn. He does not interact with other patients, and when spoken to by the hospital staff, he responds with one-word or short phrases. He was brought to the hospital by his mother and brother. Sam presents with the typical schizophrenic S posture and walks slowly with a shuffling gait with eyes downcast. He does not initiate any activities and reports that he has no energy to do anything.

Sam has been in the hospital now for 3 days. He is currently on oral 1500 mg of Depakote (valproic acid) for mood stabilization. He is also on oral 15 mg Zyprexa (olanzapine) for management of schizophrenic symptoms. The last time Sam worked was at least 1 year ago, when he worked as a plant mechanic for a company that makes carpets. When the therapist interviewed him, Sam expressed a desire to go home and resume his job as a plant mechanic.

EXERCISE 15-1: ASSESSMENT AND TREATMENT PLANNING

Based on your readings on Chapter 13 of your textbook, and working in pairs:

Explain the SP/ML assessments that you may administer to Sam and the rationale for your choice. With one student playing the role of the "client" and the other playing the "therapist," administer the suggested SP/ML assessments in about 20 minutes.

Based on findings from the assessments, make a treatment plan for Sam. Ensure that even though the treatment goals aim at enhancing sensory integration and motor control, they are related to the client's meaningful occupations and are directed toward functional outcomes (engagement in meaningful occupations).

Suggest activities that can be used for therapeutic intervention that are related to Sam's meaningful occupational functioning while at the same time addressing his sensory integration and motor-control needs (by stimulating both the vestibular and proprioceptive systems). The activities should also challenge Sam's problem-solving, sensory integration, and motor-control skills in order to facilitate CNS self-organization.

After about 45 minutes working in groups of two, combine into larger groups of about six students. Using the therapeutic goals and activities generated in the groups of two, make a group protocol for Sam and other clients with similar problems using Ross's[2-4] guidelines for a five-stage group process[1] (see Table 13-1 in Chapter 13 of your textbook). This activity should take about 15 minutes.

Now reconvene in class and discuss treatment goals and group protocols, and compare them with those of your instructor. Run a 45-minute group process in class using one of the group protocols.

REFERENCES

1. Cole MB: *Group dynamics in occupational therapy: the theoretical basis and practice application of group intervention,* ed 3, Thorofare, NJ, 2005, Slack.
2. Ross M: *Integrative group therapy: the structured five-stage approach,* ed 2, Thorofare, NJ, 1991, Slack.
3. Ross M: *Integrative group therapy: mobilizing coping abilities with the five-stage group,* Bethesda, MD, 1997, American Occupational Therapy Association.
4. Ross M, Bachner S, eds: *Adults with developmental disabilities: current approaches in occupational therapy,* ed 2, Bethesda, MD, 2004, American Occupational Therapy Association.

16
The Developmental Conceptual
Model of Practice

In Chapter 14 of your textbook, we introduced the Developmental Conceptual model of practice. This model is used by occupational therapists to guide them in the assessment of clients' adaptive skill levels, and developmental-stage–specific task accomplishment. This assessment identifies deficient adaptive skills and developmental tasks that the client needs to accomplish to adapt effectively to his or her environment according to social and cultural expectations for a person in that age-specific developmental stage. An environment that facilitates skill development and accomplishment of identified tasks is then created and relevant occupations are used to challenge the client to learn the required skills and therefore accomplish the developmental tasks. The laboratory exercise in this chapter will help you practice administering client assessment, treatment planning, and therapy implementation using the guidelines of the developmental conceptual model of practice.

After reading Chapter 3 (the developmental psychology section) and Chapter 14 of your textbook, complete Exercise 16-1. While choosing therapeutic media consistent with complexity/chaos theoretical principles, think of age-appropriate and developmental-stage–appropriate occupations and occupational tasks that can be used to provide "disequilibriating" experiences (see discussion of this construct in Chapter 14 of your textbook) that will facilitate movement of Fred's person-system from equilibrium and reorganization at a higher developmental stage. Such occupations should pose developmentally appropriate challenges in his environment to which he would need to respond in order to adapt. For example, making a scaled paper pattern of a shirt was used as such a challenging occupational task in the treatment of Ken in Chapter 14 of your textbook.

CASE STUDY: FRED

Fred was a 21-year-old African male of Tutsi ethnicity from Rwanda, Africa. He was a refugee who fled Rwanda during the horrible genocide that took place in 1994 in which his entire family was killed. He had been the firstborn of five children, including one brother and three sisters. He came into a crisis counseling center in Nairobi, Kenya, in which an occupational therapist was volunteering his services. He had been referred to the center for intervention due to increasing depression and unspecified complaints of physical illness. All medical investigations revealed nothing physically wrong with Fred.

During the initial interview, Fred presented as a well-kempt young man, polite, and appropriately responsive to questions (but not very talkative). His eyes were downcast throughout the initial interview. Fred gave the impression of a person

---

CASE STUDY: FRED—CONT'D

with very low energy. The image that came into the therapist's mind as he was looking at Fred was that of a deflated balloon. Fred expressed to the therapist that he felt lost, had no possessions that he could call his own apart from the clothes he was wearing, had no friends, and was on the verge of losing all hope. The therapist could clearly perceive this sense of hopelessness.

EXERCISE 16-1: USING THE DEVELOPMENTAL CONCEPTUAL MODEL TO GUIDE FRED'S THERAPY

Working in pairs, with one student playing the role of the client and the other the therapist, complete an occupational therapy evaluation of Fred. Refer to the outline of life developmental tasks in Table 16-1 and the *Cognitive Adaptive Skills Evaluation: Protocol Sheet* in Figure 16-1 to complete the evaluation and answer the following questions:

1. What meaningful occupation-related tasks/activities (that are personally and culturally meaningful to Fred) can you use to enable you to assess Fred's developmental level as defined in the outline of developmental tasks in Table 16-1? Explain how such an activity could help you determine Fred's developmental stage.
2. Based on your evaluation using both the outline of developmental tasks and the *Cognitive Adaptive Skills Evaluation: Protocol Sheet,* what are Fred's (a) developmental stage, (b) developmental skill deficits, and (c) task accomplishment needs?
3. Based on your evaluation findings, develop treatment goals for Fred.

Now, combine into small groups of about six students. Using the goals developed in pairs, establish a group protocol that may be used to treat Fred and other clients with similar problems. Run a 1-hour group process based on the protocol. Reconvene the class and discuss your experiences in the laboratory exercise.

While the *Cognitive Adaptive Skills Evaluation: Protocol Sheet* is a good instrument for assessing cognitive skill acquisition, the authors seem to have included some concepts whose operationalization is not clearly defined. For example, it is not clear how "moral behavior" may be evaluated from the information gleaned from this evaluation. How does a client's answer to the question, "How did you decide what materials to use?" inform the therapist about the client's sense of moral judgment about use of materials? Overall, however, it is a comprehensive assessment instrument for the purpose for which it was designed.

Table 16-1. LIFE DEVELOPMENTAL TASKS

Life Stage Process	Developmental Tasks	Psychosocial Crisis	Central Process
Infancy (birth to 2 years)	Social attachment Sensorimotor primitive intelligence causality Object permanence Maturation of motor functions	Trust versus mistrust	Mutuality with a caregiver
Toddlerhood (2 to 4 years)	Self-control Language development Fantasy and play Elaboration of locomotion	Autonomy versus shame and doubt	Imitation

Continued

Table 16-1. LIFE DEVELOPMENTAL TASKS—CONT'D

Life Stage Process	Developmental Tasks	Psychosocial Crisis	Central Process
Early school age (5 to 7 years)	Sex role identification Early moral development Concrete operations Group play	Initiative versus guilt	Identification
Middle school age (8 to 12 years)	Social cooperation Self-evaluation Skill learning Team play	Industry versus inferiority	Education
Early adolescence (13 to 17 years)	Physical maturation Formal operations Membership in a peer group Romantic relationships	Group identity versus alienation	Peer pressure
Late adolescence (18 to 22 years)	Autonomy from parents Sex role identity Internalized morality Career choice	Individual identity versus role diffusion	Role experimentation
Early adulthood (23 to 30 years)	Marriage Childbearing Work Lifestyle	Intimacy versus isolation	Mutuality among peers
Middle adulthood (31 to 50 years)	Management of a household Childbearing Management of a career	Generativity versus stagnation	Person-environment fit and creativity
Late adulthood (51 years and older)	Redirection of energy to new roles Acceptance of one's life Developing a point of view about death		

Adapted from Newman BM, Newman PR: *Development through life: a psychosocial approach,* Homewood, Illinois, 1979, Dorsey Press, pp. 30–31.

Cognitive Adaptive Skills Evaluation:
Protocol Sheet

Examinee Information:

Name: _____   Birth date/age: _____ Sex: _____

Floor/unit: _____   Admitting and discharge diagnosis: _____

Test date: _____   Indicate day of week tested: _____

Examiner:_____   Length of test time: _____

Evaluation materials:

12-inch ruler with numbers
One sheet each of $8^{1}/_{2}$ x 11 paper
  (yellow, blue, pink, white)
#2 pencil with eraser
Three pens (one blue, one red, one black)
Box of eight assorted wax crayons
A sample calender
Written directions, typed on an index card

Presentation of materials:

All materials with the exception of the sample calender listed above are to be laid out directly in front of the examinee. Writing tools and crayons are to be placed in the same general area, in a group. All sheets of paper are to be in a loose pile, with each sheet being exposed or visible to some degree, in the following order: yellow, blue, pink, white.

General introduction to be given to examinee:

Examiner states: "I am interested in how you go about doing a task. I need this information in order to help plan a program with you. We will discuss what you have done after you have completed the activity."

Turn the page and go on to specific directions and interview questions. Check behaviors as observed; note additional behaviors and comments in the Comments column.

Figure 16-1.   Cognitive Adaptive Skills Evaluation: Protocol Sheet.

(From Hemphill Pearson BJ: Cognitive adaptive skills evaluation: protocol sheet. In Hemphill Pearson BJ, ed: *Assessments in occupational therapy mental health: an integrative approach,* Thorofare, NJ, 1999, Slack, pp. 367–376.)

Continued

Directions	Behaviors and Categories	Checks	Comments/ Examinee's Responses

Directions

Present written directions to the examinee.

(Allow silent reading time.)

Examiner states: "Please read the directions aloud and begin when you are ready."

(If the examinee begins to work and completes the task, note and record behaviors and proceed with first set of interview questions and directions #2.)

(If the examinee reads directions but does not begin to work, read direction #1 to the examinee.)

Examiner states:
#1. "Here are supplies. Use what you want to make a calendar for 1 week."

(If the examinee is unable to begin working after directions are read to him or her, read directions again and proceed to direction #3.)

If the examinee can complete the task with no further directions, observe and record comments and behaviors.)

Proceed with interview questions.

Behaviors and Categories

Language
- Follows written directions
- Understands directions as given by "authority figure" (9)
- Attempts to perceive others' viewpoint; seems to know what is expected/being asked of him or her; seeks validation (8)

Cause and effect
- Seems to have a plan, works rapidly, efficiently, systematically (10)
- Trial and error behavior noted with objects, but works independently (9)
- Process seems inflexible; deliberate manipulation of objects (7-8)
- Tries to work with objects and process, seeks validation (5-6)

Images
- Seems to understand "calendar" and the steps involved in making one (9)
- Seeks validation about "what kind" of calendar (6)
- Seeks validation about own perception of "calendar" (6)

Judgment/moral behavior
- Knows the rules and agrees to follow them; engages in activity as presented (does not ask for extra materials or try to make something else) (9)
- Believes he or she knows the rules but tries to alter or refuse task (8)

Classification
- Can form classes and consider objects in several classes simultaneously (S to S=1 week; 7 days=1 week) (9)

Relations
- Has one to one correspondence; sees connection and knows S to S=7 days=1 week
- Equivalence unstable, confused by space; counting doesn't help (confuses days of week or number of days) (8)

Numbers
- Can arrange figures along some quantities dimension; seriation; can construct group of equal number and knows they are equal when spatial relations are changed or are counted in a different order (9)
- Counts repeatedly; changes size of figures to make them equal (7-8)

Figure 16-1. Cont'd.

Directions	Behaviors and Categories	Checks	Comments/ Examinee's Responses

Interview questions: First set

Examiner asks: (One question at a time)

A. "What does the word calendar mean to you?"

B. "How did you decide what materials to use?"

C. "Did you have a plan for making the calendar?"

(If response is yes, ask question C1; if no, skip to C2.)

C1. "Can you describe the plan to me?"

C2. "Were you taught to make calendars in that way or did you think of it yourself?"

D. "What came to your mind when you saw or heard the word calendar?"

D1. "Does the calendar you made look like others you have seen?"

D2. "Does your calendar look the way you had hoped it would?"

Language
- Meanings are discussed in the abstract, hypothetical (10)
- Can discuss several meanings from different perspectives (9)
- Meanings deal with the present, here and now (8)
- Word has personal meaning based on own perception, intuition, experience (7)

Judgment/decision making
- Seems to have inner value system and a sense of moral judgment about use of materials (10)
- Choice seems to be part of a systematic plan (10)
- Past experience and desires influence behavior (7)
- Random selection; no thought

Cause and effect (problem solving)
- Has a work plan; is rational, systematic flexible (10)
- Operations are concrete; apply only to objects physically present (9)
- Plan based on past experience (7-8)
- Convert trial and error; problem solved as they developed (6)
- Overt trial and error; concretely tested out solutions (5)
- Establish a goal; one scheme to deal with each goal (4)

Images
- Transformational; can change shape and position, and the intermediary steps involved (9)
- Static; lacks reversibility (7-8)
- Images used to test solutions (5)
- Trial and error variations (5)

Figure 16-1.   Cont'd.

Continued

Directions	Behaviors and Categories	Checks	Comments/ Examinee's Responses
Examiner states: #2. "Make another calendar for 1 week."	**Language** • Seems to plan work steps; rational, systematic (10) • Understands directions as given by "authority figure," verbal directions (9) • Seems to know what is expected/ being asked of him or her (8)		
(Observe and record behaviors while the examinee is working on second calendar.) (If the examinee does not begin to make second calendar, repeat direction #2.)	**Judgment** • Willingly responds to directions (9) • Ignores rules; testing, resistive (6) • Past experience influences behavior; disinterest expressed (7)		
(If there is still no response, the examiner asks: "Are there other ways to make a calendar?") (If the response is yes, the examiner states: "Please show me or tell me how.")	**Cause and effect** • Transformational images used; able to change shape, size, direction of new calendar (9) • Static; calendar identical to first; product and process (7-8) • Overt trial and error; seeking novelty, tries to make calendar different, tries possibilities; expanding schemes (5-6)		
(Note in comments section if responses are verbal only, and check appropriate boxes.)	**Classification** • Can form classes; days of week and number of days (9) • Can place into class but not rearrange; days and number of days identical to first calendar (8) • Starts to form class and becomes confused or distracted (7)		
(If response is no, go on to interview questions.) On completion of second calendar, proceed with second set of interview questions.	**Relations** • Plans how to establish equivalence; concept of week remains even if calendar is different in shape or size or made differently (9) • Equivalence is unstable, confused by space; counting doesn't help; overtly tries to pattern second calendar after first (8) • Centers; focuses on one part or aspect of an object, ignoring the rest (7)		

Figure 16-1.   Cont'd

Directions	Behaviors and Categories	Checks	Comments/ Examinee's Responses
Interview questions: Second set	**Language** • Can discuss several meanings from different perspectives (9) • Meanings deal with the present, here and now (8) • Concrete reasoning based on past experience (7)		

Directions

Interview questions: Second set

E. "What does the word *another* mean to you?"

F. "How is your calendar like or different from a monthly calendar?"

G. "How can these calendars be used?"

(Pointing to or indicating calendars examinee has made.)

H. "How is your first calendar the same or different from your second calendar?"

If the examinee is able to follow directions above and answer interview questions with no further clarification from the examiner...

Evaluation is complete—STOP.

Behaviors and Categories

Language
• Can discuss several meanings from different perspectives (9)
• Meanings deal with the present, here and now (8)
• Concrete reasoning based on past experience (7)

Relations
• Has correspondence; establishes equivalence (weeks to month) (9)
• Equivalence unstable, confused by space (8)
• Focuses on one part only and ignores other possibilities (7)

Classification
• Can form classes and consider objects in several classes simultaneously; (month/weeks) (9)
• Cannot rearrange or place in other relationships; (weeks to month)
• Starts to form a class and becomes confused or distracted (7)

Cause and effect
• Can think about abstract, hypothetical; thought is flexible, rational (10)
• Use according to previous operations performed physically by individual (9)
• Static use; stated only as individual currently uses (7-8)
• Delayed imitation; indicates he or she has seen or heard of uses in past (6)

Relations
• Can establish equivalence (9)
• Equivalence unstable; confused by space; counting doesn't help (8)

Number
• Can identify equal number and knows they are equal (9)
• Does not understand they are equal even if they are equal in number (8)

Classification
• Can consider objects simultaneously; discusses similarities and differences (9)
• Alternates discussion of similarities and/or differences; one calendar to another (7-8)
• Discusses calendars separately; does not do comparative analysis (7)

Figure 16-1.   Cont'd.

Continued

Directions	Behaviors and Categories	Checks	Comments/ Examinee's Responses

Examiner states:
#3. "Please repeat the directions to me."

(If the examinee is able to proceed after he or she states directions or after the examiner restates directions, allow to complete task and then proceed with interview questions.)

(If the examinee cannot repeat directions and/or does not engage in task even after the directions have been restated, proceed with the following.)

Examiner states:
"Do you understand what I mean by a calendar for 1 week?"

Examiner states:
"Can you tell me how to make one?"

(A positive response to both questions may indicate no problems with language or problem solving; restate reason for task to address moral judgment.)

(In the case of a negative response to either question, proceed to direction #4.)

Examiner states:
#4. "Make a calendar that looks like this."

Present sample calendar and continue to show it until the examinee stops examining it (looks away), then remove.

Language
- Is able to repeat directions (9)
- Can auditorily focus and understand the viewpoint of others including authority figures
- Is unable to repeat directions (questions written and/or auditory memory, ability to auditorily focus and/or use language)
- Words have personal meaning; own definition of words. Repeats directions in own words (7)
- Understands the viewpoint of others, including authority figures (9)
- Attempts to perceive viewpoint of others (8)
- Words have personal meaning (7)

Circular reactions (cause and effect)
- Covert trial and error problem solving; images used to test solution (describing procedure) (6)
- Perceived actions, varied, repeated varied another way, repeated (5)
- Uses two familiar schemes to establish a goal (4)
- Chance movement; magical thinking (3)
- No attempt to reach out (2)

Imitation
- Uses delayed imitation (6)
- Serial imitation; new scheme imitated and assimilated into own scheme (5)
- Action expands his or her familiar scheme (4)

Figure 16-1. Cont'd.

Directions	Behaviors and Categories	Checks	Comments/ Examinee's Responses

(If after reviewing sample, the examinee begins to work and complete task, return to direction #2. Make another calendar and interview questions following it.)

(If the examinee asks to see sample again, or to have sample continuously visible, present sample and note behaviors.)

(If the examinee completes task using sample, return to direction #2. If unable to do second calendar, go on to interview questions. If unable to do second calendar, break down activity and attempt a second calendar.)

(If unable to begin task even with sample visible, break activity down and proceed with structured direction #5.)

Examiner states:
#5. "First draw the lines, then write in the days."

(If the examinee is able to begin work and complete the calendar, go back to direction #2 and interview questions.)

(If the examinee is unable to begin working, go on to direction #6.)

Circular reaction (cause and effect)
- Images used to test solution to problem (6)
- Seeking novelty; variations in own actions (6)
- Utilizes two schemes to establish a goal (4)
- Magical thinking

Object permanence
- Explores potential of other objects and people (5)
- Object visually perceived as different from self; object has own movement, causing own effect (4)
- Objects understood in terms of own actions; action can be stopped and then resumed (3)

Time concept
- Attention focused until bored with activity (5)
- Can focus for 30-45 minutes; can anticipate future events based on interpreting signs, utilizing actions of others (4)
- Attention is action oriented (3)

Circular reaction
- Utilizes two familiar schemes to establish goal (4)

Imitation
- New learning based on old schemes (4)

Object permanence
- Object perceived as different from self; has own movement and cause (4)
- Object is permanent; action stopped and resumed (3)

Time concept
- Can focus attention 30-45 minutes (4)

Figure 16-1.   Cont'd.

Continued

Directions	Behaviors and Categories	Checks	Comments/ Examinee's Responses

Examiner states:
#6. "Do as I do..."

a. "Draw a line like this." (Line 1) (Permit the examinee to draw line.)
b. "Now draw a line like this." (Line 2)
c. "Now write Sunday over the first square."

Imitation
- Patient can imitate therapist when own familiar schemes are used (3)
- Able to use direct imitation (3)

Circular reactions
- Own actions are the cause of everything (3)
- Chance body movements, attempts to repeat (2)

Object permanence
- Patient can stop an action and then resume (3)

Time concept
- Focused attention for repetitive actions. Can remember events based on own action (3)
- Can focus attention for 2 minutes before he or she gets distracted (2)

(If the examinee seems to have difficulty with the days of the week, use abbreviations: S, M, T, W, Th, F, S.)

Continue to label the days of the week.

(If the examinee is able to complete the calendar, attempt direction #2 and/or interview questions.)

(If the examinee is unable to complete the calendar, attempt interview questions.)

End of evaluation procedure.
Review and analyze results.

References
Allen C: *Thought process and activity analysis chart,* Unpublished, 1972.
Ginsburg H, Opper S: *Piaget's theory of intellectual development,* Englewood Cliffs, NJ, 1969, Prentice-Hall.
Mosey AC: *Three frames of reference for mental health,* Thorofare, NJ, 1970, Charles B. Slack.
Singer D, Reverson T: *A Piaget primer: how a child thinks,* NY, 1978, A Plume Book, New American Library.

Figure 16-1.   Cont'd

Sunday	Monday	Tuesday	Wednesday	Thursday	Friday	Saturday

Sample for Direction #6 Only

(11)	(12)	(13)	(14)	(15)	(16)	(17)

Line #1

Sunday	Monday	Tuesday	Wednesday	Thursday	Friday	Saturday

Line #3

| Line #5 | Line #6 | Line #7 | Line #8 | Line #9 | Line #10 | Line #4 |

Line #2

For examiner use only; not to be presented to the examinee.

Figure 16-1.   Cont'd.

Continued

Cognitive Adaptive Skills Evaluation Summary Sheet

Frequency and distribution of behaviors:

	Time concept	Language	Judg-ment and moral behavior	Images	Classi-fication	Relations	Numbers	Imitation	Circular reactions	Object perman-ence
Level 3										
Level 4										
Level 5										
Level 6										
Level 7										
Level 8										
Level 9										
Level 10										

Problem identification:

Summary of assets:

Goals:

Possible learning approaches:

Figure 16-1. Cont'd.

Chapter 17

The Occupational Adaptation Conceptual Model of Practice

In Chapter 15 of your textbook, we introduced the Occupational Adaptation (OA) conceptual model of practice. You are now aware that the overarching goal for therapists using this model is to help clients develop a functional gestalt consisting of appropriate level of occupational adaptation energy, occupational adaptive response mode, adaptive response behaviors, and combination of the three person-systems (sensorimotor, cognitive, and psychosocial) and the environment so as to achieve relative mastery (ability to perform meaningful occupations effectively, efficiently, and to self-satisfaction and satisfaction of significant others). Exercises 17-1 and 17-2 will help you master the skills needed to help facilitate development of relative mastery as defined in the OA conceptual model of practice. Refer to the guidelines in Table 17-1 to help you complete the exercises.

EXERCISE 17-1: SELF-ASSESSMENT OF INTERNAL ADAPTATION PROCESS AND RELATIVE MASTERY

To complete this exercise, students should work in pairs. Using the guidelines in Table 17-1, each student should assess his or her occupational adaptation process and relative mastery with the help of his or her colleague by answering the following questions:

1. What is your current primary role?
2. What tasks/activities are associated with this role?
3. What is your current occupational environment?
4. What physical, social, and cultural aspects of your occupational environment facilitate or impede your ability to perform the role? Give examples.
5. Assess your relative mastery based on your performance of tasks associated with the current primary role by evaluating how well you perform the tasks with efficiency (appropriate use of resources, energy, and time) and effectiveness (ability to complete tasks accurately and as required), and satisfaction with yourself and from others (e.g., parents, teachers, colleagues, clients) regarding your performance.
6. What level of adaptation energy do you use most of the time when faced with challenges related to primary role activities (primary or secondary)? Explain.
7. What adaptive response mode do you use most of the time (i.e., approaches that have worked for you in the past, modified modes when methods used in the past are not effective, new approaches to solving problems associated with your role)? Give examples.
8. When faced with challenges associated with your primary role, what adaptive response behaviors do you use most of the time (primitive, transitional, or mature)? Explain.
9. How do your person-systems (sensorimotor, cognitive, and psychosocial) affect your adaptive response process and relative mastery as you respond to challenges associated with your primary role?

TABLE 17-1.   OCCUPATIONAL ADAPTATION GUIDE TO PRACTICE

Category	Questions
Occupational Adaptation Data Gathering/ Assessment	What are the client's *occupational environments* and *roles?*
	Which *role* is of primary concern to the client and his or her family?
	What occupational performance is expected in the primary *occupational environment* and *role?*
	What are the *physical, social,* and *cultural* features of the primary *occupational environment* and *role?*
	What is the client's *sensorimotor, cognitive,* and *psychosocial* status?
	What is the client's level of *relative mastery* in the primary *occupational environment* and *role?*
	What is facilitating or limiting *relative mastery* in the primary *occupational environment* and *role?*
Occupational Adaptation Programming	What combination of *occupational readiness* and *occupational activity* is needed to promote the client's *occupational adaptation process?*
	What help will the client need to *assess occupational responses* and use the results to affect the *occupational adaptation process?*
	What is the best method to engage the client in the *occupational adaptation* program?
Evaluation of the Occupational Adaptation Process	How is the program affecting the client's *occupational adaptation process?*
	Which *energy level* is used most often (*primary* or *secondary*)?
	What *adaptive response mode* is used most often (*preexisting, modified,* or *new*)?
	What is the most common *adaptive response behavior* (*primitive, transitional,* or *mature*)?
	What outcomes does the client show that reflect change in the *occupational adaptation process?* • Self-initiated adaptation • Enhanced *relative mastery* • Generalization to novel activities
	What program changes are needed to provide maximum opportunity for *occupational adaptation* to occur?

Italicized terms are constructs in the occupational adaptation model.
Adapted from Schkade JK, Schultz S: Occupational adaptation. In Kramer P, Hinojosa J, Royeen CB, eds: *Perspectives in human occupation: participation in life,* Philadelphia, 2003, Lippincott Williams & Wilkins, p. 213.

10. What do you think you can do to respond more adaptively to challenges associated with your primary role?

Take about 30 minutes to answer the above questions. Then discuss your answers with your colleague.

EXERCISE 17-2: CLIENT ASSESSMENT AND TREATMENT PLANNING

For this exercise, refer to Bret's case below.

CASE STUDY: BRET

Bret is a 65-year-old Caucasian male who was admitted to a subacute rehabilitation unit following a fall and fracture of the left hip. He had open reduction and internal fixation of the hip and was currently on toe-touch weight-bearing status, which required that he use a wheelchair and walker. Bret was referred to occupational therapy for training so that he could learn how to do basic ADLs in preparation for discharge to home with home health services.

This was the first time Bret had ever been admitted to a medical facility, and he was finding it very difficult to adjust. Up to 5 years before admission, he maintained his ranch, rode horses, mended fences, and generally took care of his cattle. His wife of 40 years had died 1 year before his fall. According to the social worker's notes in the chart, he had difficulty taking care of himself after his wife's death because he did not know how to cook, do laundry, or do general housekeeping. He had two sons who were married and lived in two different states with their own families. Therefore, Bret did not have anyone to take care of him.

At the time the therapist met Bret, he was very angry with his current status. He was confrontational when the therapist made suggestions about devices that he could use to complete his ADLs such as dressing safely. He retorted that the therapist thought that she was very smart but in fact she was not. He did not want to learn how to use any devices or new ways of doing things although clearly he could not continue to function as he had done before the fall. Instead of learning how to use assistive devices or to solve problems so that he could take care of his needs independently and safely, he insisted that he was in a hospital and it was the duty of the therapist and other hospital staff to take care of him.

Working in pairs, use the guidelines in Table 17-1 to explain how you would assess Bret's internal adaptation process and relative mastery. Based on the assessment findings, suggest short- and long-term therapy goals that you may establish in collaboration with Bret. Suggest occupations/tasks/activities that may be meaningful to Bret and that you may use to facilitate the development of his internal adaptation process. Now combine into larger groups of up to six students. Using the goals developed in pairs, establish a group protocol for client's with similar problems to those experienced by Bret. Use the protocol to run a 45-minute activity group. Then reconvene the class and discuss your experiences. (Note that the case of Bret, a condition traditionally classified in the geriatric/physical dysfunctions category is chosen to emphasize that all clients experience psychosocial upsets, even when the primary problem is physical. If occupational therapists aim at treating the "whole person" as they should, then they need to address arising psychosocial issues such as denial, anger, and grief.)

Chapter 18

The Canadian Model of Occupational Performance

In Chapter 16 of your textbook, we introduced the theoretical core and therapeutic guidelines of the Canadian Model of Occupational Performance (CMOP). You learned that the major objective of this model is to help clients to perform occupations/tasks/activities that they want, need, or are expected to perform; are age-appropriate; and are recognized in their culture to their satisfaction. Exercises 18-1 and 18-2 in this chapter will help you develop the skills necessary to apply the guidelines of this model to help clients achieve the above stated objective. To complete the exercises, students will use the Canadian Occupational Performance Measure (COPM)[2] and the scoring cards for importance, performance, and satisfaction that are usually included with the interview forms and the COPM manual. The instructor will take about 30 minutes to demonstrate administration of the COPM interview with a student volunteer.

EXERCISE 18-1: ASSESSING EACH OTHER USING THE COPM

Working in pairs, after demonstration of administration by the instructor, use the COPM to interview and calculate each other's performance and satisfaction scores. This exercise should take about 40 minutes.

Exercise 18-2: Client Assessment Using the COPM

Working in groups of two or three, use the COPM interview to evaluate Joyce (see case study below). One student will act the role of the client and the other the therapist. The third student may be an observer, making notes so as to give constructive feedback to the "therapist" regarding his or her performance in the interview.

CASE STUDY: JOYCE

Joyce is a 16-year-old Kenyan adolescent daughter of a single mother who was brought to the occupational therapist for consultation due to complaints of abdominal discomfort and poor performance in school. She is in form two (the Kenyan equivalent of tenth grade) in a public high school. Her mother became pregnant with Joyce when she was a teenager and had to drop out of high school. She did not want to discuss Joyce's father with the therapist.

Joyce had a normal childhood and completed primary school (the Kenyan equivalent of eighth grade) without any notable problems. She presented to the therapist as a young attractive woman who was neat and well-kempt. During the brief initial interview, Joyce expressed her anxiety about successfully completing high school and passing her national form four (Kenyan equivalent of twelfth grade) examination. She wanted

CASE STUDY: JOYCE—CONT'D

to attend the university to study to be either a doctor or teacher, and she needed to pass the exam with good grades (*B+* average or better) in order to gain admission to a public university. Further inquiry revealed that she did not feel that she knew how to study and that she had difficulty grasping the materials discussed in class. Furthermore, she missed class often due to her abdominal problems.

Consultation with the clinical officer (Kenyan equivalent of a physician assistant) who had treated her revealed that all laboratory tests indicated nothing physically wrong with Joyce. The clinical officer suspected that her abdominal problems were psychosomatic and probably related to anxiety about her performance in school.

Use the following questions to guide your work with Joyce:

1. What other professionals do you think you may need to consult in order to better define Joyce's problem?
2. Using the COPM interview, evaluate Joyce's ability to choose, organize, and perform with satisfaction to her and her mother occupations that are meaningful to her and that she wants, needs, or is expected to perform; are age-appropriate; and are recognized in her culture.
3. Using the findings from the COPM evaluation, establish short- and long-term goals for Joyce and an intervention plan based on the CMOP. For each intervention strategy suggested in the proposed treatment plan, identify the CMOP phase of therapy as described in Chapter 16 of your textbook.

REFERENCES

1. Law M, Baptiste S, Carswell A, et al: *Canadian occupational performance measure*, ed 3, Ottawa, ON, 1998, CAOT Publications ACE.
2. Law M, Baptiste S, Carswell A, et al: *Canadian occupational performance measure*, ed 4, Ottawa, ON, 2000, CAOT Publications ACE.

Chapter **19**

Integrating Conceptual Models of Practice

In Chapter 17 of your textbook, we presented proposed ideas for integration of conceptual models of practice for application in clinical practice. We discussed the differences between eclecticism, integrationism, and strategic eclecticism. We also proposed a framework for dynamic integration of conceptual models in psychosocial occupational therapy practice. Exercise 18-1 will help you develop the clinical reasoning skills necessary to enable you to systematically integrate conceptual models of practice to address pertinent clients' occupational performance issues. Instructors may consider giving this exercise as a semester assignment for the course.

EXERCISE 19-1: BRINGING IT ALL TOGETHER THROUGH A CASE STUDY

In groups of two, visit a psychiatric hospital, day treatment center, outpatient occupational therapy department, or another facility that offers services to individuals with psychosocial issues. Identify a client receiving services at the facility. Obtain informed consent from the client and administrative approval to interview him or her. Interview and observe him or her for at least 1 day. If you are unable to obtain approval from the facility to interview the client directly, you can interview the therapist, family members, or other health care personnel working with the client (such as the occupational therapist, nurse, social worker, psychologist, physician, and so on). In the interview, obtain the client's diagnoses (Axis I to V), detailed history of the illness, and the presenting issue(s), including occupational performance concerns.

Once you have details of the case history and presenting problem, complete a literature review focusing on what is known about the client's condition. Find research evidence that indicates what has been successful in treating the condition, especially effective methods used by occupational therapists. Choose one conceptual model of practice that best explains the client's occupational performance issues as presented in the case history. Provide a sound rationale for your choice of the model, supporting it with evidence from literature. With the model as a guide, choose assessment instruments.

With one student playing the role of the client and the other playing the role of the therapist, complete an evaluation using the chosen instruments (if you are already licensed to administer occupational therapy assessments, you may evaluate the client directly). Formulate short- and long-term goals. Choose and outline the intervention methods, strategies, and procedures that you will use to intervene, and clearly identify the conceptual models from where they are derived. Provide a detailed rationale for your choice of methods, strategies, and procedures. Explain how they are consistent with the theoretical principles of the model that you are using to organize therapeutic intervention.

Now, prepare a paper, using APA style, outlining your case study. The paper should contain the following:

1. A detailed case description and history.
2. The conceptual model of practice used to organize therapy and the rationale for its choice. Explain the theoretical core and intervention

guidelines of the model, and research evidence supporting its clinical effectiveness in treating similar conditions.

3. The occupational therapy assessment instruments and procedures used, the conceptual models of practice from which they are derived, and the rationale for their choice. If the assessment instruments and procedures are derived from models other than the organizing model, explain their compatibility with the model.

4. The findings of your assessment.

5. Short- and long-term goals.

6. A demonstration of your clinical reasoning process leading to problem identification and goal formulation (use the M-A-P-P instrument described in Chapter 6 of your textbook).

7. Outline of the intervention methods, strategies, and procedures. Explain the conceptual models of practice from which they are derived and the reason for their choice, including any research evidence available demonstrating their clinical effectiveness.

8. If you are already licensed to provide occupational therapy, implement the intervention plan. If you are not licensed or able to work with clients, imagine implementing the model and what progress you would expect.

9. Write at least one progress note, and demonstrate how you would modify your treatment plan according to the outcome of intervention.

PART IV

Occupational Therapy Across the Continuum of Care

This final section of the Lab Manual, consisting of Chapters 20 to 24, provides exercises to help the occupational therapy student heighten his or her awareness of the wide scope of occupational therapy practice. In Chapter 20, the reader will participate in laboratory activities designed to help develop skills that enhance the view of occupational therapy within the lifespan developmental perspective. The student will experientially learn that irrespective of the specific interventions used, therapy must be viewed within the context of life stages since therapeutic activities have to be meaningful to the client, and the client's developmental stage in part determines what is meaningful. In Chapter 21, the student will learn to identify psychosocial issues associated with physical disabilities and develop intervention strategies to address these issues. This chapter is designed to help develop awareness that psychosocial skills are applicable in all areas of occupational therapy practice.

In Chapter 22, the reader will practice skills that enhance the development of group interventions that address occupational performance issues of clients suffering from alcohol/substance abuse. Chapter 23 provides exercises that facilitate the development of skills for successful incorporation of family caregivers as allies in the client's rehabilitation, and skills that address the psychosocial needs of caregivers that will improve their psychosocial status and subsequently the quality of life of the client. Finally, Chapter 24 provides an exercise that will facilitate the development of skills necessary to attain community-based occupational therapy practice.

Chapter **20**
Occupational Therapy Across Ages

In Chapter 18 of your textbook, we emphasized that irrespective of the conceptual model of practice adopted by an occupational therapist, he or she has to view a client's occupational performance issues within the lifespan developmental perspective. This is because the developmental tasks that a client is required to accomplish according to his or her developmental stage and the social/cultural expectations in part determine how meaningful he or she perceives therapeutic interventions to be. Therefore, client-centered, collaborative therapy that is consistent with the dictates of the current occupational therapy paradigm is not possible without due consideration of a client's developmental stage and the developmental tasks that he or she wants or is socially and culturally required to master. The exercises in this chapter will help you improve your skills in identifying pertinent developmental tasks for clients based on an understanding of the assumptions and research evidence from the lifestyle developmental theory, as discussed in Chapter 18 of your textbook.

EXERCISE 20-1: DETERMINING YOUR DEVELOPMENTAL TASKS

After reading Chapter 18 of your textbook, in groups of two, complete the following exercise by answering the questions below:

1. What is your current developmental stage?
2. What developmental tasks are you culturally expected to accomplish at this stage?

3. Reflect on your performance of these tasks. How well are you accomplishing the developmental tasks that you are culturally expected to achieve at your developmental stage?
4. If you are not accomplishing your developmental tasks according to expectations, how is your performance affecting your ability to adapt to family, cultural, and personal expectations?
5. How could you redesign your lifestyle in order to perform better? For example, how could you change your daily routine and the occupations in which you participate in order to achieve the developmental tasks according to expectations?

Help each other answer the above questions as exhaustively and honestly as possible. This should take about 30 minutes.

Now reconvene in class, and discuss your findings with other students. This should take about 45 minutes.

EXERCISE 20-2: OCCUPATIONAL THERAPY INTERVENTIONS FOR ALL AGES

In Chapters 2 to 17 of this manual, you analyzed 10 case vignettes in order to learn how to gather clinical data, interpret them, and plan occupational therapy interventions using a variety of conceptual models of practice. Now, working in groups of two, revisit the case studies. For each case, determine the client's developmental stage and the issues related to accomplishment of developmental tasks according to his or her cultural expectations. After reflecting on each treatment plan that you developed to address the client's issues, determine the extent to which the plan addressed the identified developmental concerns. This should take about 30 minutes.

Now reconvene in class, and discuss your findings with other students. This should take about 45 minutes.

Chapter **21**

Expanded Psychosocial Occupational Therapy Practice

In Chapter 19 of your textbook, we emphasized that every physical condition that may be within the domain of concern of an occupational therapist presents with accompanying psychosocial issues that the therapist needs to address. In other words, it can be said that every occupational therapist is a psychosocial occupational therapist, irrespective of the area of specialization (e.g., pediatrics, physical disabilities, geriatrics). Exercise 21-1 in this chapter is designed to help you heighten your clinical awareness necessary to help you identify and plan interventions to address psychosocial concerns for clients with physical disabilities.

EXERCISE 21-1: PSYCHOSOCIAL OCCUPATIONAL THERAPY FOR CLIENTS WITH PHYSICAL DISABILITIES

After completing Exercise 21-1, you will be able to do the following:

1. Identify psychosocial issues of clients with a variety of psychosocial conditions
2. Establish short- and long-term goals to address the identified psychosocial issues
3. Suggest specific therapeutic interventions to address the established goals

Read the following case vignettes and complete the following exercise:

CASE STUDY: GILL

Gill is a 30-year-old African-American female with a diagnoses of lupus, myositis, and pneumonia. She was admitted to the subacute rehabilitation unit after falling at home. This is her second admission due to medical problems related to her diagnosis. About 2 months ago, Gill had been in the hospital for about 2 weeks, where she received both physical therapy and occupational therapy. She was then discharged to home where she resided with her husband and 7-year-old daughter until this admission. She has been referred to occupational therapy and physical therapy for rehabilitation to prepare her for discharge to home in about 2 weeks.

During occupational therapy evaluation, Gill complained of tingling and numbness in the area of median nerve distribution of the right upper extremity. Review of her chart reveals that she had a diagnosis of carpal tunnel syndrome (CTS) about 6 months ago. She is wearing braces on both wrists. She requires moderate assistance with transfers from low to high surfaces, and standby assistance for dynamic standing balance. Gill has difficulty maintaining head in midline, requires moderate assistance for upper-body dressing, maximum assistance for lower-body dressing, moderate assistance for toileting, and moderate assistance for grooming.

Continued

CASE STUDY: GILL—CONT'D

During the interview, Gill demonstrated appropriate interaction skills, responding appropriately to all the therapist's inquiries. She expressed concern about her husband continuing to find her attractive as she, to quote her, "withers away" and becomes disfigured. She was also frustrated because of having to ask for help to accomplish basic tasks such as dressing and grooming. She expressed concern that she is not even able to put on makeup independently in order to look nice for her husband. She was also worried about how she would continue to take care of her daughter. She stated that her husband is wonderful and very helpful, but the role of being a mother was extremely important to her and she was distressed about not being able to perform it as she thought appropriate.

CASE STUDY: ANA

Ana is a 55-year-old Caucasian female with left hemiparesis following a right cerebral vascular accident (CVA). Before the CVA and subsequent admission to the hospital, Ana lived at home with her 59-year-old husband. They have two daughters who are married and with their own families. On occupational therapy evaluation, she was found to have difficulty with bilateral coordination. As a result, Ana needs minimum assistance with basic ADLs such as grooming and toileting. She is ambulating using a walker with standby assistance. Ana requires minimum assistance for sit to stand, walker to toilet, and walker to tub transfers. She requires minimum assistance to maintain balance for cleaning after toileting.

Ana is a retired teacher who was very independent and active throughout her life. She enjoyed gardening, cooking, and hiking with her husband. During the initial interview, she expressed anxiety about her being able to continue maintaining her garden, cooking nice meals for her husband, and hiking. She was very upset that she had to ask for help even to go to the bathroom. She stated that this was the biggest assault on her dignity.

CASE STUDY: CONDY

Condy is a 27-year-old Caucasian male suffering from the early stages of symptomatic HIV infection. He was diagnosed with HIV seropositivity 2 years ago and put on retroviral medication. However, he started drinking heavily and using crack cocaine and did not observe his treatment regimen. He broke up with his girlfriend whom he had been dating for about 3 years. He stopped socializing with his friends and became more and more isolated. He lived with his parents and was unemployed. Six months ago, Condy started having persistent cough, shortness of breath, and fatigue. He also had lesions all over his chest. Two weeks ago, he was found having passed out in the bathtub by his mother. He was rushed to the hospital where he was treated for cardiopulmonary complications of opportunistic infections due to compromised immune functioning.

Condy was referred to occupational therapy for evaluation and treatment in preparation for discharge to home to live with his parents. During the initial interview, he was found to be in

---

CASE STUDY: CONDY—CONT'D

low spirits, not maintaining eye contact with the therapist, and minimally communicative. Condy answered questions in single phrases and did not elaborate on his answers until probing questions were asked by the therapist. The therapist

gathered from the interview that Condy has not disclosed to his family or the few friends that he still has his HIV status for fear that they would reject him. He has not disclosed the diagnosis to his former girlfriend either.

To complete this exercise, work in groups of three. For the cases of Gill and Ana, determine the classification of their conditions (terminal or nonterminal). For each of the three cases:

1. Describe occupational therapy instruments that you may use to assess pertinent psychosocial issues.
2. With one student playing the role of each of the three clients (Gill, Ana, and Condy, respectively) and the other student playing the therapist, administer the assessments to each other. The other student should observe and make notes so as to provide constructive feedback.
3. Identify psychosocial issues for each of the three clients.
4. In the case of Condy, use the Pizzi Assessment of Productive Living (PAPL) (Figure 21-1) in addition to other chosen occupational therapy instruments, in order to assess his psychosocial needs even more specifically.
5. For each of the three clients, make short- and long-term goals to address the identified psychosocial issues.
6. Discuss specific therapeutic interventions that you may use to address these issues and meet the established goals.

(This exercise should take 1 hour.)

Now reconvene the class and discuss the findings of your small-group exercises. Each small group will take about 15 minutes to demonstrate suggested interventions to address psychosocial issues for each of the three clients.

The reader should note that there are some shortcomings to the assessment in Figure 21-1. For instance, most of the questions seem to be addressed to the client, indicating that it is a form of structured interview. However, some of the questions seem to be addressed to the therapist (e.g., the questions pertaining to the social and physical environment). This can be confusing. The other shortcoming is that many of the questions are closed-ended, requiring yes/no types of answers. For example, "Are there certain times of day that are better for you to carry out daily tasks?" A better question would be, "What times of day are better for you to carry out daily tasks?" There are many questions phrased in this manner. A therapist using this assessment should bear in mind this shortcoming so that he or she can rephrase the questions as appropriate to encourage the client to express himself or herself more fully.

Also, there are other instruments that may be better suited to facilitate the client's development of certain insights. For instance, one of the PAPL questions is "What do you wish to accomplish with the rest of your life?" The Assessment and Intervention Instrument for Instrumentalism in Occupational Therapy (AIIIOT)[1] may be better suited to elicit that kind of information since it is designed to facilitate articulation of mission in life and establishment of goals whose achievement would lead to attaining that mission (see Figure 10-1 in Chapter 10 of this manual).

DEMOGRAPHICS

Name _____ Age _____ Sex _____

Lives with (relationship) _____

Identified caregiver _____

Race _____ Culture _____ Religion (practicing?) _____

Primary occupational roles _____

Primary diagnosis _____

Secondary diagnosis _____

Stage of HIV _____

Past medical history _____

Medications _____

ADL (USE ADL PERFORMANCE ASSESSMENT)

Are you doing these now? _____

Do you perform homemaking tasks? _____

For Areas of Difficulty

Would you like to be able to do these again like you did before? _____

Which ones? _____

Work

Job _____

When last worked _____

Describe type of activity _____

Work environment _____

If not working, would you like to be able to? _____

Do you miss being productive? _____

Play/Leisure

Types of activity engaged in _____

If not, would you like to? Which ones? _____

Would you like to try other things as well? _____

Is it important to be independent in daily living activities? _____

PHYSICAL FUNCTION

Active and passive ROM _____

Strength _____

Sensation _____

Coordination (gross and fine motor or dexterity) _____

Visual–Perceptual

Hearing _____

Balance (sit and stand) _____

Ambulation, transfers, and mobility _____

Activity tolerance and endurance _____

Figure 21-1. Pizzi Assessment of Productive Living (PAPL).
(Modified from Pizzi M: HIV infection and occupational therapy. In Mukand J, ed: *Rehabilitation for patients with HIV disease*, New York, 1991, McGraw-Hill, pp. 283–326.)

Pain

Location _____

Does it interfere with doing important activities? _____

Other

Sexual function _____

Cognition (attention span, problem solving, memory, orientation, judgment, reasoning, decision making, safety awareness)

_____

TIME ORGANIZATION

Former daily routine (before diagnosis) _____

Has this changed since diagnosis? _____

If so, how? _____

Are there certain times of day that are better for you to carry out daily tasks? _____

Do you consider yourself regimented in organizing time and activity or pretty flexible?_____

What would you change, if anything, in how your day is set up? _____

BODY IMAGE AND SELF-IMAGE

In the last 6 months, has there been a change in your physical body and how it looks?_____

How do you feel about this? _____

SOCIAL ENVIRONMENT

Describe support available and used by patient _____

PHYSICAL ENVIRONMENT

Describe environments in which the patient performs daily tasks and the level of support or impediment for function

_____

STRESSORS

What are some things, people, or situations that are/were stressful?_____

What are some current ways you manage stress?_____

SITUATIONAL COPING

How do you feel you are dealing with:

  Your diagnosis_____

  Changes in the ability to do things important to you _____

  Other psychosocial observations _____

OCCUPATIONAL QUESTIONS

What do you feel to be important to you right now? _____

Do you feel you can do things important to you now? _____

In the future?_____

Do you deal well with change?_____

What are your hopes, dreams, aspirations?_____

What are some of your goals? _____

Have these changed since you were diagnosed? How?_____

Do you feel in control of your life at this time?_____

What do you wish to accomplish with the rest of your life?_____

Figure 21-1.   Cont'd.

Continued

OCCUPATIONAL THERAPY

Plan _____

Short-term goals _____

Long-term goals _____

Frequency _____

Duration _____

Therapist _____

Figure 21-1.   Cont'd.

REFERENCE

1. Ikiugu MN: Instrumentalism in occupational therapy: guidelines for practice, *Internat J Psychosocial Rehabil* 8:165–179, 2004.

Chapter 22
Occupational Therapy for Clients with Substance Abuse Disorders

Elizabeth A. Ciaravino

Individuals with substance abuse disorders face specific challenges such as loss of life skills, a feeling of loss of control, and problems with the law that disrupt their ability to function adaptively. In this laboratory exercise, you will have the opportunity to further explore the treatment needs of substance abusers, especially females, who have special challenges due to their dependence on men, and some of whom may suffer from low self-esteem as a result of having had to engage in prostitution in order to obtain money for drugs.

As noted in the history section of Chapter 20 of your textbook, the originator of methods used to treat individuals with substance abuse problems was Father Egan. He was keenly aware of the specific needs of females leaving prisons, and helped develop halfway houses and residential treatment facilities for them. The issue of whether or not treatment facilities for males should be considered differently from those for females deserves more attention, and has been less well-researched than other aspects of treatment for substance abusers.[2] It is clear, however, that female substance abusers have special needs that require specific attention.

EXERCISE 22-1: OCCUPATIONAL THERAPY ASSESSMENT FOR FEMALE SUBSTANCE ABUSERS

Think about the types of occupational performance skills that might be particularly compromised for a female substance abuser. Within your small group, determine the types of questions that might be asked of a female client who is just beginning treatment. You may consult the Canadian Occupational Performance Measure (COPM)[3] for guidance regarding the occupational performance areas to explore.

EXERCISE 22-2: OCCUPATIONAL THERAPY INTERVENTION FOR FEMALE SUBSTANCE ABUSERS

In your small groups, use Cole's seven-step format[1] to design a small-group occupational therapy intervention for the following female clients who have recently been discharged from a detoxification facility (see Chapter 7 of your textbook for an example of group protocol). The treatment program will range from 6 to 8 months in duration. Determine the areas that should be addressed in a comprehensive occupational therapy program.

Each small group will identify the following as part of developing the small-group protocol:

1. List of performance skills to be the focus for occupational therapy interventions.
2. List of questions to evaluate and clarify issues for female clients (these could be questions used for follow-up on an individual interview, or as topics for group discussions).

3. List of group and individual interventions for clients. Provide what you would like to see as a typical schedule.
4. List of community supports or resources available to support the treatment program for clients.

The following is a description of your clientele:

Jane is a 32-year-old Caucasian female with a long history of institutionalization and limited formal education. She has only recently entered the hospital for detoxification from heroin. She had been living with a man whom she states was physically abusive and who uses cocaine. Her appearance is noteworthy for a number of missing teeth.

Mary is a 22-year-old Caucasian college student who recently had to leave college because of her extensive alcohol and amphetamine abuse. An extremely bright and talented young woman, she reports that her parents are divorced and she has not had a close relationship with them. She has no significant health issues.

Yvonne is a 27-year-old African-American female with three small children, aged 3, 5½, and 7 years old, who are currently being cared for by her mother. She has a 5-year history of PCP abuse. She graduated high school and had begun attending a beauty school program, but became pregnant and left the school. Her children's father is in and out of the picture. Yvonne has supported herself with public assistance. She reports feeling guilty that she has to rely on her mother to care for the children. She has one close female friend who is also her lover. Yvonne continues to use PCP as well as other drugs.

Jeannie is a 22-year-old Hispanic female who left high school in the eleventh grade. She has had an extensive history of barbiturate abuse, has worked as an escort, and prides herself for her physical appearance. She has continued to refuse to apply for public assistance, stating that she can earn a lot more money doing the escort service.

Danielle is a 26-year-old female from an affluent family on the west coast, who has had a long history of poly-substance abuse. She was able to remain drug free for a 6-month period when she first moved to the area, but relapsed when she began performing (sex and dancing) in clubs. Danielle has made a tremendous amount of money, but has used it on drugs. She has a history of STDs and endocarditis. She also has a history of being extremely hostile toward other women.

Maria is a 39-year-old female with a long history of involvement in abusive relationships with men. She has also had an extensive history of heroin, methadone, cocaine, and amphetamine abuse. She presents as extremely self-derogatory (she is always looking for affirmation from staff). Maria has promised to end a relationship with a man who has threatened to kill her but admits that she is very afraid to do so in the event that he will do something to hurt himself. She is also being treated for depression with Effexor. Maria has had three children, two of whom are in foster care, and a third one who died in a car accident.

Kristen is a 19-year-old female with a 4-year history of cocaine abuse; she has primarily engaged in activities based on her interest in gothic concerns. She has a large group of friends from her neighborhood. Her father left her mother and the family last year. Kristin's mother has a new boyfriend, but Kristen finds him to be a little too "pushy." Her goals are to go to college to become a writer.

Lisa is a 28-year-old African-American female with a history of heroin abuse, is HIV positive, and has recently lost her grandmother who raised her. She has agreed to come to this group facility, but states that she has no interest in interacting with anyone.

Sadie is a 39-year-old married female, with two adolescent children and a husband who has a job as a laborer. Her husband ended up in a detoxification unit for alcohol and benzodiazepine abuse. She discloses feeling overwhelmed by a chronic pain condition, as well as alienation from her family and husband. She began stealing money from the church where she volunteered as a treasurer. An extremely pleasant and affable woman, one has the sense that Sadie is harboring much resentment.

Joan is a 29-year-old single female with a son aged 9 who is currently in a boarding school. She reports an extensive history of alcohol and marijuana abuse after numerous family losses and the breakup of a relationship with her son's father. She describes having very few friends, and having put on a good face for her co-workers in the accounting office. She worries that her migraine headaches are more than just that.

Holly is a 23-year-old Caucasian female who pinpoints her difficulties with heroin following an abortion and the involvement with a former boyfriend. She admits losing a lot of money and possessions to him. Holly also admits that she began to prostitute herself after he was arrested for a fight in a bar.

REFERENCES

1. Cole MB: *Group dynamics in occupational therapy: the theoretical basis and practice application of group intervention,* ed 3, Thorofare, NJ, 2005, Slack.
2. Kaskutas L, Zhang L, French M, et al: Women's programs versus mixed-gender day treatment: results from a randomized study, *Addiction 100* (1):60–69, 2005.
3. Law M, Baptiste S, Carswell A, et al: *Canadian Occupational Performance Measure,* ed 3, Toronto, Ontario, 2000, CAOT.

Chapter 23

Integration of Caregiver Issues in Psychosocial Occupational Therapy Intervention

In Chapter 21 of your textbook, we emphasized that family caregivers are important allies in the rehabilitation process for clients with psychosocial illnesses. We also mentioned that the psychosocial status of family caregivers affects the well-being and quality of life (QOL) of clients. Thus we underscored the necessity of collaboration with caregivers in the treatment of clients with psychosocial illnesses in order to realize positive outcomes of therapy. Specifically, it is necessary to address psychosocial needs of family caregivers. Therefore caregivers may sometimes be considered to be primary occupational therapy clients. We proposed an eight-step model of integrating family caregivers in the therapeutic process. We also discussed the occupational therapist's responsibility in the case of suspected abuse of individuals with mental illness. By completing Exercise 23-1 below, you will enhance your skills necessary to involve family caregivers in occupational therapy for clients with psycho-

social diagnoses. Be sure to read Chapter 21 of your textbook before completing the exercise.

After completing Exercise 23-1, the reader will demonstrate knowledge of the following:

1. Skilled use of therapeutic relationship to engage family caregivers as allies in occupational therapy intervention for clients with psychosocial illnesses.
2. The rationale for considering the family as an occupational therapy client.
3. Skills needed to facilitate family exploration of challenges posed by the client's psychosocial illness, solutions to meet those challenges, and their role in facilitating the client's occupational performance.
4. Skills needed to plan interventions to address psychosocial needs of family caregivers so that they are better allies in the client's rehabilitation.

EXERCISE 23-1

CASE STUDY: SALLY

Sally is a 27-year-old African-American female who was diagnosed with paranoid schizophrenia. She is the fourth child in a family of eight children (four boys and four girls). Her oldest sibling, a 35-year-old brother, is a high school teacher, married, and settled with his family. Her sister, the second child in the family, is 32 years old. She got pregnant at

age 18 and dropped out of high school. Subsequently, she had two other children, after which she ran away from home. She is now a prostitute living in New York. Her three children, all boys, 15, 14, and 12 years old respectively, live with her parents. Sally's other sister, 29 years old, is married and a stay-at-home mom. Her younger siblings are three

CASE STUDY: SALLY—CONT'D

brothers, 25 years old (in graduate school studying to be a social worker), 23 years old (employed as a salesperson in a department store), and 20 years old (in the local community college studying to be an air conditioning system installer). Sally's youngest sibling is an 18-year-old sister, a freshman in college. Her father is a Baptist church minister, and her mother is a licensed vocational nurse.

Sally got pregnant with her first child when she was 18 years old and got married. She had two other children with her husband. The initial diagnosis of her condition was at age 23, when her youngest child was still an infant. She started accusing her husband of cheating on her and planning to kill her so that he could marry his mistress. She became increasingly withdrawn, locking herself and the children in the bedroom. Her husband sought help, and she was taken to the local psychiatric hospital where she was diagnosed with paranoid schizophrenia and admitted. She was discharged after 6 weeks in the hospital with antipsychotic medication (Thorazine, a dopamine receptor antagonist) to control her symptoms such as delusions. However, she stopped taking her medication after several weeks due to adverse side effects. Consequently, she had a relapse and was readmitted. Since then, she has relapsed and has been readmitted to the hospital three times. After the second readmission, Sally's husband left. When she is not in hospital, Sally and her children live at home with her mother and father, her four younger siblings, and her three nephews.

Sally's latest relapse and admission was 2 weeks ago. On interviewing her parents, the occupational therapist found that she is unemployed and financially dependent. She is withdrawn and accuses her younger brothers of planning to poison her. Consequently, she refuses to take medication because of fear of being poisoned and also because of the uncomfortable side effects, which she takes to be evidence that she is being poisoned. Sometimes, she locks herself in her room with her children, for whom she does not take

care. Sally needs constant supervision while at home for her safety and the safety of the children. She does not help with any of the house chores and has no leisure interests. Her mother had to quit work so that she can take care of Sally and her children. This is a big added burden considering that her mother also has to take care of Sally's sister's teenage boys and her own youngest teenage daughter. The family is sensitive about Sally's condition, and they tend to limit social interaction in an attempt to hide it. When Sally is in the hospital, they tell people that she is visiting relatives in another state.

Working in groups of three, discuss and explain how you would do the following:

1. Engage Sally's family so that they are allies in her rehabilitation
2. Provide the family with information about Sally's illness
3. Collaborate with the family to identify challenges posed by Sally's illness
4. Discuss how to resolve these challenges
5. Facilitate family exploration of how to facilitate Sally's occupational performance in order to enhance her sense of inclusion, control, and affection
6. Lead the family in establishing therapeutic goals
7. Use "homework" to help the family facilitate Sally's occupational performance in such a way as to enhance her sense of inclusion, control, and affection
8. Intervene to address the psychosocial needs of the family, reduce their caregiver burden, and therefore enhance their psychological well-being so that they are more effective allies in Sally's rehabilitation

Develop occupational therapy short- and long-term goals for Sally, and demonstrate to the class how you would facilitate a family therapy session to help caregivers assist Sally to achieve the established goals.

Chapter

24

Community-Based Occupational Therapy Intervention

After reading Chapter 22 of your textbook, you now realize the need and importance for occupational therapists to take initiative in establishing interventions for clients with psychosocial illness living in the community. Community-based occupational therapy practice helps facilitate integration of clients with psychosocial illness so that they are fully participating citizens of the community. Exercise 24-1 will help you develop the skills necessary for community outreach as you endeavor to help establish community-based occupational therapy practice.

EXERCISE 24-1: ESTABLISHING COMMUNITY-BASED OCCUPATIONAL THERAPY PRACTICE

Working in groups of two or three, identify a community mental health facility or agency such as a day care center, community mental health center, homeless shelter, or soup kitchen. Visit the facility. If there is an occupational therapist at the facility, interview him or her and find out the type of clients served, occupational performance issues of concern to them, and occupational therapy interventions used to address these issues. Compare the program with the occupational therapy delivery process within the six-step framework described in Chapter 22 of your textbook. If there is no occupational therapist, interview the director or any person responsible for running the facility or agency.

Find out the types of clients served by the facility, and their occupational performance needs. Identify key individuals within the community, such as the librarian, physician, dentist, or grocery store manager, whose involvement may facilitate community integration of clients served by the facility.

Write and submit to your instructor a proposal for occupational therapy intervention to help integrate clients frequenting the facility/agency into the community. Your proposal should clearly outline a detailed plan for each of the following:

1. Educating clients, other professionals, and the community regarding the role, importance, and scope of occupational therapy within the agency
2. Enlisting the cooperation of key individuals in the community, such as the bank manager, librarian, or grocery store staff, in the rehabilitation of the agency clients
3. Identifying assessment instruments that you may use to evaluate clients attending the facility based on their needs as identified by the facility official you interviewed
4. A proposed comprehensive occupational therapy program including the date when the program is expected to begin; materials, supplies, other resources needed; and so on
5. Continued evaluation and refinement of the program for quality assurance

Vocabulary of Affective Adjectives*

Kind/Helpful/Loving/Friendly/Thankful

Adaptable
Admired
Adored
Affectionate
Agreeable
Altruistic
Amiable
Amorous
Appreciative
Aroused
Benevolent
Bighearted
Brotherly
Caring
Charitable
Cherished
Comforting
Compassionate
Compatible
Congenial
Conscientious
Considerate
Cooperative
Cordial
Dedicated
Dependable
Devoted
Diligent
Empathic
Fair
Faithful
Fatherly
Fond
Forgiving
Friendly
Gallant
Generous
Gentle
Genuine
Giving
Good

Gracious
Grateful
Helpful
Honest
Honorable
Humane
Idolizing
Indebted to
Involved
Just
Kind
Long suffering
Longing for
Loving
Mellow
Merciful
Mindful
Neighborly
Nice
Obliging
Open
Optimistic
Passionate
Patient
Praiseful
Respectful
Rewarded
Sensitive
Sharing
Sincere
Softhearted
Straightforward
Sympathetic
Tender
Thoughtful
Tolerant
Treasured
Trustful
Unassuming
Understanding
Unselfish
Warmhearted

Curious/Absorbed

Absorbed
Analyzing
Attentive
Concentrating
Considering
Contemplating
Curious
Diligent
Engrossed
Imaginative
Inquiring
Inquisitive
Investigating
Occupied
Pondering
Questioning
Reasoning
Reflecting
Searching
Thoughtful
Weighing

Weak/Defeated/Shy/Belittled

All in
At the mercy of
Bashful
Bent
Broken down
Chickenhearted
Cowardly
Crippled
Crushed
Deflated
Demeaned
Dependent
Dominated
Done for
Drained
Drowsy
Exhausted
Falling

* From Walters RP: *Amity: friendship in action, part II: the skill of active listening,* Boulder, CO, 1980, Christian Helpers, pp. 41–47.

Fatigued
Feeble
Fragile
Frail
Helpless
Hungry
Imperfect
Impotent
Inadequate
Incapable
Incompetent
Ineffective
Inefficient
Inept
Inferior
Insecure
Insulted
Intimidated
Laughed at
Needy
Neglected
No good
Paralyzed
Powerless
Puny
Put down
Run down
Scoffed at
Self-conscious
Shattered
Small
Smothered
Spineless
Squelched
Stifled
Strained
Tearful
Timid
Tired
Troubled
Unable
Unambitious
Unfit
Unqualified
Unstable
Unsure of self
Unworthy
Useless
Vulnerable
Walked on
Washed up
Weak
Whipped
Worn out

Worthless
Yellow

Lonely/Forgotten/
Left Out
Abandoned
Alienated
Alone
Betrayed
Bored
Cast aside
Cheated
Deserted
Discarded
Disliked
Disowned
Empty
Excluded
Forsaken
Friendless
Hated
Hollow
Homeless
Homesick
Ignored
Isolated
Jilted
Left out
Lonesome
Lost
Neglected
Ostracized
Outcast
Overlooked
Rebuffed
Rejected
Scorned
Secluded
Shunned
Slighted
Snubbed
Stranded
Ugly
Unimportant
Uninvited
Unwelcome

Angry/Hostile/
Enraged/Irritated
Aggravated
Aggressive
Agitated
Angry
Annoyed

Aroused
Belligerent
Bitter
Boiling
Bristling
Brutal
Bullying
Burned
Contrary
Cool
Cranky
Critical
Cross
Cruel
Disagreeable
Displeased
Enraged
Exasperated
Ferocious
Fierce
Fighting
Fired up
Frenzied
Fretful
Fuming
Furious
Harsh
Hateful
Heartless
Hostile
Incensed
Indignant
Inflamed
Infuriated
Irked
Irritated
Mad
Mean
Out of sorts
Outraged
Perturbed
Provoked
Pushy
Quarrelsome
Raving
Ready to explode
Rebellious
Resentful
Revengeful
Ruffled
Sarcastic
Spiteful
Steamed
Stern

Stormy
Strung out
Unkind
Vicious
Vindictive
Violent

Interested/Excited
Active
Alert
Aroused
Attracted to
Bubbly
Bustling
Busy
Challenged
Delighted
Eager
Enchanted
Enthusiastic
Excited
Exuberant
Fascinated
Flustered
Impatient
Impressed with
Interested in
Involved
Keyed up
Quickened
Resourceful
Responsive
Spurred on
Stimulated
Tantalized
Thrilled

Confused/Surprised/
Astonished
Aghast
Amazed
Appalled
Astonished
Astounded
Awed
Awestruck
Baffled
Bewildered
Bowled over
Breathless
Changeable
Dazed
Dismayed
Disorganized
Distracted

Doubtful
Dumbfounded
Emotional
Forgetful
Gripped
Horrified
In doubt
Jarred
Jolted
Mixed up
Muddled
Mystified
Overpowered
Overwhelmed
Perplexed
Puzzled
Rattled
Ruffled
Shocked
Speechless
Staggered
Startled
Struck
Stunned
Taken aback
Torn
Trapped
Tricked
Uncertain

Sad/Depressed/
Discouraged
Below par
Bereaved
Blue
Blum
Brokenhearted
Brooding
Dejected
Demolished
Depressed
Despondent
Destroyed
Disappointed
Discouraged
Downcast
Downhearted
Dreary
Dropping
Dull
Falling apart
Forlorn
Gloomy
Grief stricken
Grieved

Heavyhearted
Hopeless
In the dumps
Let down
Lifeless
Low
Melancholy
Moody
Moping
Mournful
Oppressed
Pained
Pessimistic
Sad
Serious
Solemn
Sorrowful
Tearful
Troubled
Unhappy
Weary
Woeful
Wrecked

Vigorous/Strong/
Confident
Able bodied
Accomplished
Adequate
Adventurous
Alive
Ambitious
Assertive
Assured
Blessed
Boastful
Bold
Brave
Capable
Certain
Clever
Competent
Competitive
Confident
Courageous
Daring
Deft
Determined
Dignified
Dynamic
Effective
Efficient
Encouraged
Energetic
Equal to the task

Favored
Fearless
Firm
Fit
Forceful
Fortunate
Gifted
Hardy
Healthy
Important
In control
Independent
Intelligent
Keen
Lionhearted
Lucky
Might
Peppy
Potent
Powerful
Prosperous
Qualified
Reliable
Responsible
Robust
Secure
Self-confident
Self-reliant
Sharp
Shrewd

Skillful
Smart
Spirited
Stable
Strong
Sturdy
Successful
Suited
Sure
Together
Tough
Triumphant
Victorious
Vigorous
Well off
Well suited
Wise

**Afraid/Tense/
Worried**
Agonizing
Alarmed
Anxious
Apprehensive
Boxed in
Cautious
Concerned
Cornered
Disturbed
Dreading

Edgy
Fearful
Frantic
Frightened
Hesitant
In a cold sweat
Jittery
Jumpy
Nervous
Numb
On edge
Panicky
Petrified
Quaking
Quivering
Restless
Scared
Shaken
Suffocated
Terrified
Trembling
Troubled
Uncomfortable
Uneasy

Index

Page numbers followed by f indicate figures; t, tables; b, boxes.